SANFORD GUIDE®

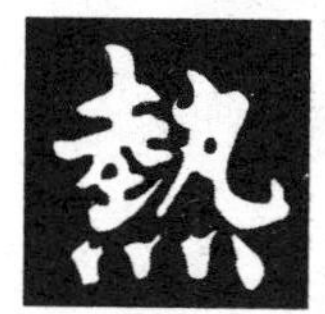

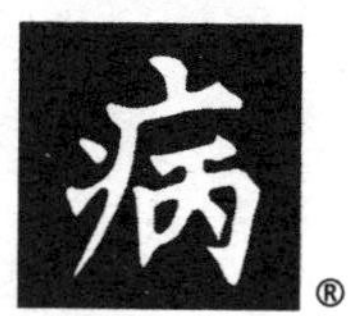

®

The Sanford Guide To Antimicrobial Therapy 2014

44th Edition

THE SANFORD GUIDE TO ANTIMICROBIAL THERAPY 2014
44TH EDITION

Editors

David N. Gilbert, M.D.
Chief of Infectious Diseases
Providence Portland Medical Center, Oregon
Professor of Medicine, Oregon Health Sciences University

Henry F. Chambers, M.D.
Professor of Medicine
Director, Clinical Research Services
UCSF Clinical and Translational Sciences Institute
University of California at San Francisco

George M. Eliopoulos, M.D.
Chief, James L. Tullis Firm,
Beth Israel Deaconess Hospital,
Professor of Medicine,
Harvard Medical School,
Boston, Massachusetts

Michael S. Saag, M.D.
Director, UAB Center for AIDS Research,
Professor of Medicine and Director,
Division of Infectious Diseases,
University of Alabama, Birmingham

Contributing Editors

Douglas Black, Pharm. D.
Associate Professor of Pharmacy,
University of Washington, Seattle

Brian S. Schwartz, M.D.
Assistant Professor of Medicine
University of California at San Francisco

David O. Freedman, M.D.
Director, Travelers Health Clinic,
Professor of Medicine,
University of Alabama, Birmingham

Andrew T. Pavia, M.D.
George & Esther Gross Presidential Professor
Chief, Division of Pediatric Infectious Diseases
University of Utah, Salt Lake City

Managing Editor

Jeb C. Sanford

Memoriam

Jay P. Sanford, M.D.
1928-1996

Merle A. Sande, M.D.
1935-2007

Robert C. Moellering, Jr., M.D.
1936-2014

Publisher

Antimicrobial Therapy, Inc.

The SANFORD GUIDES are updated annually and published by:

ANTIMICROBIAL THERAPY, INC.
P.O. Box 276, 11771 Lee Highway
Sperryville, VA 22740-0276 USA
Tel 540-987-9480 Fax 540-987-9486
Email: info@sanfordguide.com www.sanfordguide.com

Acknowledgements

Thanks to Ushuaia Solutions, SA, Argentina; Alcom Printing, Harleysville, PA and Fox Bindery, Quakertown, PA for design and production of this edition of the SANFORD GUIDE.

Note to Readers

Since 1969, the SANFORD GUIDE has been independently prepared and published. Decisions regarding the content of the SANFORD GUIDE are solely those of the editors and the publisher. We welcome questions, comments and feedback concerning the SANFORD GUIDE. All of your feedback is reviewed and taken into account in updating the content of the SANFORD GUIDE.

Every effort is made to ensure the accuracy of the content of this guide. However, current full prescribing information available in the package insert for each drug should be consulted before prescribing any product. The editors and publisher are not responsible for errors or omissions or for any consequences from application of the information in this book and make no warranty, express or implied, with respect to the currency, accuracy, or completeness of the contents of this publication. Application of this information in a particular situation remains the professional responsibility of the practitioner.

For the most current information, subscribe to webedition.sanfordguide.com or Sanford Guide mobile device applications

Check our website at for content-related notices: http://www.sanfordguide.com

Printed in the United States of America
ISBN 978-1-930808-78-2
Pocket Edition (English)

QUICK PAGE GUIDE TO THE SANFORD GUIDE

—TABLE OF CONTENTS—

ABBREVIATIONS

3TC = lamivudine
AB,% = percent absorbed
ABC = abacavir
ABCD = amphotericin B colloidal dispersion
ABLC = ampho B lipid complex
ACIP = Advisory Committee on Immunization Practices
AD = after dialysis
ADF = adefovir
AG = aminoglycoside
AIDS = Acquired Immune Deficiency Syndrome
AM-CL = amoxicillin-clavulanate
AM-CL-ER = amoxicillin-clavulanate extended release
AMK = amikacin
Amox = amoxicillin
AMP = ampicillin
Ampho B = amphotericin B
AM-SB = ampicillin-sulbactam
AP = atovaquone proguanil
AP Pen = antipseudomonal penicillins
APAG = antipseudomonal aminoglycoside (tobra, gent, amikacin)
ARDS = acute respiratory distress syndrome
ARF = acute rheumatic fever
ASA = aspirin
ATS = American Thoracic Society
ATV = atazanavir
AUC = area under the curve
Azithro = azithromycin
bid = twice a day
BL/BLI = beta-lactam/beta-lactamase inhibitor
BSA = body surface area
BW = body weight
C&S = culture & sensitivity
CAPD = continuous ambulatory peritoneal dialysis
CARB = carbapenems (DORI, ERTA, IMP, MER)
CDC = Centers for Disease Control
Cefpodox = cefpodoxime proxetil
Ceftaz = ceftazidime
Ceph= cephalosporin
CFB = ceftobiprole
CFP = cefepime
Chloro = chloramphenicol
CIP = ciprofloxacin; **CIP-ER** = CIP extended release
Clarithro = clarithromycin; **ER** = extended release
Clav = clavulanate
Clinda = clindamycin
CLO = clofazimine
Clot = clotrimazole
CMV = cytomegalovirus
CQ = chloroquine phosphate
Cobi = cobicistat
CrCl = creatinine clearance
CrCln = CrCl normalized for body surface area (BSA)
CRRT = continuous renal replacement therapy
CSD = cat-scratch disease
CSF = cerebrospinal fluid
CXR = chest x-ray
d4T = stavudine
Dapto = daptomycin
DBPCT = double-blind placebo-controlled trial
dc = discontinue
ddC = zalcitabine
ddI = didanosine
DIC = disseminated intravascular coagulation
div. = divided
DLV = delavirdine
Dori = doripenem
DOT = directly observed therapy
DOT group = B. distasonis, B. ovatus, B. thetaiotaomicron
Doxy = doxycycline
DR = delayed release
DRSP = drug-resistant S. pneumoniae
DS = double strength
EBV = Epstein-Barr virus
EES = erythromycin ethyl succinate
EFZ = efavirenz
ELV = elvitegravir
EMB = ethambutol
ENT = entecavir
ER = extended release
ERTA = ertapenem
Erythro = erythromycin
ESBLs = extended spectrum β-lactamases
ESR = erythrocyte sedimentation rate
ESRD = endstage renal disease
Flu = fluconazole
Flucyt = flucytosine
FOS-APV = fosamprenavir
FQ = fluoroquinolone (CIP, Oflox, Lome, Peflox, Levo, Gati, Moxi, Gemi)
FTC = emtricitabine
G = generic
GAS = Group A Strep
Gati = gatifloxacin
GC = gonorrhea
Gemi = gemifloxacin
Gent = gentamicin
gm = gram
GNB = gram-negative bacilli
Griseo = griseofulvin
HEMO = hemodialysis
HHV = human herpesvirus
HIV = human immunodeficiency virus
HLR = high-level resistance
H/O = history of
HSCT = hematopoietic stem cell transplant
HSV = herpes simplex virus
IA = injectable agent/anti-inflammatory drugs
ICAAC = Interscience Conference on Antimicrobial Agents & Chemotherapy
IDSA = Infectious Diseases Society of America
IDV = indinavir
IFN = interferon
IMP = imipenem-cilastatin
INH = isoniazid
Inv = investigational
IP = intraperitoneal
IT = intrathecal
Itra = itraconazole
IVDU = intravenous drug user
IVIG = intravenous immune globulin
Keto = ketoconazole
LAB = liposomal ampho B
LCM = lymphocytic choriomeningitis virus
LCR = ligase chain reaction
Levo = levofloxacin
LP/R = lopinavir/ ritonavir
Macrolides = azithro, clarithro, dirithro, erythro, roxithro
mcg = microgram
MDR = multi-drug resistant
MER = meropenem
Metro = metronidazole
mg = milligram
Mino = minocycline
Moxi = moxifloxacin
MQ = mefloquine
MSSA/MRSA = methicillin-sensitive/resistant S. aureus
MTB = Mycobacterium tuberculosis
NB = name brand
NF = nitrofurantoin
NAI = not FDA-approved (indication or dose)
NFR = nelfinavir
NNRTI = non-nucleoside reverse transcriptase inhibitor
NRTI = nucleoside reverse transcriptase inhibitor
NSAIDs = non-steroidal
NUS = not available in the U.S.
NVP = nevirapine
O Ceph 1, 2, 3 = oral cephalosporins—*see Table 10A*
Oflox = ofloxacin
P Ceph 1, 2, 3, 4 = parenteral cephalosporins—*see Table 10A*
P Ceph 3 AP = parenteral cephalosporins with antipseudomonal activity—*see Table 10A*
PCR = polymerase chain reaction
PEP = post-exposure prophylaxis
PI = protease inhibitor
PIP = piperacillin
PIP-TZ = piperacillin-tazobactam
po = per os (by mouth)
PQ = primaquine
PRCT = Prospective randomized controlled trials
PTLD = post-transplant lymphoproliferative disease

ABBREVIATIONS (2)

Pts = patients
Pyri = pyrimethamine
PZA = pyrazinamide
qid = 4 times a day
QS = quinine sulfate
Quinu-dalfo = **Q-D** = quinupristin-dalfopristin
R = resistant
RFB = rifabutin
RFP = rifapentine
Rick = Rickettsia
RIF = rifampin
RSV = respiratory syncytial virus
RTI = respiratory tract infection
RTV = ritonavir
rx = treatment
S = potential synergy in combination with penicillin, AMP, vanco, teico

SA = Staph. aureus
SD = serum drug level after single dose
Sens = sensitive (susceptible)
SM = streptomycin
SQV = saquinavir
SS = steady state serum level
STD = sexually transmitted disease
subcut = subcutaneous
Sulb = sulbactam
Sx = symptoms
Tazo = tazobactam
TBc = tuberculosis
TC-CL = ticarcillin-clavulanate
TDF = tenofovir
TEE = transesophageal echocardiography
Teico = teicoplanin
Telithro = telithromycin

Tetra = tetracycline
Ticar = ticarcillin
tid = 3 times a day
TMP-SMX = trimethoprim-sulfamethoxazole
TNF = tumor necrosis factor
Tobra = tobramycin
TPV = tipranavir
TST = tuberculin skin test
UTI = urinary tract infection
Vanco = vancomycin
VISA = vancomycin intermediately resistant S. aureus
VL = viral load
Vori = voriconazole
VZV = varicella-zoster virus
WHO = World Health Organization
ZDV = zidovudine

ABBREVIATIONS OF JOURNAL TITLES

AAC: Antimicrobial Agents & Chemotherapy
Adv PID: Advances in Pediatric Infectious Diseases
AHJ: American Heart Journal
AIDS Res Hum Retrovir: AIDS Research & Human Retroviruses
AJG: American Journal of Gastroenterology
AJM: American Journal of Medicine
AJRCCM: American Journal of Respiratory Critical Care Medicine
AJTMH: American Journal of Tropical Medicine & Hygiene
Aliment Pharmacol Ther: Alimentary Pharmacology & Therapeutics
Am J Hlth Pharm: American Journal of Health-System Pharmacy
Amer J Transpl: American Journal of Transplantation
AnEM: Annals of Emergency Medicine
AnIM: Annals of Internal Medicine
Ann Pharmacother: Annals of Pharmacotherapy
AnSurg: Annals of Surgery
Antivir Ther: Antiviral Therapy
ArDerm: Archives of Dermatology
ArIM: Archives of Internal Medicine
ARRD: American Review of Respiratory Disease
BMJ: British Medical Journal
BMT: Bone Marrow Transplantation
Brit J Derm: British Journal of Dermatology
Can JID: Canadian Journal of Infectious Diseases
Canad Med J: Canadian Medical Journal
CCM: Critical Care Medicine
CCTID: Current Clinical Topics in Infectious Disease
CDBSR: Cochrane Database of Systematic Reviews
CID: Clinical Infectious Diseases
Clin Micro Inf: Clinical Microbiology and Infection
CMN: Clinical Microbiology Newsletter
Clin Micro Rev: Clinical Microbiology Reviews
CMAJ: Canadian Medical Association Journal

COID: Current Opinion in Infectious Disease
Curr Med Res Opin: Current Medical Research and Opinion
Derm Ther: Dermatologic Therapy
Dermatol Clin: Dermatologic Clinics
Dig Dis Sci: Digestive Diseases and Sciences
DMID: Diagnostic Microbiology and Infectious Disease
EID: Emerging Infectious Diseases
EJCMID: European Journal of Clin. Micro. & Infectious Diseases
Eur J Neurol: European Journal of Neurology
Exp Mol Path: Experimental & Molecular Pathology
Exp Rev Anti Infect Ther: Expert Review of Anti-Infective Therapy
Gastro: Gastroenterology
Hpt: Hepatology
ICHE: Infection Control and Hospital Epidemiology
IDC No. Amer: Infectious Disease Clinics of North America
IDCP: Infectious Diseases in Clinical Practice
IJAA: International Journal of Antimicrobial Agents
Inf Med: Infections in Medicine
J AIDS & HR: Journal of AIDS and Human Retrovirology
J All Clin Immun: Journal of Allergy and Clinical Immunology
J Am Ger Soc: Journal of the American Geriatrics Society
J Chemother: Journal of Chemotherapy
J Clin Micro: Journal of Clinical Microbiology
J Clin Virol: Journal of Clinical Virology
J Derm Treat: Journal of Dermatological Treatment
J Hpt: Journal of Hepatology
J Inf: Journal of Infection
J Med Micro: Journal of Medical Microbiology
J Micro Immunol Inf: Journal of Microbiology, Immunology, & Infection
J Ped: Journal of Pediatrics
J Viral Hep: Journal of Viral Hepatitis

JAC: Journal of Antimicrobial Chemotherapy
JACC: Journal of American College of Cardiology
JAIDS: JAIDS Journal of Acquired Immune Deficiency Syndromes
JAMA: Journal of the American Medical Association
JAVMA: Journal of the Veterinary Medicine Association
JCI: Journal of Clinical Investigation
JCM: Journal of Clinical Microbiology
JIC: Journal of Infection and Chemotherapy
JID: Journal of Infectious Diseases
JNS: Journal of Neurosurgery
JTMH: Journal of Tropical Medicine and Hygiene
Ln: Lancet
LnID: Lancet Infectious Disease
Mayo Clin Proc: Mayo Clinic Proceedings
Med Lett: Medical Letter
Med Mycol: Medical Mycology
MMWR: Morbidity & Mortality Weekly Report
NEJM: New England Journal of Medicine
Neph Dial Transpl: Nephrology Dialysis Transplantation
Ped Ann: Pediatric Annals
Peds: Pediatrics
Pharmacother: Pharmacotherapy
PIDJ: Pediatric Infectious Disease Journal
QJM: Quarterly Journal of Medicine
Scand J Inf Dis: Scandinavian Journal of Infectious Diseases
Sem Resp Inf: Seminars in Respiratory Infections
SGO: Surgery Gynecology and Obstetrics
SMJ: Southern Medical Journal
Surg Neurol: Surgical Neurology
Transpl Inf Dis: Transplant Infectious Diseases
Transpl: Transplantation
TRSM: Transactions of the Royal Society of Medicine

TABLE 1 – CLINICAL APPROACH TO INITIAL CHOICE OF ANTIMICROBIAL THERAPY*

Treatment based on presumed site or type of infection. In selected instances, treatment and prophylaxis based on identification of pathogens. Regimens should be reevaluated based on pathogen isolated, antimicrobial susceptibility determination, and individual host characteristics. *(Abbreviations on page 2)*

ANATOMIC SITE/DIAGNOSIS/ MODIFYING CIRCUMSTANCES	ETIOLOGIES (usual)	SUGGESTED REGIMENS*		ADJUNCT DIAGNOSTIC OR THERAPEUTIC MEASURES AND COMMENTS
		PRIMARY	ALTERNATIVE§	
ABDOMEN: *See Peritoneum, page 47; Gallbladder, page 17; and Pelvic Inflammatory Disease, page 26*				
BONE: Osteomyelitis. Microbiologic diagnosis is essential. If blood culture negative, need culture of bone. Culture of sinus tract drainage not predictive of bone culture. Review: *Ln 364:369, 2004.* For comprehensive review of antimicrobial penetration into bone, see *Clinical Pharmacokinetics 48:89, 2009.*				
Hematogenous Osteomyelitis				
Empiric therapy—Collect bone and blood cultures before empiric therapy				
Newborn (<4 mos.) *See Table 16 for dose*	S. aureus, Gm-neg. bacilli, Group B strep	**MRSA possible: Vanco + (Ceftaz or CFP)**	**MRSA unlikely:** (**Nafcillin** or **oxacillin**) + (**Ceftaz or CFP**)	*Table 16 for dose.* Severe allergy or toxicity: (**Linezolid**NAI 10 mg/kg IV/po q8h + **aztreonam**).
Children (>4 mos.) — Adult: Osteo of extremity	S. aureus, Group A strep, Gm-neg. bacilli rare	**MRSA possible: Vanco**	**MRSA unlikely: Nafcillin** or **oxacillin**	Severe allergy or toxicity: **Clinda** or **TMP-SMX** or **linezolid**NAI. Adults: **ceftaz** 2 gm IV q8h, **CFP** 2 gm IV q12h. *Peds dosages in Table 16. See Table 10B for adverse reactions to drugs.*
		Add **Ceftaz or CFP** if Gm-neg. bacilli on Gram stain **Adult doses below.** *Peds Doses: Table 16.*		
Adult (>21 yrs) **Vertebral osteo ± epidural abscess**; other sites *(NEJM 355:2012, 2006)*	S. aureus most common but variety other organisms. **Blood & bone cultures essential.**	**MRSA possible: Vanco** 15-30 mg/kg IV q 8-12h for trough of 15-20 μg/mL + (**Ceftriaxone** 2 gm q24h OR **CFP** 2 gm q8h OR **Levo** 750 mg q24h)	**MRSA unlikely: Nafcillin** or **oxacillin** 2 gm IV q4h + (**Ceftriaxone** 2 gm q24h OR **CFP** 2 gm q8h OR **Levo** 750 mg q24h)	**Dx: MRI early to look for epidural abscess.** For comprehensive review of vertebral see *NEJM 362:11, 2010.* Whenever possible empirical therapy should be administered after cultures are obtained.
Specific therapy—Culture and in vitro susceptibility results known				
	MSSA	**Nafcillin** or **oxacillin** 2 gm IV q4h or **cefazolin** 2 gm IV q8h	**Vanco** 15-30 mg/kg IV q 8-12h for trough of 15-20 μg/mL OR **Dapto** 6 mg/kg q24h IV ± **RIF** 300- 450 mg po/IV bid	***Other options if susceptible in vitro and allergy/toxicity issues (see NEJM 362:11, 2010):*** 1) **TMP-SMX** 8-10 mg/kg/d po/IV div q8h + **RIF** 300-450 mg bid: limited data, particularly for MRSA *(see AAC 53:2672, 2009)*; 2) [(**CIP** 750 mg po bid or **Levo** 750 mg po q24h) + **RIF** 300 mg po bid]; 3) Linezolid assoc. with optic & peripheral neuropathy with long-term use; 4) **Fusidic acid**NUS 500 mg IV q8h + **RIF** 300 mg po bid. *(CID 42:394, 2006)*. **Ceftriaxone** 2 gm IV q24h *(CID 54:585, 2012)*
	MRSA—*See Table 6, page 79; IDSA Guidelines CID 52:e18-55, 2011; CID 52:285-92, 2011*	**Vanco** 15-30 mg/kg IV q 8-12h for trough of 15-20 μg/mL ± **RIF** 300-450 mg bid.	**Linezolid** 600 mg q12h IV/po ± **RIF** 300 mg po/IV bid OR **Dapto** 6 mg/kg 2q 24h IV ± **RIF** 300-450 mg po/IV bid	
Hemoglobinopathy: Sickle cell/thalassemia	Salmonella; other Gm-neg. bacilli	**CIP** 400 mg IV q12h OR **CIP** 750 mg PO bid	**Levo** 750 mg IV/PO q24h	Thalassemia: transfusion and iron chelation risk factors. Because of decreasing levels of susceptibility to fluoroquinolones among Salmonella spp. and growing resistance among other gram-negative bacilli, would add a second agent (e.g., third-generation cephalosporin) until susceptibility test results available.

*** DOSAGES SUGGESTED are for adults (unless otherwise indicated) with clinically severe (often life-threatening) infections. Dosages also assume normal renal function, and not severe hepatic dysfunction.**

§ ALTERNATIVE THERAPY INCLUDES these considerations: allergy, pharmacology/pharmacokinetics, compliance, costs, local resistance profiles.

TABLE 1 (2)

ANATOMIC SITE/DIAGNOSIS/ MODIFYING CIRCUMSTANCES	ETIOLOGIES (usual)	SUGGESTED REGIMENS*		ADJUNCT DIAGNOSTIC OR THERAPEUTIC MEASURES AND COMMENTS
		PRIMARY	ALTERNATIVE§	
BONE *(continued)*				
Contiguous Osteomyelitis Without Vascular Insufficiency				
Empiric therapy: Get cultures!				
Foot bone osteo due to nail through tennis shoe	P. aeruginosa	**CIP** 750 mg po bid or **Levo** 750 mg po q24h	**Ceftaz** 2 gm IV q8h or **CFP** 2 gm IV q8h	*See Skin—Nail puncture, page 56.* Need debridement to remove foreign body.
Long bone, post-internal fixation of fracture	S. aureus, Gm-neg. bacilli, P. aeruginosa	**Vanco** 15-30 mg/kg IV q 8-12h for trough of 15-20 µg/mL + [**ceftaz** or **CFP**]. *See Comment*	**Linezolid** 600 mg IV/po bid[NAI] + (**ceftaz** or **CFP**). *See Comment*	Often necessary to remove hardware after union to achieve eradication. May need revascularization. **Regimens listed are empiric.** Adjust after culture data available. If susceptible Gm-neg. bacillus, **CIP** 750 mg po bid or **Levo** 750 mg po q24h. For other *S. aureus* options: *See Hem. Osteo. Specific Therapy, page 4.*
Osteonecrosis of the jaw	Probably rare adverse reaction to bisphosphonates	Infection may be secondary to bone necrosis and loss of overlying mucosa. Treatment: minimal surgical debridement, chlorhexidine rinses, antibiotics (e.g. PIP-TZ). Evaluate for concomitant actinomycosis, for which specific long-term antibiotic treatment would be warranted *(CID 49:1729, 2009).*		
Prosthetic joint	*See prosthetic joint, page 33*			
Spinal implant infection	S. aureus, coag-neg staphylococci, gram-neg bacilli	Onset within 30 days: culture, treat for 3 mos *(CID 55:1481, 2012).*	Onset after 30 days remove implant, culture & treat	*See CID 55:1481, 2012*
Sternum, post-op	S. aureus, S. epidermidis, occasionally, gram-negative bacilli	**Vanco** 15-30 mg/kg IV q 8-12h for trough of 15-20 µg/mL recommended for serious infections.	**Linezolid** 600 mg po/IV[NAI] bid	Sternal debridement for cultures & removal of necrotic bone. For *S. aureus* options: *Hem. Osteo. Specific Therapy, page 4.* If setting or gram stain suggests possibility of gram-negative bacilli, add appropriate coverage based on local antimicrobial susceptibility profiles *(e.g., cefepime, pip-tazo).*
Contiguous Osteomyelitis With Vascular Insufficiency.				
Most pts are **diabetics** with peripheral neuropathy & infected skin ulcers *(see Diabetic foot, page 16)*	Polymicrobic [Gm+ cocci (to include MRSA) (aerobic & anaerobic) and Gm-neg. bacilli (aerobic & anaerobic)]	Debride overlying ulcer & submit bone for histology & culture. Select antibiotic based on culture results & treat for 6 weeks. **No empiric therapy unless acutely ill.** If acutely ill, *see suggestions, Diabetic foot, page 16.* Revascularize if possible.		**Diagnosis of osteo:** Culture bone biopsy (gold standard). Poor concordance of culture results between swab of ulcer and bone – need bone. *(CID 42:57, 63, 2006).* Sampling by needle puncture inferior to biopsy *(CID 48:888, 2009).* Osteo more likely if ulcer >2 cm², positive probe to bone, ESR >70 & abnormal plain x-ray *(JAMA 299:806, 2008).* **Treatment:** (1) **Revascularize if possible;** (2) Culture bone; (3) Specific antimicrobial(s). Reviews: *BMJ 339:b4905, 2006; Plast Reconstr Surg 117: (7 Suppl) 2125, 2006.*
Chronic Osteomyelitis: Specific therapy By definition, implies presence of dead bone. **Need valid cultures**	S. aureus, Enterobacteriaceae, P. aeruginosa	**Empiric rx not indicated.** Base systemic rx on results of culture, sensitivity testing. If acute exacerbation of chronic osteo, rx as acute hematogenous osteo. Surgical debridement important.		**Important adjuncts:** removal of orthopedic hardware, surgical debridement; vascularized muscle flaps, distraction osteogenesis (Ilizarov) techniques. Antibiotic-impregnated cement & hyperbaric oxygen adjunctive. **NOTE: RIF + (vanco or β-lactam)** effective in animal model and in a clinical trial of S. aureus chronic osteo. The contribution of rifampin-containing regimens in this setting is not clear, however *(AAC 53:2672, 2009).*

 **NOTE: All dosage recommendations are for adults (unless otherwise indicated) and assume normal renal function. § Alternatives consider allergy, PK, compliance, local resistance, cost*

TABLE 1 (3)

ANATOMIC SITE/DIAGNOSIS/ MODIFYING CIRCUMSTANCES	ETIOLOGIES (usual)	SUGGESTED REGIMENS*		ADJUNCT DIAGNOSTIC OR THERAPEUTIC MEASURES AND COMMENTS
		PRIMARY	ALTERNATIVE§	
BREAST: Mastitis—Obtain culture; need to know if MRSA present. Review with definitions: Review of breast infections: *BMJ 342:d396, 2011.*				
Postpartum mastitis *(Recent Cochrane Review: Cochrane Database Syst Rev 2013 Feb 28;2:CD005458; see also CID 54:71, 2012)*				
Mastitis without abscess	S. aureus; less often S. pyogenes (Gp A or B), E. coli, bacteroides species, maybe Corynebacterium sp., & selected coagulase-neg. staphylococci (e.g., S. lugdunensis)	**NO MRSA:** **Outpatient: Dicloxacillin** 500 mg po qid or **cephalexin** 500 mg po qid. **Inpatient: Nafcillin/oxacillin** 2 gm IV q4-6h	**MRSA Possible:** **Outpatient: TMP-SMX-DS** tabs 1-2 po bid or, if susceptible, **clinda** 300 mg po tid **Inpatient: Vanco** 1 gm IV q12h; if over 100 kg, 1.5 gm IV q12h.	If no abscess, ↑ freq of nursing may hasten response; discuss age-specific risks to infant of drug exposure through breast milk with pediatrician. Corynebacterium sp. assoc. with chronic granulomatous mastitis *(CID 35:1434, 2002).*
Mastitis with abscess				With abscess, d/c nursing. **I& D standard;** needle aspiration reported successful. Resume breast feeding from affected breast as soon as pain allows.
Non-puerperal mastitis with abscess	S. aureus; less often Bacteroides sp., peptostreptococcus, & selected coagulase-neg. staphylococci	*See regimens for Postpartum mastitis, page 6.*		Smoking and diabetes may be risk factors *(BMJ 342:d396, 2011)*. **If subareolar & odoriferous**, most likely anaerobes; need to **add metro** 500 mg IV/po tid. If not subareolar, staph. Need pretreatment aerobic/anaerobic cultures. Surgical drainage for abscess.
Breast implant infection	Acute: *S. aureus, S. pyogenes*. TSS reported. Chronic: Look for rapidly growing Mycobacteria	Acute: **Vanco** 1 gm IV q12h; if over 100 kg, 1.5 gm q12h.	Chronic: Await culture results. *See Table 12A* for mycobacteria treatment.	*Lancet Infect Dis 5:94, 462, 2005.* Coag-negative staph also common *(Aesthetic Plastic Surg 31:325, 2007).*
CENTRAL NERVOUS SYSTEM				
Brain abscess				
Primary or contiguous source In 51 pts, 30 positive by standard culture; using molecular diagnostics, 80 bacterial taxa & many polymicrobics *(CID 54:202, 2012).*	Streptococci (60–70%), bacteroides (20–40%), Enterobacteriaceae (25–33%), S. aureus (10–15%), S. anginosus grp. Rare: Nocardia *(below)* Listeria. *See S. aureus Comment*	**P Ceph 3** [(**cefotaxime** 2 gm IV q4h or **ceftriaxone** 2 gm IV q12h) + (**metro** 7.5 mg/kg q6h or 15 mg/kg IV q12h)]	**Pen G** 3-4 million units IV q4h + **metro** 7.5 mg/kg q6h or 15 mg/kg IV q12h	If CT scan suggests cerebritis or abscesses <2.5 cm and pt neurologically stable and conscious, start antibiotics and observe. Otherwise, surgical drainage necessary. If blood cultures or other clinical data do not yield a likely etiologic agent, aspirate even small abscesses for diagnosis if this can be done safely.
		Duration of rx unclear; treat until response by neuroimaging (CT/MRI)		Experience with Pen G (HD) + metro without ceftriaxone or nafcillin/oxacillin has been good. We use ceftriaxone because of frequency of isolation of Enterobacteriaceae. **S. aureus rare without positive blood culture; if S. aureus, use vanco until susceptibility known.** Strep. anginosus group esp. prone to produce abscess. Ceph/metro does not cover listeria.
Post-surgical, post-traumatic	S. aureus, Enterobacteriaceae	**For MSSA:** (**Nafcillin** or **oxacillin**) 2 gm IV q4h + (**ceftriaxone** or **cefotaxime**)	**For MRSA: Vanco** 15-30 mg/kg IV q 8-12h for trough of 15-20 mcg/mL + (**ceftriaxone** or **cefotaxime**)	Empirical coverage, de-escalated based on culture results. **Aspiration of abscess usually necessary for dx & rx. If P. aeruginosa suspected, substitute (Cefepime or Ceftazidime) for (Ceftriaxone or Cefotaxime).**
HIV-1 infected (AIDS)	Toxoplasma gondii	*See Table 13A, page 147*		

 **NOTE: All dosage recommendations are for adults (unless otherwise indicated) and assume normal renal function. § Alternatives consider allergy, PK, compliance, local resistance, cost*

TABLE 1 (4)

ANATOMIC SITE/DIAGNOSIS/ MODIFYING CIRCUMSTANCES	ETIOLOGIES (usual)	SUGGESTED REGIMENS*		ADJUNCT DIAGNOSTIC OR THERAPEUTIC MEASURES AND COMMENTS
		PRIMARY	ALTERNATIVE§	
CENTRAL NERVOUS SYSTEM/Brain abscess *(continued)*				
Nocardia: Haematogenous abscess	N. farcinica, N. asteroides & N. brasiliensis	**TMP-SMX:** 15 mg/kg/day of TMP & 75 mg/kg/day of SMX, IV/po div in 2-4 doses + **Imipenem** 500 mg q6h IV. If multiorgan involvement some add **amikacin** 7.5 mg/kg q12h.	**Linezolid** 600 mg IV or po q12h + meropenem 2 gm q8h	Measure peak sulfonamide levels: target 100-150 mcg/mL 2 hrs post dose. **Linezolid** 600 mg po bid reported effective. For in vitro susceptibility testing: Wallace (+1) 903-877-7680 or U.S. CDC (+1) 404-639-3158. In vitro resistance to TMP-SMX may be increasing *(Clin Infect Dis 51:1445, 2010)*, but whether this is associated with worse outcomes is not known; TMP-SMX remains a drug of choice for CNS nocardia infection. If sulfonamide resistant or sulfa-allergic, **amikacin** plus one of: **IMP**, **MER**, **ceftriaxone** or **cefotaxime**. *N. farcinica* is resistant to third-generation cephalosporins, which should not be used for treatment of infection caused by this organism.
		After 3-6 wks of IV therapy, switch to po therapy. Immunocompetent pts: **TMP-SMX**, **minocycline** or **AM-CL** x 3+ months. Immunocompromised pts: Treat with 2 drugs for at least one year.		
Subdural empyema: In adult 60–90% is extension of sinusitis or otitis media. Rx same as primary brain abscess. Surgical emergency: must drain. Review in *LnID 7:62, 2007*.				
Encephalitis/encephalopathy *IDSA Guideline: CID 47:303, 2008; Intl diagnosis consensus: CID 57:1114, 2013. (For Herpes see Table 14A, page 162 and for rabies, Table 20B, page 222)*	In 253 pts, etiol in 52%: H. simplex (42%), VZV (15%), M. TB (15%), Listeria (10%) *(CID 49:1838, 2009)*. Other: arbovirus, West Nile, rabies, Lyme, Parvo B19, Cat-scratch disease, Mycoplasma, mumps, EBV, HHV-6, and others.	Start IV **acyclovir** while awaiting results of CSF PCR for H. simplex. For amebic encephalitis *see Table 13A*. Start **Doxy** if setting suggests R. rickettsii, Anaplasma, Ehrlichia, Mycoplasma.		Review of all etiologies: *LnID 10:835, 2010*. Anti-NMDAR (N-Methyl-D-Aspartate Receptor) encephalitis, autoimmune encephalitis, more common than individual viral etiologies as a cause of encephalitis in the California Encephalitis Project cohort *(CID 54:899, 2012)*.
Meningitis, "Aseptic": Pleocytosis of up to 100s of cells, CSF glucose normal, neg. culture for bacteria *(see Table 14A, page 158)* Ref: *CID 47:783, 2008*	Enteroviruses, HSV-2, LCM, HIV, other viruses, drugs (NSAIDs, metronidazole, carbamazepine, TMP-SMX, IVIG), rarely leptospirosis	For all but leptospirosis, IV fluids and analgesics. D/C drugs that may be etiologic. For lepto (**doxy** 100 mg IV/po q12h) or (**Pen G** 5 million units IV q6h) or (**AMP** 0.5–1 gm IV q6h). Repeat LP if suspect partially-treated bacterial meningitis. **Acyclovir** 5-10 mg/kg IV q8h sometimes given for HSV-2 meningitis (Note: this entity is distinct from HSV encephalitis where early rx is mandatory).		If available, PCR of CSF for enterovirus. HSV-2 unusual without concomitant genital herpes. For lepto, positive epidemiologic history and concomitant hepatitis, conjunctivitis, dermatitis, nephritis. For list of implicated drugs: *Inf Med 25:331, 2008*.

**NOTE: All dosage recommendations are for adults (unless otherwise indicated) and assume normal renal function. § Alternatives consider allergy, PK, compliance, local resistance, cost*

TABLE 1 (5)

ANATOMIC SITE/DIAGNOSIS/ MODIFYING CIRCUMSTANCES	ETIOLOGIES (usual)	SUGGESTED REGIMENS*		ADJUNCT DIAGNOSTIC OR THERAPEUTIC MEASURES AND COMMENTS
		PRIMARY	ALTERNATIVE§	
Meningitis, Bacterial, Acute: Goal is empiric therapy, then CSF exam within 30 min. If focal neurologic deficit, give empiric therapy, then head CT, then LP. *(NEJM 354:44, 2006; Ln ID 10:32, 2010; IDSA Pract. Guid., CID 39:1267, 2004)* **NOTE:** In children, treatment caused CSF cultures to turn neg. in 2 hrs with meningococci & partial response with pneumococci in 4 hrs *(Peds 108:1169, 2001.* For distribution of pathogens by age group, *see NEJM 364:2016, 2011.*				
Empiric Therapy—CSF Gram stain is negative—immunocompetent				
Age: Preterm to <1 mo *LnID 10:32, 2010*	Group B strep 49%, E. coli 18%, listeria 7%, misc. Gm-neg. 10%, misc. Gm-pos. 10%	**AMP** 100 mg/kg IV q6h + **cefotaxime** 50 mg/kg IV q6h	**AMP** 100 mg/kg IV q6h + **gentamicin** 2.5 mg/kg IV q8h	Regimens active vs. Group B strep, most coliforms, & listeria. If premature infant with long nursery stay, S. aureus, enterococci, and resistant coliforms potential pathogens. **Optional empiric regimens (except for listeria): [nafcillin + (ceftazidime or cefotaxime)]. If high risk of MRSA,** use vanco + cefotaxime. Alter regimen after culture/sensitivity data available.
		Intraventricular treatment not recommended. Repeat CSF exam/culture 24–36 hr after start of therapy		
Age: 1 mo– 50 yrs Hearing loss is most common neurologic sequelae *(LnID 10:32, 2010).*	S. pneumo, meningococci, H. influenzae now uncommon, **listeria unlikely if young adult & immunocompetent** (add **ampicillin** if suspect listeria: 2 gm IV q4h)	Adult dosage: [(**Cefotaxime** 2 gm IV q4–6h OR **ceftriaxone** 2 gm IV q12h)] + (**dexamethasone**) + **vanco**[1].	[(**MER** 2 gm IV q8h) (Peds: 40 mg/kg IV q8h)] + IV **dexamethasone** + **vanco**[1]	Value of **dexamethasone** shown in children with H. influenzae and adults with S. pneumoniae in some studies *(NEJM 357:2431 & 2441, 2007; LnID 4:139, 2004).* In the Netherlands, adoption of dexamethasone treatment in adult pneumococcal meningitis led to reduced mortality and hearing loss compared with historical control group *(Neurology 75:1533, 2010).* For patients with severe **β-lactam allergy,** *see below (Empiric Therapy—positive gram stain and Specific Therapy)* for alternative agents that can be substituted to cover likely pathogens.
		Dexamethasone: 0.15 mg/kg IV q6h x 2–4 days. **Give with, or just before, 1st dose of antibiotic to block TNF production** *(see Comment).*		
		See footnote[1] for Vanco Adult dosage and[2] for ped. dosage		
Age: >50 yrs or alcoholism or other **debilitating assoc diseases** or **impaired cellular immunity**	S. pneumo, listeria, Gm-neg. bacilli. Note absence of meningococcus.	(**AMP** 2 gm IV q4h) + (**ceftriaxone** 2 gm IV q12h or **cefotaxime** 2 gm IV q4-6h) + **vanco** + IV **dexamethasone**	**MER** 2 gm IV q8h + **vanco** + IV **dexamethasone**. *For severe pen. Allergy, see Comment*	For patients with severe **β-lactam allergy,** *see below (Empiric Therapy—positive gram stain and Specific Therapy)* for alternative agents that can be substituted to cover likely pathogens.
		For vanco dose, *see footnote[1]*. **Dexamethasone dose:** 0.15 mg/kg IV q6h x 2–4 days; 1st dose before, or concomitant with, 1st dose of antibiotic.		
Post-neurosurgery Ventriculostomy/lumbar catheter; ventriculoperitoneal (atrial) shunt) or Penetrating trauma w/o basilar skull fracture	S. epidermidis, S. aureus, P. acnes. Facultative and aerobic gram-neg bacilli, including: P. aeruginosa & A. baumannii (may be multi-drug resistant)	**Vanco** 15 mg/kg IV q8h (to achieve trough level of 15-20 μg/mL) + (**Cefepime** or **Ceftaz** 2 gm IV q8h)	**Vanco** 15 mg/kg IV q8h (to achieve trough level of 15-20 μg/mL) + (**MER** 2 gm IV q8h)	• If possible, remove infected shunt or catheter. Logic for intraventricular therapy: goal is to achieve a 10-20 ratio of CSF concentration to MIC of infecting bacteria. For potential toxicities *see CMR 23:858, 2010.* • Use only preservative-free drug. Clamp/close catheter for 1 hr after 1st dose. • Can replace shunt once 3 serial cultures have cleared; no additional systemic Rx needed if coag-neg staph infection, diphtheroids, P. acnes; 1 additional week for other organisms *(see NEJM 362, 146, 2010).* • Acinetobacter meningitis *(LnID 9:245, 2009; AAC 57:1938, 2013).* • Review of nosocomial bacterial meningitis *(NEJM 362, 146, 2010).*
		• **If severe Pen/Ceph allergy,** for possible gram-neg, substitute either: Aztreonam 2 gm IV q6-8h or CIP 400 mg IV q8-12h. **If IV therapy inadequate, may need intraventricular therapy:** Intraventricular daily drug doses *(CID 39:1267, 2004; CMR 23:858, 2010):* **Adult: Vanco** 10-20 mg; **Amikacin** 30 mg; **Tobra** 5-20 mg; **Gent** 4-8 mg; **Colistin** 10 mg (or 5 mg q12h), **Polymyxin B** 5 mg; **Peds: Gent** 1-2 mg; **Polymyxin B** 2 mg.		
Trauma with basilar skull fracture	S. pneumoniae, H. influenzae, S. pyogenes	**Vanco** 15 mg/kg IV q8h (to achieve trough level of 15-20 μg/mL) + (**Ceftriaxone** 2 gm IV q12h or **Cefotax** 2 gm IV q6h) + [**Dexamethasone** 0.15 mg/kg IV q6h x 2-4 d (1st dose with or before 1st antibiotic dose)]. *See Clin Micro Rev 21:519, 2008.*		

[1] **Vanco adult dose:** 15 mg/kg IV q8h to achieve trough level of 15-20 μg/mL.

[2] **Dosage of drugs used to treat children ≥1 mo of age: Cefotaxime** 50 mg/kg per day IV q6h; **ceftriaxone** 50 mg/kg IV q12h; **vanco** 15 mg/kg IV q6h to achieve trough level of 15-20 μg/mL.

Abbreviations on page 2. **NOTE: All dosage recommendations are for adults (unless otherwise indicated) and assume normal renal function. § Alternatives consider allergy, PK, compliance, local resistance, cost*

TABLE 1 (6)

ANATOMIC SITE/DIAGNOSIS/ MODIFYING CIRCUMSTANCES	ETIOLOGIES (usual)	SUGGESTED REGIMENS*		ADJUNCT DIAGNOSTIC OR THERAPEUTIC MEASURES AND COMMENTS
		PRIMARY	ALTERNATIVE[§]	
CENTRAL NERVOUS SYSTEM/Meningitis, Bacterial, Acute *(continued)*				
Empiric Therapy—Positive CSF Gram stain				
Gram-positive diplococci	S. pneumoniae	(**ceftriaxone** 2 gm IV q12h or **cefotaxime** 2 gm IV q4–6h) + **vanco** 15 mg/kg IV q8h (to achieve 15-20 μg/mL trough) + timed **dexamethasone** 0.15 mg/kg q6h IV x 2–4 days.		**Alternatives: MER** 2 gm IV q8h or **Moxi** 400 mg IV q24h. **Dexamethasone** does not block penetration of vanco into CSF *(CID 44:250, 2007)*.
Gram-negative diplococci	N. meningitidis	(**Cefotaxime** 2 gm IV q4–6h or **ceftriaxone** 2 gm IV q12h)		**Alternatives: Pen G** 4 mill. units IV q4h or **AMP** 2 gm q4h or **Moxi** 400 mg IV q24h or **chloro** 1 gm IV q6h
Gram-positive bacilli or coccobacilli	Listeria monocytogenes	**AMP** 2 gm IV q4h ± **gentamicin** 2 mg/kg IV loading dose then 1.7 mg/kg IV q8h		**If pen-allergic, use TMP-SMX 5 mg/kg q6–8h or MER 2 gm IV q8h**
Gram-negative bacilli	H. influenzae, coliforms, P. aeruginosa	(**Ceftazidime** or **cefepime** 2 gm IV q8h) ± **gentamicin** 2 mg/kg IV 1st dose then 1.7 mg/kg IV q8h *(See Comment)*		**Alternatives: CIP** 400 mg IV q8–12h; **MER** 2 gm IV q8h; **Aztreonam** 2 gm IV q6-8h. Consider adding intravenous **Gentamicin** to the **β-lactam** or **CIP** if gram-stain and clinical setting suggest P. aeruginosa or resistant coliforms.
Specific Therapy—Positive culture of CSF with in vitro susceptibility results available. Interest in monitoring/reducing intracranial pressure: *CID 38:384, 2004*				
H. influenzae	β-lactamase positive	**Ceftriaxone** 2 gm IV q12h (adult), 50 mg/kg IV q12h (peds)		**Pen. allergic: Chloro** 12.5 mg/kg IV q6h (max. 4 gm/day.); **CIP** 400 mg IV q8-12h; **Aztreonam** 2 gm q6-8h.
Listeria monocytogenes *(CID 43:1233, 2006)*		**AMP** 2 gm IV q4h ± **gentamicin** 2 mg/kg IV loading dose, then 1.7 mg/kg IV q8h		**Pen. allergic: TMP-SMX** 20 mg/kg per day div. q6–12h. **Alternative: MER** 2 gm IV q8h. Success reported with **linezolid** + **RIF** *(CID 40:907, 2005)* after AMP rx for brain abscess with meningitis.
N. meningitidis	Pen MIC 0.1–1 mcg per mL	**Ceftriaxone** 2 gm IV q12h x 7 days *(see Comment)*; if β-lactam allergic, **chloro** 12.5 mg/kg (up to 1 gm) IV q6h		Rare isolates chloro-resistant. FQ-resistant isolates encountered. **Alternatives: MER** 2 gm IV q8h or **Moxi** 400 mg q24h.
S. pneumoniae	Pen G MIC <0.1 mcg/mL	**Pen G** 4 million units IV q4h or **AMP** 2 gm IV q4h		**Alternatives: Ceftriaxone** 2 gm IV q12h, **chloro** 1 gm IV q6h
NOTES:	0.1–1 mcg/mL	**Ceftriaxone** 2 gm IV q12h or **cefotaxime** 2 gm IV q4–6h		**Alternatives: Cefepime** 2 gm IV q8h or **MER** 2 gm IV q8h
1. Assumes dexamethasone just prior to 1st dose & x 4 days.	≥2 mcg/mL	**Vanco** 15 mg/kg IV q8h (15-20 μg/mL trough target) + (**ceftriaxone** or **cefotaxime** as above)		**Alternatives: Moxi** 400 mg IV q24h
2. If MIC ≥1, repeat CSF exam after 24–48h. 3. Treat for 10–14 days	Ceftriaxone MIC ≥1 mcg/mL	**Vanco** 15 mg/kg IV q8h (15-20 μg/mL trough target) + (**ceftriaxone** or **cefotaxime** as above)		**Alternatives: Moxi** 400 mg IV q24h If MIC to ceftriaxone >2 mcg/mL, add **RIF** 600 mg po/IV 1x/day to **vanco** + (**ceftriaxone** or **cefotaxime**).
E. coli, other coliforms, or P. aeruginosa	**Consultation advised**—need susceptibility results	(**Ceftazidime** or **cefepime** 2 gm IV q8h) ± **gentamicin**		**Alternatives: CIP** 400 mg IV q8–12h; **MER** 2 gm IV q8h. For intraventricular therapy: drug dosing, *see Meningitis, Post-neurosurgery, page 8.*
Prophylaxis for H. influenzae and N. meningitidis				
Haemophilus influenzae type b Household and/or day care contact: residing with index case for ≥4 hrs in a day. Day care contact or same day care facility as index case for 5-7 days before onset		**Children: RIF** 20 mg/kg po (not to exceed 600 mg) q24h x 4 doses. **Adults (non-pregnant): RIF** 600 mg q24h x 4 days		**Household:** If there is one unvaccinated contact ≤4 yrs in the household, give RIF to all household contacts except pregnant women. **Child Care Facilities:** With 1 case, if attended by unvaccinated children ≤ 2 yrs, consider prophylaxis + vaccinate susceptible. If all contacts >2 yrs: no prophylaxis. If ≥ 2 cases in 60 days & unvaccinated children attend, prophylaxis recommended for children & personnel *(Am Acad Ped Red Book 2006, page 313)*.

Abbreviations on page 2. **NOTE: All dosage recommendations are for adults (unless otherwise indicated) and assume normal renal function. § Alternatives consider allergy, PK, compliance, local resistance, cost*

TABLE 1 (7)

ANATOMIC SITE/DIAGNOSIS/ MODIFYING CIRCUMSTANCES	ETIOLOGIES (usual)	SUGGESTED REGIMENS*		ADJUNCT DIAGNOSTIC OR THERAPEUTIC MEASURES AND COMMENTS
		PRIMARY	ALTERNATIVE§	
CENTRAL NERVOUS SYSTEM/Meningitis, Bacterial, Acute/Prophylaxis for H. influenzae and N. meningitides *(continued)*				
Prophylaxis for Neisseria meningitidis exposure (close contact) **NOTE:** CDC reports **CIP-resistant group B meningococcus** from selected counties in N. Dakota & Minnesota. **Avoid CIP**. Use **ceftriaxone**, **RIF**, or single 500 mg dose of **azithro** *(MMWR 57:173, 2008)*.		[**Ceftriaxone** 250 mg IM x 1 dose (child <15 yrs 125 mg IM x 1)] **OR** [**RIF** 600 mg po q12h x 4 doses. (Children ≥1 mo 10 mg/kg po q12h x 4 doses, <1 mo 5 mg/kg q12h x 4 doses)] **OR** If not CIP-resistant, **CIP** 500 mg po x 1 dose (adult)		**Spread by respiratory droplets**, not aerosols, hence close contact req. ↑ risk if close contact for at least 4 hrs during wk before illness onset (e.g., housemates, day care contacts, cellmates) or exposure to pt's nasopharyngeal secretions (e.g., kissing, mouth-to-mouth resuscitation, intubation, nasotracheal suctioning).
Meningitis, chronic Defined as symptoms + CSF pleocytosis for ≥4 wks	MTB 40%, cryptococcosis 7%, neoplastic 8%, Lyme, syphilis, Whipple's disease	Treatment depends on etiology. No urgent need for empiric therapy, but when TB suspected treatment should be expeditious.		Long list of possibilities: bacteria, parasites, fungi, viruses, neoplasms, vasculitis, and other miscellaneous etiologies—*see Neurol Clin 28:1061, 2010*
Meningitis, eosinophilic *LnID 8:621, 2008*	Angiostrongyliasis, gnathostomiasis, baylisascaris	Corticosteroids	Not sure anthelmintic therapy works	1/3 lack peripheral eosinophilia. Need serology to confirm diagnosis. Steroid ref.: *LnID 8:621, 2008*. Automated CSF count may not correctly identify eosinophils *(CID 48: 322, 2009)*.
Meningitis, HIV-1 infected (AIDS) *See Table 11, SANFORD GUIDE TO HIV/AIDS THERAPY*	As in adults, >50 yrs: also consider cryptococci, M. tuberculosis, syphilis, HIV aseptic meningitis, Listeria monocytogenes	If etiology not identified: treat as adult >50 yrs + obtain CSF/serum cryptococcal antigen *(see Comments)*	For crypto rx, *see Table 11A, page 119*	C. neoformans most common etiology in AIDS patients. H. influenzae, pneumococci, listeria, TBc, syphilis, viral, histoplasma & coccidioides also need to be considered. Obtain blood cultures.
EAR				
External otitis				
Chronic	Usually 2° to seborrhea	Eardrops: [(**polymyxin B** + **neomycin** + **hydrocortisone** qid) + **selenium sulfide shampoo**]		Control seborrhea with dandruff shampoo containing selenium sulfide (Selsun) or [(ketoconazole shampoo) + (medium potency steroid solution, triamcinolone 0.1%)].
Fungal	Candida species	**Fluconazole** 200 mg po x 1 dose & then 100 mg po x 3-5 days.		
"Necrotizing (malignant) otitis externa" Risk groups: Diabetes mellitus, AIDS, chemotherapy.	Pseudomonas aeruginosa in >95% *(Otol & Neurotology 34:620, 2013)*	**CIP** 400 mg IV q8h; 750 mg po q8-12h only for early disease	**PIP-TZ** 3.375 gm q4h or extended infusion (3.375 gm over 4 hrs q8h) + **Tobra**	Very high ESRs are typical. Debridement usually required. R/O osteomyelitis: CT or MRI scan. If bone involved, treat for 6–8 wks. Other alternatives if P. aeruginosa is susceptible: **IMP** 0.5 gm q6h or **MER** 1 gm IV q8h or **CFP** 2 gm IV q12h or **Ceftaz** 2 gm IV q8h.
"Swimmer's ear"; occlusive devices (earphones); contact dermatitis; psoriasis *Pediatr Rev 28:77, 2007; Cochrane Database Sys Rev 2010, CD004740*	Acute infection usually 2° S. aureus (11%); other: Pseudomonas (11%), Anaerobes (2%), S. epidermidis (46%), candida (8%)	Mild: eardrops: **acetic acid** + **propylene glycol** + **HC** (**Vosol HC**) 5 gtts 3-4x/day until resolved. Moderate-severe: Eardrops **CIP** + **HC** (**Cipro HC Otic**) 3 gtts bod x 7 days		Rx includes gentle cleaning. Recurrences prevented (or decreased) by drying with alcohol drops (1/3 white vinegar, 2/3 rubbing alcohol) after swimming, then antibiotic drops or 2% acetic acid solution. Ointments should not be used in ear. Do not use neomycin or other aminoglycoside drops if tympanic membrane punctured.

**NOTE: All dosage recommendations are for adults (unless otherwise indicated) and assume normal renal function. § Alternatives consider allergy, PK, compliance, local resistance, cost*

TABLE 1 (8)

ANATOMIC SITE/DIAGNOSIS/ MODIFYING CIRCUMSTANCES	ETIOLOGIES (usual)	SUGGESTED REGIMENS*		ADJUNCT DIAGNOSTIC OR THERAPEUTIC MEASURES AND COMMENTS
		PRIMARY	ALTERNATIVE§	
EAR *(continued)*				
Otitis media—Infants, children, adults *(Cochrane review: Cochrane Database Syst Rev. Jan 31;1:CD000219, 2013)*				
Acute Two PRDB trials indicate efficacy of antibiotic rx if age < 36 mos & definite AOM *(NEJM 364:105, 116 & 168, 2011)*				
Initial empiric therapy of acute otitis media (AOM) **NOTE: Treat children <2 yrs old.** If >2 yrs old, afebrile, no ear pain, neg./questionable exam— consider analgesic treatment without antimicrobials. Favorable results in mostly afebrile pts with waiting 48hrs before deciding on antibiotic use *(JAMA 296:1235, 1290, 2006)*	Overall detection in middle ear fluid: No pathogen 4% Virus 70% Bact. + virus 66% Bacteria 92% Bacterial pathogens from middle ear: S. pneumo 49%, H. influenzae 29%, M. catarrhalis 28%. Ref.: *CID 43:1417 & 1423, 2006.* Children 6 mos-3 yrs, 2 episodes AOM/yrs & 63% are virus positive *(CID 46:815 & 824, 2008).*	**If NO antibiotics in prior month:** **Amox** po HD[3] For dosage, *see footnote*[4]. **All doses are pediatric** **Duration of rx:** <2 yrs old x 10 days; ≥2 yrs x 5–7 days. Appropriate duration unclear. 5 days may be inadequate for severe disease *(NEJM 347:1169, 2002)* **For adult dosages, see *Sinusitis, page 50, and Table 10A***	**Received antibiotics in prior month:** **Amox** HD[3] or **AM-CL** extra-strength[3] or **cefdinir** or **cefpodoxime** or **cefprozil** or **cefuroxime axetil**	**If allergic to β-lactam drugs?** If history unclear or rash, effective oral ceph OK; avoid ceph if IgE-mediated allergy, e.g., anaphylaxis. High failure rate with **TMP-SMX** if etiology is DRSP or H. influenzae; **azithro x 5 days or clarithro x 10 days** (both have ↓ activity vs. DRSP). **Up to 50% S. pneumo resistant to macrolides.** Rationale & data for single dose azithro, 30 mg per kg: *PIDJ 23:S102 & S108, 2004.* **Spontaneous resolution occurred in:** 90% pts infected with M. catarrhalis, 50% with H. influenzae, 10% with S. pneumoniae; overall 80% resolve within 2–14 days *(Ln 363:465, 2004).* Risk of DRSP ↑ if age <2 yrs, antibiotics last 3 mos, &/or daycare attendance. Selection of drug based on (1) effectiveness against β-lactamase producing H. influenzae & M. catarrhalis & (2) effectiveness against S. pneumo, inc. DRSP. **Cefaclor, loracarbef, & ceftibuten less active vs. resistant S. pneumo.** than other agents listed. No benefit of antibiotics in treatment of otitis media with effusion *(Cochrane Database Syst Rev. Sep 12;9:CD009163, 2012).*
Treatment for clinical failure after 3 days	Drug-resistant S. pneumoniae main concern	**NO antibiotics in month prior to last 3 days:** **AM-CL** high dose or **cefdinir** or **cefpodoxime** or **cefprozil** or **cefuroxime axetil** or IM **ceftriaxone** x 3 days. *For dosage, see footnote*[4] **All doses are pediatric** Duration of rx as above	**Antibiotics in month prior to last 3 days:** [(IM **ceftriaxone**) or (**clindamycin**) and/or tympanocentesis] *See clindamycin Comments*	**Clindamycin** not active vs. H. influenzae or M. catarrhalis. S. pneumo resistant to macrolides are usually also resistant to clindamycin. Definition of failure: no change in ear pain, fever, bulging TM or otorrhea after 3 days of therapy. Tympanocentesis will allow culture. **Newer FQs active vs. drug-resistant S. pneumo (DRSP), but not approved for use in children *(PIDJ 23:390, 2004).* Vanco is active vs. DRSP.** Ceftriaxone IM x 3 days superior to 1-day treatment vs. DRSP *(PIDJ 19:1040, 2000).* AM-CL HD reported successful for pen-resistant S. pneumo AOM *(PIDJ 20:829, 2001).*
After >48hrs of nasotracheal intubation	Pseudomonas sp., klebsiella, enterobacter	**Ceftazidime** or **CFP** or **IMP** or **MER** or (**PIP-TZ**) or **TC-CL** or **CIP**. *(For dosages, see Ear, Necrotizing (malignant) otitis externa, page 10)*		With nasotracheal intubation >48 hrs, about ½ pts will have otitis media with effusion.

[3] **Amoxicillin UD or HD** = amoxicillin usual dose or high dose; **AM-CL HD** = amoxicillin-clavulanate high dose. **Dosages in footnote[4].** Data supporting amoxicillin HD: *PIDJ 22:405, 2003.*

[4] **Drugs & peds dosage (all po unless specified) for acute otitis media: Amoxicillin UD** = 40 mg/kg per day div q12h or q8h. **Amoxicillin HD** = 90 mg/kg per day div q12h or q8h. **AM-CL HD** = 90 mg/kg per day of amox component. **Extra-strength AM-CL oral suspension** (Augmentin ES-600) available with 600 mg AM & 42.9 mg CL / 5 mL—dose: 90/6.4 mg/kg per day div bid. **Cefuroxime axetil** 30 mg/kg per day div q12h. **Ceftriaxone** 50 mg/kg IM x 3 days. **Clindamycin** 20–30 mg/kg per day div qid (may be effective vs. DRSP but no activity vs. H. influenzae).
Other drugs suitable for drug (e.g., penicillin) - sensitive S. pneumo: TMP-SMX 4 mg/kg of TMP q12h. **Erythro-sulfisoxazole** 50 mg/kg per day of erythro div q6–8h. **Clarithro** 15 mg/kg per day div q12h; **azithro** 10 mg/kg per day x 1 & then 5 mg/kg q24h on days 2–5. Other FDA-approved regimens: 10 mg/kg q24h x 3 days & 30 mg/kg x 1. **Cefprozil** 15 mg/kg q12h; **cefpodoxime proxetil** 10 mg/kg per day as single dose; **cefaclor** 40 mg/kg per day div q8h; **loracarbef** 15 mg/kg q12h. **Cefdinir** 7 mg/kg q12h or 14 mg/kg q24h.

TABLE 1 (9)

ANATOMIC SITE/DIAGNOSIS/ MODIFYING CIRCUMSTANCES	ETIOLOGIES (usual)	SUGGESTED REGIMENS* PRIMARY	SUGGESTED REGIMENS* ALTERNATIVE[§]	ADJUNCT DIAGNOSTIC OR THERAPEUTIC MEASURES AND COMMENTS
EAR *(continued)*				
Prophylaxis: acute otitis media *J Laryngol Otol 126:874, 2012*	Pneumococci, H. influenzae, M. catarrhalis, Staph. aureus, Group A strep *(see Comments)*	**Sulfisoxazole** 50 mg/kg po at bedtime or **amoxicillin** 20 mg/kg po q24h	**Use of antibiotics to prevent otitis media is a major contributor to emergence of antibiotic-resistant S. pneumo!** Pneumococcal protein conjugate vaccine decreases freq. AOM due to vaccine serotypes. Adenoidectomy at time of tympanostomy tubes ↓ need for future hospitalization for AOM *(NEJM 344:1188, 2001)*.	
Mastoiditis: Complication of acute or chronic otitis media. If chronic, look for cholesteatoma (Keratoma)				
Acute				
Generally too ill for outpatient therapy. Complication ref: *Otolaryng Clin No Amer 39:1237, 2006*	1st episode: S. pneumoniae H. influenzae M. catarrhalis If secondary to chronic otitis media: S. aureus P. aeruginosa S. pneumoniae	Obtain cultures, then empiric therapy. 1st episode: **Ceftriaxone** 2 gm IV once daily OR **Levofloxacin** 750 mg IV once daily	Acute exacerbation of chronic otitis media: Surgical debridement of auditory canal, then [**Vancomycin** (dose to achieve tough of 15-20 mcg/mL) + **Pip-Tazo** 3.375 gm IV q6h] OR [**Vancomycin** (dose as above) + **Ciprofloxacin** 400 mg IV q8h]	• Diagnosis: CT or MRI • Look for complication: osteomyelitis, supperative lateral sinus thrombophlebitis, purulent meningitis, brain abscess • ENT consultation for possible mastoidectomy • S. aureus *(J Otolaryng Head Neck Surg 38:483, 2009)*.
Chronic				
Generally not ill enough for parenteral antibiotics	As per 1st episode and: S. aureus P. aeruginosa Anaerobes Fungi	Culture ear drainage. May need surgical debridement. Topical Fluoroquinolone ear drops. ENT consult.		• Diagnosis: CT or MRI
EYE				
Eyelid: Little reported experience with CA-MRSA *(See Cochrane Database Syst Rev 5:CD005556, 2012)*				
Blepharitis	Etiol. unclear. Factors include Staph. aureus & Staph. epidermidis, seborrhea, rosacea, & dry eye	Lid margin care with baby shampoo & warm compresses q24h. Artificial tears if assoc. dry eye *(see Comment)*.		Usually topical ointments of no benefit. If associated rosacea, add doxy 100 mg po bid for 2 wks and then q24h.
Hordeolum (Stye)				
External (eyelash follicle)	Staph. aureus	Hot packs only. Will drain spontaneously		Infection of superficial sebaceous gland.
Internal (Meibomian glands): Can be acute, subacute or chronic.	Staph. aureus, MSSA	Oral **dicloxacillin** + hot packs		Also called acute meibomianitis. Rarely drain spontaneously; may need I&D and culture. Role of fluoroquinolone eye drops is unclear: MRSA often resistant to lower conc.; may be susceptible to higher concentration of FQ in ophthalmologic solutions of gati, levo or moxi.
	Staph. aureus, MRSA-CA	**TMP-SMX-DS**, tabs ii po bid		
	Staph. aureus, MRSA-HA	**Linezolid** 600 mg po bid possible therapy if multi-drug resistant.		
Conjunctiva: *Review: JAMA 310:1721, 2013.*				
Conjunctivitis of the newborn (**ophthalmia neonatorum**): by day of onset post-delivery—all dose pediatric				
Onset 1st day	Chemical due to silver nitrate prophylaxis	None		Usual prophylaxis is erythro ointment; hence, silver nitrate irritation rare.
Onset 2–4 days	N. gonorrhoeae	**Ceftriaxone** 25–50 mg/kg IV x 1 dose *(see Comment)*, not to exceed 125 mg		Treat mother and her sexual partners. Hyperpurulent. Topical rx inadequate. **Treat neonate for concomitant Chlamydia trachomatis.**
Onset 3–10 days	Chlamydia trachomatis	**Erythro base or ethylsuccinate syrup** 12.5 mg/kg q6h x 14 days. No topical rx needed.		Diagnosis by antigen detection. Alternative: **Azithro suspension** 20 mg/kg po q24h x 3 days. Treat mother & sexual partner.

 **NOTE: All dosage recommendations are for adults (unless otherwise indicated) and assume normal renal function. § Alternatives consider allergy, PK, compliance, local resistance, cost*

TABLE 1 (10)

ANATOMIC SITE/DIAGNOSIS/ MODIFYING CIRCUMSTANCES	ETIOLOGIES (usual)	SUGGESTED REGIMENS*		ADJUNCT DIAGNOSTIC OR THERAPEUTIC MEASURES AND COMMENTS
		PRIMARY	ALTERNATIVE§	
EYE/Conjunctiva *(continued)*				
Onset 2–16 days	Herpes simplex types 1, 2	Topical anti-viral rx under direction of ophthalmologist.		Also give Acyclovir 60 mg/kg/day IV div 3 doses *(Red Book online, accessed Jan 2011)*.
Ophthalmia neonatorum prophylaxis: **erythro** 0.5% ointment x 1 or **tetra** 1% ointment[NUS] x 1 application				
Pink eye (viral conjunctivitis) Usually unilateral	Adenovirus (types 3 & 7 in children, 8, 11 & 19 in adults)	No treatment. If symptomatic, artificial tears may help.		Highly contagious. Onset of ocular pain and photophobia in an adult suggests associated keratitis—rare.
Inclusion conjunctivitis **(adult)** Usually unilateral & concomitant genital infection	Chlamydia trachomatis	**Azithro** 1 g once	**Doxy** 100 mg po bid x 7 days	Oculogenital disease. Diagnosis NAAT. Urine NAAT for both GC & chlamydia. Treat sexual partner. May need to repeat dose of azithro.
Trachoma --a chronic bacterial keratoconjunctivitis linked to poverty	Chlamydia trachomatis	**Azithro** 20 mg/kg po single dose—78% effective in children; Adults: 1 gm po.	**Doxy** 100 mg po bid x minimum of 21 days or **tetracycline** 250 mg po qid x 14 days.	Starts in childhood and can persist for years with subsequent damage to cornea. Topical therapy of marginal benefit. Avoid doxy/tetracycline in young children. Mass treatment works *(NEJM 358:1777 & 1870, 2008; JAMA 299:778, 2008)*.
Suppurative conjunctivitis: Children and Adults (Eyedrops speed resolution of symptoms: *Cochrane Database Syst Rev. Sep 12;9:CD001211, 2012*)				
JAMA 310:1721, 2013	Staph. aureus, S. pneumoniae, H. influenzae, Viridans Strep., Moraxella sp.	FQ ophthalmic solns: **CIP** (generic); others expensive (Besi, Gati, Levo, Moxi) All 1–2 gtts q2h while awake 1st 2 days, then q4–8h up to 7 days.	**Polymyxin B + trimethoprim** solution 1–2 gtts q3–6h x 7–10 days. **Azithro** 1%, 1 gtt bid x 2 days, then 1 gtt daily x 5 days.	**FQs** best spectrum for empiric therapy. High concentrations ↑ likelihood of activity vs. S. aureus—even MRSA. **TMP** spectrum may include MRSA. Polymyxin B spectrum only Gm-neg. bacilli but no ophthal. prep of only **TMP**. Most S. pneumo resistant to **gent** & tobra. **Azithro** active vs. common gm+ pathogens.
Gonococcal (peds/adults)	N. gonorrhoeae	**Ceftriaxone** 25-50 mg/kg IV/IM (not to exceed 125 mg) as one dose in children; 1 gm IM/IV as one dose in adults		
Cornea (keratitis): Usually serious and often sight-threatening. Prompt ophthalmologic consultation essential for diagnosis, antimicrobial and adjunctive therapy! Herpes simplex most common etiology in developed countries; bacterial and fungal infections more common in underdeveloped countries.				
Viral				
H. simplex	H. simplex, types 1 & 2	**Trifluridine** ophthalmic sol'n, one drop q-2h up to 9 drops/day until re-epithelialized, then one drop q4h up to 5x/day, for total not to exceed 21 days.	**Ganciclovir** 0.15% ophthalmic gel: Indicated for acute herpetic keratitis. One drop 5 times per day while awake until corneal ulcer heals; then, one drop three times per day for 7 days. **Vidarabine** ointment— useful in children. Use 5x/day for up to 21 days (currently listed as discontinued in U.S.).	Approx 30% recurrence rate within one year; consider prophylaxis with acyclovir 400 mg bid for 12 months to prevent recurrences *(Arch Ophthal 130:108, 2012)*
Varicella-zoster ophthalmicus	Varicella-zoster virus	**Famciclovir** 500 mg po tid or **valacyclovir** 1 gm po tid x 10 days	**Acyclovir** 800 mg po 5x/day x 10 days	Clinical diagnosis most common: dendritic figures with fluorescein staining in patient with varicella-zoster of ophthalmic branch of trigeminal nerve.

Abbreviations on page 2. **NOTE: All dosage recommendations are for adults (unless otherwise indicated) and assume normal renal function. § Alternatives consider allergy, PK, compliance, local resistance, cost*

TABLE 1 (11)

ANATOMIC SITE/DIAGNOSIS/ MODIFYING CIRCUMSTANCES	ETIOLOGIES (usual)	SUGGESTED REGIMENS*		ADJUNCT DIAGNOSTIC OR THERAPEUTIC MEASURES AND COMMENTS
		PRIMARY	ALTERNATIVE§	
EYE/Cornea (keratitis) *(continued)*				
Bacterial		**All treatment listed for bacterial, fungal, protozoan is topical unless otherwise indicated**		
Acute: No comorbidity	*S. aureus, S. pneumo., S. pyogenes, Haemophilus sp.*	**Moxi:** ophthalmic 0.5%: 1 drop q1h for the first 48h then taper according to response	**Gati:** ophthalmic 0.3%: 1 drop q1h for the first 48h then taper according to response	Regimens vary: some start rx by appling drops q5 min for 5 doses; some apply drops q15-30 min for several hours; some extend interval to q2h during sleep. In a clinical trial, drops were applied q1h for 48-72h, then q2h through day 6; then q2h during waking hours on days 7-9; then q6h until healing *(Cornea 29:751, 2010)*. **Note:** despite high concentrations, may fail vs. MRSA. Prior use of fluoroquinolones associated with increased MICs (*JAMA Ophthalmol. 131:310, 2013*); high MICs associated with poorer outcome (*Clin Infect Dis 54:1381, 2012*).
Contact lens users	P. aeruginosa	**CIP** 0.3% ophthalmic solution or **LEVO** 0.5% ophthalmic solution 1-2 gtts hourly x24-72h, taper based on response.	**Gent** or **Tobra** 0.3% ophthalmic solution 1-2 gtts hourly x24h then taper based on clinical response.	Recommend alginate swab culture and susceptibility testing; refer to ophthalmologist. **Cornea abrasions:** treated with Tobra, Gent, or CIP gtts qid for 3-5 days; referral to ophthalmologist recommended cornea infiltrate or ulcer, visual loss, lack of improvement or worsening symptoms *(Am Fam Physician. 87:114, 2013)*.
Dry cornea, diabetes, immunosuppression	Staph. aureus, S. epidermidis, S. pneumoniae, S. pyogenes, Enterobacteriaceae, listeria	**CIP** 0.3% ophthalmic solution 1-2 gtts hourly x24–72 hrs, then taper based on clinical response.	**Vanco** (50 mg/mL) + **Ceftaz** (50 mg/mL) hourly for 24-72h, taper depending upon response. *See Comment.*	Specific therapy guided by results of alginate swab culture.
Fungal	Aspergillus, fusarium, candida and others.	**Natamycin** (5%): 1 drop every 1-2 h for several days; then q3-4h for several days; can reduce frequency depending upon response.	**Amphotericin B** (0.15%): 1 drop every 1-2 hours for several days; can reduce frequency depending upon response.	Obtain specimens for fungal wet mount and cultures. Numerous other treatment options (1% topical Itra for 6 wks, oral Itra 100 mg bid for 3 wks, topical voriconazole 1% hourly for 2 wks, topical miconazole 1% 5x a day, topical silver sulphadiazine 0.5-1.0% 5x a day) appear to have similar efficacy *(Cochrane Database Syst Rev 2:004241, 2012)*
Mycobacteria: Post-refractive eye surgery	*Mycobacterium chelonae*	**Gati** or **Moxi** eye drops: 1 gtt qid, probably in conjunction with other active antimicrobials		Used in conjunction with other topical and/or systemic anti-mycobacterial agents *(J Cataract Refract Surg 33:1978, 2007; Ophthalmology 113:950, 2006)*.
Protozoan Soft contact lens users. Ref: *CID 35:434, 2002.*	Acanthamoeba, sp.	Optimal regimen uncertain. Suggested regimen: [(**Chlorhexidine** 0.02% or Polyhexamethylene biguanide 0.02%) + (Propamidine isethionate 0.1% or Hexamidine 0.1%)] drops. Apply one drop every hour for 48h, then one drop every hour only while awake for 72h, then one drop every two hours while awake for 3-4 weeks, then reducing frequency based on response *(Ref: Am J Ophthalmol 148:487, 2009; Curr Op Infect Dis 23:590, 2010)*.		Uncommon. Trauma and soft contact lenses are risk factors. To obtain suggested drops: Leiter's Park Ave Pharmacy (800-292-6773; www.leiterrx.com). Cleaning solution outbreak: *MMWR 56: 532, 2007.*

**NOTE: All dosage recommendations are for adults (unless otherwise indicated) and assume normal renal function. § Alternatives consider allergy, PK, compliance, local resistance, cost*

TABLE 1 (12)

ANATOMIC SITE/DIAGNOSIS/ MODIFYING CIRCUMSTANCES	ETIOLOGIES (usual)	SUGGESTED REGIMENS*		ADJUNCT DIAGNOSTIC OR THERAPEUTIC MEASURES AND COMMENTS
		PRIMARY	ALTERNATIVE§	
EYE *(continued)*				
Lacrimal apparatus				
Canaliculitis	Actinomyces most common. Rarely, Arachnia, fusobacterium, nocardia, candida	Remove granules & irrigate with **pen G** (100,000 mcg/mL)	If fungi, irrigate with **nystatin** approx. 5 mcg/mL: 1 gtt tid	Digital pressure produces exudate at punctum; Gram stain confirms diagnosis. Hot packs to punctal area qid. M. chelonae reported after use of intracanalic plugs *(Ophth Plast Reconstr Surg 24: 241, 2008).*
		Child: AM-CL or **cefprozil or cefuroxime** *(See dose on Table 16)*		
Dacryocystitis (lacrimal sac)	S. pneumo, S. aureus, H. influenzae, S. pyogenes, P. aeruginosa	Often consequence of obstruction of lacrimal duct. Empiric systemic antimicrobial therapy based on Gram stain of aspirate—*see Comment*.		Need ophthalmologic consultation. Surgery may be required. Can be acute or chronic. Culture to detect MRSA.
Endophthalmitis: Endogenous (secondary to bacteremia or fungemia) and exogenous (post-injection, post-operative) types				
Bacterial: Haziness of vitreous key to diagnosis. Needle aspirate of both vitreous and aqueous humor for culture prior to therapy. Intravitreal administration of antimicrobials essential.				
Postocular surgery (cataracts)				
Early, acute onset (incidence 0.05%)	S. epidermidis 60%, Staph. aureus, streptococci, & enterococci each 5–10%, Gm-neg. bacilli 6%	**Immediate ophthal. consult.** If only light perception or worse, immediate vitrectomy + intravitreal vanco 1 mg & intravitreal ceftazidime 2.25 mg. No clear data on intravitreal steroid. May need to repeat intravitreal antibiotics in 2–3 days. Can usually leave lens in. Adjunctive systemic antibiotics (e.g., Vancomycin, Ceftazidime, Moxifloxacin or Gatifloxacin[NUS]) not of proven value, but recommended in endogenous infection.		
Low grade, chronic	Propionibacterium acnes, S. epidermidis, S. aureus (rare)	Intraocular **vanco**. Usually requires vitrectomy, lens removal.		
Post filtering blebs for glaucoma	Strep. species (viridans & others), H. influenzae	Intravitreal agent (e.g., **Vanco** 1 mg + **Ceftaz** 2.25 mg) and a topical agent. Consider a systemic agent such as **Amp-Sulb** or **Cefuroxime** or **Ceftaz** (add **Vanco** if MRSA is suspected)		
Post-penetrating trauma	Bacillus sp., S. epiderm.	Intravitreal agent as above + systemic **clinda** or **vanco**. Use topical antibiotics post-surgery (tobra & cefazolin drops).		
None, suspect hematogenous	S. pneumoniae, N. meningitidis, Staph. aureus, Grp B Strep, K. pneumo	(**cefotaxime** 2 gm IV q4h or **ceftriaxone** 2 gm IV q24h) + **vanco** 30-60 mg/kg/day in 2-3 div doses to achieve target trough serum concentration of 15-20 mcg/mL pending cultures. Intravitreal antibiotics as with early post-operative.		
IV heroin abuse	Bacillus cereus, Candida sp.	Intravitreal agent + systemic agent based on etiology and antimicrobial susceptibility.		
Mycotic (fungal): Broad-spectrum antibiotics, often corticosteroids, indwelling venous catheters	Candida sp., Aspergillus sp.	Intravitreal **ampho B** 0.005–0.01 mg in 0.1 mL. *Also see Table 11A, page 117 for concomitant systemic therapy. See Comment.*		Patients with *Candida* spp. chorioretinitis usually respond to systemically administered antifungals *(Clin Infect Dis 53:262, 2011)*. Intravitreal amphotericin and/or vitrectomy may be necessary for those with vitritis or endophthalmitis *(Br J Ophthalmol 92:466, 2008; Pharmacotherapy 27:1711, 2007).*
Retinitis				
Acute retinal necrosis	Varicella zoster, Herpes simplex	IV **acyclovir** 10–12 mg/kg IV q8h x 5–7 days, then 800 mg po 5x/day x 6 wks		Strong association of VZ virus with atypical necrotizing herpetic retinopathy.
HIV+ (AIDS) CD4 usually <100/mm³	Cytomegalovirus	*See Table 14A, page 160*		Occurs in 5–10% of AIDS patients

Abbreviations on page 2. *NOTE: *All dosage recommendations are for adults (unless otherwise indicated) and assume normal renal function. § Alternatives consider allergy, PK, compliance, local resistance, cost*

TABLE 1 (13)

ANATOMIC SITE/DIAGNOSIS/ MODIFYING CIRCUMSTANCES	ETIOLOGIES (usual)	SUGGESTED REGIMENS*		ADJUNCT DIAGNOSTIC OR THERAPEUTIC MEASURES AND COMMENTS
		PRIMARY	ALTERNATIVE§	
EYE/Retinitis *(continued)*				
Progressive outer retinal necrosis	VZV, H. simplex, CMV (rare)	**Acyclovir** 10-12 mg/kg IV q8h for 1-2 weeks, then (**valacyclovir** 1000 mg po tid, or **famciclovir** 500 mg po tid, or **acyclovir** 800 mg po tid). Ophthalmology consultation imperative: approaches have also included intra-vitreal injection of anti-virals (foscarnet, ganciclovir implant). In rare cases due to CMV use **ganciclovir/valganciclovir** *(see CMV retinitis, Table 14A).*		Most patients are highly immunocompromised (HIV with low CD4 or transplantation). In contrast to Acute Retinal Necrosis, lack of intraocular inflammation or arteritis. May be able to stop oral antivirals when CD4 recovers with ART *(Ocul Immunol Inflammation 15:425, 2007).*
Orbital cellulitis *(see page 54 for erysipelas, facial)*	S. pneumoniae, H. influenzae, M. catarrhalis, S. aureus, anaerobes, group A strep, occ. Gm-neg. bacilli post-trauma	**Vancomycin** 15-20 mg/kg IV q8-12h (target **vancomycin** trough serum concentrations of 15-20 μg/mL) + ([**Ceftriaxone** 2 gm IV q24h + **Metronidazole** 1 gm IV q12h] OR **Piperacillin-Tazobactam** 4.5 gm IV q8h)		**If penicillin/ceph allergy: Vanco** + **levo** 750 mg IV once daily + **metro** IV. Problem is frequent inability to make microbiologic diagnosis. Image orbit (CT or MRI). Risk of cavernous sinus thrombosis. If vanco intolerant, another option for s. aureus is dapto 6 mg/kg IV q24h.
FOOT				
"Diabetic foot"—Two thirds of patients have triad of neuropathy, deformity and pressure-induced trauma. IDSA Guidelines *CID 54:e132, 2012.*				
Ulcer without inflammation	Colonizing skin flora	No antibacterial therapy. Moderate strength evidence for improved healing with biologic skin equivalent or negative pressure wound therapy. Low strength evidence for platelet derived growth factor and silver cream *(AnIM 159:532, 2013).*		**General:** 1. Glucose control, eliminate pressure on ulcer 2. **Assess for peripheral vascular disease** 3. Caution in use of TMP-SMX in patients with diabetes, as many have risk factors for hyperkalemia (e.g., advanced age, reduced renal function, concomitant medications) *(Arch Intern Med 170:1045, 2010).* **Principles of empiric antibacterial therapy:** 1. Obtain culture; cover for MRSA in moderate, more severe infections pending culture data, local epidemiology. 2. Severe limb and/or life-threatening infections require initial parenteral therapy with predictable activity vs. Gm-positive cocci, coliforms & other aerobic Gm-neg. rods, & anaerobic Gm-neg. bacilli. 3. **NOTE:** The regimens listed are suggestions consistent with above principles. Other alternatives exist & may be appropriate for individual patients. 4. Is there an associated osteomyelitis? Risk increased if ulcer area >2 cm^2, positive probe to bone, ESR >70 and abnormal plain x-ray. Negative MRI reduces likelihood of osteomyelitis *(JAMA 299:806, 2008).* MRI is best imaging modality *(CID 47:519 & 528, 2008).*
Mild infection	*S. aureus (assume MRSA), S. agalactiae (Gp B), S. pyogenes predominate*	**Oral therapy:** Diclox or cephalexin or AM-CL (not MRSA) Doxy or TMP-SMX-DS (MRSA) CLINDA (covers MSSA, MRSA, strep) *Dosages in footnote*[5]		
Moderate infection. **Osteomyelitis** *See Comment.*	As above, plus coliforms possible	**Oral:** As above **Parenteral therapy:** [based on prevailing susceptibilities: (**AM-SB** or **TC-CL** or **PIP-TZ** or **ERTA** or other carbapenem)] plus [**vanco** (or alternative anti-MRSA drug as below) until MRSA excluded]. *Dosages in footnotes*[6,7]		
Extensive local inflammation plus systemic toxicity.	As above, plus anaerobic bacteria. Role of enterococci unclear.	**Parenteral therapy:** (**Vanco** plus **β-lactam/β-lactamase inhibitor**) or (**vanco** plus [**Dori** or **IMP** or **MER**]). Other alternatives: 1. **Dapto** or **linezolid** for vanco 2. (**CIP** or **Levo** or **Moxi** or **aztreonam**) plus **metronidazole** for β-lactam/β-lactamase inhibitor *Dosages in footnote*[7] **Assess for arterial insufficiency!**		

[5] **TMP-SMX-DS** 1-2 tabs po bid, **minocycline** 100 mg po bid, **Pen VK** 500 mg po qid, (O Ceph 2, 3: **cefprozil** 500 mg po q12h, **cefuroxime axetil** 500 mg po q12h, **cefdinir** 300 mg po q12h or 600 mg po q24h, **cefpodoxime** 200 mg po q12h), **CIP** 750 mg po bid. **Levo** 750 mg po q24h. **Diclox** 500 mg qid. **Cephalexin** 500 mg qid. **AM-CL** 875/125 bid. **Doxy** 100 mg bid. **CLINDA** 300-450 mg tid

[6] **AM-CL-ER** 2000/125 mg po bid, **TMP-SMX-DS** 1-2 tabs po bid, **CIP** 750 mg po bid, **Levo** 750 mg po q24h, **Moxi** 400 mg po q24h, **linezolid** 600 mg po bid.

[7] **Vanco** 1 gm IV q12h, (**parenteral β-lactam/β-lactamase inhibitors**; **AM-SB** 3 gm IV q6h, **PIP-TZ** 3.375 gm IV q6h or 4.5 gm IV q8h or 4 hr infusion of 3.375 gm q8h;TC-CL 3.1 gm IV q6h); **carbapenems: Doripenem** 500 mg (1-hr infusion) q8h, **ERTA** 1 gm IV q24h, **IMP** 0.5 gm IV q6h, **MER** 1 gm IV q8h, **daptomycin** 6 mg per kg IV q24h, **linezolid** 600 mg IV q12h, **aztreonam** 2 gm IV q8h. **CIP** 400 mg IV q12h, **Levo** 750 mg IV q24h, **Moxi** 400 mg IV q24h, **metro** 1 gm IV loading dose & then 0.5 gm IV q6h or 1 gm IV q12h.

 **NOTE: All dosage recommendations are for adults (unless otherwise indicated) and assume normal renal function. § Alternatives consider allergy, PK, compliance, local resistance, cost*

TABLE 1 (14)

ANATOMIC SITE/DIAGNOSIS/ MODIFYING CIRCUMSTANCES	ETIOLOGIES (usual)	SUGGESTED REGIMENS*		ADJUNCT DIAGNOSTIC OR THERAPEUTIC MEASURES AND COMMENTS
		PRIMARY	ALTERNATIVE§	
FOOT *(continued)*				
Onychomycosis: *See Table 11, page 121, fungal infections*				
Puncture wound: Nail/Toothpick	P. aeruginosa	Cleanse. Tetanus booster. Observe.		*See page 4. 1–2% evolve to osteomyelitis*. After toothpick injury *(PIDJ 23:80, 2004)*: S. aureus, Strep sp, and mixed flora.
GALLBLADDER				
Cholecystitis, cholangitis, biliary sepsis, or common duct obstruction (partial: 2nd to tumor, stones, stricture). Cholecystitis Ref: *NEJM 358:2804, 2008.*	Enterobacteriaceae 68%, enterococci 14%, bacteroides 10%, Clostridium sp. 7%, rarely candida	(**PIP-TZ** or **AM-SB** or **TC-CL**) If life-threatening: **IMP** or **MER** or **Dori** *Dosages in footnote[7] on page 16.* * Add vanco for empiric activity vs. enterococci	(**P Ceph 3*** + **metro**) or (**Aztreonam*** + **metro**) or (**CIP***+ **metro**) or **Moxi**	In severely ill pts, antibiotic therapy complements adequate biliary drainage. 15-30% pts will require decompression: surgical, percutaneous or ERCP-placed stent.
GASTROINTESTINAL				
Gastroenteritis—Empiric Therapy (laboratory studies not performed or culture, microscopy, toxin results NOT AVAILABLE)				
Premature infant with necrotizing enterocolitis	Associated with intestinal flora	Antibiotic treatment should cover broad range of intestinal organisms, using regimens appropriate to age and local susceptibility patterns, rationale as in diverticulitis/peritonitis, *page 22. See Table 16, page 209 for pediatric dosages.*		Pneumatosis intestinalis, if present on x-ray confirms diagnosis. Bacteremia-peritonitis in 30–50%. If Staph. epidermidis isolated, add vanco (IV). For review and general management, *see NEJM 364:255, 2011.*
Mild diarrhea (≤3 unformed stools/day, minimal associated symptomatology)	Bacterial *(see Severe, below)*, viral (norovirus), parasitic. Viral usually causes mild to moderate disease. For traveler's diarrhea, *see page 20*	Fluids only + lactose-free diet, avoid caffeine		**Rehydration: For po fluid replacement,** *see Cholera, page 19.* **Antimotility** (Do not use if fever, bloody stools, or suspicion of HUS): Loperamide (Imodium) 4 mg po, then 2 mg after each loose stool to max. of 16 mg per day. Bismuth subsalicylate (Pepto-Bismol) 2 tablets (262 mg) po qid. **Hemolytic uremic syndrome (HUS):** Risk in **children** infected with E. coli 0157:H7 is 8–10%. Early treatment with TMP-SMX or FQs ↑ risk of HUS. **Norovirus:** Etiology of over 90% of non-bacterial diarrhea (± nausea/vomiting). Lasts 12-60 hrs. Hydrate. No effective antiviral. **Other potential etiologies:** Cryptosporidia—no treatment in immunocompetent host. Cyclospora—usually chronic diarrhea, responds to TMP-SMX *(see Table 13A)*. Klebsiella oxytoca identified as cause of antibiotic-associated hemorrhagic colitis (cytotoxin positive): *NEJM 355:2418, 2006.*
Moderate diarrhea (≥4 unformed stools/day &/or systemic symptoms)		Antimotility agents *(see Comments)* + fluids		
Severe diarrhea (≥6 unformed stools/day, &/or temp ≥101°F, tenesmus, blood, or fecal leukocytes) **NOTE: Severe afebrile bloody diarrhea should ↑ suspicion of Shiga-toxin E. coli 0157:H7 & others** *(MMWR 58 (RR-12):1, 2009).*	Shigella, salmonella, C. jejuni, Shiga toxin + E. coli, toxin-positive C. difficile, Klebsiella oxytoca, E. histolytica. *For typhoid fever, see page 61*	**FQ** (**CIP** 500 mg po q12h or **Levo** 500 mg q24h) times 3–5 days	**TMP-SMX-DS** po bid times 3–5 days. Campylobacter resistance to TMP-SMX common in tropics.	
		If recent antibiotic therapy (C. difficile toxin colitis possible) **add:**		
		Metro 500 mg po tid times 10–14 days	**Vanco** 125 mg po qid times 10–14 days	

Abbreviations on page 2. **NOTE: All dosage recommendations are for adults (unless otherwise indicated) and assume normal renal function. § Alternatives consider allergy, PK, compliance, local resistance, cost*

TABLE 1 (15)

ANATOMIC SITE/DIAGNOSIS/ MODIFYING CIRCUMSTANCES	ETIOLOGIES (usual)	SUGGESTED REGIMENS* PRIMARY	SUGGESTED REGIMENS* ALTERNATIVE§	ADJUNCT DIAGNOSTIC OR THERAPEUTIC MEASURES AND COMMENTS
GASTROINTESTINAL *(continued)*				
Gastroenteritis—Specific Therapy (results of culture, microscopy, toxin assay AVAILABLE) (Ref.: *NEJM 361:1560, 2009*)				
If culture negative, probably **Norovirus (Norwalk)** other virus *(EID 17:1381, 2011) — see Norovirus, page 168* **NOTE:** WBC > 15,000 suggestive of C. difficile in hospitalized patient.	**Aeromonas/Plesiomonas**	**CIP** 750 mg po bid x3 days.	**TMP-SMX DS** tab 1 po bid x 3 days	Although no absolute proof, increasing evidence for Plesiomonas as cause of diarrheal illness *(NEJM 361:1560, 2009)*.
	Amebiasis (Entamoeba histolytica, Cyclospora, Cryptosporidia and **Giardia)**, *see Table 13A*			
	Campylobacter jejuni History of fever in 53-83%. Self-limited diarrhea in normal host.	**Azithro** 500 mg po q24h x 3 days.	**Erythro stearate** 500 mg po qid x 5 days or **CIP** 500 mg po bid (CIP resistance increasing).	**Post-Campylobacter Guillain-Barré;** assoc. 15% of cases *(Ln 366:1653, 2005)*. Assoc. with small bowel lymphoproliferative disease; may respond to antimicrobials *(NEJM 350:239, 2004)*. **Reactive arthritis** another potential sequelae. *See Traveler's diarrhea, page 20.*
	Campylobacter fetus Diarrhea uncommon. More systemic disease in debilitated hosts	**Gentamicin** *(see Table 10D)*	**AMP** 100 mg/kg/day IV div q6h or **IMP** 500 mg IV q6h	Draw blood cultures. In bacteremic pts, 32% of C. fetus resistant to FQs *(CID 47:790, 2008)*. Meropenem inhibits C. fetus at low concentrations in vitro.
Differential diagnosis of toxin-producing diarrhea: • C. difficile • Klebsiella oxytoca • S. aureus • Shiga toxin producing E. coli (STEC) • Enterotoxigenic B. fragilis *(CID 47:797, 2008)* More on C. difficile: *Treatment review: CID 51:1306, 2010.* *SHEA/IDSA treatment guidelines: ICHE 31:431, 2010; ESCMID guidelines: Clin Microbiol Infect 15:1067, 2009; AnIM 155:839, 2011.* *(Continued on next page)*	**C. difficile** toxin positive antibiotic-associated colitis. **Probiotics:** (lactobacillus or saccharomyces) inconsistent results *(AnIM 157:878, 2012; Lancet 382:1249, 2013)*.			
	po meds okay; WBC <15,000; no increase in serum creatinine.	**Metro** 500 mg po tid or 250 mg qid x 10-14 days	**Vanco** 125 mg po qid x 10-14 days **Teicoplanin**[NUS] 400 mg po bid x 10 days	**D/C antibiotic if possible; avoid antimotility agents, hydration, enteric isolation.** Recent review suggests antimotility agents can be used cautiously in certain pts with mild disease who are receiving rx *(CID 48: 598, 2009)*. **Relapse in 10-20%.**
	po meds okay; Sicker; WBC >15,000; ≥ 50% increase in baseline creatinine	**Vanco** 125 mg po qid x 10-14 days. To use IV **vanco po**, *see* Table 10A, *page 96.*	**Fidaxomicin** 200 mg po bid x 10 days	Vanco superior to metro in sicker pts. Relapse in 10-20%. Fidaxomicin had lower rate of recurrence than Vanco for diarrhea with non-NAP1strains *(N Engl J Med 364:422, 2011)*.
	Post-treatment relapse	**1st relapse** **Metro** 500 mg po tid x 10 days	**2nd relapse** **Vanco** 125 mg po qid x 10-14 days, then immediately start taper *(See Comments)*	**Vanco** taper (all doses 125 mg po): week 1– bid, week 2 – q24h; week 3 – qod; then every 3rd day for 5 doses *(NEJM 359, 1932, 2008)*. Another option: After initial vanco, **rifaximin**[NAI] 400-800 mg po daily divided bid or tid x 2 wks. **Fecal transplant** more efficacious than vancomycin (15/16 [93%] versus 7/26 [27%]) in curing recurrent C. difficile infection *(New Engl J Med 368:407, 2013)*
	Post-op ileus; severe disease with toxic megacolon *(NEJM 359:1932, 2008)*.	**Metro** 500 mg IV q6h + **vanco** 500 mg q6h via nasogastric tube (or naso-small bowel tube) ± retrograde via catheter in cecum. *See comment* for dosage.		For vanco instillation into bowel, add 500 mg vanco to 1 liter of saline and perfuse at 1-3 mL/min to maximum of 2 gm in 24 hrs *(CID 690, 2002)*. **Note: IV vanco not effective.** Indications for colectomy, *see ICHE 31:431, 2010*. Reported successful use of tigecycline[NAI] IV to treat severe C. diff refractory to standard rx *(CID 48:1732, 2009)*.
	Enterohemorrhagic E. coli (EHEC). Some produce **Shiga toxin E. coli (STEC)** and cause **hemolytic uremic syndrome (HUS).** Strains: 0157:H7, 0104:H4 and others. Classically bloody diarrhea and afebrile	**Hydration:** avoid antiperistaltic drugs. 25% increased risk of precipitating HUS in children < age 10 yrs given TMP-SMX, beta lactam, metronidazole or azithromycin for diarrhea *(CID 55:33, 2012)*. In uncontrolled study, antibiotic treatment of STEC outbreak, shorter excretion of E. coli, fewer seizures, lower mortality *(BMJ 345:e4565, 2012)*. If on empiric antibiotics, then Dx of STEC, reasonable to discontinue antibiotics. Avoid all antibiotics in children age < 10 yrs with bloody diarrhea. If antibiotics used, azithromycin may be the safest choice *(JAMA 307:1046, 2012)*.		• HUS more common in children, 15% in age < 10 yrs; 6-9% overall. • Diagnosis: EIA for Shiga toxins 1 & 2 in stool *(MMWR 58(RR-12), 2009)*. • Treatment: In vitro and in vivo data, that exposure of STEC to TMP-SMX and CIP causes burst of HUS toxin production as bacteria die *(JID 181:664, 2000)*. • HUS bad disease: 10% mortality; 50% some degree of permanent renal damage *(CID 38:1298, 2004)*.

 **NOTE: All dosage recommendations are for adults (unless otherwise indicated) and assume normal renal function. § Alternatives consider allergy, PK, compliance, local resistance, cost*

TABLE 1 (16)

ANATOMIC SITE/DIAGNOSIS/ MODIFYING CIRCUMSTANCES	ETIOLOGIES (usual)	SUGGESTED REGIMENS*		ADJUNCT DIAGNOSTIC OR THERAPEUTIC MEASURES AND COMMENTS
		PRIMARY	ALTERNATIVE[§]	
GASTROINTESTINAL/Gastroenteritis—Specific Therapy *(continued)*				
(Continued from previous page)	**Klebsiella oxytoca—antibiotic-associated diarrhea**	Responds to stopping antibiotic		Suggested that stopping NSAIDs helps. Ref.: *NEJM 355:2418, 2006.*
	Listeria monocytogenes	Usually self-limited. Value of oral antibiotics (e.g., ampicillin or TMP-SMX) unknown, but their use might be reasonable in populations at risk for serious listeria infections. Those with bacteremia/meningitis require parenteral therapy: *see pages 9 & 60.*		Recognized as a cause of food-associated febrile gastroenteritis. Not detected in standard stool cultures. Populations at ↑ risk of severe systemic disease: pregnant women, neonates, the elderly, and immunocompromised hosts *(MMWR 57:1097, 2008).*
	Salmonella, non-typhi— For typhoid (enteric) fever, *see page 61* Fever in 71–91%, history of bloody stools in 34%	If pt asymptomatic or illness mild, antimicrobial therapy not indicated. **Treat if** <1 yr old or >50 yrs old, if immunocompromised, if vascular grafts or prosthetic joints, bacteremic, hemoglobinopathy, or hospitalized with fever and severe diarrhea *(see typhoid fever, page 61).*		
		(**CIP** 500 mg bid) or (**Levo** 500 mg q24h) x 7-10 days (14 days if immunocompromised).	**Azithro** 500 mg po once daily x 7 days (14 days if immunocompromised).	↑ resistance to TMP-SMX and chloro. Ceftriaxone, cefotaxime usually active if IV therapy required *(see footnote, page 25, for dosage).* CLSI has established new interpretive breakpoints for susceptibility to CIP: susceptible strains, MIC < 0.06 μg/mL *(Clin Infect Dis 55:1107, 2012).* **Primary treatment of enteritis is fluid and electrolyte replacement.**
	Shigella Fever in 58%, history of bloody stools 51%	**CIP** 750 mg po bid x 3 days *See Comment for peds rx per dose*	**Azithro** 500 mg po once daily x 3 days	Recent expert review recommended adult CIP dose of 750 mg once daily for 3 days *(NEJM 361:1560, 2009).* Infection due to S. flexneri resistant to CIP, ceftriaxone and cefotaxime has been reported *(MMWR 59:1619, 2010).* **Peds doses: Azithro** 10 mg/kg/day once daily x 3 days. For severe disease, ceftriaxone 50–75 mg/kg per day x 2–5 days. CIP suspension 10 mg/kg bid x 5 days. CIP superior to ceftriaxone in children *(LnID 3:537, 2003).* **Immunocompromised children & adults: Treat for 7–10 days.** Azithro superior to cefixime in trial in children *(PIDJ 22:374, 2003).*
	Spirochetosis (Brachyspira pilosicoli)	Benefit of treatment unclear. Susceptible to **metro**, **ceftriaxone**, and **Moxi**.		Anaerobic intestinal spirochete that colonizes colon of domestic & wild animals plus humans. Case reports of diarrhea with large numbers of the organism present *(JCM 39:347, 2001; Am J Clin Path 120:828, 2003).* Rarely, *B. pilosicoli* has been isolated from blood culture *(Ann Clin Micro Antimicrob 7:19, 2008).*
	Vibrio cholerae Treatment decreases duration of disease, volume losses, & duration of excretion	**Primary therapy is rehydration.** Select antibiotics based on susceptibility of locally prevailing isolates. Options include: **Doxycycline** 300 mg po single dose **OR Azithromycin** 1 gm po single dose **OR Tetracycline** 500 mg po qid x 3 days **OR Erythromycin** 500 mg po qid x 3 days (these options are based on CDC recommendations for 2010 Haiti epidemic)	**For pregnant women: Azithromycin** 1 gm po single dose **OR Erythromycin** 500 mg po qid x 3 days **For children: Azithromycin** 20 mg/kg po as single dose; for other age-specific alternatives, *see CDC website http://www.cdc.gov/haiticholera/hcp_goingtohaiti.htm*	Antimicrobial therapy shortens duration of illness, but rehydration is paramount. When IV hydration is needed, use Ringer's lactate. Switch to PO repletion with Oral Rehydration Salts (ORS) as soon as able to take oral fluids. ORS are commercially available for reconstitution in potable water. If not available, WHO suggests a substitute can be made by dissolving ½ teaspoon salt and 6 level teaspoons of sugar per liter of potable water *(http://www.who.int/cholera/technical/en/).* CDC recommendations for other aspects of management developed for Haiti outbreak can be found at *http://www.cdc.gov/haiticholera/hcp_goingtohaiti.htm* Isolates from this outbreak demonstrate reduced susceptibility to ciprofloxacin and resistance to sulfisoxazole, nalidixic acid and furazolidone.

Abbreviations on page 2. **NOTE: All dosage recommendations are for adults (unless otherwise indicated) and assume normal renal function. § Alternatives consider allergy, PK, compliance, local resistance, cost*

TABLE 1 (17)

ANATOMIC SITE/DIAGNOSIS/ MODIFYING CIRCUMSTANCES	ETIOLOGIES (usual)	SUGGESTED REGIMENS*		ADJUNCT DIAGNOSTIC OR THERAPEUTIC MEASURES AND COMMENTS
		PRIMARY	ALTERNATIVE§	
GASTROINTESTINAL/Gastroenteritis—Specific Therapy *(continued)*				
	Vibrio parahaemolyticus	Antimicrobial rx does not shorten course. Hydration.		Shellfish exposure common. Treat severe disease: **FQ, doxy, P Ceph 3**
	Vibrio vulnificus	Usual presentation is skin lesions & bacteremia; life-threatening; treat early: **ceftaz** + **doxy**—*see page 54; levo.*		
	Yersinia enterocolitica Fever in 68%, bloody stools in 26%	No treatment unless severe. If severe, combine **doxy** 100 mg IV bid + (**tobra** or **gent** 5 mg/kg per day once q24h). **TMP-SMX** or **FQs** are alternatives.		Mesenteric adenitis pain can mimic acute appendicitis. Lab diagnosis difficult: requires "cold enrichment" and/or yersinia selective agar. Desferrioxamine therapy increases severity, discontinue if pt on it. Iron overload states predispose to yersinia.
Gastroenteritis—Specific Risk Groups–Empiric Therapy				
Anoreceptive intercourse				
Proctitis (distal 15 cm only)	Herpes viruses, gonococci, chlamydia, syphilis *See Genital Tract, page 22*			
Colitis	Shigella, salmonella, campylobacter, E. histolytica *(see Table 13A)*			*See specific GI pathogens, Gastroenteritis, above.*
HIV-1 infected (AIDS): >10 days diarrhea	G. lamblia			*See Table 13A*
Acid-fast organisms:	Cryptosporidium parvum, Cyclospora cayetanensis			
Other:	Isospora belli, microsporidia (Enterocytozoon bieneusi, Septata intestinalis)			
Neutropenic enterocolitis or "typhlitis" *(CID 56:711, 2013)*	Mucosal invasion by **Clostridium septicum**. Occasionally caused by C. sordellii or P. aeruginosa	Appropriate agents include PIP-TZ, IMP, MER, DORI plus bowel rest.		Tender right lower quadrant may be clue, but tenderness may be diffuse or absent in immunocompromised host. Need surgical consult. Surgical resection controversial but may be necessary. **NOTE:** Resistance of clostridia to clindamycin reported. Broad-spectrum agents such as PIP-TZ, IMP, MER, DORI should cover most pathogens.
Traveler's diarrhea, self-medication. Patient often afebrile	**Acute**: 60% due to diarrheagenic E. coli; shigella, salmonella, or campylobacter. C. difficile, amebiasis *(see Table 13A)*. **If chronic**: cyclospora, cryptosporidia, giardia, isospora	**CIP** 750 mg po bid for 1-3 days **OR** **Levo** 500 mg po q24h for 1-3 days **OR** **Oflox** 300 mg po bid for 3 days **OR** **Rifaximin** 200 mg po tid for 3 days **OR** **Azithro** 1000 mg po once or 500 mg po q24h for 3 days		**For pediatrics:** Azithro 10 mg/kg/day as a single dose for 3 days or Ceftriaxone 50 mg/kg/day as single dose for 3 days. Avoid FQs. **For pregnancy:** Use Azithro. Avoid FQs. **Antimotility agent:** For non-pregnant adults with no fever or blood in stool, add loperamide 4 mg po x 1, then 2 mg po after each loose stool to a maximum of 16 mg per day. **Comments:** Rifaximin approved only for ages 12 and older. Works only for diarrhea due to non-invasive E. coli; do not use if fever or bloody stool. **References:** *NEJM 361:1560, 2009; BMJ 337: a1746, 2008; http://wwwnc.cdc.gov/travel/yellowbook/2012/chapter-2-the-pre-travel-consultation/travelers-diarrhea.htm.*
Prevention of Traveler's diarrhea	Not routinely indicated. Current recommendation is to take **FQ** + **Imodium** with 1st loose stool.			

 **NOTE: All dosage recommendations are for adults (unless otherwise indicated) and assume normal renal function. § Alternatives consider allergy, PK, compliance, local resistance, cost*

TABLE 1 (18)

ANATOMIC SITE/DIAGNOSIS/ MODIFYING CIRCUMSTANCES	ETIOLOGIES (usual)	SUGGESTED REGIMENS*		ADJUNCT DIAGNOSTIC OR THERAPEUTIC MEASURES AND COMMENTS
		PRIMARY	ALTERNATIVE§	
GASTROINTESTINAL *(continued)*				
Gastrointestinal Infections by Anatomic Site: Esophagus to Rectum				
Esophagitis	Candida albicans, HSV, CMV	See SANFORD GUIDE TO HIV/AIDS THERAPY and Table 11A.		
Duodenal/Gastric ulcer; gastric cancer, MALT lymphomas (not 2° NSAIDs) *Ref: Gut 61:646, 2012; Med Lett 9:55, 2012.*	**Helicobacter pylori** *See Comment* Prevalence of pre-treatment resistance increasing	**Sequential therapy:** (**Rabeprazole** 20 mg + **amox** 1 gm) bid x 5 days, then (**rabeprazole** 20 mg + **clarithro** 500 mg + **tinidazole** 500 mg) bid for another 5 days. *See footnote*[8]. Can modify by substituting Levo for Clarithro *(JAMA 309:578, 2013; Ln 381:205, 2013).*	**Quadruple therapy (10-14 days): Bismuth** *(see footnote*[9]*)*, bismuth subsalicylate 2 tabs qid + **tetracycline** 500 mg qid + **metro** 500 mg tid + **omeprazole** 20 mg bid.	**Comment:** In many locations, 20% failure rates with previously recommended *triple* regimens **(PPI + Amox + Clarithro)** are not acceptable. With 10 days of quadruple therapy [(**omeprazole** 20 mg po twice daily) + (3 capsules po four times per day, each containing **Bismuth subcitrate potassium** 140 mg + **Metro** 125 mg + **Tetracycline** 125 mg)], eradication rates were 93% in a per protocol population and 80% in an intention-to-treat population, both significantly better than with 7-day triple therapy regimen (PPI + Amox + Clarithro) *(Lancet 377:905, 2011)*. Exercise caution regarding potential interactions with other drugs, contraindications in pregnancy and warnings for other special populations. **Dx: Stool antigen**—Monoclonal EIA >90% sens. & 92% specific. Other tests: if endoscoped, rapid urease &/or histology &/or culture; urea breath test, but some office-based tests underperform. Testing ref: *BMJ 344:44, 2012.* **Test of cure:** Repeat stool antigen and/or urea breath test >8 wks post-treatment. **Treatment outcome:** Failure rate of triple therapy 20% due to clarithro resistance. Cure rate with sequential therapy 90%.
Small intestine: Whipple's disease *(NEJM 356:55, 2007; LnID 8:179, 2008)* Treatment: *JAC 69:219, 2014.* *See Infective endocarditis, culture-negative, page 30.*	Tropheryma whipplei	(**Doxycycline** 100 mg po bid + **Hydroxychloroquine** 200 mg pot id) x 1 year, then **Doxycycline** 100 mg po bid for life Immune reconstitution inflammatory response (IRIS) reactions occur: Thalidomide therapy may be better than steroids *(J Infect 60:79, 2010)*		In vitro susceptibility testing and collected clinical experience *(JAC 69:219, 2014)*. In vitro resistance to TMP-SMX plus frequent clinical failures & relapses. Frequent in vitro resistance to carbapenems. Complete in vitro resistance to Ceftriaxone.

[8] Can substitute other proton pump inhibitors for omeprazole or rabeprazole--all bid: **esomeprazole** 20 mg (FDA-approved), **lanzoprazole** 30 mg (FDA-approved), **pantoprazole** 40 mg (not FDA-approved for this indication).

[9] **Bismuth preparations:** (1) In U.S., **bismuth subsalicylate (Pepto-Bismol)** 262 mg tabs; adult dose for helicobacter is 2 tabs (524 mg) qid. (2) Outside U.S., colloidal bismuth subcitrate (De-Nol) 120 mg chewable tablets; dose is 1 tablet qid. In the U.S., bismuth subcitrate is available in combination cap only (Pylera: each cap contains bismuth subcitrate 140 mg + Metro 125 mg + Tetracycline 125 mg), given as 3 caps po 4x daily for 10 days **together with** a twice daily PPI.

  **NOTE: All dosage recommendations are for adults (unless otherwise indicated) and assume normal renal function. § Alternatives consider allergy, PK, compliance, local resistance, cost*

TABLE 1 (19)

ANATOMIC SITE/DIAGNOSIS/ MODIFYING CIRCUMSTANCES	ETIOLOGIES (usual)	SUGGESTED REGIMENS*		ADJUNCT DIAGNOSTIC OR THERAPEUTIC MEASURES AND COMMENTS
		PRIMARY	ALTERNATIVE§	
GASTROINTESTINAL/Gastrointestinal Infections by Anatomic Site: Esophagus to Rectum *(continued)*				
Diverticulitis, perirectal abscess, peritonitis *Also see Peritonitis, page 47*	Enterobacteriaceae, occasionally P. aeruginosa, Bacteroides sp., enterococci	**Outpatient rx—mild diverticulitis, drained perirectal abscess:**		Must "cover" both Gm-neg. aerobic & Gm-neg. anaerobic bacteria. **Drugs active only vs. anaerobic Gm-neg. bacilli:** clinda, metro. **Drugs active only vs. aerobic Gm-neg. bacilli:** APAG[10], P Ceph 2/3/4 *(see Table 10A, page 92)*, aztreonam, AP Pen, CIP, Levo. **Drugs active vs. both aerobic/anaerobic Gm-neg. bacteria:** cefoxitin, cefotetan, TC-CL, PIP-TZ, AM-SB, ERTA, Dori, IMP, MER, Moxi, & tigecycline. **Increasing resistance of B. fragilis group** % Resistant: **Moxi** 42-80; **Cefoxitin** 34-45; **Cefotetan** 48-60; **Clindamycin** 19-35 *Ref: Anaerobe 17:147, 2011; AAC 56:1247, 2012; Surg Infect 10:111, 2009.*
		[(**TMP-SMX-DS** bid) or (**CIP** 750 mg bid or **Levo** 750 mg q24h)] + **metro** 500 mg q6h. All po x 7–10 days.	**AM-CL-ER** 1000/62.5 mg 2 tabs po bid x 7–10 days **OR Moxi** 400 mg po q24h x 7-10 days	
		Mild-moderate disease—Inpatient—Parenteral Rx: (e.g., focal periappendiceal peritonitis, peridiverticular abscess, endomyometritis)		**Resistance:** Resistance to metro, PIP-TZ rare. Resistance to FQ increased in enteric bacteria, particularly if any FQ used recently. **Ertapenem** poorly active vs. P. aeruginosa/Acinetobacter sp.
		PIP-TZ 3.375 gm IV q6h **or** 4.5 gm IV q8h **or TC-CL** 3.1 gm IV q6h **or ERTA** 1 gm IV q24h **or MOXI** 400 mg IV q24h	[(**CIP** 400 mg IV q12h) or (**Levo** 750 mg IV q24h)] + (**metro** 500 mg IV q6h or 1 gm IV q12h) **OR Moxi** 400 mg IV q24h	
		Severe life-threatening disease, ICU patient:		**Concomitant surgical management important**, esp. with moderate-severe disease. **Role of enterococci remains debatable**. Probably pathogenic in infections of biliary tract. Probably need drugs active vs. enterococci in pts with valvular heart disease. **Severe penicillin/cephalosporin allergy:** (**aztreonam** 2 gm IV q6h to q8h) + [**metro** (500 mg IV q6h) or (1 gm IV q12h)] **OR** [(**CIP** 400 mg IV q12h) or (**Levo** 750 mg IV q24h) + **metro**]. **Tigecycline: Black Box Warning:** All cause mortality higher in pts treated with tigecycline (2.5%) than comparators (1.8%) in meta-analysis of clinical trials. Cause of mortality risk difference of 0.6% (95% CI 0.1, 1.2) not established. Tigecycline should be reserved for use in situations when alternative treatments are not suitable *(FDA MedWatch Sep 27, 2013)*
		IMP 500 mg IV q6h **or MER** 1 gm IV q8h **or Dori** 500 mg q8h (1-hr infusion).	**AMP** + **metro** + (**CIP** 400 mg IV q12h or **Levo** 750 mg IV q24h) **OR** [**AMP** 2 gm IV q6h + **metro** 500 mg IV q6h + **aminoglycoside**[10] *(see Table 10D, page 109)*]	
GENITAL TRACT: Mixture of empiric & specific treatment. Divided by sex of the patient. For sexual assault (rape), *see Table 15A, page 197 & MMWR 59 (RR-12), 2010.* **See Guidelines for Dx of Sexually Transmitted Diseases,** *MMWR 59 (RR-12), 2010 www.cdc.gov/std/treatment.*				
Both Women & Men:				
Chancroid	H. ducreyi	**Ceftriaxone** 250 mg IM single dose OR **azithro** 1 gm po single dose	**CIP** 500 mg bid po x 3 days OR **erythro base** 500 mg qid po x 7 days.	In HIV+ pts, failures reported with single dose azithro *(CID 21:409, 1995)*. Evaluate after 7 days, ulcer should objectively improve. Symptoms improve in 7 days. All patients treated for chancroid should be tested for HIV and syphilis. All sex partners of pts with chancroid should be examined and treated if they have evidence of disease or have had sex with index pt within the last 10 days.

[10] **Aminoglycoside = antipseudomonal aminoglycosidic aminoglycoside, e.g., amikacin, gentamicin, tobramycin**

 **NOTE: All dosage recommendations are for adults (unless otherwise indicated) and assume normal renal function. § Alternatives consider allergy, PK, compliance, local resistance, cost*

TABLE 1 (20)

ANATOMIC SITE/DIAGNOSIS/ MODIFYING CIRCUMSTANCES	ETIOLOGIES (usual)	SUGGESTED REGIMENS*		ADJUNCT DIAGNOSTIC OR THERAPEUTIC MEASURES AND COMMENTS
		PRIMARY	ALTERNATIVE§	
GENITAL TRACT/Both Women & Men *(continued)*				
Chlamydia, et al. non-gonococcal or post-gonococcal urethritis, cervicitis **NOTE: Assume concomitant N. gonorrhoeae** Chlamydia conjunctivitis, *see page 12*.	Chlamydia 50%, Mycoplasma genitalium (30%). Other known etiologies (10–15%): trichomonas, herpes simplex virus, *see JID 206:357, 2012*.	(**Doxy** 100 mg bid po x 7 days) or (**azithro** 1 gm po as single dose). Evaluate & treat sex partner **In pregnancy: Azithromycin** 1 gm po single dose OR **amox** 500 mg po tid x 7 days.	(**Erythro base** 500 mg qid po x 7 days) or (**Oflox** 300 mg q12h po x 7 days) or (**Levo** 500 mg q24h x 7 days) **In pregnancy: Erythro** base 500 mg po qid for 7 days **Doxy & FQs contraindicated**	**Diagnosis:** Nucleic acid amplification tests for C. trachomatis & N. gonorrhoeae on urine samples equivalent to cervix or urethra specimens *(AnIM 142:914, 2005)*. Test all urethritis/cervicitis pts for HIV & syphilis. For additional erythromycin regimens, *see MMWR (RR-11), 2006*. **Evaluate & treat sex partners.** Re-test for cure in pregnancy. Azithromycin 1 gm was superior to doxycycline for M. genitalium male urethritis *(CID 48:1649, 2009)*, but may select resistance leading to ↑ failure of multi-dose azithromycin retreatment regimens *(CID 48:1655, 2009)*.
Recurrent/persistent urethritis	**C. trachomatis** (43%), **M. genitalium** (30%), **T. vaginalis** (13%) *(CID 52:163, 2011)*.	**Metro** 2 gm po x 1 dose + Azithro 1 gm po x 1 dose	**Tinidazole** 2 gm po X 1 + **Azithromycin** 1 gm po X 1	High failure rate of Azithro if M. genitalium *(CID 56:934, 2013)*. Can try Moxi 400 mg po once daily x 10 days if Azithro failure *(PLoS One 3:e3618, 2008)*.
Gonorrhea *(MMWR 59 (RR-12): 49, 2010)*. **FQs no longer recommended for treatment of gonococcal infections** *(MMWR 59 (RR-12):49, 2010)*. **Cephalosporin resistance:** *JAMA 309:163 & 185, 2013.*				
Conjunctivitis (adult)	N. gonorrhoeae	**Ceftriaxone** 1 gm IM or IV single dose		Consider one-time saline lavage of eye.
Disseminated gonococcal infection (DGI, dermatitis-arthritis syndrome)	N. gonorrhoeae	**Ceftriaxone** 1 gm IV q24h—*see Comment*	(**Cefotaxime** 1 gm q8h IV) or (**Ceftizoxime** 1 gm q8h IV) —*see Comment*. FQs may be effective if susceptible organism.	Continue IM or IV regimen for 24hr after symptoms ↓; reliable pts may be discharged 24hr after sx resolve to complete 7 days rx with **cefixime**[11] **400 mg po bid.** R/O meningitis/ endocarditis. **Treat presumptively for concomitant C. trachomatis.**
Endocarditis	N. gonorrhoeae	**Ceftriaxone** 1–2 gm IV q24h x 4 wks		Ref: *JID 157:1281, 1988.*
Pharyngitis Dx: NAAT	N. gonorrhoeae	**Ceftriaxone** 250 mg IM x 1 PLUS (**Azithro** 1 gm po x 1) or (**doxy** 100 mg po bid x 7 days).	Due to resistance concerns, **do not use FQs**.	Pharyngeal GC more difficult to eradicate. Some suggest test of cure culture after 1 wk. **Spectinomycin**[NUS]**, cefixime, cefpodoxime & cefuroxime not effective**
Urethritis, cervicitis, proctitis (uncomplicated) For prostatitis, *see page 27*. **Diagnosis:** Nucleic acid amplification test (NAAT) on vaginal swab, urine or urethral swab *MMWR 59 (RR-12):49, 2010.*	N. gonorrhoeae (50% of pts with urethritis, cervicitis have concomitant C. trachomatis — **treat for both unless NAAT indicates single pathogen**). Risk of MDR gonorrhea greatest in MSM *(MMWR 62:103, 2013; AnIM 158:321, 2013)*.	[(**Ceftriaxone** 250 mg IM x 1) **+** [(**Azithro** 1 gm po x 1) or (**doxy** 100 mg po bid x 7 days)]. Add **Azithro** or **Doxy** even if chlamydia ruled out. **Alternative: Azithro** 2 gm po x 1 **Rx failure: Ceftriaxone** 500 mg IM x 1 + **Azithro** 2 gm po x 1; treat partner; NAAT for test of cure one week post-treatment Severe pen/ceph allergy? Maybe **Azithro**—see azithro comment. Understanding risk of FQ-resistance, could try FQ therapy with close follow-up.		Screen for syphilis. **Other alternatives for GC (Test of Cure recommended one week after Rx for ALL of these approaches listed below):** • **Cefixime** 400 mg po x1 OR **Cefpodoxime** 400 mg po x 1 (Note: not effective for pharyngeal disease); oral cephalosporin use is no longer recommended as primary therapy owing to emergence of resistance, *MMWR 61:590, 2012*. • Other single-dose cephalosporins: ceftizoxime 500 mg IM, cefotaxime 500 mg IM, cefoxitin 2 gm IM + probenecid 1 gm po. • **Azithro** 1 gm po x 1 effective for chlamydia but need 2 gm po for GC; not recommended for GC due to GI side-effects, expense & rapid emergence of resistance.
Granuloma inguinale (Donovanosis)	Klebsiella (formerly Calymmatobacterium) granulomatis	**Doxy** 100 mg po bid x 3–4 wks	**TMP-SMX** one DS tablet bid x 3 wks **OR Erythro** 500 mg po qid x 3 wks OR **CIP** 750 mg po bid x 3 wks OR **Azithro** 1 gm po q wk x 3 wks	Clinical response usually seen in 1 wk. **Rx until all lesions healed,** may take 4 wks. Treatment failures & recurrence seen with doxy & TMP-SMX. Report of efficacy with FQ and chloro. Ref.: *CID 25:24, 1997.* Relapse can occur 6-18 months after apparently effective Rx. If improvement not evidence in first few days, some experts add gentamicin 1 mg/kg IV q8h.

[11] Cefixime oral preparations now available as oral suspension, 200 mg/5 mL, and 400 mg tablets (Lupine Pharmaceuticals, (+1) 866-587-4617). *(MMWR 57:435, 2008).*

TABLE 1 (21)

ANATOMIC SITE/DIAGNOSIS/ MODIFYING CIRCUMSTANCES	ETIOLOGIES (usual)	SUGGESTED REGIMENS*		ADJUNCT DIAGNOSTIC OR THERAPEUTIC MEASURES AND COMMENTS
		PRIMARY	ALTERNATIVE§	
GENITAL TRACT/Both Women & Men *(continued)*				
Herpes simplex virus	*See Table 14A, page 162*			
Human papilloma virus (HPV)	*See Table 14A, page 168*			
Lymphogranuloma venereum	Chlamydia trachomatis, serovars. L1, L2, L3	**Doxy** 100 mg po bid x 21 days	**Erythro** 0.5 gm po qid x 21 days or **Azithro** 1 gm po qwk X 3 weeks (clinical data lacking)	Dx based on serology; biopsy contraindicated because sinus tracts develop. Nucleic acid ampli tests for *C. trachomatis* will be positive. In MSM, presents as fever, rectal ulcer, anal discharge *(CID 39:996, 2004; Dis Colon Rectum 52:507, 2009)*.
Phthirus pubis **(pubic lice, "crabs")** & scabies	Phthirus pubis & Sarcoptes scabiei		*See Table 13A, page 153*	
Syphilis *(JAMA 290:1510, 2003)*; **Syphilis & HIV:** *MMWR 59 (RR-12):26, 2010; Review JCI 121:4584, 2011.*				
Early: primary, secondary, or latent <1 yr. Screen with treponema-specific antibody or RPR/VDRL, see JCM 50:2 & 148, 2012.	T. pallidum NOTE: Test all pts with syphilis for HIV; test all HIV patients for latent syphilis.	**Benzathine pen G (Bicillin L-A)** 2.4 million units IM x 1 or **Azithro** 2 gm po x 1 dose *(See Comment)*	(**Doxy** 100 mg po bid x 14 days) or (**tetracycline** 500 mg po qid x 14 days) or (**ceftriaxone** 1 gm IM/IV q24h x 10–14 days). Follow-up mandatory.	If early or congenital syphilis, **quantitative VDRL at 0**, 3, 6, 12 & 24 mos after rx. If 1° or 2° syphilis, VDRL should ↓ 2 tubes at 6 mos, 3 tubes 12 mos, & 4 tubes 24 mos. Update on congenital syphilis *(MMWR 59:413, 2010)*. Early latent: 2 tubes ↓ at 12 mos. With 1°, 50% will be RPR seronegative at 12 mos, 24% neg. FTA/ABS at 2–3 yrs *(AnIM 114:1005, 1991)*. If titers fail to fall, examine CSF; if CSF (+), treat as neurosyphilis; if CSF is negative, retreat with benzathine Pen G 2.4 mu IM weekly x 3 wks. **Azithro** 2 gm po x 1 dose (equivalent to **benzathine Pen** 2.4 M x 1 dose in early syphilis *(J Infect Dis 201:1729, 2010)*. **Azithro-resistant syphilis** documented in California, Ireland, & elsewhere *(CID 44:S130, 2007; AAC 54:583, 2010)*. NOTE: Use of **benzathine procaine penicillin** is inappropriate!!
More than 1 yr's duration (latent of indeterminate duration, cardiovascular, late benign gumma)	For penicillin desensitization method, *see Table 7, page 80* and *MMWR 59 (RR-12): 26, 2010.*	**Benzathine pen G (Bicillin L-A)** 2.4 million units IM q week x 3 = 7.2 million units total	**Doxy** 100 mg po bid x 28 days or **tetracycline** 500 mg po qid x 28 days; **Ceftriazone** 1 gm IV or IM daily for 10-14 days MAY be an alternative (No clinical data; consult an ID specialist)	No published data on efficacy of alternatives. **Indications for LP (CDC): neurologic symptoms, treatment failure, any eye or ear involvement, other evidence of active syphilis (aortitis, gumma, iritis).**
Neurosyphilis—Very difficult to treat. Includes ocular (retrobulbar neuritis) syphilis **All need CSF exam.**		**Pen G** 18-24 million units per day either as continuous infusion or as 3–4 million units IV q4h x 10–14 days.	(**Procaine pen G** 2.4 million units IM q24h + **probenecid** 0.5 gm po qid) both x 10–14 days—*See Comment*	**Ceftriaxone** 2 gm (IV or IM) q24h x 14 days. 23% failure rate reported *(AJM 93:481, 1992)*. For penicillin allergy: either desensitize to penicillin or obtain infectious diseases consultation. **Serologic criteria for response to rx: 4-fold or greater ↓ in VDRL titer over 6–12 mos.** *[CID 28 (Suppl. 1):S21, 1999]*.
HIV infection (AIDS) *CID 44:S130, 2007.*		Treatment same as HIV uninfected with closer follow-up. Treat early neurosyphilis for 10-14 days regardless of CD4 count: *MMWR 56:625, 2007.*		*See Syphilis discussion in MMWR 59 (RR-12), 2010.* Treat for neurosyphilis if CSF VDRL negative but >20 CSF WBCs *(STD 39:291, 2012)*.
Pregnancy and syphilis		Same as for non-pregnant, some recommend 2nd dose (2.4 million units) **benzathine pen G** 1 wk after initial dose esp. in 3rd trimester or with 2° syphilis	Skin test for penicillin allergy. Desensitize if necessary, as parenteral pen G is only therapy with documented efficacy!	Monthly quantitative VDRL or equivalent. If 4-fold ↑, re-treat. Doxy, tetracycline contraindicated. Erythro not recommended because of high risk of failure to cure fetus.

 **NOTE: All dosage recommendations are for adults (unless otherwise indicated) and assume normal renal function. § Alternatives consider allergy, PK, compliance, local resistance, cost*

TABLE 1 (22)

ANATOMIC SITE/DIAGNOSIS/ MODIFYING CIRCUMSTANCES	ETIOLOGIES (usual)	SUGGESTED REGIMENS*		ADJUNCT DIAGNOSTIC OR THERAPEUTIC MEASURES AND COMMENTS
		PRIMARY	ALTERNATIVE§	
GENITAL TRACT/Both Women & Men *(continued)*				
Congenital syphilis *(Update on Congenital Syphilis: MMWR 59 (RR-12): 36, 2010)*	T. pallidum	**Aqueous crystalline pen G** 50,000 units/kg per dose IV q12h x 7 days, then q8h for 10 day total.	**Procaine pen G** 50,000 units/kg IM q24h for 10 days	Another alternative: Ceftriaxone ≤30 days old, 75 mg/kg IV/IM q24h (use with caution in infants with jaundice) or >30 days old 100 mg/kg IV/IM q24h. Treat 10–14 days. If symptomatic, ophthalmologic exam indicated. If more than 1 day of rx missed, restart entire course. **Need serologic follow-up!**
Warts, anogenital	*See Table 14A, page 168*			
Women:				
Amnionitis, septic abortion	Bacteroides, esp. Prevotella bivius; Group B, A strepto-cocci; Enterobacteriaceae; C. trachomatis	[(**Cefoxitin** or **TC-CL** or **Dori**[NAI] or **IMP** or **MER** or **AM-SB** or **ERTA** or **PIP-TZ**) + **doxy**] **OR** [**Clinda** + (**aminoglycoside** or **ceftriaxone**)] *Dosage: see footnote*[12] **Note:** in US and Europe, 1/3 of Grp B Strep resistant to clindamycin.		D&C of uterus. **In septic abortion,** Clostridium perfringens may cause fulminant intravascular hemolysis. **In postpartum patients** with enigmatic fever and/or pulmonary emboli, **consider septic pelvic vein thrombophlebitis** *(see Vascular septic pelvic vein thrombophlebitis, page 67)*. After discharge: doxy or clinda for C. trachomatis.
Cervicitis, mucopurulent Treatment based on results of nucleic acid amplification test	N. gonorrhoeae	Treat for Gonorrhea, *page 23*		Criteria for diagnosis: 1) (muco) purulent endocervical exudate and/or 2) sustained endocervical bleeding after passage of cotton swab. >10 WBC/hpf of vaginal fluid is suggestive. Intracellular gram-neg diplococci are specific but insensitive. If in doubt, send swab or urine for culture, EIA or nucleic acid amplification test and treat for both.
	Chlamydia trachomatis	Treat for non-gonococcal urethritis, *page 23*		
Endomyometritis/septic pelvic phlebitis				
Early postpartum (1st 48 hrs) (usually after C-section)	Bacteroides, esp. Prevotella bivius; Group B, A strepto-cocci; Enterobacteriaceae; C. trachomatis	[(**Cefoxitin** or **TC-CL** or **ERTA** or **IMP** or **MER** or **AM-SB** or **PIP-TZ**) + **doxy**] or [**Clinda** + (**aminoglycoside** or **ceftriaxone**)] *Dosage: see footnote*[12]		*See Comments under Amnionitis, septic abortion, above*
Late postpartum (48 hrs to 6 wks) (usually after vaginal delivery)	Chlamydia trachomatis, M. hominis	**Doxy** 100 mg IV or po q12h times 14 days		Tetracyclines not recommended in nursing mothers; discontinue nursing. M. hominis sensitive to tetra, clinda, not erythro.
Fitzhugh-Curtis syndrome	C. trachomatis, N. gonorrhoeae	Treat as for pelvic inflammatory disease immediately below.		Perihepatitis (violin-string adhesions)
Pelvic actinomycosis; usually tubo-ovarian abscess	A. Israelii most common	**AMP** 50 mg/kg/day IV div 3-4 doses x 4-6 wks, then **Pen VK** 2-4 gm/day po x 3-6 mos.	**Doxy** or **ceftriaxone** or **clinda** or **erythro**	Complication of intrauterine device (IUD). Remove IUD. Can use **Pen G** 10-20 million units/day IV instead of **AMP** x 4-6 wks.

[12] **P Ceph 2** (**cefoxitin** 2 gm IV q6–8h, **cefotetan** 2 gm IV q12h, **cefuroxime** 750 mg IV q8h); **TC-CL** 3.1 gm IV q4–6h; **AM-SB** 3 gm IV q6h; **PIP-TZ** 3.375 gm q6h or for nosocomial pneumonia: 4.5 gm IV q6h or 4-hr infusion of 3.375 gm q8h; **doxy** 100 mg IV/po q12h; **clinda** 450–900 mg IV q8h; **aminoglycoside** (**gentamicin**, *see Table 10D, page 109*); **P Ceph 3** (**cefotaxime** 2 gm IV q8h, **ceftriaxone** 2 gm IV q24h); **doripenem** 500 mg IV q8h (1-hr infusion); **ertapenem** 1 gm IV q24h; **IMP** 0.5 gm IV q6h; **MER** 1 gm IV q8h; **azithro** 500 mg IV q24h; **linezolid** 600 mg IV/po q12h; **vanco** 1 gm IV q12h

Abbreviations on page 2. **NOTE: All dosage recommendations are for adults (unless otherwise indicated) and assume normal renal function. § Alternatives consider allergy, PK, compliance, local resistance, cost*

TABLE 1 (23)

ANATOMIC SITE/DIAGNOSIS/ MODIFYING CIRCUMSTANCES	ETIOLOGIES (usual)	SUGGESTED REGIMENS*		ADJUNCT DIAGNOSTIC OR THERAPEUTIC MEASURES AND COMMENTS
		PRIMARY	ALTERNATIVE[§]	
Pelvic Inflammatory Disease (PID), salpingitis, tubo-ovarian abscess				
Outpatient rx: limit to pts with temp <38°C, WBC <11,000 per mm^3, minimal evidence of peritonitis, active bowel sounds & able to tolerate oral nourishment *CID 44:953 & 961, 2007; MMWR 59 (RR-12):63, 2010 & www.cdc.gov/std/treatment*	N. gonorrhoeae, chlamydia, bacteroides, Enterobacteriaceae, streptococci, especially S. agalactiae Less commonly: G. vaginalis, Haemophilus influenzae, cytomegalovirus (CMV), M. genitalium, U. urealyticum	**Outpatient rx:** [(**ceftriaxone** 250 mg IM or IV x 1) (± **metro** 500 mg po bid x 14 days) + (**doxy** 100 mg po bid x 14 days)]. **OR** (**cefoxitin** 2 gm IM with **probenecid** 1 gm po both as single dose) plus (**doxy** 100 mg po bid with **metro** 500 mg bid—both times 14 days)	**Inpatient regimens:** [(**Cefotetan** 2 gm IV q12h or **cefoxitin** 2 gm IV q6h) + (**doxy** 100 mg IV/po q12h)] (**Clinda** 900 mg IV q8h) + (**gentamicin** 2 mg/kg loading dose, then 1.5 mg/kg q8h or 4.5 mg/kg once per day), then **doxy** 100 mg po bid x 14 days	Another alternative parenteral regimen: **AM-SB** 3 gm IV q6h + **doxy** 100 mg IV/po q12h Remember: Evaluate and treat sex partner. FQs not recommended due to increasing resistance *(MMWR 59 (RR-12), 2010 & www.cdc.gov/std/treatment)*. Suggest initial inpatient evaluation/therapy for pts with tubo-ovarian abscess. For inpatient regimens, continue treatment until satisfactory response for ≥ 24-hr before switching to outpatient regimen.
Vaginitis—*MMWR 59 (RR-12):63, 2010*				
Candidiasis Pruritus, thick cheesy discharge, pH <4.5 *See Table 11A, page 117*	Candida albicans 80–90%. C. glabrata, C. tropicalis may be increasing—they are less susceptible to azoles	**Oral azoles: Fluconazole** 150 mg po x 1; **itraconazole** 200 mg po bid x 1 day. For milder cases, Topical Therapy with one of the over the counter preparations usually is successful (e.g., clotrimazole, butoconazole, miconazole, or tioconazole) as creams or vaginal suppositories.	**Intravaginal azoles:** variety of strengths—from 1 dose to 7–14 days. Drugs available (all end in -azole): butocon, clotrim, micon, tiocon, tercon *(doses: Table 11A)*	Nystatin vag. tabs times 14 days less effective. Other rx for azole-resistant strains: gentian violet, boric acid. If recurrent candidiasis (4 or more episodes per yr): 6 mos. suppression with: fluconazole 150 mg po q week or itraconazole 100 mg po q24h or clotrimazole vag. suppositories 500 mg q week.
Trichomoniasis Copious foamy discharge, pH >4.5 Treat sexual partners—see *Comment*	Trichomonas vaginalis **Dx:** NAAT & PCR available; wet mount not sensitive, but can try	**Metro** 2 gm as single dose or 500 mg po bid x 7 days OR **Tinidazole** 2 gm po single dose **Pregnancy:** *See Comment*	**For rx failure:** Re-treat with metro 500 mg po bid x 7 days; if 2nd failure: metro 2 gm po q24h x 3–5 days. If still failure, **Tinidazole** 2 gm po q24h x 5 days	**Treat male sexual partners (2 gm metronidazole as single dose).** Nearly 20% men with NGU are infected with trichomonas *(JID 188:465, 2003)*. For alternative option in refractory cases, *see CID 33:1341, 2001*. **Pregnancy:** No data indicating metro teratogenic or mutagenic. For discussion of treating trichomonas, including issues in pregnancy, *see MMWR 59 (RR-12), 2010*.
Bacterial vaginosis (BV) Malodorous vaginal discharge, pH >4.5	Etiology unclear: associated with Gardnerella vaginalis, mobiluncus, , Mycoplasma hominis, Prevotella sp., & Atopobium vaginae et al.	**Metro** 0.5 gm po bid x 7 days or **metro vaginal gel**[13] (1 applicator intravaginally) 1x/day x 5 days OR **Tinidazole** (2 gm po once daily x 2 days or 1 gm po once daily x 5 days) 2% **clinda vaginal cream** 5 gm intravaginally at bedtime x 7 days	**Clinda** 0.3 gm bid po x 7 days or **clinda ovules** 100 mg intravag-inally at bedtime x 3 days.	Reported 50% ↑ in cure rate if abstain from sex or use condoms: *CID 44:213 & 220, 2007*. Treatment of male sex partner **not** indicated unless balanitis present. Metro extended release tabs 750 mg po q24h x 7 days available; no published data. **Pregnancy:** Oral **metro** or oral **clinda** 7-day regimens *(see Canadian OB GYN practice guidelines in JObstetGynCan 30:702, 2008)*. If recurrent BV, can try adding **boric acid** to suppressive regimen: Metro 0.5 gm po bid x 7 days, then vaginal boric acid gelatin capsule 600 mg hs x 21 days, followed by Metro vaginal gel 2x/week x 16 weeks *(Sex Trans Dis 36:732, 2009)*.

[13] 1 applicator contains 5 gm of gel with 37.5 mg metronidazole

[illegible] are for adults (unless otherwise indicated) and assume normal renal function. § *Alternatives consider allergy, PK, compliance, local resistance, cost*

TABLE 1 (24)

ANATOMIC SITE/DIAGNOSIS/ MODIFYING CIRCUMSTANCES	ETIOLOGIES (usual)	SUGGESTED REGIMENS*		ADJUNCT DIAGNOSTIC OR THERAPEUTIC MEASURES AND COMMENTS
		PRIMARY	ALTERNATIVE§	
GENITAL TRACT *(continued)*				
Men:				
Balanitis	Candida 40%, Group B strep, gardnerella	**Metro** 2 gm po as a single dose OR **Fluc** 150 mg po x1 OR **Itra** 200 mg po bid x 1 day.		Occurs in 1/4 of male sex partners of women infected with candida. Exclude circinate balanitis (Reiter's syndrome). Plasma cell balanitis (non-infectious) responds to hydrocortisone cream.
Epididymo-orchitis *Reviews in Brit J Urol Int 87:747, 2001; Andrologia 40:76, 2008.*				
Age <35 years	N. gonorrhoeae, Chlamydia trachomatis	**Ceftriaxone** 250 mg IM x 1 + **doxy** 100 mg po bid x 10 days		Also: bed rest, scrotal elevation, and analgesics. Enterobacteriaceae occasionally encountered. All patients treated for epididymo-orchitis < 35 yrs of age should be tested for HIV and syphilis.
Age >35 years or homosexual men (insertive partners in anal intercourse)	Enterobacteriaceae (coliforms)	[**Levo** 500-750 mg IV/po once daily] OR [(**cipro** 500 mg po bid) or (400 mg IV twice daily)] for 10-14 days.	**AM-SB**, **P Ceph 3**, **TC-CL**, **PIP-TZ** *(Dosage: see footnote page 25)*	Midstream pyuria and scrotal pain and edema. Also: bed rest, scrotal elevation, and analgesics. NOTE: Do urine NAAT (nucleic acid amplification test) to ensure absence of N. gonorrhoeae with concomitant risk of FQ-resistant gonorrhoeae or of chlamydia if using agents without reliable activity. Other causes include: mumps, brucella, TB, intravesicular BCG, B. pseudomallei, coccidioides, Behcet's *(see Brit J Urol Int 87:747, 2001)*.
Non-gonococcal urethritis	*See Chlamydia et al, Non-gonococcal urethritis, Table 1(20), page 23*			
Prostatitis—Review: *CID 50:1641, 2010.*				
Acute Uncomplicated (with risk of STD; age < 35 yrs)	N. gonorrhoeae, C. trachomatis	(**ceftriaxone** 250 mg IM x 1 OR **cefixime** 400 mg po X 1) then **doxy** 100 mg bid x 10 days.		FQs no longer recommended for gonococcal infections. Test for HIV. In AIDS pts, prostate may be focus of Cryptococcus neoformans.
Uncomplicated with low risk of STD	Enterobacteriaceae (coliforms)	**FQ** *(dosage: see Epididymo-orchitis, >35 yrs, above)* or **TMP-SMX** 1 DS tablet (160 mg TMP) po bid x 10–14 days (minimum). Some authorities recommend 4 weeks of therapy.		Treat as acute urinary infection, 14 days (not single dose regimen). Some authorities recommend 3–4 wks therapy. If uncertain, do urine test for C. trachomatis and of N. gonorrhoeae. If resistant enterobacteriaceae, use ERTA 1 gm IV qd. If resistant pseudomonas, use IMP or MER (500 mg IV q6 or q8 respectively)
Chronic bacterial	Enterobacteriaceae 80%, enterococci 15%, P. aeruginosa	**FQ** (**CIP** 500 mg po bid x 4-6 wks, **Levo** 750 mg po q24h x 4 wks—*see Comment*)	**TMP-SMX-DS** 1 tab po bid x 1–3 mos	With treatment failures consider infected prostatic calculi. FDA approved dose of levo is 500 mg; editors prefer higher dose.
Chronic prostatitis/chronic pain syndrome (New NIH classification, *JAMA 282:236, 1999*)	The most common prostatitis syndrome. Etiology is unknown, molecular probe data suggest infectious etiology *(Clin Micro Rev 11: 604, 1998)*.	**α-adrenergic blocking agents are controversial** *(AnIM 133:367, 2000)*.		Pt has sx of prostatitis but negative cultures and no cells in prostatic secretions. Rev.: *JAC 46:157, 2000*. In randomized double-blind study, CIP and an alpha-blocker of no benefit *(AnIM 141:581 & 639, 2004)*.

Abbreviations on page 2. **NOTE: All dosage recommendations are for adults (unless otherwise indicated) and assume normal renal function. § Alternatives consider allergy, PK, compliance, local resistance, cost*

TABLE 1 (25)

ANATOMIC SITE/DIAGNOSIS/ MODIFYING CIRCUMSTANCES	ETIOLOGIES (usual)	SUGGESTED REGIMENS*		ADJUNCT DIAGNOSTIC OR THERAPEUTIC MEASURES AND COMMENTS
		PRIMARY	ALTERNATIVE[§]	
HAND *(Bites: See Skin)*				
Paronychia				
Nail biting, manicuring	Staph. aureus (maybe MRSA)	Incision & drainage; do culture	**TMP-SMX-DS** 1-2 tabs po bid while waiting for culture result.	*See Table 6 for alternatives*. Occasionally--candida, gram-negative rods.
Contact with oral mucosa—dentists, anesthesiologists, wrestlers	Herpes simplex (Whitlow)	**Acyclovir** 400 mg tid po x 10 days	**Famciclovir** or **valacyclovir** should work, *see Comment*	Gram stain and routine culture negative. Famciclovir/valacyclovir doses used for primary genital herpes should work; *see Table 14A, page 162*
Dishwasher (prolonged water immersion)	Candida sp.	**Clotrimazole** (topical)		Avoid immersion of hands in water as much as possible.
HEART				
Infective endocarditis—Native valve—empirical rx awaiting cultures—No IV illicit drugs	**NOTE: Diagnostic criteria** include evidence of continuous bacteremia (multiple positive blood cultures), new murmur (worsening of old murmur) of valvular insufficiency, definite emboli, and echocardiographic (transthoracic or transesophageal) evidence of valvular vegetations. Refs.: *Circulation 111:3167, 2005; Eur Heart J 30:2369, 2009*. For antimicrobial prophylaxis, *see Table 15C, page 202*.			
Valvular or congenital heart disease but no modifying circumstances *See Table 15C, page 202 for prophylaxis*	Viridans strep 30–40%, "other" strep 15–25%, enterococci 5–18%, staphylococci 20-35% (including coag-neg staphylococci--*CID 46:232, 2008*).	[(**Pen G** 20 million units IV q24h, continuous or div. q4h) or (**AMP** 12 gm IV q24h, continuous or div. q4h) + (**nafcillin** or **oxacillin** 2 gm IV q4h) + **gentamicin** 1 mg/kg IM or IV q8h *(see Comment)*]	Vanco 30-60 mg/kg/d in 2-3 divided doses to achieve trough of 15-20 mcg/mL+ **gentamicin** 1 mg/kg[14] IM or IV q8h **OR dapto** 6 mg/kg IV q24h	If patient not acutely ill and not in heart failure, wait for blood culture results. If initial 3 blood cultures neg. after 24–48 hrs, obtain 2–3 more blood cultures before empiric therapy started. **Nafcillin/oxacillin + gentamicin** may not cover enterococci, hence addition of penicillin G pending cultures. When blood cultures +, modify regimen to specific therapy for organism. **Gentamicin** used for synergy; peak levels need not exceed 4 mcg per mL. **Surgery indications:** *See NEJM 368:1425, 2013*. Role of surgery in pts with left-sided endocarditis & large vegetation *(NEJM 366:2466, 2012)*.
Infective endocarditis—Native valve—IV illicit drug use ± evidence rt-sided endocarditis — empiric therapy	S. aureus*(MSSA & MRSA)*. All others rare	**Vanco** 30-60 mg/kg per day in 2-3 divided doses to achieve target trough concentrations of 15-20 mcg/mL recommended for serious infections.	**Dapto** 6 mg/kg IV q24h Approved for right-sided endocarditis.	
Infective endocarditis—Native valve—culture positive				
Viridans strep, S. bovis *(S. gallolyticus)* with **penicillin G MIC ≤0.12 mcg/mL**	**Viridans strep, S. bovis (S. gallolyticus subsp. gallolyticus)**	[(**Pen G** 12–18 million units/day IV, divided q4h **x 2 wks**) PLUS (**gentamicin** IV 1 mg/kg q8h IV **x 2 wks**)] **OR** (**Pen G** 12–18 million units/day IV, divided - q4h **x 4 wks**) **OR** (**ceftriaxone** 2 gm IV q24h **x 4 wks**)	(**Ceftriaxone** 2 gm IV q24h + **gentamicin** 1 mg per kg IV q8h both **x 2 wks**). If allergy pen G or ceftriax, use **vanco** 15 mg/kg IV q12h to 2 gm/day max unless serum levels measured **x 4 wks**	Target **gent levels:** peak 3 mcg/mL, trough <1 mcg/mL. If very obese pt, recommend consultation for dosage adjustment. Infuse vanco over ≥1 hr to avoid "red man" syndrome. **S. bovis suggests occult bowel pathology (new name: S. gallolyticus).** Since relapse rate may be greater in pts ill for >3 mos. prior to start of rx, the penicillin-gentamicin synergism theoretically may be advantageous in this group.
Viridans strep, S. bovis (S. gallolyticus) with **penicillin G MIC >0.12 to ≤0.5 mcg/mL**	**Viridans strep, S. bovis, nutritionally variant streptococci, (e.g. S. abiotrophia) tolerant strep[14]**	**Pen G** 18 million units/day IV (divided q4h) **x 4 wks PLUS Gent** 1 mg/kg IV q8h **x 2 wks NOTE: Low dose of Gent**	**Vanco** 15 mg/kg IV q12h to max. 2 gm/day unless serum levels documented **x 4 wks**	Can use cefazolin for pen G in pt with allergy that is not IgE-mediated (e.g., anaphylaxis). Alternatively, can use vanco. *(See Comment above on gent and vanco)*. **NOTE: If necessary to remove infected valve & valve culture neg., 2 weeks antibiotic treatment post-op sufficient** *(CID 41:187, 2005)*.

[14] Tolerant streptococci = MBC 32-fold greater than MIC

normal renal function. § Alternatives consider allergy, PK, compliance, local resistance, cost

TABLE 1 (26)

ANATOMIC SITE/DIAGNOSIS/ MODIFYING CIRCUMSTANCES	ETIOLOGIES (usual)	SUGGESTED REGIMENS*		ADJUNCT DIAGNOSTIC OR THERAPEUTIC MEASURES AND COMMENTS
		PRIMARY	ALTERNATIVE[§]	
HEART/Infective endocarditis—Native valve—culture positive *(continued)*				
For viridans strep or S. bovis with **pen G MIC >0.5** and enterococci susceptible to AMP/pen G, vanco, gentamicin (synergy positive) **NOTE:** Inf. Dis. consultation suggested	**"Susceptible" enterococci, viridans strep, S. bovis, nutritionally variant streptococci** (new names are: Abiotrophia sp. & Granulicatella sp.)	[(**Pen G** 18–30 million units per 24h IV, divided q4h **x 4–6 wks**) **PLUS** (**gentamicin** 1 mg/kg q8h IV **x 4–6 wks**)] **OR** (**AMP** 12 gm/day IV, divided q4h + **gent** as above **x 4–6 wks**)	**Vanco** 15 mg/kg IV q12h to max of 2 gm/day unless serum levels measured **PLUS gentamicin** 1 mg/kg q8h IV **x 4–6 wks** **NOTE: Low dose of gent**	**4 wks of rx if symptoms <3 mos.; 6 wks of rx if symptoms >3 mos.** Vanco for pen-allergic pts; do not use cephalosporins. Do **not** give gent once-q24h for enterococcal endocarditis. Target gent levels: peak 3 mcg/mL, trough <1 mcg/mL. Vanco target serum levels: peak 20–50 mcg/mL, trough 5–12 mcg/mL. **NOTE:** Because of ↑ frequency of resistance *(see below)*, all enterococci causing endocarditis should be tested in vitro for susceptibility to penicillin, gentamicin and vancomycin plus β lactamase production.
Enterococci: MIC streptomycin >2000 mcg/mL; MIC gentamicin >500-2000 mcg/mL; no resistance to penicillin	**Enterococci, high-level aminoglycoside resistance**	**E. faecium: Pen G** or **AMP** IV as above **x 8–12 wks** (approx. 50% cure) Rx success in single pt: **AMP** + **Dapto** *(AAC 56:6064, 2012; Eur J CLin Micro Inf Dis 30:807, 2011).*	**E. faecalis:** (**Ceftriaxone** 2 gm IV q12h + **AMP** 2 gm IV q4h) x 7-8 wks *(CID 56:1261, 2013)*	10–25% E. faecalis and 45–50% E. faecium resistant to high gent levels. May have to consider surgical removal of infected valve. Theory of efficacy of combination: sequential blocking of PBPs 4&5 (Amp) and 2&3 (ceftriaxone).
Enterococci: pen G MIC >16 mcg/mL; no gentamicin resistance	**Enterococci, intrinsic pen G/AMP resistance** (E. faecium or E. faecalis)	(**Vanco** 15 mg/kg IV q12h (check levels if >2 gm) + **Gent** 1 mg/kg q8h x 6 wks *(see Comment).* Vanco alternative: **AM-SB** 3 gm IV q6h		Desired vanco serum levels: trough 5–12 mcg/mL. **Gentamicin** used for synergy; peak levels need not exceed 4 mcg/mL.
Enterococci: Pen/AMP resistant + high-level gent/strep resistant + vanco resistant; usually VRE **Consultation suggested**	**Enterococci, vanco-resistant, usually E. faecium**	**E. faecium: Linezolid** 600 mg IV/po q12h x 8 wks or **Quinu-dalfo** 7.5 mg/kg IV (central line) q8h x min 8 wks	**E. faecalis:** (**IMP** 500 mg IV q6h + **AMP** 2 gm IV q4h) or **Ceftriaxone** 2 gm IV q12h + **AMP** 2 gm IV q4h) x min 8 wks *(CID 56:1261, 2013)*	**Synercid** not active vs. E. faecalis. Linezolid bacteriostatic; failures have occurred. Dapto bactericidal in vitro but sparse clinical data *(CID 41:1134, 2005).* Cure of single E. faecalis pt: AMP + Dapto *(AAC:56:6064, 2012; Eur J Clin Micro Infect Dis 30:807, 2011).* Teicoplanin active vs. subset of vanco-resist enterococci, but NUS.
Staphylococcal endocarditis **Aortic &/or mitral valve infection—MSSA** Surgery indications: *see Comment page 28.*	**Staph. aureus, methicillin-sensitive** **Note: Low dose of gentamicin for only 3-5 days**	**Nafcillin** (**oxacillin**) 2 gm IV q4h **x 4–6 wks**	[(**Cefazolin** 2 gm IV q8h **x 4–6 wks**) **OR** **Vanco** 30-60 mg/kg/d in 2-3 divided doses to achieve trough of 15-20 mcg/mL **x 4–6 wks**	If IgE-mediated penicillin allergy, 10% cross-reactivity to cephalosporins *(AnIM 141:16, 2004).* Gentamicin optional. The benefit of low dose gentamicin in improving outcome is unproven and even low-dose gentamicin for only a few days is nephrotoxic *(CID 48:713, 2009);* if used at all it should be administered **for no more than 3-5 days**. **Cefazolin** and **Nafcillin** probably similar in efficacy and Cefazolin better tolerated *(AAC 55:5122, 2011)*
Aortic and/or mitral valve—MRSA	**Staph. aureus, methicillin-resistant**	**Vanco** 30-60 mg/kg per day in 2-3 divided doses to achieve target trough concentrations of 15-20 mcg/mL recommended for serious infections.	**Dapto** 8-10 mg/kg q24h IV (NOT FDA approved for this indication or dose)	In clinical trial *(NEJM 355:653, 2006)*, high failure rate with both vanco and dapto in small numbers of pts. For other alternatives, *see Table 6, pg 79.* Daptomycin references: *JAC 68:936 & 2921, 2013.* Case reports of success with Telavancin *(JAC 65:1315, 2010; AAC 54 5376, 2010; JAC (Jun 8), 2011)* and ceftaroline *(JAC 67:1267, 2012; J Infect Chemo online 7/14/12).*
Tricuspid valve infection (usually IVDUs): MSSA	**Staph. aureus, methicillin-sensitive**	**Nafcillin** (**oxacillin**) 2 gm IV q4h **PLUS gentamicin** 1 mg/kg IV q8h **x 2 wks.** **NOTE: low dose of gent**	**If penicillin allergy:** **Vanco** 30-60 mg/kg/d in 2-3 divided doses to achieve trough of 15-20 mcg/mL x 4 wks **OR** **Dapto** 6 mg/kg IV q24h (avoid if concomitant left-sided endocarditis). 8-12 mg/kg IV q24h used in some cases, but not FDA approved.	**2-week regimen not long** enough if metastatic infection (e.g., osteo) or left-sided endocarditis. If **Dapto** is used treat for at least 4 weeks. **Dapto** resistance can occur de novo, after or during vanco, or after/during dapto therapy. **Dapto** resistant MRSA killed by combination of **dapto** + **TMP/SMX** or nafcillin *(AAC 54:5187, 2010, AAC 56:6192, 2012; worked in 7 pts, CID 53:158, 2011).*

Abbreviations on page 2. **NOTE: All dosage recommendations are for adults (unless otherwise indicated) and assume normal renal function. § Alternatives consider allergy, PK, compliance, local resistance, cost*

TABLE 1 (27)

ANATOMIC SITE/DIAGNOSIS/ MODIFYING CIRCUMSTANCES	ETIOLOGIES (usual)	SUGGESTED REGIMENS*		ADJUNCT DIAGNOSTIC OR THERAPEUTIC MEASURES AND COMMENTS
		PRIMARY	ALTERNATIVE§	
HEART/Infective endocarditis—Native valve—culture positive *(continued)*				
Tricuspid valve--MRSA	**Staph. aureus, methicillin-resistant**	**Vanco** 30-60 mg/kg per day in 2-3 divided doses to achieve target trough concentrations of 15-20 mcg/mL recommended for serious infections **x 4–6 wks**	**Dapto** 6 mg/kg IV q24h x 4-6 wks equiv to **vanco** for rt-sided endocarditis; both vanco & dapto did poorly if lt-sided endocarditis *(NEJM 355: 653, 2006). (See Comments & table 6, page 79)*	**Linezolid:** Limited experience *(see JAC 58:273, 2006)* in patients with few treatment options; 64% cure rate; clear failure in 21%; thrombocytopenia in 31%. **Dapto** dose of 8-12 mg/kg may help in selected cases, but not FDA-approved.
Slow-growing fastidious Gm-neg. bacilli--any valve	**HACEK group** *(see Comments).*	**Ceftriaxone** 2 gm IV q24h **x 4 wks** OR **CIP** 400 mg IV q12h x 4 wks (Bartonella resistant – *see below).*	**AM-SB** 3 gm IV q6h x 4 wks or **CIP** (400 mg IV q12h or 500 mg po bid) x 4 wks	**HACEK (acronym for Haemophilus parainfluenzae, H. (aphrophilus) aggregatibacter, Actinobacillus, Bartonella, Cardiobacterium, Eikenella, Kingella).** Penicillinase-positive HACEK organisms should be susceptible to AM-SB + gentamicin. *Ref: Circulation 111:e394, 2005.*
Bartonella species--any valve	B. henselae, B. quintana	[**Ceftriaxone** 2 gm IV q24h x 6 wks + **gentamicin** 1 mg/kg IV q8h x 14 days] + **doxy** 100 mg IV/po bid x 6 wks. If Gent toxicity precludes its use, substitute **Rifampin** 300 mg IV/po bid.		**Dx:** Immunofluorescent antibody titer ≥1:800; blood cultures only occ. positive, or PCR of tissue from surgery. **Surgery:** Over ½ pts require valve surgery; relation to cure unclear. B. quintana transmitted by body lice among homeless.
Infective endocarditis— "culture negative"				
Fever, valvular disease, and ECHO vegetations ± emboli and neg. cultures.		Etiology in 348 cases studied by serology, culture, histopath, & molecular detection: C. burnetii 48%, Bartonella sp. 28%, and rarely (Abiotrophia elegans (nutritionally variant strep), Mycoplasma hominis, Legionella pneumophila, Tropheryma whipplei—together 1%), & rest without etiology identified (most on antibiotic). *See CID 51:131, 2010 for approach to work-up.*		
Infective endocarditis—Prosthetic valve—empiric therapy (cultures pending) S. aureus now most common etiology *(JAMA 297:1354, 2007).*				
Early (<2 mos post-op)	S. epidermidis, S. aureus. Rarely, Enterobacteriaceae, diphtheroids, fungi	**Vanco** 15 mg/kg IV q12h + **gentamicin** 1 mg/kg IV q8h + **RIF** 600 mg po q24h		Early surgical consultation advised especially if etiology is S. aureus, evidence of heart failure, presence of diabetes and/or renal failure, or concern for valve ring abscess *(JAMA 297:1354, 2007; CID 44:364, 2007).*
Late (>2 mos post-op)	S. epidermidis, viridans strep, enterococci, S. aureus			
Infective endocarditis— Prosthetic valve—positive blood cultures Treat for 6 weeks, even if suspect Viridans Strep. **Surgical consultation advised:** Indications for surgery: severe heart failure, S. aureus infection, prosthetic dehiscence, resistant organism, emboli due to large vegetation *(JACC 48:e1, 2006). See also, Eur J Clin Micro Infect Dis 38:528, 2010.*	Staph. epidermidis	(**Vanco** 15 mg /kg IV q12h + **RIF** 300 mg po q8h) **x 6 wks** + **gentamicin** 1 mg/kg IV q8h **x 14 days**.		If S. epidermidis is susceptible to nafcillin/oxacillin in vitro (not common), then substitute nafcillin (or oxacillin) for vanco.
	Staph. aureus	Methicillin sensitive: (**Nafcillin** 2 gm IV q4h + **RIF** 300 mg po q8h) **times 6 wks** + **gentamicin** 1 mg per kg IV q8h **times 14 days.** Methicillin resistant: (**Vanco** 1 gm IV q12h + **RIF** 300 mg po q8h) **times 6 wks** + **gentamicin** 1 mg per kg IV q8h **times 14 days.**		
	Viridans strep, enterococci	*See infective endocarditis, native valve, culture positive, page* 28. Treat for 6 weeks.		
	Enterobacteriaceae or P. aeruginosa	**Aminoglycoside** (**tobra** if P. aeruginosa) + (**AP Pen** or **P Ceph 3 AP** or **P Ceph 4**)		In theory, could substitute CIP for aminoglycoside, but no clinical data.
	Candida, aspergillus	*Table 11, page 114*		High mortality. Valve replacement plus antifungal therapy standard therapy but some success with antifungal therapy alone.

*NOTE: All dosage recommendations are for adults (unless otherwise indicated) and assume normal renal function. § Alternatives consider allergy, PK, compliance, local resistance, cost

TABLE 1 (28)

ANATOMIC SITE/DIAGNOSIS/ MODIFYING CIRCUMSTANCES	ETIOLOGIES (usual)	SUGGESTED REGIMENS*		ADJUNCT DIAGNOSTIC OR THERAPEUTIC MEASURES AND COMMENTS
		PRIMARY	ALTERNATIVE§	
HEART *(continued)*				
Infective endocarditis—Q fever *LnID 10:527, 2010; NEJM 356:715, 2007.*	Coxiella burnetii	**Doxy** 100 mg po bid + **hydroxychloroquine** 600 mg/day for at least 18 mos *(Mayo Clin Proc 83:574, 2008). Pregnancy: Need long term* **TMP-SMX** *(see CID 45:548, 2007).*		**Dx:** Phase I IgG titer >800 plus clinical evidence of endocarditis. Treatment duration: 18 mos for native valve, 24 mos for prosthetic valve. Monitor serologically for 5 yrs.
Pacemaker/defibrillator infections	S. aureus (40%), S. epidermidis (40%), Gram-negative bacilli (5%), fungi (5%).	**Device removal** + **vanco** 1 gm IV q12h + **RIF** 300 mg po bid	**Device removal** + **dapto** 6 mg per kg IV q24h[NAI] ± **RIF** *(no data)* 300 mg po bid	**Duration of rx after device removal:** For "pocket" or subcutaneous infection, 10–14 days; if lead-assoc. endocarditis, 4–6 wks depending on organism. Device removal and absence of valvular vegetation assoc. with significantly higher survival at 1 yr *(JAMA 307:1727, 2012).*
Pericarditis, purulent— empiric therapy *Ref: Medicine 88: 52, 2009.*	Staph. aureus, Strep. pneumoniae, Group A strep, Enterobacteriaceae	**Vanco + CIP** *(Dosage, see footnote[15])*	**Vanco + CFP** *(see footnote[15])*	Drainage required if signs of tamponade. Forced to use empiric vanco due to high prevalence of MRSA.
Rheumatic fever with carditis Ref.: *Ln 366:155, 2005*	Post-infectious sequelae of Group A strep infection (usually pharyngitis)	ASA, and usually prednisone 2 mg/kg po q24h for symptomatic treatment of fever, arthritis, arthralgia. May not influence carditis.		Clinical features: Carditis, polyarthritis, chorea, subcutaneous nodules, erythema marginatum. *Prophylaxis: see page 61*
Ventricular assist device-related infection *CID 57:1438, 2013*	S. aureus, S. epidermidis, aerobic gm-neg bacilli, Candida sp	After culture of blood, wounds, drive line, device pocket and maybe pump: **Vanco** 15-20 mg/kg IV q8-12h + (**Cip** 400 mg IV q12h or **levo** 750 mg IV q24h) + **fluconazole** 800 mg IV q24h.		Can substitute **daptomycin** 10 mg/kg/d[NAI] for **vanco, cefepime** 2 gm IV q12h for FQ, and (**vori, caspo, micafungin or anidulafungin**) for **fluconazole**. Modify regimen based on results of culture and susceptibility tests. Higher than FDA-approved Dapto dose because of potential emergence of resistance.
JOINT—*Also see Lyme Disease, page 58*				
Reactive arthritis				
Reiter's syndrome *(See Comment for definition)*	Occurs wks after infection with C. trachomatis, Campylobacter jejuni, Yersinia enterocolitica, Shigella/Salmonella sp.	Only treatment is non-steroidal anti-inflammatory drugs		Definition: Urethritis, conjunctivitis, arthritis, and sometimes uveitis and rash. Arthritis: asymmetrical oligoarthritis of ankles, knees, feet, sacroiliitis. Rash: palms and soles—keratoderma blennorrhagica; circinate balanitis of glans penis. HLA-B27 positive predisposes to Reiter's.
Poststreptococcal reactive arthritis *(See Rheumatic fever, above)*	Immunologic reaction after strep pharyngitis: (1) arthritis onset in <10 days, (2) lasts months, (3) unresponsive to ASA	Treat strep pharyngitis and then NSAIDs (prednisone needed in some pts)		A reactive arthritis after a β-hemolytic strep infection in absence of sufficient Jones criteria for acute rheumatic fever. Ref.: *Mayo Clin Proc 75:144, 2000.*
Septic arthritis: Treatment requires both adequate drainage of purulent joint fluid and appropriate antimicrobial therapy. **There is no need to inject antimicrobials into joints.** Empiric therapy after collection of blood and joint fluid for culture; review Gram stain of joint fluid.				
Infants <3 mos (neonate)	Staph. aureus, Enterobacteriaceae, Group B strep	**If MRSA not a concern:** (**Nafcillin** or **oxacillin**) + **P Ceph 3** *(Dosage, see Table 16, page 209)*	**If MRSA a concern: Vanco + P Ceph 3**	Blood cultures frequently positive. Adjacent bone involved in 2/3 pts. Group B strep and gonococci most common community-acquired etiologies.

[15] **Aminoglycosides** *(see Table 10D, page 109)*, **IMP** 0.5 gm IV q6h, **MER** 1 gm IV q8h, **nafcillin** or **oxacillin** 2 gm IV q4h, **TC-CL** 3.1 gm IV q6h, **PIP-TZ** 3.375 gm IV q6h or 4.5 gm q8h, **AM-SB** 3 gm IV q6h, **P Ceph** 1 (cephalothin 2 gm IV q4h or cefazolin 2 gm IV q8h), **CIP** 750 mg po bid or 400 mg IV bid, **vanco** 1 gm IV q12h, **RIF** 600 mg po q24h, **aztreonam** 2 gm IV q8h, **CFP** 2 gm IV q12h

 **NOTE: All dosage recommendations are for adults (unless otherwise indicated) and assume normal renal function. § Alternatives consider allergy, PK, compliance, local resistance, cost*

TABLE 1 (29)

ANATOMIC SITE/DIAGNOSIS/ MODIFYING CIRCUMSTANCES	ETIOLOGIES (usual)	SUGGESTED REGIMENS*		ADJUNCT DIAGNOSTIC OR THERAPEUTIC MEASURES AND COMMENTS
		PRIMARY	ALTERNATIVE§	
JOINT/Septic arthritis *(continued)*				
Children (3 mos–14 yrs)	Staph. aureus 27%, S. pyogenes & S. pneumo 14%, H. influenzae 3%, Gm-neg. bacilli 6%, other (GC, N. meningitidis) 14%, unknown 36%	**Vanco** + **(Cefotaxime, ceftizoxime or ceftriaxone)** until culture results available *See Table 16 for dosage* Steroids—*see Comment*		Marked ↓ in H. influenzae since use of conjugate vaccine. **NOTE:** Septic arthritis due to salmonella has no association with sickle cell disease, unlike salmonella osteomyelitis. 10 days of therapy as effective as a 30-day treatment course if there is a good clinical response and CRP levels normalize quickly *(CID 48:1201, 2009)*.
Adults *(review Gram stain): See page 58 for Lyme Disease and page 58 for gonococcal arthritis*				
Acute monoarticular				
At risk for sexually-transmitted disease	**N. gonorrhoeae** *(see page 23)*, S. aureus, streptococci, rarely aerobic Gm-neg. bacilli	**Gram stain negative: Ceftriaxone** 1 gm IV q24h or **cefotaxime** 1 gm IV q8h or **ceftizoxime** 1 gm IV q8h	If Gram stain shows Gm+ cocci in clusters: **vanco** 1 gm IV q12h; if >100 kg, 1.5 gm IV q12h.	For treatment comments, *see Disseminated GC, page 23*
Not at risk for sexually-transmitted disease	S. aureus, streptococci, Gm-neg. bacilli	**All empiric choices guided by Gram stain** **Vanco** + **P Ceph 3** *For treatment duration, see Table 3, page 71* *For dosage, see footnote page 34*	**Vanco**+ (**CIP** or **Levo**)	Differential includes gout and chondrocalcinosis (pseudogout). **Look for crystals in joint fluid.** **NOTE:** *See Table 6 for MRSA treatment.*
Chronic monoarticular	Brucella, nocardia, mycobacteria, fungi	*See Table 2 & Table 12*		
Polyarticular, usually acute	**Gonococci,** B. burgdorferi, acute rheumatic fever; viruses, e.g., hepatitis B, rubella vaccine, parvo B19	Gram stain usually negative for GC. If sexually active, culture urethra, cervix, anal canal, throat, blood, joint fluid, and then: **ceftriaxone** 1 gm IV q24h		If GC, usually associated petechiae and/or pustular skin lesions and tenosynovitis. Consider Lyme disease if exposure areas known to harbor infected ticks. *See page 58.* Expanded differential includes gout, pseudogout, reactive arthritis (HLA-B27 pos.).
Septic arthritis, post intra-articular injection	MSSE/MRSE 40%, MSSA/ MRSA 20%, P. aeruginosa, Propionibacteria, mycobacteria	**NO empiric therapy.** Arthroscopy for culture/sensitivity, crystals, washout		Treat based on culture results x 14 days (assumes no foreign body present).

 **NOTE: All dosage recommendations are for adults (unless otherwise indicated) and assume normal renal function. § Alternatives consider allergy, PK, compliance, local resistance, cost*

TABLE 1 (30)

ANATOMIC SITE/DIAGNOSIS/ MODIFYING CIRCUMSTANCES	ETIOLOGIES (usual)	SUGGESTED REGIMENS*		ADJUNCT DIAGNOSTIC OR THERAPEUTIC MEASURES AND COMMENTS
		PRIMARY	ALTERNATIVE§	
JOINT *(continued)*				
Infected prosthetic joint (PJI) • Suspect infection if sinus tract or wound drainage; acutely painful prosthesis; chronically painful prosthesis; or high ESR/CRP assoc. w/painful prosthesis. • **Empiric therapy is NOT recommended.** Treat based on culture and sensitivity results. • **3 surgical options:** 1) debridement and prosthesis retention (if sx < 3 wks or implantation < 30 days); 2) 1 stage, direct exchange; 3) 2 stage: debridement, removal, reimplantation • **IDSA Guidelines:** *CID 56:e1, 2013.* • Data do not allow assessment of value of adding antibacterial cement to temporary joint spacers *(CID 55:474, 2012).*	MSSA/MSSE	**Debridement/Retention**: [(**Nafcillin** 2 gm IV q4h or **Oxacillin** 2 gm IV q4h IV) + **Rifampin** 300 mg po bid] OR (**Cefazolin** 2 gm IV q8h + **Rifampin** 300 mg po bid) x 2-6 weeks followed by [(**Ciprofloxacin** 750 mg po bid OR **Levofloxacin** 750 mg po q24h) + **Rifampin** 300 mg po bid] for 3-6 months (shorter duration for total hip arthroplasty) **1-stage exchange:** IV/PO regimen as above for 3 mos **2-stage exchange:** regimen as above for 4-6 wks	(**Daptomycin** 6-8 mg/kg IV q24h OR **Linezolid** 600 mg po/IV bid) ± **Rifampin** 300 mg po bid	• **Confirm isolate susceptibility to fluoroquinolone and rifampin:** for fluoroquinolone-resistant isolate consider using other active highly bioavailable agent, e.g., TMP-SMX, Doxy, Minocycline, Amoxicillin-Clavulanate, Clindamycin, or Linezolid • Enterococcal infection: addition of aminoglycoside optional. • *P. aeruginosa* infection: consider adding aminoglycoside if isolate is susceptible, (but if this improves outcome unclear). • Prosthesis retention most important risk factor for treatment failure *(Clin Microbiol Infect 16:1789, 2010).* (Linezolid 600 mg + Rifampin 300 mg) may be effective as salvage therapy if device removal not possible *(Antimicrob Agents Chemother 55:4308, 2011)* • If prosthesis is retained, consider long-term, suppressive therapy, particularly for staphylococcal infections: depending on in vitro susceptibility options include TMP-SMX, Doxycycline, Minocycline, Amoxicillin, Ciprofloxacin, Cephalexin. • Culture yield may be increased by sonication of prosthesis *(N Engl J Med 357:654, 2007).* • Other treatment consideration: Rifampin is bactericidal vs. biofilm-producing bacteria. Never use Rifampin alone due to rapid development of resistance. Rifampin 300 mg po/IV bid + Fusidic acid[NUS] 500 mg po/IV tid is another option *(Clin Micro Inf 12(S3):93, 2006).* • Watch for toxicity if Linezolid is used for more than 2 weeks of therapy.
	MRSA/MRSE	**Debridement/Retention:** (**Vancomycin** 15-20 mg/kg IV q8-12h + **Rifampin** 300 mg po bid) x 2-6 weeks *followed by* [(**Ciprofloxacin** 750 mg po bid OR **Levofloxacin** 750 mg po q24h) + **Rifampin** 300 mg po bid] for 3-6 months (shorter duration for total hip arthroplasty) **1-stage exchange:** IV/PO regimen as above for 3 mos **2-stage exchange:** regimen as above for 4-6 wks	(**Daptomycin** 6-8 mg/kg IV q24h OR **Linezolid** 600 mg po/IV bid) ± **Rifampin** 300 mg po bid	
	Streptococci (Grps A, B, C, D, viridans, other)	**Debridement/Retention: Penicillin** G 20 million units IV continuous infusion q24h or in 6 divided doses OR **Ceftriaxone** 2 gm IV q24h x 4-6 weeks **1 or 2 stage exchange:** regimen as above for 4-6 wks	**Vancomycin** 15 mg/kg IV q12h	
	Enterococci	**Debridement/Retention: Pen-susceptible: Ampicillin** 12 gm IV OR **Penicillin** G 20 million units IV continuous infusion q24h or in 6 divided doses x 4-6 weeks **Pen-resistant: Vancomycin** 15 mg/kg IV q12h x 4-6 weeks **1 or 2 stage exchange:** regimen as above for 4-6 wks	**Daptomycin** 6-8 mg/kg IV q24h OR **Linezolid** 600 mg po/IV bid	
	Propionibacterium acnes	**Debridement/Retention: Penicillin** G 20 million units IV continuous infusion or in 6 divided doses OR **Ceftriaxone** 2 gm IV q24h x 4-6 weeks **1 or 2 stage exchange:** regimen as above for 4-6 wks	**Vancomycin** 15 mg/kg IV q12h OR **Clindamycin** 300-450 mg po qid	
	Gm-neg enteric bacilli	**Debridement/Retention: Ertapenem** 1 gm q24h IV OR other beta-lactam (e.g., **Ceftriaxone** 2 gm IV q24h OR **Cefepime** 2 gm IV q12h, based on susceptibility) x 4-6 weeks **1 or 2 stage exchange:** regimen as above for 4-6 wks	**Ciprofloxacin** 750 mg po bid	
	P. aeruginosa	**Debridement/Retention: Cefepime** 2 gm IV q12h OR **Meropenem** 1 gm IV q8h + **Tobramycin** 5.1 mg/kg once daily IV **1 or 2 stage exchange:** regimen as above for 4-6 wks	**Ciprofloxacin** 750 mg po bid or 400 mg IV q8h	
Rheumatoid arthritis	**TNF inhibitors** (adalimumab, certolizumab, etanercept, golimumab, infliximab) and other anti-inflammatory biologics (tofacitinib, rituximab, tocilizumab, abatacept) ↑ risk of TBc, fungal infection, legionella, listeria, and malignancy. *See Med Lett 55:1, 2013 for full listing.*			
Septic bursitis: Olecranon bursitis; prepatellar bursitis	Staph. aureus >80%, M. tuberculosis (rare), M. marinum (rare)	(**Nafcillin** or **oxacillin** 2 gm IV q4h or **dicloxacillin** 500 mg po qid) if **MSSA** *Other doses, see footnote page 34*	(**Vanco** 15-20 mg/kg IV q8-12h or **linezolid** 600 mg po bid) if **MRSA**	Empiric MRSA coverage recommended if risk factors are present and in high prevalence areas. Immunosuppression, not duration of therapy, is a risk factor for recurrence; 7 days of therapy may be sufficient for immunocompetent patients undergoing one-stage bursectomy *(JAC 65:1008, 2010).*

Abbreviations on page 2. **NOTE: All dosage recommendations are for adults (unless otherwise indicated) and assume normal renal function. § Alternatives consider allergy, PK, compliance, local resistance, cost*

TABLE 1 (31)

ANATOMIC SITE/DIAGNOSIS/ MODIFYING CIRCUMSTANCES	ETIOLOGIES (usual)	SUGGESTED REGIMENS*		ADJUNCT DIAGNOSTIC OR THERAPEUTIC MEASURES AND COMMENTS
		PRIMARY	ALTERNATIVE§	
KIDNEY, BLADDER AND PROSTATE				
Acute uncomplicated urinary tract infection (cystitis-urethritis) in females: ***NEJM 366:1028, 2012; CID 57:719, 2013; CID 52:e103, 2011.***				
NOTE: Resistance of E. coli to TMP-SMX approx. 15–20% & correlates with microbiological/ clinical failure. **Recent reports of E. coli resistant to FQs.**	Enterobacteriaceae (E. coli), Staph. saprophyticus. Enterococci and/or Strep agalactiae in midstream urine often result in false positive results *(NEJM 369:1883 & 1959, 2013).*	**<20% of Local E. coli resistant to TMP-SMX & no allergy: TMP-SMX-DS** bid x 3 days; if sulfa allergy, **nitrofurantoin** 100 mg po bid x 5 days or **fosfomycin** 3 gm po x one dose. All plus **Pyridium**	**>20% Local E. coli resistant to TMP-SMX or sulfa allergy:** then 3 days of **CIP** 250 mg bid, **CIP-ER** 500 mg q24h, **Levo** 250 mg q24h OR **Moxi** 400 mg q24h **OR Nitrofurantoin** 100 mg bid OR single 3 gm dose of **fosfomycin.** All plus **Pyridium**	7-day rx recommended **in pregnancy** [discontinue or do not use sulfonamides (TMP-SMX) near term (2 weeks before EDC) because of potential ↑ in kernicterus]. If failure on 3-day course, culture and rx 2 weeks. **Fosfomycin** 3 gm po times 1 less effective vs. E. coli than multi-dose TMP-SMX or FQ. Fosfo active vs. E. faecalis; poor activity vs. other coliforms. **Moxifloxacin:** Not approved for UTIs. Moxi equivalent to comparator drugs in unpublished clinical trials (on file with Bayer). Therapy of **ESBL producing E. coli and Klebsiella spp.** problematic because of multiple drug resistances: ESBL producers susceptible to fosfomycin, ertapenem, and combo of amox-clav + cefdinir in vitro *(AAC 53:1278, 2009).* Amox-Clav or an oral cephalosporin are options, but generally less efficacious. **Phenazopyridine (Pyridium)** —non-prescription— may relieve dysuria: 200 mg po tid times 2 days. Hemolysis if G6PD deficient.
Risk factors for STD, Dipstick: positive leukocyte esterase or hemoglobin, neg. Gram stain	C. trachomatis	**Azithro** 1 gm po single dose	**Doxy** 100 mg po bid 7 days	Pelvic exam for vaginitis & herpes simplex, urine LCR/PCR for GC and C. trachomatis.
Recurrent (3 or more episodes/ year) in young women	Any of the above bacteria	Eradicate infection, then **TMP-SMX** 1 single-strength tab po q24h long term		A cost-effective alternative to continuous prophylaxis is self-administered single dose rx (TMP-SMX DS, 2 tabs, 320/1600 mg) at symptom onset. Another alternative: 1 DS tablet TMP-SMX post-coitus.
Child: ≤5 yrs old & grade 3–4 reflux	Coliforms	[**TMP-SMX** 8-12 mg/kg/day (based on TMP comp) div q12h] or (**nitrofurantoin** 2 mg per kg po q24h). **CIP** approved as alternative drug ages 1–17 yrs.		
Recurrent UTI in postmenopausal women	E. coli & other Enterobacteriaceae, enterococci, S. saprophyticus	Treat as for uncomplicated UTI. Evaluate for potentially correctable urologic factors—*see Comment.* **Nitrofurantoin** more effective than vaginal cream in decreasing frequency, but Editors worry about pulmonary fibrosis with long-term NF rx.		Definition: ≥3 culture + symptomatic UTIs in 1 year or 2 UTIs in 6 months. Urologic factors: (1) cystocele, (2) incontinence, (3) ↑ residual urine volume (≥50 mL).
Acute uncomplicated pyelonephritis (usually women 18–40 yrs, temperature >102°F, definite costovertebral tenderness) [NOTE: Culture of urine and blood indicated prior to therapy]. **If male, look for obstructive uropathy or other complicating pathology.**				
Moderately ill (outpatient) **NOTE:** May need one IV dose due to nausea.	Enterobacteriaceae (most likely E. coli), enterococci (Gm stain of **uncentrifuged** urine may allow identification of Gm-neg. bacilli vs. Gm+ cocci)	**FQ** po times 5-7 days: **CIP** 500 mg bid or **CIP-ER** 1000 mg q24h, **Levo** 750 mg q24h, **Oflox** 400 mg bid, **Moxi** NAI 400 mg q24h possibly ok—see comment.	**AM-CL, O Ceph,** or **TMP-SMX-DS po.** Treat for 14 days. Dosage in footnote[16] Beta-lactams less effective than FQs.	7 day course of **Cipro** 500 mg bid as effective as 14 day course in women *(Lancet 380:484, 2012)* **Levo** 750 mg FDA-approved for 5 days. Ertapenem 1 gm IV q24h or other carbapenem for suspected ESBL-producing organism. Ref: *NEJM 366:1028, 2012.*

[16] **AM-CL** 875/125 mg po q12h or 500/125 mg po tid or 2000 /125 mg po bid; *Antipseudomonal penicillins*: **AM-SB** 3 gm IV q6h; **PIP** 3 gm IV q4-6h; **PIP-TZ** 3.375 gm IV q4-6h (4.5 gm IV q6h for pseudomonas pneumonia); **TC-CL** 3.1 gm IV q6h; *Antipseudomonal cephalosporins*: **ceftaz** 2 gm IV q8h; **CFP** 2 gm IV q12h; **aztreonam** 2 gm IV q8h; *Carbapenems*: **DORI** 500 mg IV q8h (1 hr infusion); **ERTA** 1 gm IV q24h; **IMP** 0.5 gm IV q12h (max 4 gm/day); **MER** 1 gm IV q8h; *Parenteral cephalosporins*: **cefotaxime** 1 gm IV q12h (2 gm IV q4h for severe infection); **cefoxitin** 2 gm IV q8h; **ceftriaxone** 1-2 gm IV q24h; *Oral cephalosporins-- see, Table 10A page 95*; **dicloxacillin** 500 mg po q6h; *FQs*: **CIP** 400 mg IV q12h; **Gati**NUS 400 mg IV q24h; **levo** 750 mg IV q24h; **gentamicin**-- *see Table 10D, page 109*; **linezolid** 600 mg IV/po q12h; **metro** 500 mg po q6h or 15 mg/kg IV q12h (max 4 gm/day); **nafcillin/oxacillin** 2 gm IV q4h; **TMP-SMX** 2 mg/kg (TMP component) IV q6h; **vanco** 1 gm IV q12h (if over 100 kg, 1.5 gm IV q12h).

Abbreviations on page 2. **NOTE: All dosage recommendations are for adults (unless otherwise indicated) and assume normal renal function. § Alternatives consider allergy, PK, compliance, local resistance, cost*

TABLE 1 (32)

ANATOMIC SITE/DIAGNOSIS/ MODIFYING CIRCUMSTANCES	ETIOLOGIES (usual)	SUGGESTED REGIMENS*		ADJUNCT DIAGNOSTIC OR THERAPEUTIC MEASURES AND COMMENTS
		PRIMARY	ALTERNATIVE§	
KIDNEY, BLADDER AND PROSTATE/Acute uncomplicated pyelonephritis *(continued)*				
Acute pyelonephritis-- Hospitalized	E. coli most common, enterococci 2nd in frequency	**FQ** (IV) or (**AMP** + **gentamicin**) or **ceftriaxone** or **PIP-TZ**. Treat for 14 days.	**TC-CL** or **AM-SB** or **PIP-TZ** or **ERTA** or **DORI**. Treat for 14 days.	Treat IV until pt afebrile 24–48 hrs, then complete 2-wks course with oral drugs *(as Moderately ill, above)*. **DORI** approved for 10 day treatment. Ertapenem 1 gm IV q24h or other carbapenem for suspected ESBL-producing organism.
		Dosages in footnote[16] on page 34. Do not use cephalosporins for suspect or proven enterococcal infection		**If pt hypotensive, prompt imaging (Ultrasound or CT) is recommended to ensure absence of obstructive uropathy. NOTE: Cephalosporins & ertapenem not active vs. enterococci.**
Complicated UTI/catheters Obstruction, reflux, azotemia, transplant, **Foley catheter-related, R/O obstruction; multi-drug resistant gram-neg bacilli.** *For IDSA Guidelines: CID 50:625, 2010.*	Enterobacteriaceae, P. aeruginosa, enterococci, rarely S. aureus	(**AMP** + **gent**) or **PIP-TZ** or **TC-CL** or **DORI** or **IMP** or **MER** for up to 2–3 wks	(IV **FQ**: **CIP**, **Gati**, **Levo**) or **Ceftaz** or **CFP** for up to 2–3 wks	Not all listed drugs predictably active vs. enterococci or *P. aeruginosa*. **CIP** approved in children (1-17 yrs) as alternative. Not 1st choice secondary to increased incidence joint adverse effects. Peds dose: 6-10 mg/kg (400 mg max) **IV** q8h or 10-20 mg/kg (750 mg max) **po** q12h.
		Switch to po **FQ** or **TMP-SMX** when possible *For dosages, see footnote[16] on page 34.*		Treat for 7 days for catheter-associated UTI if prompt resolution of symptoms and 10-14 days if delayed response; a 3-day course of therapy may be consider for women < 65 years of age *(CID 50:625, 2010)*
Asymptomatic bacteriuria. IDSA Guidelines: *CID 40:643, 2005; U.S. Preventive Services Task Force AnIM 149:43, 2008.*				
Preschool children		Base regimen on C&S, not empirical		Diagnosis requires ≥10[5] CFU per mL urine of same bacterial species in 2 specimens obtained 3–7 days apart.
Pregnancy	Aerobic Gm-neg. bacilli & Staph. hemolyticus	Screen 1st trimester. If positive, rx 3–7 days with **amox**, **nitrofurantoin**, **O Ceph**, **TMP-SMX**, or **TMP** alone		Screen monthly for recurrence. Some authorities treat continuously until delivery (stop TMP-SMX 2 wks before EDC). ↑ resistance of E. coli to TMP-SMX.
Before and after invasive urologic intervention, e.g., Foley catheter	Aerobic Gm-neg. bacilli	Obtain urine culture and then rx 3 days with **TMP-SMX DS,** bid. For prevention of UTI: Consider removal after 72 hrs *(CID 46:243 & 251, 2008)*.		Clinical benefit of antimicrobial-coated Foley catheters is uncertain *(AnIM 144:116, 2006)*. *(CID 60:625, 2010)*.
Neurogenic bladder – see "spinal cord injury" below		No therapy in asymptomatic patient; intermittent catheterization if possible		Ref.: *AJM 113(1A):67S, 2002*—Bacteriuria in spinal cord injured patient.
Asymptomatic, advanced age, male or female Ref: *CID 40:643, 2005*		No therapy indicated unless in conjunction with surgery to correct obstructive uropathy; measure residual urine vol. in females; prostate exam/PSA in males. No screening recommended in men and non-pregnant women *(AnIM 149:43, 2008; CID 55:771, 2012)*.		
Malacoplakia	E. coli	**Bethanechol chloride** + (**CIP** or **TMP-SMX**)		Chronic pyelo with abnormal inflammatory response.
Perinephric abscess				
Associated with staphylococcal bacteremia	Staph. aureus	If **MSSA, Nafcillin/ oxacillin** or **cefazolin** *(Dosage, see footnote page 34)*	If **MRSA: Vanco** 1 gm IV q12h **OR dapto** 6 mg/kg IV q24h	Drainage, surgical or image-guided aspiration
Associated with pyelonephritis	Enterobacteriaceae	*See pyelonephritis, complicated UTI, above*		Drainage, surgical or image-guided aspiration
Post Renal Transplant Obstructive Uropathy *(CID 46:825, 2008)*	Corynebacterium urealyticum	**Vanco** or **Teicoplanin**[NUS]		Organism can synthesize struvite stones. Requires 48-72 hr incubation to detect in culture
Prostatitis		*See prostatitis, page 27*		
Spinal cord injury pts with UTI	E. coli, Klebsiella sp., enterococci	**CIP** 250 mg po bid x 14 days		If fever, suspect assoc. pyelonephritis. Microbiologic cure greater after 14 vs. 3 days of CIP *(CID 39:658 & 665, 2004)*; for asymptomatic bacteriuria see *AJM 113(1A):675, 2002.*

Abbreviations on page 2. **NOTE: All dosage recommendations are for adults (unless otherwise indicated) and assume normal renal function. § Alternatives consider allergy, PK, compliance, local resistance, cost*

TABLE 1 (33)

ANATOMIC SITE/DIAGNOSIS/ MODIFYING CIRCUMSTANCES	ETIOLOGIES (usual)	SUGGESTED REGIMENS*		ADJUNCT DIAGNOSTIC OR THERAPEUTIC MEASURES AND COMMENTS
		PRIMARY	ALTERNATIVE[§]	
LIVER *(for spontaneous bacterial peritonitis, see page 47)*				
Cholangitis		*See Gallbladder, page 17*		
Cirrhosis & variceal bleeding	Esophageal flora	(**Norfloxacin** 400 mg po bid or **CIP** 400 mg IV q12h) x max. of 7 days	**Ceftriaxone** 1 gm IV once daily for max. of 7 days	Short term prophylactic antibiotics in cirrhotics with G-I hemorr, with or without ascites, decreases rate of bacterial infection & ↑ survival *(Hepatology 46:922, 2007)*.
Hepatic abscess Klebsiella liver abscess ref.: *Ln ID 12:881, 2012*	Enterobacteriaceae (esp. Klebsiella sp.), bacteroides, enterococci, Entamoeba histolytica, Yersinia enterocolitica (rare), Fusobacterium necrophorum *(Lemierre's)*. *For echinococcus, see Table 13, page 152. For cat-scratch disease (CSD), see pages 45 & 57*	**Metro** + (**ceftriaxone** or **cefoxitin** or **TC-CL** or **PIP-TZ** or **AM-SB** or **CIP** or **levo**. *(Dosage, see footnote[16] on page 34)*	**Metro** (for amoeba) + either **IMP**, **MER** or **Dori** *(Dosage, see footnote[16] on page 34)*	**Serological tests for amebiasis should be done on all patients;** if neg., surgical drainage or percutaneous aspiration. In pyogenic abscess, ½ have identifiable GI source or underlying biliary tract disease. If amoeba serology positive, treat with **metro** alone without surgery. Empiric **metro** included for both E. histolytica & bacteroides. **Hemochromatosis** associated with Yersinia enterocolitica liver abscess; regimens listed are effective for yersinia. Klebsiella pneumonia genotype K1 associated ocular & CNS Klebsiella infections.
Hepatic encephalopathy	Urease-producing gut bacteria	**Rifaximin** 550 mg po bid (take with lactulose)		Refs: *NEJM 362:1071, 2010; Med Lett 52:87, 2010.*
Leptospirosis	Leptospirosis, *see page 60*			
Peliosis hepatis in AIDS pts	Bartonella henselae and B. quintana	*See page 57*		
Post-transplant infected "biloma"	Enterococci (incl. VRE), candida, Gm-neg. bacilli (P. aeruginosa 8%), anaerobes 5%	**Linezolid** 600 mg IV bid + **CIP** 400 mg IV q12h + **fluconazole** 400 mg IV q24h	**Dapto** 6 mg/kg per day + **Levo** 750 mg IV q24h + **fluconazole** 400 mg IV q24h	Suspect if fever & abdominal pain post-transplant. Exclude hepatic artery thrombosis. Presence of candida and/or VRE bad prognosticators.
Viral hepatitis	Hepatitis A, B, C, D, E, G	*See Table 14F and Table 14G*		
LUNG/Bronchi				
Bronchiolitis/wheezy bronchitis (expiratory wheezing)				
Infants/children (≤ age 5) *See RSV, Table 14A page 169* Ref: *Ln 368:312, 2006*	**Respiratory syncytial virus** (RSV) 50%, parainfluenza 25%, human metapneumovirus	Antibiotics not useful, mainstay of therapy is oxygen. Ribavirin for severe disease: 6 gm vial (20 mg/mL) in sterile H_2O by SPAG-2 generator over 18-20 hrs daily times 3-5 days.		RSV most important. Rapid diagnosis with antigen detection methods. For prevention a humanized mouse monoclonal antibody, **palivizumab**. *See Table 14A, page 169*. RSV immune globulin is no longer available. Review: *Red Book of Peds 2006, 27th Ed.*
Bronchitis				
Infants/children (≤ age 5)	< Age 2: Adenovirus; age 2–5: Respiratory syncytial virus, parainfluenza 3 virus, human metapneumovirus		Antibiotics indicated only with associated sinusitis or heavy growth on throat culture for S. pneumo., Group A strep, H. influenzae or no improvement in 1 week. Otherwise rx is symptomatic.	
Adolescents and adults with acute tracheobronchitis (Acute bronchitis) Ref.: *NEJM 355:2125, 2006*	Usually viral. M. pneumoniae 5%; C. pneumoniae 5%. *See Persistent cough (Pertussis)*	**Antibiotics not indicated.** Antitussive ± inhaled bronchodilators. Throat swab PCR available for Dx of mycoplasma or chlamydia.		Purulent sputum alone not an indication for antibiotic therapy. Expect cough to last 2 weeks. If fever/rigors, get chest x-ray. **If mycoplasma documented, prefer doxy over macrolides due to increasing macrolide resistance (*JAC 68:506, 2013*).**

 **NOTE: All dosage recommendations are for adults (unless otherwise indicated) and assume normal renal function. § Alternatives consider allergy, PK, compliance, local resistance, cost*

TABLE 1 (34)

ANATOMIC SITE/DIAGNOSIS/ MODIFYING CIRCUMSTANCES	ETIOLOGIES (usual)	SUGGESTED REGIMENS*		ADJUNCT DIAGNOSTIC OR THERAPEUTIC MEASURES AND COMMENTS
		PRIMARY	ALTERNATIVE[§]	
LUNG/Bronchi/Bronchitis *(continued)*				
Persistent cough (>14 days), afebrile during community outbreak: Pertussis (whooping cough) 10–20% adults with cough >14 days have pertussis *(MMWR 54 (RR-14), 2005)*. Review: *Chest 130:547, 2006*	Bordetella pertussis & occ. Bordetella parapertussis. Also consider asthma, gastroesophageal reflux, post-nasal drip, mycoplasma and also chlamydia.	**Peds doses: Azithro/ clarithro** OR **erythro estolate**[17] OR **erythro base**[17] OR **TMP-SMX** *(doses in footnote[17])*	**Adult doses: Azithro** po 500 mg day 1, 250 mg q24h days 2–5 OR **erythro estolate** 500 mg po qid times 14 days OR **TMP-SMX-DS** 1 tab po bid times 14 days OR (**clarithro** 500 mg po bid or 1 gm **ER** q24h times 7 days)	**3 stages of illness:** catarrhal (1–2 wks), paroxysmal coughing (2–4 wks), and convalescence (1–2 wks). Treatment may abort or eliminate pertussis in catarrhal stage, but does not shorten paroxysmal stage. **Diagnosis:** PCR on nasopharyngeal secretions or ↑ pertussis-toxin antibody. **Rx aimed at eradication of NP carriage.** In non-outbreak setting, likelihood of pertussis increased if post-tussive emesis or inspiratory whoop present *(JAMA 304:890, 2010)*.
Pertussis: Prophylaxis of household contacts	Drugs and doses as per treatment immediately above			Recommended by Am. Acad. Ped. Red Book 2006 for all household or close contacts; community-wide prophylaxis not recommended.
Acute bacterial exacerbation of chronic bronchitis (ABECB), adults (almost always smokers with COPD) Ref: *NEJM 359:2355, 2008.*	Viruses 20–50%, C. pneumoniae 5%, M. pneumoniae <1%; role of S. pneumo, H. influenzae & M. catarrhalis controversial. Tobacco use, air pollution contribute.	**Severe ABECB** = ↑ dyspnea, ↑ sputum viscosity/purulence, ↑ sputum volume. For severe ABECB: (1) consider chest x-ray, esp. if febrile &/or low O_2 sat.; (2) inhaled anticholinergic bronchodilator; (3) oral corticosteroid; taper over 2 wks *(Cochrane Library 3, 2006)*; (4) D/C tobacco use; (5) non-invasive positive pressure ventilation. **Role of antimicrobial therapy is debated even for severe disease, but recent study of >80,000 patients shows value of antimicrobial therapy in patients hospitalized with severe disease *(JAMA 303(20):2035, 2010)*. For mild or moderate disease, no antimicrobial treatment** or maybe **amox**, **doxy**, **TMP-SMX**, or **O Ceph. For severe disease, AM-CL, azithro/clarithro**, or **O Ceph** or FQs with enhanced activity vs. drug-resistant S. pneumo (**Gemi**, **Levo**, or **Moxi**). *Drugs & doses in footnote.* **Duration** varies with drug: range 3–10 days. Limit **Gemi** to 5 days to decrease risk of rash. **Azithro** 250 mg daily x 1 yr modestly reduced frequency of acute exacerbations in pts with milder disease *(NEJM 365:689, 2011)*.		
Fever, cough, myalgia during influenza season *(See NEJM 360:2605, 2009 regarding novel H1N1 influenza A)*	Influenza A & B	*See Influenza, Table 14A, page 166.*		**Complications: Influenza pneumonia, secondary bacterial pneumonia** Community MRSA and MSSA, *S. pneumoniae, H. influenzae.*
Bronchiectasis. Thorax 65(suppl 1): i1, 2010; *Am J Respir Crit Care Med 188:647, 2013.* Acute exacerbation	H. influ., P. aeruginosa, and rarely S. pneumo.	**Gemi**, **levo**, or **moxi** x 7-10 days. *Dosage in footnote[17].*		Many potential etiologies: obstruction, ↓ immune globulins, cystic fibrosis, dyskinetic cilia, tobacco, prior severe or recurrent necrotizing bronchitis: e.g. pertussis.
Prevention of exacerbation	Not applicable	Two randomized trials of **Erythro** 250 mg bid *(JAMA 309:1260, 2013)* or **Azithro** 250 mg qd *(JAMA 309:1251, 2013)* x 1 year showed significant reduction in the rate of acute exacerbations, better preservation of lung function, and better quality of life versus placebo in adults with non-cystic fibrosis bronchiectasis.		**Caveats:** higher rates of macrolide resistance in oropharyngeal flora; potential for increased risk of a) cardiovascular deaths from macrolide-induced QTc prolongation, b) liver toxicity, or c) hearing loss *(see JAMA 309:1295, 2013)*. **Pre-treatment screening:** baseline liver function tests, electrocardiogram; assess hearing; sputum culture to exclude mycobacterial disease.
Specific organisms	Aspergillus *(see Table 11)* MAI *(Table 12)* and P. aeruginosa *(Table 5A)*.			

[17] **ADULT DOSAGE: AM-CL** 875/125 mg po bid or 500/125 mg po q8h or 2000/125 mg po bid; **azithro** 500 mg po x 1 dose, then 250 mg q24h x 4 days or 500 mg po q24h x 3 days; *Oral cephalosporins*: **cefaclor** 500 mg po q8h or 500 mg extended release q12h; **cefdinir** 300 mg po q12h or 600 mg po q24h; **cefditoren** 200 mg tabs—2 tabs bid; **cefixime** 400 mg po q24h; **cefpodoxime proxetil** 200 mg po q12h; **cefprozil** 500 mg po q12h; **ceftibuten** 400 mg po q24h; **cefuroxime axetil** 250 or 500 mg q12h; **loracarbef** 400 mg po q12h; **clarithro** extended release 1000 mg po q24h; **doxy** 100 mg po bid; **erythro base** 40 mg/kg/day po div q6h; **erythro estolate** 40 mg/kg/day po div qid; *FQs*: **CIP** 750 mg po q12h; **gemi** 320 mg po q24h; **levo** 500 mg po q24h; **moxi** 400 mg po q24h; **TMP-SMX** 1 DS tab po bid.
PEDS DOSAGE: azithro 10 mg/kg/day po on day 1, then 5 mg/kg po q24h x 4 days; **clarithro** 7.5 mg/kg po q12h; **erythro base** 40 mg/kg/day div q6h; **erythro estolate** 40 mg/kg/day div q8-12h; **TMP-SMX** (>6 mos. of age) 8 mg/kg/day (TMP component) div bid.

Abbreviations on page 2. **NOTE: All dosage recommendations are for adults (unless otherwise indicated) and assume normal renal function. § Alternatives consider allergy, PK, compliance, local resistance, cost*

TABLE 1 (35)

ANATOMIC SITE/DIAGNOSIS/ MODIFYING CIRCUMSTANCES	ETIOLOGIES (usual)	SUGGESTED REGIMENS*		ADJUNCT DIAGNOSTIC OR THERAPEUTIC MEASURES AND COMMENTS
		PRIMARY	ALTERNATIVE§	
LUNG/Bronchi *(continued)*				
Pneumonia: CONSIDER TUBERCULOSIS IN ALL PATIENTS; ISOLATE ALL SUSPECT PATIENTS				
Neonatal: Birth to 1 month	**Viruses:** CMV, rubella, H. simplex **Bacteria:** Group B strep, listeria, coliforms, S. aureus, P. aeruginosa **Other:** Chlamydia trachomatis, syphilis	**AMP** + **gentamicin** ± **cefotaxime**. Add **vanco** if MRSA a concern. For chlamydia therapy, **erythro** 12.5 mg per kg po or IV qid times 14 days.		Blood cultures indicated. Consider C. trachomatis if afebrile pneumonia, staccato cough, IgM >1:8; therapy with erythro or sulfisoxazole. If MRSA documented, **vanco**, **TMP-SMX**, & **linezolid** alternatives. **Linezolid** dosage from birth to age 11 yrs is **10 mg per kg q8h**.
Age 1–3 months Pneumonitis syndrome. Usually afebrile	C. trachomatis, RSV, parainfluenza virus 3, human metapneumovirus, Bordetella, S. pneumoniae, S. aureus (rare)	**Outpatient: po erythro** 12.5 mg/kg q6h x 14 days or po **azithro** 10 mg/kg x dose, then 5 mg/kg x 4 days.	**Inpatient: If afebrile erythro** 10 mg/kg IV q6h or **azithro** 2.5 mg/kg IV q12h *(see Comment)*. **If febrile**, add **cefotaxime** 200 mg/kg per day div q8h	Pneumonitis syndrome: Cough, tachypnea, dyspnea, diffuse infiltrates, afebrile. Usually requires hospital care. Reports of hypertrophic pyloric stenosis after erythro under age 6 wks; not sure about azithro; bid azithro dosing theoretically might ↓ risk of hypertrophic pyloric stenosis. If lobar pneumonia, give AMP 200–300 mg per kg per day for S. pneumoniae. No empiric coverage for S. aureus, as it is rare etiology.
		For **RSV**, *see Bronchiolitis, page 36*		
Infants and Children, age > 3 months to 18 yrs (IDSA Treatment Guidelines: *CID 53:617, 2011*).				
Outpatient	RSV, human metapneumovirus, rhinovirus, influenza virus, adenovirus, parainfluenza virus, Mycoplasma, H. influenzae, S. pneumoniae, S. aureus (rare)	**Amox** 90 mg/kg in 2 divided doses x 5 days	**Azithro** 10 mg/kg x 1 dose(max 500 mg), then 5 mg/kg (max 250 mg) x 4 days OR **Amox-Clav** 90 mg/kg (Amox) in 2 divided doses x 5 days	Antimicrobial therapy not routinely required for preschool-aged children with CAP as most infections are viral etiologies.
Inpatient	As above	Fully immunized: **AMP** 50 mg/kg IV q6h Not fully immunized: **Cefotaxime** 150 mg/kg IV divided q8h	Fully immunized: **Cefotaxime** 150 mg/kg IV divided q8h	If atypical infection suspected, add **Azithro** 10 mg/kg x 1 dose (max 500 mg), then 5 mg/kg (max 250 mg) x 4 days. If community MRSA suspected, add **Vanco** 40-60 mg/kg/day divided q6-8h OR **Clinda** 40 mg/kg/day divided q6-8h. Duration of therapy: 10-14 days. Depending on clinical response, may switch to oral agents as early as 2-3 days.

 **NOTE: All dosage recommendations are for adults (unless otherwise indicated) and assume normal renal function. § Alternatives consider allergy, PK, compliance, local resistance, cost*

TABLE 1 (36)

ANATOMIC SITE/DIAGNOSIS/ MODIFYING CIRCUMSTANCES	ETIOLOGIES (usual)	SUGGESTED REGIMENS*		ADJUNCT DIAGNOSTIC OR THERAPEUTIC MEASURES AND COMMENTS
		PRIMARY	ALTERNATIVE[§]	
LUNG/Bronchi/Pneumonia *(continued)*				
Adults (over age 18) — IDSA/ATS Guideline for CAP in adults: ***CID 44 (Suppl 2): S27-S72, 2007.***				
Community-acquired, not hospitalized **Prognosis prediction: CURB-65** *(Thorax 58:377, 2003)* C: confusion = 1 pt U: BUN >19 mg/dl = 1 pt R: RR >30 min = 1 pt B: BP <90/60 = 1 pt Age ≥65 = 1 pt **If score = 1, ok for outpatient therapy; if >1, hospitalize.** The higher the score, the higher the mortality. Lab diagnosis of invasive pneumococcal disease: *CID 46:926, 2008.*	Varies with clinical setting. **No co-morbidity:** Atypicals—M. pneumoniae, et al.[18], S. pneumo, viral **Co-morbidity:** Alcoholism: S. pneumo, anaerobes, coliforms Bronchiectasis: *see Cystic fibrosis, page 43* COPD: H. influenzae, M. catarrhalis, S. pneumo IVDU: Hematogenous S. aureus Post-CVA aspiration: Oral flora, incl. S. pneumo Post-obstruction of bronchi: S. pneumo, anaerobes Post- influenza: S. pneumo. and S. aureus	**No co-morbidity:** **Azithro** 0.5 gm po times 1, then 0.25 gm per day **OR azithro-ER** 2 gm times 1 **OR clarithro** 500 mg po bid or **clarithro-ER** 1 gm po q24h **OR doxy** 100 mg po bid **OR if prior antibiotic within 3 months:** (**azithro** or **clarithro**) + (**amox** 1 gm po tid or high dose **AM-CL OR Respiratory FQ**	**Co-morbidity present:** **Respiratory FQ** *(see footnote[19])* OR [(**azithro** or **clarithro**) + (high dose **amox**, high dose **AM-CL**, **cefdinir**, **cefpodoxime**, **cefprozil**)] *Doses in footnote[20]*	**Azithro/clarithro:** Pro: appropriate spectrum of activity; q24h dosing; better tolerated than erythro. Con: Overall S. pneumo resistance in vitro 20–30%, higher if pen G resist. Slightly higher risk of cardiovascular events found in retrospective studies *(BMJ 346:f1235, 2013)*; consider alternative regimen in setting of cardiovascular disease. **Amoxicillin:** Pro: Active 90–95% S. pneumo at 3–4 gm per day. Con: No activity atypicals or β-lactamase positive organisms. **AM-CL:** Pro: Spectrum of activity includes β-lactamase positive organisms. Con: No activity atypicals. **Cephalosporins—po:** Cefditoren, cefpodoxime, cefprozil, cefuroxime & others—*see footnote[20]*. Pro: Active 75–85% S. pneumo & H. influenzae. Cefuroxime least active & higher mortality rate when S. pneumo resistant. Con: Inactive vs. atypical pathogens. **Doxycycline:** Pro: Active vs. S. pneumo but resistance may be increasing. Active vs. H. influenzae, atypicals, & bioterrorism agents (anthrax, plague, tularemia). Con: Resistance of S. pneumo 18–20%. Sparse clinical data. **FQs—Respiratory FQs:** Moxi, levo & gemi Pro: In vitro & clinically effective vs. pen-sensitive & pen-resistant S. pneumo. **NOTE: dose of Levo is 750 mg q24h.** Q24H dosing. Gemi only available po. Con: Geographic pockets of resistance with clinical failure. Important Drug-drug interactions *(see Table 22A, page 224)*. Reversible rash in young females given Gemi for >7 days. **Ceftriaxone/cefotaxime:** Pro: Drugs of choice for pen-sens. S. pneumo, active H. influenzae, M. catarrhalis, & MSSA Con: Not active atypicals or pneumonia due to bioterrorism pathogens. Add macrolide for atypicals and perhaps their anti-inflammatory activity. **Ceftaroline:** (FDA approved at a dose of 600 mg q12h IV for 5-7 days for hospitalized patients with CAP): Pro: Clinical response rates at day 4 and clinical cure rates at days 8-15 post-treatment were similar for ceftaroline and ceftriaxone *(see ceftaroline package insert)*. Con: More expensive; no data for MRSA yet.
		Duration of rx: S. pneumo—Not bacteremic: until afebrile 3 days—Bacteremic: 10–14 days reasonable C. pneumoniae—Unclear. Some reports suggest 21 days. Some bronchitis pts required 5–6 wks of clarithro *(J Med Micro 52:265, 2003)* Legionella—10–21 days Necrotizing pneumonia 2° to coliforms, S. aureus, anaerobes: ≥2 weeks **Cautions:** **1. If local macrolide resistance to S. pneumoniae >25%, use alternative empiric therapy.** **2. Esp. during influenza season, look for S. aureus.**		
Community-acquired, hospitalized—NOT in the ICU Empiric therapy Treat for minimum of 5 days, afebrile for 48-72 hrs, with stable BP, adequate oral intake, and room air O_2 saturation of >90% *(COID 20:177, 2007)*.	Etiology by co-morbidity & risk factors *as above*. Culture sputum & blood. S. pneumo, urine antigen reported helpful *(CID 40: 1608, 2005)*. Legionella urine antigen indicated. In general, the sicker the pt, the more valuable culture data. Look for S. aureus if precedent/concomitant influenza or IVDU.	**Ceftriaxone** 1 gm IV q24h + **azithro** 500 mg IV q24h OR **Ertapenem** 1 gm q24h plus **azithro** 500 mg IV q24h	**Levo** 750 mg IV q24h or **Moxi** 400 mg IV q24h **Gati** 400 mg IV q24h (gati no longer marketed in US due to hypo- and hyperglycemic reactions)	
		Administration of antibiotic within 6h associated with improved survival in pneumonia and severe sepsis *(Eur Respir J 39:156, 2012)*; if in ER, first dose in ER. If diagnosis of pneumonia vague, OK for admitting diagnosis of "uncertain." *(Chest 130:16, 2006)*.		

[18] Atypical pathogens: Chlamydophila pneumoniae, C. psittaci, Legionella sp., M. pneumoniae, C. burnetii (Q fever) (Ref.: *LnID 3:709, 2003*)

[19] Respiratory FQs with enhanced activity vs. S. pneumo with high-level resistance to penicillin: **Gati**[NUS] 400 mg IV/po q24h (no longer marketed in US due to hypo- and hyperglycemic reactions), **Gemi** 320 mg po q24h, **Levo** 750 mg IV/po q24h, **Moxi** 400 mg IV/po q24h. Ketolide: **telithro** 800 mg po q24h (physicians warned about rare instances of hepatotoxicity).

[20] **O Ceph** dosage: **Cefdinir** 300 mg po q12h, **cefditoren pivoxil** 200 mg, 2 tabs po bid, **cefpodoxime proxetil** 200 mg po q12h, **cefprozil** 500 mg po q12h, **high dose amox** 1 gm po tid; **high dose AM-CL**—use **AM-CL-ER** 1000/62.5 mg, 2 tabs po bid.

TABLE 1 (37)

ANATOMIC SITE/DIAGNOSIS/ MODIFYING CIRCUMSTANCES	ETIOLOGIES (usual)	SUGGESTED REGIMENS*		ADJUNCT DIAGNOSTIC OR THERAPEUTIC MEASURES AND COMMENTS
		PRIMARY	ALTERNATIVE§	
LUNG/Bronchi/Pneumonia/Adults (over age 18) *(continued)*				
Community-acquired, hospitalized—IN ICU Empiric therapy 4 clinical settings: • **Severe COPD** • **Post-influenza** • **Suspect gm-neg bacilli** • **Risk of Pen G-resistant S. pneumo**	**Severe COPD:** S. pneumoniae (8-38%), H. influenzae, Moraxella sp., S. aureus (0-5%) (rare). If admitted to ICU: S. pneumo (15-23%), S. aureus (1.2-8.3%), GNB/P. aeruginosa (0.6-5.5%). *Refs: Chest 133:610, 2008; Thorax 66:340, 2011; CID 50:202, 2010; Isr Med Assn 12:477, 2010; Int J Antimicrob Agts 31:107, 2008.* **Severe COPD pt with pneumonia:** S. pneumoniae, H. influenzae, Moraxella sp., Legionella sp. Rarely S. aureus. Culture sputum, blood and maybe pleural fluid. Look for respiratory viruses. Urine antigen for both Legionella and S. pneumoniae. Sputum PCR for Legionella.	(**Levo** 750 mg IV q24h or **Moxi** 400 mg IV q24h) + **Azithro** *(see Comment)* **Gati** not available in US due to hypo- and hyperglycemic reactions **Procalcitonin:** Several clinical trials and meta-analyses indicate that normalization of procalcitonin levels can be used to guide duration of antibiotic therapy: Safe to discontinue antibiotics when procalcitonin level has decreased to 0.1-0.2 mcg/mL *(CID 55:651, 2012; JAMA 309:717, 2013)*.	[**Ceftriaxone** 1 gm IV q24h + **azithro** 500 mg IV q24h] or **ERTA** 1 gm q24h IV + **azithro** 500 mg IV q24h *(see Comment)*	Improved outcome with β-lactam/macrolide combo vs. β-lactam alone (patients treated with fluoroquinolones were excluded) in hospitalized CAP of moderate- or high- but not low-severity *(Thorax 68:493, 2013)*. **Ertapenem** could substitute for ceftriaxone; need azithro for atypical pathogens. Do not use if suspect P. aeruginosa. **Legionella:** Not all Legionella species detected by urine antigen; if suspicious do PCR on airway secretions. *(CID 57:1275, 2013)*. In patients with normal sinus rhythm and not receiving beta-blockers, relative bradycardia suggests Legionella, psittacosis, Q-fever, or typhoid fever.
	Post/concomitant influenza: S. aureus, S. pneumoniae	**Vanco** 15 mg/kg q8-12h + (**Levo** 750 mg IV q24h or **moxi** 400 mg IV q24h)	**Linezolid** 600 mg IV bid + (**levo** or **moxi**)	Sputum gram stain or PCR may help. *S. aureus* post-influenza ref: *EID 12:894, 2006* Empiric therapy vs. MRSA decreases risk of mortality *(CCM 34:2069, 2006)*
	Suspect aerobic gm-neg bacilli: Risk factors (see *Comment*), Hypoxic and/or hypotensive "Cover" S. pneumo & GNB	Anti-pseudomonal beta-lactam[21] + (respiratory **FQ or aminoglycoside**). Add **azithro** if no FQ *Drugs and doses in footnote[21]*. Empiric Vanco + PIP-TZ: advantage is activity vs. S. aureus; disadvantage: only one agent active vs. GNB	If severe IgE-mediated beta-lactam allergy: **aztreonam** + **FQ** or (**aztreonam + aminoglycoside + azithro**).	**Risk factors:** alcoholism with necrotizing pneumonia, underlying chronic bronchiectasis (e.g. cystic fibrosis), chronic tracheostomy and/or mechanical ventilation, febrile neutropenia and pulmonary infiltrates, septic shock, underlying malignancy, or organ failure. **P. aeruginosa:** need higher doses of **CIP** (400 mg IV q8h) and/or **PIP-TZ** 3.375 gm IV q4h.
	Risk of Pen G-resistant S. pneumoniae: 2° antibiotic use in last 3 months.	High dose IV **amp (or Pen G)** + **azithro** + **respiratory FQ**	Beta-lactam allergy: **vanco** + **respiratory FQ**	If Pen G MIC>4 mg/mL, vanco. Very rare event.
Health care-associated pneumonia (HCAP) *Ref: CID 46 (Suppl 4): S296, 2008.*	HCAP used to designate large diverse population of pts with many co-morbidities who reside in nursing homes, other long-term care facilities, require home IV therapy or are dialysis pts. Pneumonia in these pts frequently resembles hospital-acquired pneumonia *(below)*. Higher frequency of resistant bacteria than pts with CAP; MRSA (11.5%); MDR enterobacteriaceae (7.8%); P. aeruginosa (6.9%) *(CID 57:1373, 2013)*.			

[21] *Antipseudomonal beta-lactams:* **Aztreonam** 2 gm IV q6h; **piperacillin** 3 gm IV q4h; **piperacillin/tazobactam** 3.375 gm IV q4h or 4.5 gm IV q6h or 4-hr infusion of 3.375 gm q8h(high dose for Pseudomonas); **cefepime** 2 gm IV q12h; **ceftazidime** 2 gm IV q8h; **doripenem** (do NOT use to treat pneumonia); **imipenem/cilastatin** 500 mg IV q6h; **meropenem** 1 gm IV q8h; **gentamicin or tobramycin** *(see Table 10D, page 109)*. FQ dose for P. aeruginosa: **CIP** 400 mg IV q8h or **levo** 750 mg IV once daily. **Respiratory FQs: levofloxacin** 750 mg IV q24h or **moxifloxacin** 400 mg IV q24h; **high-dose ampicillin** 2 gm IV q6h; **azithromycin** 500 mg IV q24h; **vanco** 15-20 mg/kg (based on actual body wt) IV q8-12h (to achieve traget trough concentration of 15-20 μg/mL).

Abbreviations on page 2. **NOTE: All dosage recommendations are for adults (unless otherwise indicated) and assume normal renal function. § Alternatives consider allergy, PK, compliance, local resistance, cost*

TABLE 1 (38)

ANATOMIC SITE/DIAGNOSIS/ MODIFYING CIRCUMSTANCES	ETIOLOGIES (usual)	SUGGESTED REGIMENS*		ADJUNCT DIAGNOSTIC OR THERAPEUTIC MEASURES AND COMMENTS
		PRIMARY	ALTERNATIVE[§]	
LUNG/Bronchi/Pneumonia/Adults (over age 18) *(continued)*				
Hospital-acquired—usually with mechanical ventilation (VAP) (empiric therapy) Refs: *U.S. Guidelines: AJRCCM 171:388, 2005; U.S. Review: JAMA 297:1583, 2007; Canadian Guidelines: Can J Inf Dis Med Micro 19:19, 2008; British Guidelines: JAC 62:5, 2008*	Highly variable depending on clinical setting: S. pneumo, S. aureus, Legionella, coliforms, P. aeruginosa, Stenotrophomonas, Acinetobacter sp. (susceptibility to IMP/MER may be discordant) *(CID 41:758, 2005)*, anaerobes all possible. In some locales, GNB that produce extended spectrum beta-lactamase (ESBL) and/or carbapenemases *Diagnosis: see Comment*	(**IMP** 0.5 gm IV q6h or **MER** 1 gm IV q8h) plus, if suspect legionella or bioterrorism, **respiratory FQ (Levo or Moxi)** + **Vanco** for MRSA *Dosages: See footnote[21] on page 40.* Duration of therapy, *see footnote[23]*	If suspect P. aeruginosa, empirically start 2 drugs to increase likelihood that at least one will be active, e.g.: (**IMP** or **CFP** or **PIP-TZ**)[22] + (**CIP** or **tobra**). Ref: *CCM 35:1888, 2007*	**Dx of ventilator-associated pneumonia:** Fever & lung infiltrates often **not** pneumonia. Quantitative cultures helpful: bronchoalveolar lavage (>10^4 per mL pos.) or protect. spec. brush (>10^3 per mL pos.) Ref.: *AJRCCM 165:867, 2002; AnIM 132:621, 2000.* **Microbial etiology:** No empiric regimen covers all possibilities. Regimens listed active majority of **S. pneumo**, **legionella**, & **most coliforms**. Regimens **not active vs. MRSA, Stenotrophomonas & others;** *see below: Specific therapy when culture results known.* **Ventilator-associated pneumonia—Prevention:** Keep head of bed elevated 30° or more. Remove N-G, endotracheal tubes as soon as possible. If available, continuous subglottic suctioning. Chlorhexidine oral care. Silver-coated endotracheal tubes reported to reduce incidence of VAP *(JAMA 300:805 & 842, 2008).*
Hospital- or community-acquired, neutropenic pt (<500 neutrophils per mm³)	Any of organisms listed under community- & hospital-acquired + fungi (aspergillus). *See Table 11.*	*See Hospital-acquired, immediately above.* Vanco not included in initial therapy unless high suspicion of infected IV access or drug-resistant S. pneumo. Ampho not used unless still febrile after 3 days or high clinical likelihood. *See Comment*		IDSA guidelines: *Clin Infect Dis 52:e56, 2011.*
Adults—Selected specific therapy after culture results (sputum, blood, pleural fluid, etc.) available. *Also see Table 2, page 68*				
Acinetobacter baumannii *(See also Table 5A);* Ref: *NEJM 358:1271, 2008*	Patients with VAP	Use **IMP**, or **MER** if susceptible	If **IMP** resistant: **colistin** + (**IMP** or **MER**). Colistin Dose: *Table 10A, page 100.*	Sulbactam portion of AM-SB often active; dose: 3 gm IV q6h. For second-line agents: *see Pharmacother 30:1279, 2010; J Inten Care Med 25:343, 2010*
Burkholderia (Pseudomonas) pseudomallei (etiology of melioidosis) Can cause primary or secondary skin infection *See NEJM 367:1035, 2012*	Gram-negative	**Initial parenteral rx:** **Ceftazidime** 30–50 mg per kg IV q8h or **IMP** 20 mg per kg IV q8h. Rx minimum 10 days & improving, then po therapy → *see Alternative column*	**Post-parenteral po rx:** **Adults** *(see Comment for children)*: **TMP-SMX** 5 mg/kg (TMP component) bid + **Doxy** 2 mg/kg bid x 3 mos.	**Children ≤8 yrs old & pregnancy:** For oral regimen, use **AM-CL-ER** 1000/62.5, 2 tabs po bid times 20 wks. Even with compliance, relapse rate is 10%. Max. daily ceftazidime dose: 6 gm. Tigecycline: No clinical data but active in vitro *(AAC 50:1555, 2006)*
Haemophilus influenzae	β-lactamase negative β-lactamase positive	**AMP** IV, **amox** po, **TMP-SMX**, **azithro/clarithro**, **doxy** **AM-CL**, **O Ceph 2/3**, **P Ceph 3**, **FQ** Dosage: *Table 10A*		25–35% strains β-lactamase positive. ↑ resistance to both TMP-SMX and doxy. *See Table 10A, page 92 for dosages.* High % of commensal H. hemolyticus misidentified as H. influenza *(JID 195:81, 2007).*
Klebsiella sp.—ESBL pos. & other coliforms[23]	β-lactamase positive	**IMP** or **MER**; if resistant, **Colistin** + (**IMP** or **MER**)		ESBL inactivates all cephalosporins, β-lactam/β-lactamase inhibitor drug activ. not predictable; co-resistance to all FQs & often aminoglycosides.
Legionella species Relative bradycardia common feature	**Hospitalized/ immunocompromised**	**Azithro** 500 mg **IV** or **Levo** 750 mg **IV** or **Moxi** 400 mg **IV**. *See Table 10A, pages 97 & 99 for dosages.* Treat for 7–14 days *(CID 39:1734, 2004)*		Legionella website: www.legionella.org. Two studies support superiority of **Levo** over macrolides *(CID 40:794 & 800, 2005), although not FDA-approved.*

[22] **PIP-TZ** for P. aeruginosa pneumonia: 3.375 gm IV over 4 hrs & repeat q8h *(CID 44:357, 2007)* plus **tobra**.

[23] Dogma on duration of therapy not possible with so many variables: i.e. certainty of diagnosis, infecting organism, severity of infection and number/severity of co-morbidities. Agree with efforts to de-escalate & shorten course. Treat at least 7-8 days. Need clinical evidence of response: fever resolution, improved oxygenation, falling WBC. Refs: *AJRCCM 171:388, 2005; CID 43:S75, 2006; COID 19:185, 2006.*

Abbreviations on page 2. **NOTE: All dosage recommendations are for adults (unless otherwise indicated) and assume normal renal function. § Alternatives consider allergy, PK, compliance, local resistance, cost*

TABLE 1 (39)

ANATOMIC SITE/DIAGNOSIS/ MODIFYING CIRCUMSTANCES	ETIOLOGIES (usual)	SUGGESTED REGIMENS*		ADJUNCT DIAGNOSTIC OR THERAPEUTIC MEASURES AND COMMENTS
		PRIMARY	ALTERNATIVE§	
LUNG/Pneumonia/Adults— Selected specific therapy after culture results (sputum, blood, pleural fluid, etc.) available *(continued)*				
Moraxella catarrhalis	93% β-lactamase positive	**AM-CL**, **O Ceph 2/3**, **P Ceph 2/3**, **macrolide**[24], **FQ**, **TMP-SMX**. **Doxy** another option. *See Table 10A, page 92 for dosages*		
Pseudomonas aeruginosa Combination rx controversial: superior in animal model *(AAC 57:2788, 2013)* but no benefit in observational trials *(AAC 57:1270, 2013; CID 57:208, 2013)*.	Often ventilator-associated	(**PIP-TZ** 3.375 gm IV q4h or prefer 4-hr infusion of 3.375 gm q8h) + **tobra** 5 mg/kg IV once q24h *(see Table 10D, page 109)*. Could substitute anti-pseudomonal **cephalosporin** or **carbapenem** (**IMP**, **MER**) for **PIP-TZ** if pt. strain is susceptible.		Options: **CFP** 2 gm IV q8h; **CIP** 400 mg IV q8h + **PIP-TZ**; **IMP** 500 mg IV q6h + **CIP** 400 mg IV q8h; if multi-drug resistant, **Colistin** IV + **(IMP or MER) + Colistin** by inhalation 80 mg bid (controversial, *CID 52:1278, 2011*). Also available for inhalation rx: **tobra** and **aztreonam**.
Q Fever Acute atypical pneumonia. *See MMWR 62 (3):1, 2013.*	Coxiella burnetii	No valvular heart disease: **Doxy** 100 mg po bid x 14 days	Valvular heart disease: (**Doxy** 100 mg po bid + **hydroxychloroquine** 200 mg tid) x 12 months (CID 57:836, 2013)	In pregnancy: **TMP-SMX DS** 1 tab po bid throughout pregnancy.
Staphylococcus aureus Duration of treatment: 2-3 wks if just pneumonia; 4-6 wks if concomitant endocarditis and/or osteomyelitis. *IDSA Guidelines, CID 52 (Feb 1):1, 2011.*	Nafcillin/oxacillin susceptible	**Nafcillin/oxacillin** 2 gm IV q4h	**Vanco** 30-60 mg/kg/d iv in 2-3 divided doses or **linezolid** 600 mg IV q12h	Adjust dose of vancomycin to achieve target trough concentrations of 15-20 mcg/mL. Some authorities recommend a 25-30 mg/kg loading dose (actual body weight) in severely ill patients *(CID 49:325, 2009)*. Prospective trial for MRSA pneumonia: cure rate with Linezolid (58%), Vanco (47%), p = 0.042; no difference in mortality *(CID 54:621, 2012)*. **Telavancin** 10 mg/kg IV x 60 min q24h another option.
	MRSA	**Vanco** 30-60 mg/kg/d IV in 2-3 divided doses or **Linezolid** 600 mg IV/po q12h	**Dapto** not an option; pneumonia developed during dapto rx *(CID 49:1286, 2009)*.	
Stenotrophomonas maltophilia		**TMP-SMX** up to 20 mg/kg/day div q8h	**TC-CL** 3.1 gm IV q4h	Potential synergy: **TMP-SMX** + **TC-CL** *(JAC 62:889, 2008)*. Tigecycline may be another option *(J Chemother 24:150, 2012)*.
Streptococcus pneumoniae	Penicillin-susceptible	**AMP** 2 gm IV q6h, **amox** 1 gm po tid, **macrolide**[24], **pen G** IV[25], **doxy**, **O Ceph 2**, **P Ceph 2/3**. *See Table 10A, page 92 for other dosages.* Treat until afebrile, 3-5 days (min. of 5 days).		
	Penicillin-resistant, high level	**FQs** with enhanced activity: **Gemi**, **Levo**, **Moxi**; **P Ceph 3** (resistance rare); high-dose IV **AMP**; **vanco** IV—*see Table 5A, page 78 for more data*. If all options not possible (e.g., allergy), **linezolid** active: 600 mg IV or po q12h. *Dosages Table 10A.* Treat until afebrile, 3-5 days (min. of 5 days). In CAP trial, **Ceftaroline** 600 mg IV q12h superior to Ceftriaxone *(CID 51:641, 2010)*.		
Yersinia pestis (Plague) *CID 49:736, 2009*	Aerosol Y. pestis.	**Gentamicin** 5 mg/kg IV q24h	**Doxy** 200 mg IV times 1, then 100 mg IV bid	TMP-SMX used as prophylaxis for plague pneumonia *(CID 40:1166, 2005)*. Chloro effective but potentially toxic. Cephalosporins and FQs effective in animal models.
Actinomycosis	A. Israelii and rarely others	**AMP** 50 mg/kg/day IV div in 3-4 doses x 4-6 wks, then **Pen VK** 2-4 gm/day po x 3-6 wks	**Doxy** or **ceftriaxone** or **clinda** or **erythro**	Can use **Pen G** instead of AMP: 10-20 million units/day IV x 4-6 wks.

[24] **Macrolide** = azithromycin, clarithromycin and erythromycin.
[25] **IV Pen G dosage:** no meningitis, 2 million units IV q4h. If concomitant meningitis, 4 million units IV q4h.

Abbreviations on page 2. **NOTE: All dosage recommendations are for adults (unless otherwise indicated) and assume normal renal function. § Alternatives consider allergy, PK, compliance, local resistance, cost*

TABLE 1 (40)

ANATOMIC SITE/DIAGNOSIS/ MODIFYING CIRCUMSTANCES	ETIOLOGIES (usual)	SUGGESTED REGIMENS*		ADJUNCT DIAGNOSTIC OR THERAPEUTIC MEASURES AND COMMENTS
		PRIMARY	ALTERNATIVE§	
LUNG—Other Specific Infections				
Anthrax **Inhalation** (applies to oropharyngeal & gastrointestinal forms): **Treatment** (Cutaneous: *See page 51*) Ref: *www.bt.cdc.gov*	Bacillus anthracis **To report possible bioterrorism event: 770-488-7100** Plague, tularemia: *See page 45.* Chest x-ray: mediastinal widening & pleural effusion	**Adults (including pregnancy):** (**CIP** 400 mg IV q12h) or (**Levo** 500 mg IV q24h) or (**doxy** 100 mg IV q12h) **plus** (**clindamycin** 900 mg IV q8h &/or **RIF** 300 mg IV q12h + **raxibacumab** 40 mg/kg IV over 2 hrs). Switch to po antibiotic when able & lower CIP to 500 mg po bid; clinda to 450 mg po q8h; & RIF 300 mg po bid. Treat times 60 days.	**Children:** (**CIP** 10 mg/kg IV q12h or 15 mg/kg po q12h) or (**Doxy**: >8 y/o & >45 kg: 100 mg IV q12h; >8 y/o & ≤45 kg: 2.2 mg/kg IV q12h; ≤8 y/o: 2.2 mg/kg IV q12h) **plus clindamycin** 7.5 mg/kg IV q6h **and/or RIF** 20 mg/kg (max. 600 mg) IV q24h + **raxibacumab** 40-80 mg/kg IV over 2 hrs. See package insert. Treat times 60 days. *See Table 16, page 209 for oral dosage.*	1. Clinda may block toxin production 2. Rifampin penetrates CSF & intracellular sites. 3. If isolate shown penicillin-susceptible: a. **Adults: Pen G** 4 million units IV q4h b. **Children: Pen G** <12 y/o: 50,000 units per kg IV q6h; >12 y/o: 4 million units IV q4h c. Constitutive & inducible β-lactamases—do not use pen or amp alone. 4. Do not use cephalosporins or TMP-SMX. 5. Erythro, azithro activity borderline; clarithro active. 6. No person-to-person spread. 7. Monoclonal antitoxin antibody approved: **raxibacumab** single 2 hr IV infusion. 8. Moxi should work, but no clinical data 9. Case report of survival with use of anthrax immunoglobulin (*CID 44:968, 2007; CID 54:1848, 2012*).
Anthrax, prophylaxis	Info: www.bt.cdc.gov	**Adults (including pregnancy) or children >50 kg:** (**CIP** 500 mg po bid or **Levo** 500 mg po q24h) x 60 days. **Children <50 kg: CIP** 20–30 mg/kg per day div q12h x 60 days or **levo** 8 mg/kg q12h x 60 days	**Adults (including pregnancy): Doxy** 100 mg po bid x 60 days. **Children** (*see Comment*): **Doxy** >8 y/o & >45 kg: 100 mg po bid; >8 y/o & ≤45 kg: 2.2 mg/kg po bid; ≤8 y/o: 2.2 mg/kg po bid. All for 60 days.	1. Once organism shows suscept. to penicillin, switch to amoxicillin 80 mg per kg per day div. q8h (max. 500 mg q8h); pregnant pt to amoxicillin 500 mg po tid. 2. Do **not** use cephalosporins or TMP-SMX. 3. Other FQs (Gati, Moxi) & clarithro should work but no clinical experience.
Aspiration pneumonia/anaerobic lung infection/lung abscess	Transthoracic culture in 90 pts—% of total isolates: anaerobes 34%, Gm-pos. cocci 26%, S. milleri 16%, Klebsiella pneumoniae 25%, nocardia 3%	**Clindamycin** 300-450 mg po tid OR **Ampicillin-sulbactam** 3 g IV q6h OR **A carbapenem** (e.g., ertapenem 1 g IV q24h)	**Ceftriaxone** 1 gm IV q24h plus **metro** 500 mg IV q6h or 1 gm IV q12h	Typically anaerobic infection of the lung: aspiration pneumonitis, necrotizing pneumonia, lung abscess and empyema (*REF: Anaerobe 18:235, 2012*) Other treatment options: PIP-TZ 3.325 g IV q6h (for mixed infections with resistant Gram-negative aerobes) or Moxi 400 mg IV/po q24h (*CID 41:764, 2005*).
Chronic pneumonia with fever, night sweats and weight loss	M. tuberculosis, coccidioidomycosis, histoplasmosis	*See Table 11, Table 12.* For risk associated with TNF inhibitors, *see CID 41(Suppl.3):S187, 2005.*		HIV+, foreign-born, alcoholism, contact with TB, travel into developing countries
Cystic fibrosis **Acute exacerbation of pulmonary symptoms** *BMC Medicine 9:32, 2011* (*continued on next page*)	S. aureus or H. influenzae early in disease; P. aeruginosa later in disease Nontuberculous mycobacteria emerging as an important pathogen (*Semin Respir Crit Care Med 34:124, 2013*)	**For P. aeruginosa:** (Peds doses) **Tobra** 3.3 mg/kg q8h or 12 mg/kg IV q24h. Combine tobra with (**PIP** or **ticarcillin** 100 mg/kg q6h) **or ceftaz** 50 mg/kg IV q8h to max of 6 gm per day. If resistant to above, **CIP/Levo** used if P. aeruginosa susceptible. *See footnote[26] & Comment*	**For S. aureus: (1) MSSA—oxacillin/nafcillin** 2 gm IV q4h (*Peds dose, Table 16*). **(2) MRSA—vanco** 15 mg/kg (actual wt) IV q8-12h (to achieve target trough concentration of 15-20 μg/mL.	Cystic Fibrosis Foundation Guidelines: 1. Combination therapy for P. aeruginosa infection. 2. Once-daily dosing for aminoglycosides. 3. Need more data on continuous infusion beta-lactam therapy. 4. Routine use of steroid not recommended. Inhalation options (P. aeruginosa suppression): 1) Nebulized tobra 300 mg bid x 28 days, no rx for 28 days, repeat; 2) Inhaled tobra powder-hand held: 4-28 mg cap bid x 28 days, no rx for 28 days, repeat; Nebulized aztreonam (Cayston): 75 mg tid after pre-dose bronchodilator. *Ref: Med Lett 55:51, 2013.*

[26] Other options: (Tobra + aztreonam 50 mg per kg IV q8h); (IMP 15–25 mg per kg IV q6h + tobra); **CIP commonly used in children**, e.g., CIP IV/po + ceftaz IV (*LnID 3:537, 2003*).

 **NOTE: All dosage recommendations are for adults (unless otherwise indicated) and assume normal renal function. § Alternatives consider allergy, PK, compliance, local resistance, cost*

TABLE 1 (41)

ANATOMIC SITE/DIAGNOSIS/ MODIFYING CIRCUMSTANCES	ETIOLOGIES (usual)	SUGGESTED REGIMENS*		ADJUNCT DIAGNOSTIC OR THERAPEUTIC MEASURES AND COMMENTS
		PRIMARY	ALTERNATIVE§	
LUNG—Other Specific Infections *(continued)*				
(continued from previous page)	Burkholderia (Pseudomonas) cepacia	**TMP-SMX** 5 mg per kg (TMP) IV q6h	**Chloro** 15–20 mg per kg IV/po q6h	B. cepacia has become a major pathogen. Patients develop progressive respiratory failure, 62% mortality at 1 yr. **Fail to respond to aminoglycosides,** piperacillin, & ceftazidime. Patients with B. cepacia should be isolated from other CF patients.
		For other alternatives, see Table 2		
Empyema. Refs.: Pleural effusion review: *CID 45:1480, 2007; IDSA Treatment Guidelines for Children, CID 53:617, 2011.*				
Neonatal	Staph. aureus	*See Pneumonia, neonatal, page 38*		Drainage indicated.
Infants/children (1 month–5 yrs)	Staph. aureus, Strep. pneumoniae, H. influenzae	*See Pneumonia, age 1 month–5 years, page 38*		Drainage indicated.
Child >5 yrs to ADULT—Diagnostic thoracentesis; chest tube for empyemas				
Acute, usually parapneumonic *For dosage, see Table 10B or footnote page 25*	Strep. pneumoniae, Group A strep	**Cefotaxime** or **ceftriaxone** *(Dosage, see footnote[12] page 25)*	**Vanco**	Tissue Plasminogen Activator (10 mg) + DNase (5 mg) bid x 3 days via chest tube improves outcome *(NEJM 365:518, 2011)*.
	Staph. aureus: Check for MRSA	**Nafcillin** or **oxacillin** if MSSA	**Vanco** or **linezolid** if MRSA.	Usually complication of S. aureus pneumonia &/or bacteremia.
	H. influenzae	**Ceftriaxone**	**TMP-SMX** or **AM-SB**	Pleomorphic Gm-neg. bacilli. ↑ resistance to TMP-SMX.
Subacute/chronic	Anaerobic strep, Strep. milleri, Bacteroides sp., Enterobacteriaceae, M. tuberculosis	**Clinda** 450–900 mg IV q8h + **ceftriaxone**	**Cefoxitin** or **IMP** or **TC-CL** or **PIP-TZ** or **AM-SB** *(Dosage, see footnote[12] page 25)*	Intrapleural administration tissue plasminogen activator (t-PA) 10 mg + DNase 5 mg via chest tube twice daily for 3 days improved fluid drainage, reduced frequency of surgery, and reduced duration of the hospital stay; neither agent was effective alone *(N Engl J Med 365:518, 2011)*. If organisms not seen, treat as subacute; drain fluid. Pleural biopsy with culture for mycobacteria and histology if TBc suspected.
Human immunodeficiency virus infection (HIV+): *See SANFORD GUIDE TO HIV/AIDS THERAPY*				
CD4 T-lymphocytes <200 per mm³ or clinical AIDS Dry cough, progressive dyspnea, & diffuse infiltrate **Prednisone first if suspect pneumocystis** *(see Comment)*	Pneumocystis carinii most likely; also MTB, fungi, Kaposi's sarcoma, & lymphoma NOTE: AIDS pts may develop pneumonia due to DRSP or other pathogens—*see next box below*	*Rx listed here is for* **severe** *pneumocystis; see Table 11A, page 123 for po regimens for* **mild** *disease.* **Prednisone 1st** *(see Comment),* **then:** **TMP-SMX** [IV: 15 mg per kg per day div q8h (TMP component) or po: 2 DS tabs q8h], total of 21 days	(**Clinda** 600 mg IV q8h + **primaquine** 30 mg po q24h) or (**pentamidine isethionate** 4 mg per kg per day IV) times 21 days. *See Comment*	**Diagnosis (induced sputum or bronchial wash) for:** histology or monoclonal antibody strains or PCR. Serum beta-glucan (Fungitell) levels under study *(CID 46:1928 & 1930, 2008)*. **Prednisone 40 mg bid po times 5 days then 40 mg q24h po times 5 days then 20 mg q24h po times 11 days is indicated with PCP (pO_2 <70 mmHg), should be given at initiation of anti-PCP rx; don't wait until pt's condition deteriorates.** If PCP studies negative, consider bacterial pneumonia, TBc, cocci, histo, crypto, Kaposi's sarcoma or lymphoma. **Pentamidine not active vs. bacterial pathogens.** **NOTE: Pneumocystis resistant to TMP-SMX, albeit rare, does exist.**
CD4 T-lymphocytes normal Acute onset, purulent sputum & pulmonary infiltrates ± pleuritic pain. **Isolate pt until TBc excluded: Adults**	Strep. pneumoniae, H. influenzae, aerobic Gm-neg. bacilli (including P. aeruginosa), Legionella rare, MTB.	Ceftriaxone 1 gm IV q24h (over age 65 1 gm IV q24h) + **azithro**. Could use **Levo,** or **Moxi** IV as alternative *(see Comment)*		If Gram stain of sputum shows Gm-neg. bacilli, options include **P Ceph 3 AP**, **TC-CL**, **PIP-TZ**, **IMP**, or **MER**. **FQs: Levo** 750 mg po/IV q24h; **Moxi** 400 mg po/IV q24h. Gati not available in US due to hypo- & hyperglycemic reactions.
As above: Children	Same as adult with HIV + lymphoid interstitial pneumonia (LIP)	As for HIV+ adults with pneumonia. If diagnosis is LIP, rx with steroids.		In children with AIDS, LIP responsible for 1/3 of pulmonary complications, usually >1 yr of age vs. PCP, which is seen at <1 yr of age. Clinically: clubbing, hepatosplenomegaly, salivary glands enlarged (take up gallium), lymphocytosis.

 **NOTE: All dosage recommendations are for adults (unless otherwise indicated) and assume normal renal function. § Alternatives consider allergy, PK, compliance, local resistance, cost*

TABLE 1 (42)

ANATOMIC SITE/DIAGNOSIS/ MODIFYING CIRCUMSTANCES	ETIOLOGIES (usual)	SUGGESTED REGIMENS*		ADJUNCT DIAGNOSTIC OR THERAPEUTIC MEASURES AND COMMENTS
		PRIMARY	ALTERNATIVE§	
LUNG—Other Specific Infections *(continued)*				
Nocardia pneumonia Expert Help: Wallace Lab (+1) 903-877-7680; CDC (+1) 404-639-3158 Ref: *Medicine 88:250, 2009.*	N. asteroides, N. brasiliensis	**TMP-SMX** 15 mg/kg/day IV/po in 2-4 divided doses + **Imipenem** 500 mg IV q6h for first 3-4 weeks then **TMP-SMX** 10 mg/kg/day in 2-4 divided doses x 3-6 mos.	**IMP** 500 mg IV q6h + **amikacin** 7.5 mg/kg IV q12h x 3-4 wks & then po **TMP-SMX**	**Duration:** 3 mos. if immunocompetent; 6 mos. if immunocompromised. **Measure peak sulfonamide levels:** Target is 100-150 mcg/mL 2 hrs post po dose. **Linezolid** active in vitro *(Ann Pharmacother 41:1694, 2007)*. In vitro resistance to TMP-SMX may be increasing *(Clin Infect Dis 51:1445, 2010)*, but whether this is associated with worse outcomes is not known.
Tularemia **Inhalational tularemia** Ref.: *JAMA 285:2763, 2001 & www.bt.cdc.gov*	Francisella tularemia **Treatment**	(**Streptomycin** 15 mg per kg IV bid) or (**gentamicin** 5 mg per kg IV qd) times 10 days	**Doxy** 100 mg IV or po bid times 14–21 days or **CIP** 400 mg IV (or 750 mg po) bid times 14–21 days	For pediatric doses, *see Table 16, page 209*. Pregnancy: *as for non-pregnant adults*. **Tobramycin** should work.
	Postexposure prophylaxis	**Doxy** 100 mg po bid times 14 days	**CIP** 500 mg po bid times 14 days	For pediatric doses, *see Table 16, page 209*. Pregnancy: *As for non-pregnant adults*
Viral (interstitial) pneumonia suspected *See Influenza, Table 14A, page 166.* Ref: *Chest 133:1221, 2008.*	Consider: **Influenza**, adenovirus, coronavirus (SARS), hantavirus, metapneumovirus, parainfluenza virus, respiratory syncytial virus	**Oseltamivir** 75 mg po bid for 5 days or **zanamivir** two 5 mg inhalations twice a day for 5 days.		No known efficacious drugs for adenovirus, coronavirus (SARS), hantavirus, metapneumovirus, parainfluenza or RSV. Need travel (SARS) & exposure (Hanta) history. RSV and human metapneumovirus as serious as influenza in the elderly *(NEJM 352:1749 & 1810, 2005; CID 44:1152 & 1159, 2007)*.
LYMPH NODES (approaches below apply to lymphadenitis without an obvious primary source)				
Lymphadenitis, acute **Generalized**	Etiologies: EBV, early HIV infection, syphilis, toxoplasma, tularemia, Lyme disease, sarcoid, lymphoma, systemic lupus erythematosus, **Kikuchi-Fujimoto** disease and others. For differential diagnosis of fever and lymphadenopathy see *NEJM 369:2333, 2013.*			
Regional				
Cervical—see cat-scratch disease (CSD), below	CSD (B. henselae), Grp A strep, Staph. aureus, anaerobes, MTB (scrofula), M. avium, M. scrofulaceum, M. malmoense, toxo, tularemia		History & physical exam directs evaluation. If nodes fluctuant, aspirate and base rx on Gram & acid-fast stains. **Kikuchi-Fujimoto** disease causes fever and benign self-limited adenopathy; the etiology is unknown *(CID 39:138, 2004)*.	
Inguinal Sexually transmitted	HSV, chancroid, syphilis, LGV			
Not sexually transmitted	GAS, SA, tularemia, CSD, Y. pestis (plague)		Consider bubonic plague & glandular tularemia.	
Axillary	GAS, SA, CSD, tularemia, Y. pestis, sporotrichosis		Consider bubonic plague & glandular tularemia.	
Extremity, with associated nodular lymphangitis	Sporotrichosis, leishmania, Nocardia brasiliensis, Mycobacterium marinum, Mycobacterium chelonae, tularemia		Treatment varies with specific etiology	A distinctive form of lymphangitis characterized by subcutaneous swellings along inflamed lymphatic channels. Primary site of skin invasion usually present; regional adenopathy variable.
Nocardia lymphadenitis & skin abscesses	N. asteroides, N. brasiliensis	**TMP-SMX** 5-10 mg/kg/day based on TMP IV/po div in 2-4 doses	**Sulfisoxazole** 2 gm po qid or **minocycline** 100-200 mg po bid.	**Duration:** 3 mos. if immunocompetent; 6 mos. if immunocompromised. **Linezolid:** 600 mg po bid reported effective *(Ann Pharmacother 41:1694, 2007)*.
Cat-scratch disease—immunocompetent patient Axillary/epitrochlear nodes 46%, neck 26%, inguinal 17%. Ref: *Amer Fam Physician 83:152, 2011.*	Bartonella henselae	**Azithro** dosage—**Adults** (>45.5 kg): 500 mg po x 1, then 250 mg/day x 4 days. **Children** (<45.5 kg): liquid azithro 10 mg/kg x 1, then 5 mg/kg per day x 4 days. Rx is controversial	No therapy; resolves in 2–6 mos. Needle aspiration relieves pain in suppurative nodes. Avoid I&D.	**Clinical:** Approx. 10% nodes suppurate. Atypical presentation in <5% pts, i.e., lung nodules, liver/spleen lesions, Parinaud's oculoglandular syndrome, CNS manifestations in 2% of pts (encephalitis, peripheral neuropathy, retinitis), FUO. **Dx:** Cat exposure. Positive IFA serology. Rarely need biopsy.

Abbreviations on page 2. **NOTE: All dosage recommendations are for adults (unless otherwise indicated) and assume normal renal function. § Alternatives consider allergy, PK, compliance, local resistance, cost*

TABLE 1 (43)

ANATOMIC SITE/DIAGNOSIS/ MODIFYING CIRCUMSTANCES	ETIOLOGIES (usual)	SUGGESTED REGIMENS*		ADJUNCT DIAGNOSTIC OR THERAPEUTIC MEASURES AND COMMENTS
		PRIMARY	ALTERNATIVE§	
MOUTH				
Aphthous stomatitis, recurrent	Etiology unknown	Topical steroids (Kenalog in Orabase) may ↓ pain and swelling; if AIDS, *see SANFORD GUIDE TO HIV/AIDS THERAPY*.		
Buccal cellulitis Children <5 yrs	H. influenzae	**Cefuroxime** or **ceftriaxone**	**AM-CL** or **TMP-SMX**	With Hib immunization, invasive H. influenzae infections have ↓ by 95%. Now occurring in infants prior to immunization.
		Dosage: see Table 16, page 209		
Candida Stomatitis ("Thrush")	C. albicans	**Fluconazole**	Echinocandin	*See Table 11, page 114.*
Herpetic stomatitis	Herpes simplex virus 1 & 2	*See Table 14*		
Submandibular space infection, bilateral (Ludwig's angina)	Oral anaerobes, facultative streptococci, S. aureus (rare)	(**PIP-TZ** or **TC-CL**) or (**Pen G** IV + **Metro** IV)	**Clinda** 600 mg IV q6-8h (for Pen-allergic pt)	**Ensure adequate airway** and early surgical debridement. Add Vanco IV if gram-positive cocci on gram stain.
Ulcerative gingivitis (Vincent's angina or Trench mouth)	Oral anaerobes + vitamin deficiency	**Pen G** po/IV + **Metro** po/IV	**Clinda**	Replete vitamins (A-D). Can mimic scurvy. Severe form is NOMA (Cancrum oris) *(Ln 368:147, 2006)*
MUSCLE				
"Gas gangrene". Contaminated traumatic wound. Can be spontaneous without trauma.	C. perfringens, other histotoxic Clostridium sp.	(**Clinda** 900 mg IV q8h) + (**pen G** 24 million units/day div. q4–6h IV)	**Ceftriaxone** 2 gm IV q12h or **erythro** 1 gm q6h IV (not by bolus)	Surgical debridement primary therapy. **Hyperbaric oxygen** adjunctive: efficacy debated, consider if debridement not complete or possible. Clinda given to decrease toxin production.
Pyomyositis	Staph. aureus, Group A strep, (rarely Gm-neg. bacilli), variety of anaerobic organisms	(**Nafcillin** or **oxacillin** 2 gm IV q4h) or [**P Ceph 1** (**cefazolin** 2 gm IV q8h)] if **MSSA**	**Vanco** 1 gm IV q12h if **MRSA**	Common in tropics; rare, but occurs, in temperate zones. Follows exercise or muscle injury, *see Necrotizing fasciitis*. Now seen in HIV/AIDS. Add **metro** if anaerobes suspected or proven.
PANCREAS: Review: *NEJM 354:2142, 2006.*				
Acute alcoholic (without necrosis) (idiopathic) pancreatitis	Not bacterial	None No necrosis on CT	1–9% become infected but prospective studies show no advantage of prophylactic antimicrobials. Observe for pancreatic abscesses or necrosis which require therapy.	
Post-necrotizing pancreatitis; infected pseudocyst; pancreatic abscess	Enterobacteriaceae, enterococci, S. aureus, S. epidermidis, anaerobes, candida	Need culture of abscess/infected pseudocyst to direct therapy; **PIP-TZ** is reasonable empiric therapy		Can often get specimen by fine-needle aspiration. **Moxi**, **MER**, **IMP**, **ERTA** are all options *(AAC 56:6434, 2012)*.
Antimicrobic prophylaxis, necrotizing pancreatitis	As above	If > 30% pancreatic necrosis on CT scan (with contrast), initiate antibiotic therapy: **IMP** 0.5-1 gm IV q6h or **MER** 1 gm IV q8h. No need for empiric Fluconazole. If patient worsens CT guided aspiration for culture & sensitivity. Controversial: *Cochrane Database Sys Rev 2003: CD 002941; Gastroenterol 126:977, 2004; Ann Surg 245:674, 2007.*		
PAROTID GLAND				
"Hot" tender parotid swelling	S. aureus, S. pyogenes, oral flora, & aerobic Gm-neg. bacilli (rare), mumps, rarely enteroviruses/ influenza: **Nafcillin** or **oxacillin** 2 gm IV q4h if MSSA; **vanco** if MRSA; **metro** or **clinda** for anaerobes			Predisposing factors: stone(s) in Stensen's duct, dehydration. Therapy depends on ID of specific etiologic organism.
"Cold" non-tender parotid swelling	Granulomatous disease (e.g., mycobacteria, fungi, sarcoidosis, Sjögren's syndrome), drugs (iodides, et al.), diabetes, cirrhosis, tumors			History/lab results may narrow differential; may need biopsy for diagnosis

 **NOTE: All dosage recommendations are for adults (unless otherwise indicated) and assume normal renal function. § Alternatives consider allergy, PK, compliance, local resistance, cost*

TABLE 1 (44)

ANATOMIC SITE/DIAGNOSIS/ MODIFYING CIRCUMSTANCES	ETIOLOGIES (usual)	SUGGESTED REGIMENS* PRIMARY	ALTERNATIVE[§]	ADJUNCT DIAGNOSTIC OR THERAPEUTIC MEASURES AND COMMENTS
PERITONEUM/PERITONITIS: *Reference—CID 50:133, 2010*				
Primary (spontaneous bacterial peritonitis, SBP) *Hepatology 49:2087, 2009.* Dx: Pos. culture & ≥ 250 neutrophils/μL of ascitic fluid	Enterobacteriaceae 63%, S. pneumo 9%, enterococci 6–10%, anaerobes <1%. Extended β-lactamase (ESBL) positive Klebsiella species.	[**Cefotaxime** 2 gm IV q8h (if life-threatening, q4h)] or [**TC-CL** or **PIP-TZ**] OR [**ceftriaxone** 2 gm IV q24h] or [**ERTA** 1 gm IV q24h] **If resistant E. coli/Klebsiella species (ESBL+), then:** (**DORI**, **ERTA**, **IMP** or **MER**) or (**FQ: CIP**, **Levo**, **Moxi**) *(Dosage in footnote[27])*. Check in vitro susceptibility.		One-year **risk of SBP** in pts with ascites and cirrhosis as high as 29% *(Gastro 104: 1133, 1993)*. Diagnosis of SBP: 30–40% of pts have neg. cultures of blood and ascitic fluid. % pos. cultures ↑ if 10 mL of pt's ascitic fluid added to blood culture bottles *(JAMA 299:1166, 2008)*. **Duration of rx unclear.** Treat for at least 5 days, perhaps longer if pt bacteremic *(Pharm & Therapeutics 34:204, 2009)*. **IV albumin** (1.5 gm/kg at dx & 1 gm/kg on day 3) may ↓ frequency of renal impairment (p 0.002) & ↓ hospital mortality (p 0.01) *(NEJM 341:403, 1999)*.
Prevention of SBP *(Amer J Gastro 104:993, 2009)*: Cirrhosis & ascites *For prevention after UGI bleeding, see Liver, page 36*		**TMP-SMX-DS** 1 tab po 5 days/wk or **CIP** 750 mg po q wk		**TMP-SMX** ↓ peritonitis or spontaneous bacteremia from 27% to 3% *(AnIM 122:595, 1995)*. Ref. for CIP: *Hepatology 22:1171, 1995*
Secondary (bowel perforation, ruptured appendix, ruptured diverticula) Ref: *CID 50:133, 2010 (IDSA Guidelines)* **Antifungal rx?** No need if successful uncomplicated 1st surgery for viscus perforation. Treat for candida if: recurrent surg. perforation(s), anastomotic leaks, necrotizing pancreatitis, liver/pancreas transplant, pure peritoneal culture, candidemia *(Ln 2:1437, 1989; Am Surg 76:197, 2010)*. Detection of beta-D-glucan antigen in serum of limited value due to low sensitivity/specificity and many false positives *(JCM 51:3478, 2013)*.	Enterobacteriaceae, Bacteroides sp., enterococci, P. aeruginosa (3-15 %). C. albicans (may contribute with recurrent perforation/multiple surgeries) If VRE documented, dapto may work *(Int J Antimicrob Agents 32:369, 2008)*.	**Mild-moderate disease—Inpatient—parenteral rx:** (e.g., focal periappendiceal peritonitis, peridiverticular abscess). **Usually need surgery for source control.** **PIP-TZ** 3.375 gm IV q6h or 4.5 gm IV q8h or 4-hr infusion of 3.375 gm q8h **OR** **TC-CL** 3.1 gm IV q6h **OR** **ERTA** 1 gm IV q24h **OR** **MOXI** 400 mg IV q24h **Severe life-threatening disease—ICU patient: Surgery for source control +** **IMP** 500 mg IV q6h or **MER** 1 gm IV q8h or **DORI** 500 mg IV q8h (1-hr infusion). *See Comments.* **Concomitant surgical management important.**	[(**CIP** 400 mg IV q12h or **Levo** 750 mg IV q24h) + (**metro** 1 gm IV q12h)] or (**CFP** 2 gm q12h + **metro**) Note: avoid tigecycline unless no other alternative due to increased mortality risk (FDA warning) [**AMP** + **metro** + (**CIP** 400 mg IV q8h or **Levo** 750 mg IV q24h)] **OR** [**AMP** 2 gm IV q6h + **metro** 500 mg IV q6h + **aminoglycoside** *(see Table 10D, page 109)*]	Must "cover" both Gm-neg. aerobic & Gm-neg. anaerobic bacteria. Empiric coverage of MRSA, enterococci and candida not necessary unless culture indicates infection. Cover enterococci if valvular heart disease. **Drugs active only vs. anaerobic Gm-neg. bacilli:** metro. **Drugs active only vs. aerobic Gm-neg. bacilli:** aminoglycosides, P Ceph 2/3/4, aztreonam, AP Pen, CIP, Levo. **Drugs active vs. both aerobic/anaerobic Gm-neg. bacteria:** cefoxitin, TC-CL, PIP-TZ, Dori, IMP, MER, Moxi. Increasing resistance (R) of Bacteroides species *(Anaerobe 17:147, 2013; AAC 56:1247, 2012)*: **Cefoxitin / Cefotetan / Clindamycin** **% R** 5-30 / 17–87 / 19-35 Essentially no resistance of Bacteroides to: **metro**, **PIP-TZ.** Case report of B. fragilis resistant to all drugs except minocycline, tigecycline & linezolid *(MMWR 62:694, 2013)*. **Ertapenem** not active vs. P. aeruginosa/ Acinetobacter species. If absence of ongoing fecal contamination, **aerobic/anaerobic culture** of peritoneal exudate/abscess may be of help in guiding specific therapy. Less need for aminoglycosides. **With severe pen allergy,** can "cover" Gm-neg. aerobes with **CIP** or **aztreonam. Remember DORI/IMP/MER are β-lactams.** IMP dose increased to 1 gm q6h if suspect P. aeruginosa and pt. is critically ill. If VRE documented, daptomycin may work *(Int J Antimicrobial Agents 32:369, 2008)*.

[27] Parenteral **IV therapy** for peritonitis: **TC-CL** 3.1 gm q6h, **PIP-TZ** 3.375 gm q6h or 4.5 gm q8h or 4-hr infusion of 3.375 gm q8h *(See Table 10)*, **Dori** 500 mg IV q8h (1-hr infusion), **IMP** 0.5-1 gm q6h, **MER** 1 gm q8h, **FQ** [**CIP** 400 mg q12h, **Oflox** 400 mg q12h, **Levo** 750 mg q24h, **Moxi** 400 mg q24h], **AMP** 1 gm q6h, **aminoglycoside** *(see Table 10D, page 109)*, **cefotetan** 2 gm q12h, **cefoxitin** 2 gm q8h, **P Ceph 3** (**cefotaxime** 2 gm q4–8h, **ceftriaxone** 1–2 gm q24h, **ceftizoxime** 2 gm q4–8h), **P Ceph 4** (**CFP** 2 gm q12h, **cefpirome**[NUS] 2 gm q12h), **clinda** 600–900 mg q8h, **Metronidazole** 1 gm (15 mg/kg) loading dose IV, then 1 gm IV q12h (Some data supports once-daily dosing, *see Table 10A, page 101*), **AP Pen** (**ticarcillin** 4 gm q6h, **PIP** 4 gm q6h, **aztreonam** 2 gm q8h)

 **NOTE: All dosage recommendations are for adults (unless otherwise indicated) and assume normal renal function. § Alternatives consider allergy, PK, compliance, local resistance, cost*

TABLE 1 (45)

ANATOMIC SITE/DIAGNOSIS/ MODIFYING CIRCUMSTANCES	ETIOLOGIES (usual)	SUGGESTED REGIMENS*		ADJUNCT DIAGNOSTIC OR THERAPEUTIC MEASURES AND COMMENTS
		PRIMARY	ALTERNATIVE[§]	
PERITONEUM/PERITONITIS *(continued)*				
Abdominal actinomycosis	A. Israelii and rarely others	**AMP** 50 mg/kg/day IV div in 3-4 doses x 4-6 wks, then **Pen VK** 2-4 gm/day po x 3-6 mos.	**Doxy** or **ceftriaxone** or **clinda**	Presents as mass +/- fistula tract after abdominal surgery, e.g., for ruptured appendix. Can use IV Pen G instead of AMP: 10-20 million units/day IV x 4-6 wks.
Associated with chronic ambulatory peritoneal dialysis (Abdominal pain, cloudy dialysate, dialysate WBC >100 cell/μL with >50% neutrophils; normal = <8 cells/μL. Ref: *Perit Dial Int 30:393, 2010.*)	Gm+ 45%, Gm- 15%, Multiple 1%, Fungi 2%, MTB 0.1% *(Perit Dial Int 24:424, 2004)*.	**Empiric therapy:** Need activity vs. MRSA **(Vanco)** & aerobic gram-negative bacilli (**Ceftaz**, **CFP**, **Carbapenem**, **CIP**, **Aztreonam**, **Gent**). Add **Fluconazole** if gram stain shows yeast. Use intraperitoneal dosing, unless bacteremia (rare). For bacteremia, IV dosing. For dosing detail, *see Table 19, page 220.*		**For diagnosis:** concentrate several hundred mL of removed dialysis fluid by centrifugation. Gram stain concentrate and then inject into aerobic/anaerobic blood culture bottles. A positive Gram stain will guide initial therapy. If culture shows Staph. epidermidis and no S. aureus, good chance of "saving" dialysis catheter; **if multiple Gm-neg. bacilli cultured, consider catheter-induced bowel perforation and need for catheter removal.** *See Perit Dialysis Int 29:5, 2009.* Other indications for catheter removal: relapsing/refractory peritonitis, fungal peritonitis, catheter tunnel infection.
PHARYNX				
Pharyngitis/Tonsillitis				
Exudative or Diffuse Erythema				
Associated cough, rhinorrhea, hoarseness and/or oral ulcers suggest viral etiology. IDSA Guidelines on Group A Strep: *CID 55:1279, 2012; CID 55:e86, 2012.*	Group A, C, G Strep.; Fusobacterium (in research studies); EBV; Primary HIV; *N. gonorrhea*; Respiratory viruses	**For Strep pharyngitis:** (**Pen V** po x 10 days or **Benzathine Pen** 1.2 million units IM x 1 dose) OR (**Cefdinir** or **Cefpodoxime**) x 5 days. **Cephalosporin doses in footnote**[28] (adult and peds) (Durations are FDA-approved).	**For Strep pharyngitis: Pen allergic: Clinda** 300-450 mg po q8h x 10 days. **Azithro**, **Clarithro** are alternatives, but resistant *S. pyogenes* reported *(JAC 63:42, 2009)*. Sulfonamides and Tetracyclines have questionable efficacy.	Dx: Rapid Strep test. No need for post-treatment test of cure rapid strep test or culture. Complications of Strep pharyngitis: 1) Acute rheumatic fever 48 – follows Grp A *S. pyogenes* infection, rare after Grp C/G infection. *See footnote*[29]. For prevention, start treatment within 9 days of onset of symptoms. 2) Children age < 7 yrs at risk for post-streptococcal glomerulonephritis. 3) Pediatric autoimmune neuropsychiatric disorder associated with Grp A Strep (PANDAS) infection. 4) Peritonsillar abscess; Suppurative phlebitis are potential complications.
	Gonococcal pharyngitis	**Ceftriaxone** 250 mg IM x 1 dose + (**Azithro** 1 gm po x 1 dose) or **Doxy** 100 mg po bid x 7 days	FQs not recommended due to resistance	Not effective for pharyngeal GC: spectinomycin, cefixime, cefpodoxime and cefuroxime. Ref: *MMWR 61:590, 2012.*
(Continued on the page)	Proven *S. pyogenes* recurrence	**Cefdinir** or **Cefpodoxime**	**AM-CL** or **Clinda**	

[28] **Treatment of Group A, C & G strep: Treatment durations are from approved package inserts. Subsequent studies indicate efficacy of shorter treatment courses. All po unless otherwise indicated. PEDIATRIC DOSAGE; Benzathine penicillin** 25,000 units per kg IM to max. 1.2 million units; **Pen V** 25–50 mg per kg per day div. q6h x 10 days; **amox** 1000 mg po once daily x 10 days; **AM-CL** 45 mg per kg per day div. q12h x 10 days; **cephalexin** 20 mg/kg/dose bid (max 500 mg/dose) x 10 days; **cefuroxime axetil** 20 mg per kg per day div. bid x 10 days; **cefpodoxime proxetil** 10 mg per kg div. bid x 10 days; **cefdinir** 7 mg per kg q12h x 5–10 days or 14 mg per kg q24h x 10 days; **cefprozil** 15 mg per kg per day div. bid x 10 days; **cefadroxil** 30 mg/kg once daily (max 1 gm/day) x 10 days; **clarithro** 15 mg per kg per day div. bid x bid or 250 mg qid x 10 days; **azithro** 12 mg per kg once daily x 5 days; clinda 20–30 mg per kg per day div. q8h x 10 days. **ADULT DOSAGE; Benzathine** penicillin 1.2 million units IM x 1; **Pen V** 500 mg bid or 250 mg qid x 10 days;**cefditoren** 200 mg bid x 10 days; **cefuroxime axetil** 250 mg bid x 4 days; **cefpodoxime proxetil** 100 mg bid x 5 days; **cefdinir** 300 mg q12h x 5–10 days or 600 mg q24h x 10 days; **cefditoren** 200 mg bid; **cefprozil** 500 mg q24h x 10 days; **NOTE:** All **O Ceph 2** drugs approved for 10-day rx of strep. pharyngitis; increasing number of studies show efficacy of 4–6 days; **clarithro** 250 mg bid x 10 days; **azithro** 500 mg x 1 and then 250 mg q24h x 4 days or 500 mg q24h x 3 days.

[29] Primary rationale for therapy is eradication of Group A strep (GAS) and prevention of acute rheumatic fever (ARF). Benzathine penicillin G has been shown in clinical trials to ↓ rate of ARF from 2.8 to 0.2%. This was associated with clearance of GAS on pharyngeal cultures *(CID 19:1110, 1994)*. Subsequent studies have been based on cultures, not actual prevention of ARF. Treatment decreases duration of symptoms.

 **NOTE: All dosage recommendations are for adults (unless otherwise indicated) and assume normal renal function. § Alternatives consider allergy, PK, compliance, local resistance, cost*

TABLE 1 (46)

ANATOMIC SITE/DIAGNOSIS/ MODIFYING CIRCUMSTANCES	ETIOLOGIES (usual)	SUGGESTED REGIMENS* PRIMARY	SUGGESTED REGIMENS* ALTERNATIVE§	ADJUNCT DIAGNOSTIC OR THERAPEUTIC MEASURES AND COMMENTS
PHARYNX/Pharyngitis/Tonsillitis/Exudative or Diffuse Erythema *(continued)*				
(continued from previous page)	Grp A infections: 6 in 1 yr; 4 in 2 consecutive yrs	Tonsillectomy not recommended to decrease Strep infections		Hard to distinguish true Grp A Strep infection from chronic Grp A Strep carriage and/or repeat viral infections.
Peritonsillar abscess – Sometimes a serious complication of exudative pharyngitis ("Quinsy") *(JAC 68:1941, 2013)*	**F. necrophorum** (44%) Grp A Strep (33%) Grp C/G Strep (9%) Strep anginosus grp	**Surgical drainage plus** **PIP-TZ** 3.375 gm IV q6h or (**Metro** 500 mg IV/po q6-8h+ **Ceftriaxone** 2 gm IV q24h)	Pen allergic: **Clinda** 600-900 mg IV q6-8h	**Avoid macrolides: Fusobacterium is resistant.** Reports of beta-lactamase production by oral anaerobes *(Anaerobe 9:105, 2003)*. *See jugular vein suppurative phlebitis, page 50. See JAC 68:1941, 2013. Etiologies ref: CID 49:1467, 2009.*
Other complications	*See parapharyngeal space infection and jugular vein suppurative phlebitis (see next page)*			
Membranous pharyngitis: due to **Diphtheria** Respiratory isolation, nasal & pharyngeal cultures (special media), obtain antitoxin. **Place pt in respiratory droplet isolation.**	*C. diphtheriae* (human to human), *C. ulcerans* and *C. pseudotuberculosis* (animal to human) (rare)	**Treatment: antibiotics + antitoxin** **Antibiotic therapy: Erythro** 500 mg IV qid OR **Pen G** 50,000 units/kg (max 1.2 million units) IV q12h. Can switch to Pen VK 250 mg po qid when able. Treat for 14 days	**Diphtheria antitoxin:** Horse serum. Obtain from CDC, +1 404-639-2889. Do scratch test before IV therapy. Dose depends on stage of illness: < 48hrs: 20,000-40,000 units; if NP membranes: 40,000-60,000 units; > 3 days & bull neck: 80,000-120,000 units	**Ensure adequate airway.** EKG & cardiac enzymes. F/U cultures 2 wks post-treatment to document cure. Then, diphtheria toxoid immunization. Culture contacts; treat contacts with either single dose of **Pen G** IM: 600,000 units if age < 6 yrs, 1.2 million units if age ≥ 6 yrs. If Pen-allergic, **Erythro** 500 mg po qid x 7-10 days. Assess immunization status of close contacts: toxoid vaccine as indicated. In vitro, C. diphtheriae suscept. to clarithro, azithro, clinda, FQs, TMP/SMX.
Vesicular, ulcerative pharyngitis (viral)	Coxsackie A9, B1-5, ECHO (multiple types), Enterovirus 71, Herpes simplex 1,2	Antibacterial agents not indicated. For HSV-1, 2: **acyclovir** 400 mg tid po x 10 days.		Small vesicles posterior pharynx suggests enterovirus. Viruses are most common etiology of acute pharyngitis. Suspect viral if concurrent conjunctivitis, coryza, cough, skin rash, hoarseness.
Epiglottitis (Supraglottis): Concern in life-threatening obstruction of the airway				
Children	H. influenzae (rare), S. pyogenes, S. pneumoniae, S. aureus (includes MRSA), viruses	**Peds dosage: (Cefotaxime** 50 mg per kg IV q8h or **ceftriaxone** 50 mg per kg IV q24h) + **Vanco**	**Peds dosage: Levo** 10 mg/kg IV q24h + **Clinda** 7.5 mg/kg IV q6h	Have tracheostomy set "at bedside." **Levo** use in children is justified as emergency empiric therapy in pts with severe beta-lactam allergy. *Ref: Ped Clin No Amer 53:215, 2006.* Use of steroids is controversial; do not recommend.
Adults	Group A strep, H. influenzae (rare) & many others	Same regimens as for children. **Adult dosage:** *See footnote*[30]		
Parapharyngeal space infection [Spaces include: sublingual, submandibular (Ludwig's angina), *(see page 46)* lateral pharyngeal, retropharyngeal, pretracheal]				
Poor dental hygiene, dental extractions, foreign bodies (e.g., toothpicks, fish bones) Ref: *CID 49:1467, 2009*	Polymicrobic: Strep sp., anaerobes, Eikenella corrodens. Anaerobes outnumber aerobes 10:1.	[(**Clinda** 600–900 mg IV q8h) or (**pen G** 24 million units/day by cont. infusion or div. q4–6h IV]+ **metro** 1 gm load and then 0.5 gm IV q6h)	**PIP-TZ** 3.375 gm IV q6h or **AM-SB** 3 gm IV q6h	Close observation of airway, 1/3 require intubation. MRI or CT to identify abscess; **surgical drainage. Metro** may be given 1 gm IV q12h. Complications: infection of carotid (rupture possible) & jugular vein phlebitis.

[30] Parapharyngeal space infection: **Ceftriaxone** 2 gm IV q24h; **cefotaxime** 2 gm IV q4–8h; **PIP-TZ** 3.375 gm IV q6h or 4-hr infusion of 3.375 gm q8h; **TC-CL** 3.1 gm IV q4–6h; **TMP-SMX** 8–10 mg per kg per day (based on TMP component) div q6h, q8h, or q12h ; **Clinda** 600-900 mg IV q6-8h; **Levo** 750 mg IV q24h; **vanco** 15 mg/kg IV q12h.

TABLE 1 (47)

ANATOMIC SITE/DIAGNOSIS/ MODIFYING CIRCUMSTANCES	ETIOLOGIES (usual)	SUGGESTED REGIMENS*		ADJUNCT DIAGNOSTIC OR THERAPEUTIC MEASURES AND COMMENTS
		PRIMARY	ALTERNATIVE§	
PHARYNX/Parapharyngeal space infection *(continued)*				
Jugular vein suppurative phlebitis (Lemierre's syndrome) *LnID 12:808, 2012.*	Fusobacterium necrophorum in vast majority	**PIP-TZ** 4.5 gm IV q8h or **IMP** 500 mg IV q6h or (**Metro** 500 mg po/IV q8h + **ceftriaxone** 2 gm IV once daily)	**Clinda** 600–900 mg IV q8h. **Avoid macrolides: fusobacterium are resistant**	Emboli: pulmonary and systemic common. Erosion into carotid artery can occur. Lemierre described F. necrophorum in 1936; other anaerobes & Gm-positive cocci are less common etiologies of suppurative phlebitis post-pharyngitis.
Laryngitis (hoarseness)	Viral (90%)	Not indicated		
SINUSES, PARANASAL				
Sinusitis, acute *(Ref: CID 54:e72, 2012). Guidelines: Pediatrics 132:e262 & 284, 2013 (American Academy of Pediatrics)*				
Treatment goals: • Speed resolution • Prevent bacterial complications (see Comment) • Prevent chronic sinusitis • Avoid unnecessary use of antibiotics	S. pneumonia 33% H. influenza 32% M. catarrhalis 9% Anaerobes 6% Grp A strep 2% Viruses 15-18% S. aureus 10% *(see Comment)*	Most common: obstruction of sinus ostia by inflammation from virus or allergy. Treatment: Saline irrigation **Antibiotics for bacterial sinusitis if:** 1) fever, pain, purulent nasal discharge; 2) still symptomatic after 10 days with no antibiotic; 3) clinical failure despite antibiotic therapy		**Treatment:** • Clinda: Haemophilus & Moraxella sp. are resistant; may need 2nd drug • Duration of rx: 5-7 days *(IDSA Guidelines)*, 10-14 days (*Amer Acad Ped Guidelines)* • Adjunctive rx: 1) do not use topical decongestant for > 3 days; 2) no definite benefit from nasal steroids & antihistamines; 3) saline irrigation may help • Avoid macrolides & TMP-SMX due to resistance • Empiric rx does not target S. aureus: incidence same in pts & controls *(CID 45:e121, 2007)* Potential complications: transient hyposmia, orbital infection, epidural abscess, brain abscess, meningitis, cavernous sinus thrombosis. For other adult drugs and doses, *see footnote*[31].
		No penicillin allergy **Peds: Amox** 90 mg/kg/day divided q12h or **Amox-Clav** suspension 90 mg/kg/day (Amox comp) divided q12h. Treat for 10-14 days **Adult: Amox-Clav** 1000/62.5-2 tabs po bid x 5-7 days	*Penicillin allergy* **Peds (if anaphylaxis): Clinda** 30-40 mg/kg/day divided tid or qid x 10-14 days (see Comment) **Peds (no anaphylaxis): Cefpodoxime** 10 mg/kg/day po div q12h **Adult (if anaphylaxis): Levo** or doxy. Adult (no anaphylaxis): **Cefpodoxime** 200 mg po bid	
Clinical failure after 3 days	As above; consider diagnostic tap/aspirate	**Mild/Mod. Disease: AM-CL-ER** OR (**cefpodoxime**, **cefprozil**, or **cefdinir**)	**Severe Disease: Gati**[NUS]**, Gemi, Levo, Moxi**	
		Treat 5-10 days. Adult doses in footnote[31]		
Diabetes mellitus with acute keto-acidosis; neutropenia; deferox-amine rx: Mucormycosis	Rhizopus sp., (mucor), aspergillus	*See Table 11, pages 112 & 123.*		

[31] **Adult doses for sinusitis (all oral): AM-CL-ER** 2000/125 **mg** bid, **amox high-dose (HD)** 1 gm tid, **clarithro** 500 mg bid or **clarithro ext. release** 1 gm q24h, **doxy** 100 mg bid, **respiratory FQs** (**Gati** 400 mg q24hNUS due to hypo/hyperglycemia; **Gemi** 320 mg q24h *(not FDA indication but should work)*, **Levo** 750 mg q24h x 5 days, **Moxi** 400 mg q24h); **O Ceph** (**cefdinir** 300 mg q12h or 600 mg q24h, **cefpodoxime** 200 mg bid, **cefprozil** 250–500 mg bid, **cefuroxime** 250 mg bid), **TMP-SMX** 1 double-strength (TMP 160 mg) bid (results after 3- and 10-day rx similar).

 **NOTE: All dosage recommendations are for adults (unless otherwise indicated) and assume normal renal function. § Alternatives consider allergy, PK, compliance, local resistance, cost*

TABLE 1 (48)

ANATOMIC SITE/DIAGNOSIS/ MODIFYING CIRCUMSTANCES	ETIOLOGIES (usual)	SUGGESTED REGIMENS*		ADJUNCT DIAGNOSTIC OR THERAPEUTIC MEASURES AND COMMENTS
		PRIMARY	ALTERNATIVE§	
SINUSES, PARANASAL *(continued)*				
Hospitalized + nasotracheal or nasogastric intubation	Gm-neg. bacilli 47% (pseudomonas, acinetobacter, E. coli common), Gm+ (S. aureus) 35%, yeasts 18%. Polymicrobial in 80%	Remove nasotracheal tube: if fever persists and ENT available, recommend sinus aspiration for C/S prior to empiric therapy **IMP** 0.5 gm IV q6h or **MER** 1 gm IV q8h. Add vanco for MRSA if Gram stain suggestive.	(**Ceftaz** 2 gm IV q8h + **vanco**) or (**CFP** 2 gm IV q12h + **vanco**).	After 7 days of nasotracheal or nasogastric tubes, 95% have x-ray "sinusitis" (fluid in sinuses), but on transnasal puncture only 38% culture + *(AJRCCM 150:776, 1994)*. For pts requiring mechanical ventilation with nasotracheal tube for ≥1 wk, bacterial sinusitis occurs in <10% *(CID 27:851, 1998)*. May need fluconazole if yeast on Gram stain of sinus aspirate.
Sinusitis, chronic **Adults** **Defined:** (drainage, blockage, facial pain, ↓ sense of smell) + (mucopurulence on endoscopy or CT scan changes) *(Rhinology 50:1, 2012)*.	4 categories (alone or in combination): allergy, infection, dental, idiopathic	No persuasive evidence of benefit from antibiotics, but amox-clav or clinda often given for 3-10 wks *(Curr Opin Otolaryngol Head Neck Surg 21:61, 2013)*.	Otolaryngology consultation. If acute exacerbation, treat as acute sinusitis. Steroid inhalers help if allergic. Sinus irrigation may help.	Pathogenesis unclear and may be polyfactorial: damage to ostiomeatal complex during acute bacterial disease, allergy ± polyps, occult immunodeficiency, and/or odontogenic disease (periodontitis in maxillary teeth). Serum IgE levels if suspect allergy *(Allergy 68:1, 2012)*. CT scan of maxillary bone if suspect odontogenic source.
SKIN				
Acne vulgaris *(Med Lett Treatment Guidelines 11 (Issue 125): 1, 2013)*.				
Comedonal acne, "blackheads," "whiteheads," earliest form, no inflammation	Excessive sebum production & gland obstruction. No Propionibacterium acnes	Once-q24h: Topical **tretinoin** (cream 0.025 or 0.05%) or (gel 0.01 or 0.025%)	All once-q24h: Topical **adapalene** 0.1% gel OR **azelaic acid** 20% cream or **tazarotene** 0.1% cream	Goal is prevention, ↓ number of new comedones and create an environment unfavorable to P. acnes. Adapalene causes less irritation than tretinoin. Azelaic acid less potent but less irritating than retinoids. **Tazarotene: Do not use in pregnancy.**
Mild inflammatory acne: small papules or pustules	Proliferation of P. acnes + abnormal desquamation of follicular cells	Topical **erythro** 3% + **benzoyl peroxide** 5%, bid	Can substitute **clinda** 1% gel for erythro	In random. controlled trial, topical benzoyl peroxide + erythro of equal efficacy to oral minocycline & tetracycline and not affected by antibiotic resistance of propionibacteria *(Ln 364:2188, 2004)*.
Inflammatory acne: comedones, papules & pustules. Less common: deep nodules (cysts)	Progression of above events. Also, drug induced, e.g., glucocorticoids, phenytoin, lithium, INH & others.	(Topical **erythro** 3% + **benzoyl peroxide** 5% bid) ± oral antibiotic. *See Comment for mild acne*	Oral drugs: (**doxy** 50 mg bid) or (**minocycline** 50 mg bid). Others: **tetracycline**, **erythro**, **TMP-SMX**, **clinda.** Expensive extended release **once-daily minocycline** (Solodyn) 1 mg/kg/d	Systemic **isotretinoin** reserved for pts with severe widespread nodular cystic lesions that fail oral antibiotic rx; 4–5 mos. course of 0.1–1 mg per kg per day. Aggressive/violent behavior reported. **Tetracyclines** stain developing teeth. **Doxy** can cause photosensitivity. **Minocycline** side-effects: urticaria, vertigo, pigment deposition in skin or oral mucosa. Rare induced autoimmunity in children: fever; polyarthralgia, positive ANCA *(J Peds 153:314, 2008)*.
Acne rosacea Ref: *NEJM 352:793, 2005.*	Skin mite: Demadex folliculorum *(Arch Derm 146:896, 2010)*	Facial erythema: Brimonidine gel (Mirvaso) applied to affected area bid *(J Drugs Dermatol 12:650, 2013)*	Papulopustular rosacea: **Azelaic acid** gel bid, topical or **Metro** topical cream once daily or q24h	Avoid activities that provoke flushing, e.g., alcohol, spicy food, sunlight.
Anthrax, **cutaneous**, inhalation **To report bioterrorism event: 770-488-7100;** **For info: www.bt.cdc.gov** *See JAMA 281:1735, 1999; MMWR 50:909, 2001.* Treat as inhalation anthrax if systemic illness.	B. anthracis Spores are introduced into/under the skin by contact with infected animals/animal products. *See Lung, page 43.*	**Adults (including pregnancy) and children >50 kg:** (**CIP** 500 mg po bid or **Levo** 500 mg IV/po q24h) x 60 days. **Children <50 kg:** [**CIP** 30 mg/kg day div q12h po (to max. 1 gm per day) or **levo** 8 mg/kg po q12h] x 60 days	**Adults (including pregnancy): Doxy** 100 mg po bid x 60 days. **Children: Doxy** >8 y/o & >45 kg: 100 mg po bid; >8 y/o & ≤45 kg: 2.2 mg/kg po bid; ≤8 y/o: 2.2 mg/kg po bid All for 60 days.	1. If penicillin susceptible, then: **Adults: Amox** 500 mg po q8h times 60 days. **Children: Amox** 80 mg per kg per day div. q8h (max. 500 mg q8h) 2. **Usual treatment of cutaneous anthrax is 7–10 days; 60 days in setting of bioterrorism with presumed aerosol exposure.** 3. Other **FQs** (Levo, Moxi) should work based on in vitro susceptibility data 4. Outbreak among heroin users in Europe *(Emerg Infect Dis 18:1307, 2012)* 5. Anthrax vaccine absorbed recommended at 0, 2, 4 wks postexposure for postexposure prophylaxis.

Abbreviations on page 2. **NOTE: All dosage recommendations are for adults (unless otherwise indicated) and assume normal renal function. § Alternatives consider allergy, PK, compliance, local resistance, cost*

TABLE 1 (49)

ANATOMIC SITE/DIAGNOSIS/ MODIFYING CIRCUMSTANCES	ETIOLOGIES (usual)	SUGGESTED REGIMENS*		ADJUNCT DIAGNOSTIC OR THERAPEUTIC MEASURES AND COMMENTS
		PRIMARY	ALTERNATIVE§	
SKIN *(continued)*				
Bacillary angiomatosis: For other Bartonella infections, *see Cat-scratch disease lymphadenitis, page 45, and Bartonella systemic infections, page 57*				
In immunocompromised (HIV-1, bone marrow transplant) patients *Also see SANFORD GUIDE TO HIV/AIDS THERAPY*	Bartonella henselae and quintana	**Clarithro** 500 mg po bid or ext. release 1 gm po q24h or **azithro** 250 mg po q24h *(see Comment)*	**Erythro** 500 mg po qid or **doxy** 100 mg po bid or (**Doxy** 100 mg po bid + **RIF** 300 mg po bid)	For AIDS pts, continue suppressive therapy until HIV treated and CD > 200 cells/μL for 6 mos.
Bite: Remember tetanus prophylaxis— *See Table 20B, page 222 for rabies prophylaxis.* For extensive review of microbiology of animal bite caused infections, *see CMR 24:231, 2011.*				
Bat, raccoon, skunk	Strep & staph from skin; rabies	**AM-CL** 875/125 mg po bid or 500/125 mg po tid	**Doxy** 100 mg po bid	In Americas, **anti-rabies rx indicated:** rabies immune globulin + vaccine. *(See Table 20B, page 222)*
Camel	S. aureus, P. aeruginosa, Other Gm-neg bacilli	**Diclox** 250-500 mg po q6h + **CIP** 750 mg po bid	**Cephalexin** 500 mg po qid + **CIP** 750 mg po bid	*See EJCMID 18:918, 1999.*
Cat: 80% get infected, culture & treat empirically. Cat-scratch disease: *page 45*	**Pasteurella multocida**, Streptococci, Staph. aureus, Neisseria, Moraxella	**AM-CL** 875/125 mg po bid or 500/125 mg po tid	**Cefuroxime axetil** 0.5 gm po q12h or **doxy** 100 mg po bid. **Do not use cephalexin.** Sens. to FQs in vitro.	**P. multocida resistant to dicloxacillin, cephalexin, clinda; many strains resistant to erythro** (most sensitive to azithro but no clinical data). P. multocida infection develops within 24 hrs. Observe for osteomyelitis. If culture + for only P. multocida, can switch to pen G IV or pen VK po. See Dog Bite
Catfish sting	Toxins	*See Comments*		Presents as immediate pain, erythema and edema. Resembles strep cellulitis. May become secondarily infected; AM-CL is reasonable choice for prophylaxis
Dog: Only 5% get infected; treat only if bite severe or bad co-morbidity (e.g. diabetes).	**Pasteurella canis**, S. aureus, Streptococci, Fusobacterium sp., Capnocytophaga canimorsus	**AM-CL** 875/125 mg po bid or 500/125 mg po tid	**Clinda** 300 mg po qid + FQ (adults) or **clinda** + **TMP-SMX** (children)	Consider anti-rabies prophylaxis: rabies immune globulin + vaccine *(see Table 20B)*. Capnocytophaga in splenectomized pts may cause local eschar, sepsis with DIC. **P. canis resistant to diclox, cephalexin, clinda and erythro;** sensitive to ceftriaxone, cefuroxime, cefpodoxime and FQs.
Human For bacteriology, *see CID 37:1481, 2003*	Viridans strep 100%, Staph epidermidis 53%, corynebacterium 41%, **Staph. aureus 29%, eikenella 15%,** bacteroides 82%, peptostrep 26%	**Early** (not yet infected): **AM-CL** 875/125 mg po bid times 5 days. **Later:** Signs of infection (usually in 3–24 hrs): (**AM-SB** 1.5 gm IV q6h or **cefoxitin** 2 gm IV q8h) or (**TC-CL** 3.1 gm IV q6h) or (**PIP-TZ** 3.375 gm IV q6h or 4.5 gm q8h or 4-hr infusion of 3.375 gm q8h). Pen allergy: **Clinda** + (either **CIP** or **TMP-SMX**)		**Cleaning, irrigation and debridement most important.** For clenched fist injuries, x-rays should be obtained. Bites inflicted by hospitalized pts, consider aerobic Gm-neg. bacilli. **Eikenella resistant to clinda, nafcillin/oxacillin, metro, P Ceph 1, and erythro; susceptible to FQs and TMP-SMX.**
Leech (Medicinal) *(Ln 381:1686, 2013)*	Aeromonas hydrophila	**CIP** (400 mg IV or 750 mg po) bid	**TMP-SMX DS** 1 tab po bid	Aeromonas found in GI tract of leeches. Some use prophylactic antibiotics when leeches used medicinally, but not universally accepted or necessary.
Pig (swine)	Polymicrobic: Gm+ cocci, Gm-neg. bacilli, anaerobes, Pasteurella sp.	**AM-CL** 875/125 mg po bid	**P Ceph 3** or **TC-CL** or **AM-SB** or **IMP**	Information limited but infection is common and serious *(Ln 348:888, 1996)*.
Prairie dog	Monkeypox	*See Table 14A, page 168.* No rx recommended		
Primate, non-human	Microbiology. Herpesvirus simiae	**Acyclovir:** *See Table 14B, page 172*		*CID 20:421, 1995*
Rat	Spirillum minus & Streptobacillus moniliformis	**AM-CL** 875/125 mg po bid	**Doxy**	Anti-rabies rx not indicated. Causes rat bite fever (Streptobacillus moniliformis): Pen G or doxy, alternatively erythro or clinda.
Seal	Marine mycoplasma	Tetracycline times 4 wks		Can take weeks to appear after bite *(Ln 364:448, 2004)*.
Snake: pit viper (Ref.: *NEJM 347:347, 2002)*	Pseudomonas sp., Enterobacteriaceae, Staph. epidermidis, Clostridium sp.		**Primary therapy is antivenom**. Penicillin generally used but would not be effective vs. organisms isolated. Ceftriaxone should be more effective. Tetanus prophylaxis indicated. Ref: *CID 43:1309, 2006.*	

 **NOTE: All dosage recommendations are for adults (unless otherwise indicated) and assume normal renal function. § Alternatives consider allergy, PK, compliance, local resistance, cost*

TABLE 1 (50)

ANATOMIC SITE/DIAGNOSIS/ MODIFYING CIRCUMSTANCES	ETIOLOGIES (usual)	SUGGESTED REGIMENS*		ADJUNCT DIAGNOSTIC OR THERAPEUTIC MEASURES AND COMMENTS
		PRIMARY	ALTERNATIVE§	
SKIN/Bite *(continued)*				
Spider bite: Most necrotic ulcers attributed to spiders are probably due to another cause, e.g., cutaneous anthrax *(Ln 364:549, 2004)* or **MRSA infection** (spider bite painful; anthrax not painful.)				
Widow (Latrodectus)	Not infectious	None	May be confused with "acute abdomen." Diazepam or calcium gluconate helpful to control pain, muscle spasm. Tetanus prophylaxis.	
Brown recluse (Loxosceles) *NEJM 352:700, 2005*	Not infectious. Overdiagnosed! Spider distribution limited to S. Central & desert SW of US	Bite usually self-limited & self-healing. No therapy of proven efficacy.	**Dapsone** 50 mg po q24h often used despite marginal supportive data	Dapsone causes hemolysis (check for G6PD deficiency). Can cause hepatitis; baseline & weekly liver panels suggested.
Boils—Furunculosis—Subcutaneous abscesses in drug addicts ("skin poppers"). Carbuncles = multiple connecting furuncles; Emergency Dept Perspective *(IDC No Amer 22:89, 2008)*.				
Active lesions *See Table 6, page 79*	Staph. aureus, both MSSA & MRSA *IDSA Guidelines: CID 52 (Feb 1):1, 2011.*	**Boils and abscesses** < 5 cm, outpatient setting, no diabetes, immunosuppression, most will respond to simple I&D. For larger or multiple abscesses, systemic inflammatory response syndrome antibiotics may provide added benefit to I&D: Options include **TMP/SMX** 1-2 DS bid (higher dose if BMI > 40), **Clinda** 300-450 mg po tid (higher dose if BMI > 40), or **Doxy** 100 mg po bid or **Minocycline** 100 mg po bid, for 5-10 days. **Incision and Drainage mainstay of therapy!**		Other options: (1) **Linezolid** 600 mg po bid x 10 days; (2) **Fusidic acid**[NUS] 250-500 mg po q8-12h ± **RIF** *(CID 42:394, 2006)*; (3) cephalexin 500 mg po tid-qid or dicloxacillin 500 mg po tid-qid, only in low prevalence setting for MRSA.
To lessen number of furuncle recurrences --decolonization *For surgical prophylaxis, see Table 15B, page 198.*	MSSA & MRSA. *IDSA Guidelines, CID 52 (Feb 1):1, 2011; AAC 56:1084, 2012.*	7-day therapy: **Chlorhexidine** (2%) washes daily; 2% **mupirocin ointment** anterior nares 2x daily + (**rifampin** 300 mg bid + **doxy** 100 mg bid).	**Mupirocin ointment** in anterior nares bid x 7 days + **chlorhexidine** (2%) washes daily x 7 days + (**TMP-SMX DS** 1 tab po bid + **RIF** 300 mg po bid) x 7 days	Optimal regimen uncertain. Can substitute bleach baths for chlorhexidine *(Inf Control Hosp Epidemiol 32:872, 2011)*. Bacitracin oint. inferior to Mupirocin *(ICHE 20:351, 1999)*.
Hidradenitis suppurativa Not infectious disease, but bacterial superinfection occurs	Lesions secondarily infected: S. aureus, Enterobacteriaceae, pseudomonas, anaerobes	Clinda 1% topical cream **Adalimumab** 40 mg once weekly beneficial *(AnIM 157:846, 2012)*	Tetracycline 500 mg po bid x 3 months	Caused by keratinous plugging of apocrine glands of axillary, inguinal, perianal, perineal, infra-mammary areas. Other therapy: antiperspirants, loose clothing and anti-androgens. *Dermatol Clin 28:779, 2010.*
Burns. Overall management: *NEJM 350:810, 2004 – step-by-step case outline*				
Initial wound care Use burn unit, if available Topical rx options *(NEJM 359:1037, 2008; Clin Plastic Surg 36:597, 2009)*	**Not infected** Prophylaxis for potential pathogens: Gm-pos cocci Gm-neg bacilli Candida	Early excision & wound closure. Variety of skin grafts/substitutes. Shower hydrotherapy. Topical antimicrobials	**Silver sulfadiazine** cream 1% applied 1-2 x daily. Minimal pain. Transient reversible neutropenia due to margination in burn – not marrow toxicity	Mafenide acetate cream is an alternative but painful to apply. Anti-tetanus prophylaxis indicated.
Burn wound sepsis Proposed standard def: *J Burn Care Res 28:776, 2007.* Need quantitative wound cultures	Strep. pyogenes, Enterobacter sp., S. aureus, S. epidermidis, E. faecalis, E. coli, P. aeruginosa. Fungi (rare). Herpesvirus (rare).	**Vanco** high dose to rapidly achieve trough concentration of 15-20 µg/mL + (**MER** 1 gm IV q8h or **cefepime** 2 gm IV q8h) + **Fluconazole** 6 mg/kg IV qd *See Comments for alternatives*		Vanco allergic/intolerant: **Dapto** 6-12 mg/kg IV qd IgE mediated allergy to beta lactams: **Aztreonam** 2 gm IV q6h. ESBL- or carbapenemase-producing MDR gm-neg bacilli: only option is **Colistin** + (**MER** or **IMP**)

 **NOTE: All dosage recommendations are for adults (unless otherwise indicated) and assume normal renal function. § Alternatives consider allergy, PK, compliance, local resistance, cost*

TABLE 1 (51)

ANATOMIC SITE/DIAGNOSIS/ MODIFYING CIRCUMSTANCES	ETIOLOGIES (usual)	SUGGESTED REGIMENS*		ADJUNCT DIAGNOSTIC OR THERAPEUTIC MEASURES AND COMMENTS
		PRIMARY	ALTERNATIVE§	
SKIN *(continued)*				
Cellulitis, erysipelas: Be wary of macrolide (erythro-resistant) Streptococcus sp.. Review: *NEJM 350:904, 2004*. **NOTE:** Consider diseases that masquerade as cellulitis *(AnIM 142:47, 2005)*				
Extremities, non-diabetic *For diabetes, see below.* Practice guidelines: *CID 41:1373, 2005.*	Streptococcus sp., Groups A, B, C & G. Staph. aureus, including MRSA (but rare).	Inpatients: Elevate legs. **Pen G** 1–2 million units IV q6h or **cefazolin** 1 gm IV q8h. If Pen-allergic: **Vanco** 15 mg/kg IV q12h. When afebrile: **Pen VK** 500 mg po qid ac & hs. Total therapy: 10 days.	Outpatient: Elevate legs. **Pen VK** 500 mg po qid ac & hs x 10 days. If Pen-allergic: **Azithro** 500 mg po x 1 dose, then 250 mg po once daily x 4 days (total 5 days). Rarely, might need **Linezolid** 600 mg po bid (expensive).	Look for tinea pedis as portal of entry. Treat if present. If S. aureus suspected due to fluctuance or positive gram stain: MSSA: **Diclox** 500 mg po qid or **Nafcillin/Oxacillin** 2 gm IV q4h; MRSA: **Doxy** 100 mg po bid or **TMP-SMX-DS** 1 tab po bid or **Vanco** 1 gm IV q12h (inpatient). If S. aureus confirmed, usually need I&D. **Leg elevation is helpful. Note**: TMP-SMX for MRSA but not S. pyogenes; S. pyogenes may fail in vivo even if active in vitro *(Eur J Clin Micro 3:424, 1984)*.
Facial, adult (erysipelas)	Strep. sp. (Grp A, B, C & G), Staph. aureus (to include MRSA), S. pneumo	**Vanco** 15 mg/kg (actual wt) IV q8-12h (to achieve target trough concentration of 15-20 µg/mL	**Dapto** 4 mg/kg IV q 24h **or Linezolid** 600 mg IV q 12h	**Choice of empiric therapy must have activity vs. S. aureus**. S. aureus erysipelas of face can mimic streptococcal erysipelas of an extremity. Forced to treat empirically for MRSA until in vitro susceptibilities available.
Diabetes mellitus and erysipelas *(See Foot, "Diabetic", page 16)*	Strep. sp. (Grp A, B, C & G), Staph. aureus, Enterobacteriaceae; Anaerobes	**Early mild: TMP-SMX-DS** 1-2 tabs po bid + (**Pen VK** 500 mg po qid or **cephalexin** 500 mg po qid). **For severe disease: IMP**, **MER**, **ERTA** or **Dori** IV + (**linezolid** 600 mg IV/po bid or **vanco** IV or **dapto** 4 mg/kg IV q 24h). *Dosage, see page 16, Diabetic foot*		Prompt surgical debridement indicated to rule out necrotizing fasciitis and to obtain cultures. If septic, consider x-ray of extremity to demonstrate gas. **Prognosis dependent on blood supply: assess arteries.** *See diabetic foot, page 16.* For severe disease, use regimen that targets both aerobic gram-neg bacilli & MRSA.
Erysipelas 2° to lymphedema (congenital = Milroy's disease); post-breast surgery with lymph node dissection	Streptococcus sp., Groups A, C, G	**Benzathine pen G** 1.2 million units IM q4 wks or **Pen VK** 500 mg po bid or **azithro** 250 mg po qd		Indicated only if pt is having frequent episodes of cellulitis. Benefit in controlled clinical trial *(NEJM 368:1695, 2013)*.
Dandruff (seborrheic dermatitis)	Malassezia species	**Ketoconazole shampoo** 2% or **selenium sulfide** 2.5% *(see page 10, chronic external otitis)*		
Erythema multiforme	H. simplex type 1, mycoplasma, Strep. pyogenes, drugs (sulfonamides, phenytoin, penicillins)			**Rx: Acyclovir** if due to H. simplex *(Dermatology 207:349, 2003)*.
Erythema nodosum	Sarcoidosis, inflammatory bowel disease, MTB, coccidioidomycosis, yersinia, sulfonamides, Whipple's disease.			**Rx: NSAIDs; glucocorticoids** if refractory. Identify and treat precipitant disease if possible.
Erythrasma	Corynebacterium minutissimum	Localized infection: **Topical Clinda** 2-3 x daily x 7-14 days	Widespread infection: **Clarithro** 500 mg po bid or **Erythro** 250 mg po bid) x 14 days	Dx: Coral red fluorescence with Wood's lamp. If infection recurs, prophylactic bathing with anti-bacterial soap or wash with benzyl peroxide.
Folliculitis	S. aureus, candida, P. aeruginosa common	Usually self-limited, no Rx needed. Could use topical mupirocin for Staph and topical antifungal for Candida.		
Furunculosis	Staph. aureus	*See Boils, page 53*		
Hemorrhagic bullous lesions				
Hx of sea water-contaminated abrasion or eating raw seafood in cirrhotic pt.	**Vibrio vulnificus** *(CID 52:788, 2011; JAC 67:488, 2012)*	**Ceftriaxone** 1-2 gm IV q24h + (**Doxy** or **Minocycline**) 100 mg po/IV bid	**CIP** 750 mg po bid or 400 mg IV bid	Wound infection in healthy hosts, but bacteremia mostly in cirrhotics. Pathogenesis: Open wound exposure to contaminated seawater. Can cause necrotizing fasciitis *(JAC 67:488, 2012)*. Surgical debridement *(Am J Surg 206:32, 2013)*.
Herpes zoster (shingles): *See Table 14*				

 **NOTE: All dosage recommendations are for adults (unless otherwise indicated) and assume normal renal function. § Alternatives consider allergy, PK, compliance, local resistance, cost*

TABLE 1 (52)

ANATOMIC SITE/DIAGNOSIS/ MODIFYING CIRCUMSTANCES	ETIOLOGIES (usual)	SUGGESTED REGIMENS* PRIMARY	SUGGESTED REGIMENS* ALTERNATIVE§	ADJUNCT DIAGNOSTIC OR THERAPEUTIC MEASURES AND COMMENTS
SKIN *(continued)*				
Impetigo—children, military				
"Honey-crust" lesions (non-bullous). Ecthyma is closely related. Causes "punched out" skin lesions.	**Group A strep impetigo** (rarely Strept. sp. Groups B, C or G); crusted lesions can be Staph. aureus + streptococci. Staph. aureus may be secondary colonizer.	Mupirocin ointment 2% tid or fusidic acid cream[NUS] 2%, times 7–12 days or retapamulin ointment, 1% bid times 5 days *For dosages, see Table 10A for adults and Table 16, page 209 for children*	Should be no need for oral antibiotics.	In meta-analysis that combined strep & staph impetigo, mupirocin had higher cure rates than placebo. Mupirocin superior to oral erythro. Penicillin inferior to erythro. Few placebo-controlled trials. Ref.: *Cochrane Database Systemic Reviews, 2004 (2): CD003261.* 46% of USA-300 CA-MRSA isolates carry gene encoding resistance to Mupirocin *(Ln 367:731, 2006).* **Note:** While resistance to Mupirocin continues to evolve, over-the-counter triple antibiotic ointment (Neomycin, polymyxin B, Bacitracin) remains active in vitro *(DMID 54:63, 2006).* **Ecthyma:** Infection deeper into epidermis than impetigo. May need parenteral penicillin. Military outbreaks reported: *CID 48: 1213 & 1220, 2009 (good images).*
Bullous (if ruptured, thin "varnish-like" crust)	**Staph. aureus** MSSA & MRSA: strains that produce exfoliative toxin A.	**For MSSA:** po therapy with **dicloxacillin**, **oxacillin**, **cephalexin**, **AM-CL**, **azithro**, **clarithro**, or **mupirocin** ointment or **retapamulin** ointment *For dosages, see Table 10A*	**For MRSA: Mupirocin** ointment or po therapy with, **TMP-SMX-DS, minocycline, doxy, clinda**	
Infected wound, extremity —Post-trauma *(for bites, see page 52; for post-operative, see below)*— **Gram stain negative**				
Mild to moderate; uncomplicated Debride wound, if necessary.	Polymicrobic: S. aureus (MSSA & MRSA), aerobic & anaerobic strep, Enterobacteriaceae, C. perfringens, C. tetani; if water exposure, Pseudomonas sp., Aeromonas sp. Acinetobacter in soldiers in Iraq *(see CID 47:444, 2008).*	**TMP-SMX-DS** 1-2 tabs po bid or **clinda** 300–450 mg po tid *(see Comment)*	**Minocycline** 100 mg po bid or **linezolid** 600 mg po bid *(see Comment)*	**Culture & sensitivity, check Gram stain. Tetanus toxoid if indicated.** **Mild infection:** Suggested drugs focus on S. aureus & Strep species. If suspect Gm-neg. bacilli, add **AM-CL-ER** 1000/62.5 two tabs po bid. If MRSA is erythro-resistant, may have inducible resistance to clinda. **Fever—sepsis:** Another alternative is **linezolid** 600 mg IV/po q12h. If Gm-neg. bacilli & severe pen allergy, **CIP** 400 mg IV q12h (q8h if P. aeruginosa) or **Levo** 750 mg IV q24h. Why 1-2 **TMP-SMX-DS?** *See discussion in footnote 1 of Table 6 (MRSA)* **TMP-SMX** not predictably active vs. strep species.
Febrile with sepsis—hospitalized Debride wound, if necessary.		[**TC-CL** or **PIP-TZ** or **DORI**[NAI] or **IMP** or **MER** or **ERTA** *(Dosage, page 25)*] + **vanco** 1 gm IV q12h (1.5 gm if > 100 kg)	(**Vanco** 1 gm IV q12h or **dapto** 6 mg/kg IV q 24h or **ceftaroline** 600 mg IV q12h or **telavancin** 10 mg/kg IV q24h) + (**CIP** or **Levo** IV—*dose in Comment)*	
Infected wound, post-operative—Gram stain negative: for Gram stain positive cocci – see below				
Surgery not involving GI or female genital tract				
Without sepsis (mild, afebrile)	Staph. aureus, Group A, B, C or G strep sp.	**TMP-SMX-DS** 1 tab po bid	**Clinda** 300–450 mg po tid	Check Gram stain of exudate. If Gm-neg. bacilli, **add** β-lactam/β-lactamase inhibitor: **AM-CL-ER** po or (**ERTA** or **PIP-TZ** or **TC-CL**) IV. *Dosage on page 25.* Why 1-2 **TMP-SMX-DS?** *See discussion in footnote 1 of Table 6 (MRSA).* **TMP-SMX** not predictably active vs. strep species.
With sepsis (severe, febrile)		**Vanco** 15 mg/kg (actual wt) IV q8-12h (to achieve target trough concentration of 15-20 µg/mL	**Dapto** 6 mg per kg IV q24h or **telavancin** 10 mg/kg IV q24h	
Surgery involving GI tract (includes oropharynx, esophagus) or female genital tract—fever, neutrophilia	MSSA/MRSA, coliforms, bacteroides & other anaerobes	[**PIP-TZ** or (**P Ceph 3** + **metro**) or **DORI** or **ERTA** or **IMP** or **MER**] + (**vanco** 1 gm IV q12h or **dapto** 6 mg/kg IV q 24h) **if severely ill.** **Mild infection: AM-CL-ER** 1000/62.5 mg 2 tabs po bid + **TMP-SMX-DS** 1-2 tabs po bid if Gm+ cocci on Gram stain. *Dosages Table 10A & footnote 33, page 62.*		For all treatment options, *see Peritonitis, page 47.* Most important: Drain wound & get cultures. Can sub **linezolid** for vanco. Can sub **CIP or Levo** for β-lactams. Why 2 **TMP-SMX-DS?** *See discussion in footnote 1 of Table 6 (MRSA)*
Meleney's synergistic gangrene	*See Necrotizing fasciitis, page 56*			

Abbreviations on page 2. **NOTE: All dosage recommendations are for adults (unless otherwise indicated) and assume normal renal function. § Alternatives consider allergy, PK, compliance, local resistance, cost*

TABLE 1 (53)

ANATOMIC SITE/DIAGNOSIS/ MODIFYING CIRCUMSTANCES	ETIOLOGIES (usual)	SUGGESTED REGIMENS*		ADJUNCT DIAGNOSTIC OR THERAPEUTIC MEASURES AND COMMENTS
		PRIMARY	ALTERNATIVE§	
SKIN/Infected wound, post-operative—Gram stain negative *(continued)*				
Infected wound, post-op, febrile patient— Positive gram stain: Gram-positive cocci in clusters	S. aureus, possibly MRSA	**Do culture & sensitivity; open & drain wound** **Oral: TMP-SMX-DS** 1 tab po bid or **clinda** 300–450 mg po tid *(see Comment)*	**IV: Vanco** 1 gm IV q12h or **dapto** 4-6 mg/kg IV q24h or **ceftaroline** 600 mg IV q12h or **telavancin** 10 mg/kg IV q24h	Need culture & sensitivity to verify MRSA. Other po options for CA-MRSA include minocycline 100 mg po q12h or **Doxy** 100 mg po bid (inexpensive) & linezolid 600 mg po q12h (expensive). If MRSA clinda-sensitive but erythro-resistant, watch out for inducible clinda resistance.
Necrotizing fasciitis ("flesh-eating bacteria")				
Post-surgery, trauma, or streptococcal skin infections *See Gas gangrene, page 46, & Toxic shock, page 64.* Refs: *CID 44:705, 2007; NEJM 360:281, 2009.*	**5 types:** (1) Strep sp., Grp A, C, G; (2) Clostridia sp.; (3) polymicrobic: aerobic + anaerobic (if S. aureus + anaerobic strep = Meleney's synergistic gangrene); (4) Community- associated MRSA; (5) K. pneumoniae *(CID 55:930 & 946, 2012)*	*For treatment of clostridia, see Muscle, gas gangrene, page 46.* The terminology of **polymicrobic** wound infections is not precise: Meleney's synergistic gangrene, Fournier's gangrene, necrotizing fasciitis have common pathophysiology. **All require prompt surgical debridement** + antibiotics. Dx of necrotizing fasciitis req incision & probing. If no resistance to probing subcut with fascial plane involvement. (fascial plane), diagnosis = necrotizing fasciitis. **Need Gram stain/culture** to determine if etiology is strep, clostridia, polymicrobial, or S. aureus. **Treatment: Pen G** if strep or clostridia; **DORI**[NAI], **IMP** or **MER** if polymicrobial, add **vanco OR dapto** if MRSA suspected. **NOTE:** If strep necrotizing fasciitis, reasonable to treat with penicillin & clinda; if clostridia ± gas gangrene, add clinda to penicillin *(see page 46)*. MRSA ref.: *NEJM 352:1445, 2005.* ***See toxic shock syndrome, streptococcal, page 64.***		
Puncture wound—nail, toothpick	Through tennis shoe: P. aeruginosa	Local debridement to remove foreign body & tetanus prophylaxis; no antibiotic therapy.		Osteomyelitis evolves in only 1–2% of plantar puncture wounds. Consider x-ray if chance of radio-opaque foreign body.
Staphylococcal scalded skin syndrome Ref.: *PIDJ 19:819, 2000*	Toxin-producing S. aureus	**Nafcillin** or **oxacillin** 2 gm IV q4h (children: 150 mg/kg/ day div. q6h) x 5–7 days for MSSA; **vanco** 1 gm IV q12h (children 40–60 mg/kg/day div. q6h) for MRSA		Toxin causes **intraepidermal split** and positive Nikolsky sign. Biopsy differentiates: drugs cause epidermal/dermal split, **called toxic epidermal necrolysis**—more serious.
Ulcerated skin lesions: Differential Dx	Consider: anthrax, tularemia, P. aeruginosa (ecthyma gangrenosum), plague, blastomycosis, spider (rarely), mucormycosis, mycobacteria, leishmania, YAWS, arterial insufficiency, venous stasis, and others.			
Ulcerated skin: venous/arterial insufficiency; pressure with secondary infection (infected decubiti) Care of non-healing, non-infected ulcers *(AnIM 159:532, 2013).*	Polymicrobic: Streptococcus sp. (Groups A, C, G), enterococci, anaerobic strep, Enterobacteriaceae, Pseudomonas sp., Bacteroides sp., Staph. aureus	Severe local or possible bacteremia: **IMP** or **MER** or **DORI** or **TC-CL** or **PIP-TZ** or **ERTA.** If Gm-pos cocci on gram stain, add **Vanco**. *Dosages, see footnotes* [5, 6, 7, 12, 15, 33]	[(**CIP** or **Levo**) + **Metro**] or [(**CFP** or **Ceftaz**) + **Metro**]. If Gm-pos cocci on gram stain, add **Vanco**.	If ulcer clinically inflamed, treat IV with no topical rx. If not clinically inflamed, consider debridement, removal of foreign body, lessening direct pressure for weight-bearing limbs & leg elevation (if no arterial insufficiency). Topical rx to reduce bacterial counts: silver sulfadiazine 1% or combination antibiotic ointment. **Chlorhexidine & povidone iodine may harm "granulation tissue"–Avoid.** If not inflamed, healing improved on air bed, protein supplement, radiant heat, electrical stimulation *(AnIM 159:39, 2013).*
Whirlpool: (Hot Tub) folliculitis	Pseudomonas aeruginosa	Usually self-limited, treatment not indicated		Decontaminate hot tub: drain and chlorinate. Also associated with exfoliative beauty aids (loofah sponges).
Whirlpool: Nail Salon, soft tissue infection	Mycobacterium (fortuitum or chelonae)	**Minocycline**, **doxy** or **CIP**		Ref: *CID 38:38, 2004.*
SPLEEN. For post-splenectomy prophylaxis, *see Table 15A, page 197-198; for Septic Shock Post-Splenectomy, see Table 1, pg 63.*				
Splenic abscess				
Endocarditis, bacteremia	Staph. aureus, streptococci	**Nafcillin** or **oxacillin** 2 gm IV q4h if MSSA	**Vanco** 15 mg/kg (actual wt) IV q8-12h (to achieve target trough concentration of 15-20 μg/mL).	Burkholderia (Pseudomonas) pseudomallei is common cause of splenic abscess in SE Asia. Presents with fever and LUQ pain. Usual treatment is antimicrobial therapy and splenectomy.
Contiguous from intra-abdominal site	Polymicrobic	*Treat as Peritonitis, secondary, page 47*		
Immunocompromised	Candida sp.	**Amphotericin B** *(Dosage, see Table 11, page 114)*	**Fluconazole, caspofungin**	

 NOTE: All dosage recommendations are for adults (unless otherwise indicated) and assume normal renal function. § Alternatives consider allergy, PK, compliance, local resistance, cost

ANATOMIC SITE/DIAGNOSIS/ MODIFYING CIRCUMSTANCES	ETIOLOGIES (usual)	SUGGESTED REGIMENS* PRIMARY	SUGGESTED REGIMENS* ALTERNATIVE§	ADJUNCT DIAGNOSTIC OR THERAPEUTIC MEASURES AND COMMENTS
SYSTEMIC SYNDROMES (FEBRILE/NON-FEBRILE)				
Spread by infected **TICK, FLEA, or LICE**: Epidemiologic history crucial. **Babesiosis, Lyme disease, & Anaplasma (Ehrlichiosis)** have same reservoir & tick vector.				
Babesiosis: *see NEJM 366:2397, 2012.* Do not treat if asymptomatic, young, has spleen, and immunocompetent; can be fatal in lymphoma pts.	Etiol.: B. microti et al. Vector: Usually Ixodes ticks Host: White-footed mouse & others	[(**Atovaquone** 750 mg po q12h) + (**azithro** 600 mg po day 1, then 500-1000 mg per day) times 7-10 days]. If severe infection [**clinda** 1.2 gm IV bid or 600 mg po tid times 7 days + **quinine** 650 mg po tid times 7 days. **Ped. dosage: Clinda** 20–40 mg per kg per day and **quinine** 25 mg per kg per day]. **Exchange transfusion**-- *See Comment*		**Seven diseases where pathogen visible in peripheral blood smear:** African/American trypanosomiasis; babesia; bartonellosis; filariasis; malaria; relapsing fever. **Dx:** Giemsa-stained blood smear; antibody test available. PCR if available. **Rx: Exchange transfusions successful adjunct if used early, in severe disease.** May need treatment for 6 or more wks if immunocompromised. Look for Lyme and/or Anaplasma co-infection.
Bartonella infections: Review *EID 12:389, 2006*				
Bacteremia, asymptomatic	B. quintana, B. henselae	**Doxy** 100 mg po/IV times 15 days		Can lead to endocarditis &/or trench fever: found in homeless, alcoholics, esp. if lice/leg pain. Often missed since asymptomatic.
Cat-scratch disease	B. henselae	**Azithro** 500 mg po x 1 dose, then 250 mg/day po x 4 days. **Or** symptomatic only—*see Lymphadenitis, page 45:* usually lymphadenitis, hepatitis, splenitis, FUO, neuroretinitis, transverse myelitis, oculoglandular syndrome.		
Bacillary angiomatosis; Peliosis hepatis—pts with AIDS *MMWR 58(RR-4):39, 2009; AAC 48:1921, 2004.*	B. henselae, B. quintana	**Erythro** 500 mg po qid or **Doxy** 100 mg po bid x 3 months or longer. If CNS involvement: **Doxy** 100 mg IV/po bid + **RIF** 300 mg po bid Regardless of CD4 count, DC therapy after 3-4 mos. & observe. If no relapse, no suppressive rx. If relapse, **doxy**, **azithro** or **erythro** x 3 mos. Stop when CD4 >200 x 6 mos.	**Azithro** 250 mg po once daily x 3 months or longer	**Do not use:** TMP-SMX, CIP, Pen, Ceph. **Manifestations of Bartonella infections:** **HIV/AIDS Patient:** Bacillary angiomatosis; Bacillary peliosis; Bacteremia/endocarditis/FUO **Immunocompetent Patient:** Bacteremia/endocarditis/FUO/ encephalitis; Cat scratch disease; Vertebral osteo; Trench fever; Parinaud's oculoglandular syndrome
Endocarditis (*see page 28*) (*Circ 111:3167, 2005; AAC 48:1921, 2004*)	B. henselae, B. quintana	Surgical removal of infected valve *If suspect endocarditis:* **Ceftriaxone** 2 gm IV once daily x 6 weeks + **Gent** 1 mg/kg IV q8h x 14 days + **Doxy** 100 mg IV/po bid x 6 wks	*If proven endocarditis:* **Doxy** 100 mg IV/po bid x 6 wks + **Gent** 1 mg/kg IV q8h x 11 days	**Gentamicin toxicity:** If Gent toxicity, substitute Rifampin 300 mg IV/po bod x 14 days. Role of valve removal surgery to cure unclear. Presents as SBE. Diagnosis: ECHO, serology & PCR of resected heart valve.
Oroya fever (acute) & Verruga peruana (chronic) (*AAC 48:1921, 2004*)	B. bacilliformis	**Oroya fever:** (**CIP** 500 mg po bid or **Doxy** 100 mg po bid) x 14 d. Alternative: **Chloro** 500 mg IV/po q6h + (**beta lactam** or **Doxy** 100 mg po bid) x 14 days	**Verruga peruana: RIF** 10 mg/kg po once daily x 14 d or **Streptomycin** 15-20 mg/kg IM/IV once daily x 10 days or **Azithro** 500 mg po q24h x 7 days	Oroya fever transmitted by sand-fly bite in Andes Mtns. Related Bartonella (B. rochalimae) caused bacteremia, fever and splenomegaly (*NEJM 356:2346 & 2381, 2007*). **CIP and Chloro preferred due to prevention of secondary Salmonella infections.**
Trench fever (FUO) (*AAC 48:1921, 2004*)	B. quintana	No endocarditis: **Doxy** 100 mg po bid x 4 wks; If endocarditis: **Doxy** + **Gentamicin** 3 mg/kg once daily for 1st 2 wks of therapy (*AAC 48:1921, 2004*).		Vector is body louse. Do not use: TMP-SMX, FQs, cefazolin or Pen

 **NOTE: All dosage recommendations are for adults (unless otherwise indicated) and assume normal renal function. § Alternatives consider allergy, PK, compliance, local resistance, cost*

TABLE 1 (55)

ANATOMIC SITE/DIAGNOSIS/ MODIFYING CIRCUMSTANCES	ETIOLOGIES (usual)	SUGGESTED REGIMENS*		ADJUNCT DIAGNOSTIC OR THERAPEUTIC MEASURES AND COMMENTS
		PRIMARY	ALTERNATIVE§	
SYSTEMIC SYNDROMES (FEBRILE/NON-FEBRILE) *(continued)*				
Ehrlichiosis[32]. CDC def. is one of: (1) 4x ↑ IFA antibody, (2) detection of Ehrlichia DNA in blood or CSF by PCR, (3) visible morulae in WBC and IFA ≥1:64. New species in *WI, MN (NEJM 365:422, 2011)*.				
Human monocytic ehrlichiosis (HME) *(MMWR 55(RR-4), 2006; CID 43:1089, 2006)*	Ehrlichia chaffeensis (Lone Star tick is vector)	**Doxy** 100 mg po/IV bid times 7–14 days	**Tetracycline** 500 mg po qid x 7–14d. No current rec. for children or pregnancy	30 states: mostly SE of line from NJ to Ill. to Missouri to Oklahoma to Texas. History of outdoor activity and tick exposure. April-Sept. Fever, rash (36%), leukopenia and thrombocytopenia. Blood smears no help. PCR for early dx.
Human Anaplasmosis (formerly known as Human granulocytic ehrlichiosis)	Anaplasma (Ehrlichia) phagocytophilum (Ixodes sp. ticks are vector). Dog variant is Ehrlichia ewingii *(NEJM 341:148 & 195, 1999)*	**Doxy** 100 mg bid po or IV times 7–14 days	**Tetracycline** 500 mg po qid times 7–14 days. Not in children or pregnancy. *See Comment*	Upper Midwest, NE, West Coast & Europe. H/O tick exposure. April-Sept. Febrile flu-like illness after outdoor activity. No rash. Leukopenia/ thrombocytopenia common. **Dx:** Up to 80% have + blood smear. Antibody test for confirmation. **Rx:** RIF active in vitro *(IDCNA 22:433, 2008)* but worry about resistance developing. Minocycline should work if doxy not available.
Lyme Disease NOTE: Think about concomitant tick-borne disease—e.g., babesiosis and ehrlichiosis. **Guidelines:** *CID 51:1, 2010; Med Lett 52:53, 2010.*				
Bite by ixodes-infected tick in an endemic area -- **Postexposure prophylaxis**	Borrelia burgdorferi **IDSA guidelines:** *CID 43:1089, 2006; CID 51:1, 2010* Western blot diagnostic criteria: **IgM**—Need 2 of 3 positive of kilodaltons (KD): 23, 39, 41 **IgG**—Need 5 of 10 positive of KD: 18, 21, 28, 30, 39, 41, 45, 58, 66, 93 Interest in 2 tier diagnostic approach: 1) standard lyme ELISA & if positive; 2) C6 peptide ELISA. Better sensitivity/specificity. Applicable to European cases *(CID 57:333 & 341, 2013)*.	**If endemic area,** if nymphal partially engorged deer tick: **doxy** 200 mg po times 1 dose with food	**If not endemic area,** not engorged, not deer tick: No treatment	Prophylaxis study in endemic area: erythema migrans developed in 3% of the control group and 0.4% doxy group *(NEJM 345:79 & 133, 2001)*.
Early (erythema migrans) *See Comment*		**Doxy** 100 mg po bid. or **amoxicillin** 500 mg po tid or **cefuroxime axetil** 500 mg po bid or **erythro** 250 mg po qid. All regimens for 14–21 days. (10 days as good as 20: *AnIM 138:697, 2003*) *See Comment for peds doses*		High rate of clinical failure with azithro & erythro *(Drugs 57:157, 1999)*. **Peds** (all po for 14–21 days): **Amox** 50 mg per kg per day in 3 div. doses or **cefuroxime axetil** 30 mg per kg per day in 2 div. doses or **erythro** 30 mg per kg per day in 3 div. doses. Lesions usually homogenous—not target-like *(AnIM 136:423, 2002)*.
Carditis *See Comment*		(**Ceftriaxone** 2 gm IV q24h) or (**cefotaxime** 2 gm IV q4h) or (**Pen G** 3 million units IV q4h) times 14–21 days	**Doxy** *(see Comments)* 100 mg po bid times 14–21 days or **amoxicillin** 500 mg po tid times 14–21 days.	First degree AV block: Oral regimen. Generally self-limited. High degree AV block (PR >0.3 sec.): IV therapy—permanent pacemaker not necessary.
Facial nerve paralysis (isolated finding, early)		(**Doxy** 100 mg po bid) or (**amoxicillin** 500 mg po) tid times 14–21 days	**Ceftriaxone** 2 gm IV q24h times 14–21 days	LP suggested excluding central neurologic disease. If LP neg., oral regimen OK. If abnormal or not done, suggest parenteral Ceftriaxone.
Meningitis, encephalitis *For encephalopathy, see Comment*		**Ceftriaxone** 2 gm IV q24h times 14–28 days	(**Pen G** 20 million units IV q24h in div. dose) or (**cefotaxime** 2 gm IV q8h) times 14–28 days	Encephalopathy: memory difficulty, depression, somnolence, or headache, CSF abnormalities. 89% had objective CSF abnormalities. 18/18 pts improved with ceftriaxone 2 gm per day times 30 days *(JID 180:377, 1999)*. No compelling evidence that prolonged treatment has any benefit in post-Lyme syndrome *(Neurology 69:91, 2007)*.
Arthritis		(**Doxy** 100 mg po bid) or (**amoxicillin** 500 mg po tid), both times 30–60 days	(**Ceftriaxone** 2 gm IV q24h) or (**pen G** 20–24 million units per day IV) times 14–28 days	Start with 1 mo of therapy; if only partial response, treat for a second mo.
Pregnancy		Choice should **not** include doxy; **amoxicillin** 500 mg po tid times 21 days.	**If pen. allergic:** (**azithro** 500 mg po q24h times 7–10 days) or (**erythro** 500 mg po qid times 14–21 days)	
Post-Lyme Disease Syndromes		None indicated		No benefit from treatment *(AJM 126:665, 2013; CID 51:1, 2010; NEJM 345:85, 2001)*.

[32] In endemic area (New York), high % of both adult ticks and nymphs were jointly infected with both Anaplasma (HGE) and B. burgdorferi *(NEJM 337:49, 1997)*.

Abbreviations on page 2. **NOTE: All dosage recommendations are for adults (unless otherwise indicated) and assume normal renal function. § Alternatives consider allergy, PK, compliance, local resistance, cost*

TABLE 1 (56)

ANATOMIC SITE/DIAGNOSIS/ MODIFYING CIRCUMSTANCES	ETIOLOGIES (usual)	SUGGESTED REGIMENS*		ADJUNCT DIAGNOSTIC OR THERAPEUTIC MEASURES AND COMMENTS
		PRIMARY	ALTERNATIVE§	
SYSTEMIC SYNDROMES (FEBRILE/NON-FEBRILE)/Spread by infected TICK, FLEA, or LICE *(continued)*				
Relapsing fever				
Louse-borne (LBRF)	*Borrelia recurrentis* Reservoir: human Vector: Louse pediculus humanus	**Tetracycline** 500 mg IV/po x 1 dose	**Erythro** 500 mg IV/po x 1 dose	Jarisch-Herxheimer (fever, ↑ pulse, ↑ resp., ↓ blood pressure) in most patients (occurs in ~2 hrs). Not prevented by prior steroids. **Dx: Examine peripheral blood smear during fever for spirochetes.** Can relapse up to 10 times. Postexposure **doxy** pre-emptive therapy highly effective *(NEJM 355:148, 2006)* *B. miyamoto ref: EIN 17:816, 2011.* Meningoencephalitis in lymphoma patient *(NEJM 368:240, 2013; AnIM 159:21, 2013).*
Tick-borne (TBRF)	No Amer: *B. hermsii, B. turicata;* Africa: *B. hispanica, B. crocidurae, B. duttonii;* Russia: *B. miyamoto*	**Doxy** 100 mg po bid x 7-10 days	**Erythro** 500 mg po qid x 7-10 days	
Rickettsial diseases. Review—Disease in travelers *(CID 39:1493, 2004)*				
Spotted fevers (NOTE: Rickettsial pox not included)				
Rocky Mountain spotted fever (RMSF) *(LnID 8:143, 2008 and MMWR 55 (RR-4), 2007)*	R. rickettsii (Dermacentor tick vector)	**Doxy** 100 mg po/IV bid times 7 days or for 2 days after temp. normal. Do not use in pregnancy. Some suggest single 200 mg loading dose.	**Chloro** 50 mg/kg/day in 4 div doses. Use in pregnancy.	Fever, rash (88%), petechiae 40–50%. **Rash spreads from distal extremities to trunk.** Rash in <50% pts in 1st 72 hrs. Dx: Immunohistology on skin biopsy; confirmation with antibody titers. Highest incidence in SE and South Central states; also seen in Oklahoma, S. Dakota, Montana. Cases reported from 42 U.S. states. **NOTE: Only 3–18% of pts present with fever, rash, and hx of tick exposure; many early deaths in children & empiric doxy reasonable** *(MMWR 49: 885, 2000).*
NOTE: Can mimic ehrlichiosis. Pattern of rash important—*see Comment*				
Other spotted fevers, e.g., Rickettsial pox, African tick bite fever	At least 8 species on 6 continents *(CID 45 (Suppl 1) S39, 2007).*	**Doxy** 100 mg po bid times 7 days	**Chloro** 500 mg po/IV qid times 7 days Children <8 y.o.: **azithro** or **clarithro** *(if mild disease)*	Clinical diagnosis suggested by: 1) fever, intense myalgia, headache; 2) exposure to mites or ticks; 3) localized eschar (tache noire) or rash. Definitive Dx: PCR of blood, skin biopsy or sequential antibody tests.
Typhus group—Consider in returning travelers with fever				
Louse-borne: epidemic typhus Ref: *LnID 8:417, 2008.*	R. prowazekii (vector is body or head louse)	**Doxy** 100 mg IV/po bid times 7 days; single 200 mg dose 95% effective.	**Chloro** 500 mg IV/po qid times 5 days	**Brill-Zinsser disease** *(Ln 357:1198, 2001)* is a relapse of typhus acquired during WWII. Truncal rash (64%) spreads centrifugally—opposite of RMSF. Louse borne typhus is a winter disease. Diagnosis by serology. R. prowazekii found in flying squirrels in SE US. Delouse clothing of infected pt.
Murine typhus (cat flea typhus): *EID 14:1019, 2008.*	R. typhi (rat reservoir and flea vector): *CID 46:913, 2008*	**Doxy** 100 mg IV/po bid times 7 days	**Chloro** 500 mg IV/po qid times 5 days	Rash in 20-54%, not diagnostic. Without treatment most pts recover in 2 wks. Faster recovery with treatment. Dx based on suspicion; confirmed serologically.
Scrub typhus	O. tsutsugamushi [rodent reservoir; vector is larval stage of mites (chiggers)]	**Doxy** 100 mg po/IV bid x 7 days. In pregnancy: **Azithro** 500 mg po x one dose	**Chloro** 500 mg po/IV qid x 7 days	Asian rim of Pacific. Suspect Dx in endemic area. Confirm with serology. If Doxy resistance suspected, alternatives are **Doxy** + **RIF** 900 or 600 mg once daily *(Ln 356:1057, 2000)* or **Azithro**.
Tularemia, typhoidal type Ref. **bioterrorism**: *see JAMA 285:2763, 2001; ID Clin No Amer 22:489, 2008; MMWR 58:744, 2009.*	Francisella tularensis. (Vector depends on geography: ticks, biting flies, mosquitoes identified)	Moderate/severe: [(**Gentamicin** or **tobra** 5 mg per kg per day div. q8h IV) or (**Streptomycin** 10 mg/kg IV/IM q12h)] x 10 days	Mild: [**CIP** 400 mg IV (or 750 mg po) bid or **Doxy** 100 mg IV/po bid] x 14-21 days	Diagnosis: Culture on cysteine-enriched media & serology. Dangerous in the lab. Hematogenous meningitis is a complication: treatment is **Streptomycin** + **Chloro** 50-100 mg/kg/day IV in 4 divided doses *(Arch Neurol 66:523, 2009).*

Abbreviations on page 2. **NOTE: All dosage recommendations are for adults (unless otherwise indicated) and assume normal renal function. § Alternatives consider allergy, PK, compliance, local resistance, cost*

TABLE 1 (57)

ANATOMIC SITE/DIAGNOSIS/ MODIFYING CIRCUMSTANCES	ETIOLOGIES (usual)	SUGGESTED REGIMENS*		ADJUNCT DIAGNOSTIC OR THERAPEUTIC MEASURES AND COMMENTS
		PRIMARY	ALTERNATIVE§	
SYSTEMIC SYNDROMES (FEBRILE/NON-FEBRILE) *(continued)*				
Other Zoonotic Systemic Bacterial Febrile Illnesses: Obtain careful epidemiologic history				
Brucellosis Refs: *NEJM 352:2325, 2005; CID 46:426, 2008; MMWR 57:603, 2008; BMJ 336:701, 2008; PLoS One 7:e32090, 2012.*	B. abortus–cattle B. suis–swine B. melitensis–goats B canis–dogs	**Non focal disease:** [**Doxy** 100 mg po bid x 6 wks + **Gent** 5 mg/kg once daily for 1st 7 days	(**Doxy** 100 mg po bid + **RIF** 600-900 mg po once daily) x 6 wks. Less optimal: **CIP** 500 mg po bid + (**Doxy** or **RIF**) x 6 wks	Bone involvement, esp. sacroiliitis in 20-30%. **Neurobrucellosis:** Usually meningitis. 1% of all pts with brucellosis. Role of corticosteroids unclear; not recommended. **Endocarditis:** Rare but most common cause of death. Need surgery + antimicrobials. **Pregnancy:** TMP-SMX may cause kernicterus if given during last week of pregnancy.
		Spondylitis, Sacroiliitis: [**Doxy** + **Gent** (as above) + **RIF**] x min 3 mos	(**CIP** 750 mg po bid + **RIF** 600-900 mg po once daily) x min 3 mos	
		Neurobrucellosis: [**Doxy** + **RIF** (as above) + **ceftriaxone** 2 gm IV q12h until CSF returned to normal *(AAC 56:1523, 2012)*		
		Endocarditis: Surgery + **[(RIF + Doxy + TMP-SMX)** x 1-1/2 to 6 mos + **Gent** for 2-4 wks *(CID 56:1407, 2013)*		
		Pregnancy: Not much data. **RIF** 900 mg po once daily x 6 wks	**RIF** 900 mg po once daily + **TMP-SMX** 5 mg/kg (TMP comp) po bid x 4 wks.	
Leptospirosis *(CID 36:1507 & 1514, 2003; LnID 3:757, 2003)*	Leptospira—in urine of domestic livestock, dogs, small rodents	Severe illness: **Pen G** 1.5 million units IV q6h or **ceftriaxone** 2 gm q24h. Duration: 7 days	Mild illness: (**Doxy** 100 mg IV/po q12h **Amoxicillin** 500 mg po tid x 7 days	**Severity varies**. Two-stage mild anicteric illness to severe icteric disease (Weil's disease) with renal failure and myocarditis. **Rx:** Azithro 1 gm once, then 500 mg daily x 2 days: non-inferior to, and fewer side effects than, doxy in standard dose *(AAC 51:3259, 2007)*. Jarisch-Herxheimer reaction can occur post-Pen therapy.
Salmonella bacteremia other than S. typhi–non-typhoidal)	Salmonella enteritidis—a variety of serotypes from animal sources	If NOT acquired in Asia: (**CIP** 400 mg IV q12h or **Levo** 750 mg po once daily) x 14 days *(See Comment)*	If acquired in Asia: **Ceftriaxone** 2 gm IV q24h or **Azithro** 1 gm po x 1 dose, then 500 mg po once daily x 5-7 days. Do NOT use FQs until susceptibility determined. *(See Comment)*	In vitro resistance to nalidixic acid indicates relative resistance to FQs. Bacteremia can infect any organ/tissue: look for infection of atherosclerotic aorta, osteomyelitis in sickle cell pts. Rx duration range 14 days (immunocompetent) to ≥6 wks if mycotic aneurism or endocarditis. Alternative, if susceptible: **TMP-SMX** 8-10 mg/kg/day (TMP comp) divided q8h.
Miscellaneous Systemic Febrile Syndromes				
Fever in Returning Travelers Etiology by geographic exposure & clinical syndrome *(AnIM 158:456, 2013).*	Dengue	Flavivirus	Supportive care; *see Table 14A, page 158*	Average incubation period 4 days; serodiagnosis.
	Malaria	Plasmodia sp.	Diagnosis: peripheral blood smear	*See Table 13A, page 145*
	Typhoid fever	Salmonella sp.	*See Table 1, page 60.*	Average incubation 7-14 days; diarrhea in 45%.

 **NOTE: All dosage recommendations are for adults (unless otherwise indicated) and assume normal renal function. § Alternatives consider allergy, PK, compliance, local resistance, cost*

TABLE 1 (58)

ANATOMIC SITE/DIAGNOSIS/ MODIFYING CIRCUMSTANCES	ETIOLOGIES (usual)	SUGGESTED REGIMENS*		ADJUNCT DIAGNOSTIC OR THERAPEUTIC MEASURES AND COMMENTS
		PRIMARY	ALTERNATIVE§	
SYSTEMIC SYNDROMES (FEBRILE/NON-FEBRILE) *(continued)*				
Kawasaki syndrome 6 weeks to 12 yrs of age, peak at 1 yr of age; 85% below age 5. Ref: *Pediatrics 124:1, 2009.*	Acute self-limited vasculitis with ↑ temp., rash, conjunctivitis, stomatitis, cervical adenitis, red hands/feet & coronary artery aneurysms (25% if untreated)	**IVIG** 2 gm per kg over 8-12 hrs x 1 + **ASA** 20-25 mg per kg qid THEN **ASA** 3–5 mg per kg per day po q24h times 6–8 wks	If still febrile after 1st dose of IVIG, some give 2nd dose. In Japan: **IVIG** + prednisolone 2 mg/kg/day. Continue steroid until CRP normal for 15 days *(Lancet 379:1571, 2012).*	IV gamma globulin (2 gm per kg over 10 hrs) in pts rx before 10th day of illness ↓ coronary artery lesions. See *Table 14A, page 169* for IVIG adverse effects. In children, wait until 11+ months after IVIG before giving live virus vaccines.
Rheumatic Fever, acute Ref.: *Ln 366:155, 2005*	Post-Group A strep pharyngitis (not Group B, C, or G)	(1) Symptom relief: **ASA** 80–100 mg per kg per day in children; 4–8 gm per day in adults. (2) Eradicate Group A strep: **Pen** times 10 days *(see Pharyngitis, page 48).* (3) Start prophylaxis: *see below*		
Prophylaxis				
Primary prophylaxis: Treat S. pyogenes pharyngitis	**Benzathine pen G** 1.2 million units IM *(see Pharyngitis, p. 48)*		**Penicillin** for 10 days prevents rheumatic fever even when started 7–9 days after onset of illness *(see page 48).* **Alternative: Penicillin V** 250 mg po bid or **sulfadiazine (sulfisoxazole)** 1 gm po q24h or **erythro** 250 mg po bid.	
Secondary prophylaxis (previous documented rheumatic fever)	**Benzathine pen G** 1.2 million units IM q3–4 wks		**Duration?** No carditis: 5 yrs or until age 21, whichever is longer; carditis without residual heart disease: 10 since last attack; carditis with residual valvular disease: 10 yrs since last episode or until age 40 whichever is longer *(PEDS 96:758, 1995).*	
Typhoidal syndrome (typhoid fever, enteric fever) Global susceptibility results: *CID 50:241, 2010. Treatment: BMJ 338:b1159 & b1865, 2009.*	Salmonella typhi, S. paratyphi A, B, C & S. choleraesuis. **NOTE: In vitro resistance to nalidixic acid predicts clinical failure of CIP (FQs).** Do not use empiric FQs if Asia-acquired infection. Need susceptibility results.	**If NOT acquired in Asia:** (**CIP** 400 mg IV q12h or **Levo** 750 mg po/IV q24h) x 7-10 d. *(See Comment)* In children, azithro 10 mg/kg once daily x 7 days *(AAC 51:819, 2007).*	**If acquired in Asia:** (**Ceftriaxone** 2 gm IV daily x 7-14 d) or (**Azithro** 1 gm po x 1 dose, then 500 mg po daily x 5-7 d) or (**Chloro** 500 mg po/IV q6h x 14 d) *(See Comment)*	**Dexamethasone: Use in severely ill pts: 1st dose just prior to antibiotic, 3 mg/kg IV, then 1 mg/kg q6h x 8 doses.** **Complications:** perforation of terminal ileum &/or cecum, osteo, septic arthritis, **mycotic aneurysm**, meningitis, hematogenous pneumonia. FQs, including Gati, remain best treatment if isolate susceptible *(BMJ 338:b1159 & 1865, 2009; LnID 11:445, 2011).*
Sepsis: Following suggested **empiric** therapy assumes pt is bacteremic; mimicked by viral, fungal, rickettsial infections and pancreatitis *(Intensive Care Medicine 34:17, 2008; IDC No Amer 22:1, 2008).*				
Neonatal—early onset <1 week old	Group B strep, E. coli, klebsiella, enterobacter, Staph. aureus (uncommon), listeria (rare in U.S.)	**AMP** 25 mg/kg IV q8h + **cefotaxime** 50 mg/kg q12h	(**AMP** + **gent** 2.5 mg/kg IV/IM q12h) or (**AMP** + **ceftriaxone** 50 mg/kg IV/IM q24h)	Blood cultures are key but only 5–10% +. Discontinue antibiotics after 72 hrs if cultures and course do not support diagnosis. In Spain, listeria predominates; in S. America, salmonella. If Grp B Strep infection + severe beta-lactam allergy, alternatives include: erythro & clinda; report of clinda resistance at 38% & erythro resistance at 51% *(AAC 56:739, 2012).*
Neonatal—late onset 1–4 weeks old	As above + H. influenzae & S. epidermidis	(**AMP** 25 mg/kg IV q6h + **cefotaxime** 50 mg/kg q8h) or (**AMP** + **ceftriaxone** 75 mg/kg IV q24h)	**AMP** + **gent** 2.5 mg/kg q8h IV or IM	**If MSSA/MRSA a concern, add vanco.**

 **NOTE: All dosage recommendations are for adults (unless otherwise indicated) and assume normal renal function. § Alternatives consider allergy, PK, compliance, local resistance, cost*

TABLE 1 (59)

ANATOMIC SITE/DIAGNOSIS/ MODIFYING CIRCUMSTANCES	ETIOLOGIES (usual)	SUGGESTED REGIMENS*		ADJUNCT DIAGNOSTIC OR THERAPEUTIC MEASURES AND COMMENTS
		PRIMARY	ALTERNATIVE§	
SYSTEMIC SYNDROMES (FEBRILE/NON-FEBRILE)/Sepsis *(continued)*				
Child; not neutropenic	Strep. pneumoniae, meningococci, Staph. aureus (MSSA & MRSA), H. influenzae now rare	(**Cefotaxime** 50 mg/kg IV q8h or **ceftriaxone** 100 mg/kg IV q24h) + **vanco** 15 mg/kg IV q6h	**Aztreonam** 7.5 mg/kg IV q6h + **linezolid** *(see Table 16, page 209 for dose)*	Major concerns are S. pneumoniae & community-associated MRSA. Coverage for Gm-neg. bacilli included but H. influenzae infection now rare. Meningococcemia mortality remains high *(Ln 356:961, 2000)*.
Adult; not neutropenic; NO HYPOTENSION but LIFE-THREATENING!—***For Septic shock, see page 63***				Systemic inflammatory response syndrome **(SIRS):** 2 or more of the following: 1. Temperature >38°C or <36°C 2. Heart rate >90 beats per min. 3. Respiratory rate >20 breaths per min. 4. WBC >12,000 per mcL or >10% bands **Sepsis:** SIRS + a documented infection (+ culture) **Severe sepsis:** Sepsis + organ dysfunction: hypotension or hypoperfusion abnormalities (lactic acidosis, oliguria, ↓ mental status) **Septic shock:** Sepsis-induced hypotension (systolic BP <90 mmHg) not responsive to 500 mL IV fluid challenge + peripheral hypoperfusion.
Source unclear—consider primary bacteremia, intra-abdominal or skin source. May be **Life-threatening.** Survival greater with quicker, effective empiric antibiotic Rx *(CCM 38:1045 & 1211, 2010)*.	Aerobic Gm-neg. bacilli; S. aureus; streptococci; others	(**IMP** or **MER**) + **vanco**] or (**PIP-TZ** + **vanco**) If ESBL and/or carbapenemase-producing GNB. Empiric options pending clarification of clinical syndrome/culture results: **Low prevalence: Vanco + PIP-TZ** **High prevalence: Colistin +** (**MER** or **IMP**) *Dosages in footnote*[33] For Colistin combination dosing, *see Table 10A, page 100.*	(**Dapto** 6 mg/kg IV q24h) + (**cefepime** or **PIP-TZ** or **TC-CL**)	
If suspect biliary source *(see* Gallbladder *p.17)*	Enterococci + aerobic Gm-neg. bacilli	**PIP-TZ** or **TC-CL**	**Ceftriaxone** + **metro** or (**CIP** or **Levo**) + **metro** *Dosages–footnote*[33]	If enterococci a concern, add ampicillin or vanco to metro regimens
If community-acquired pneumonia *(see page 39 and following pages)*	**S. pneumoniae; MRSA, Legionella, Gm-neg. bacillus, others**	(**Levo** or **moxi**) + (**PIP-TZ**) + **Vanco**	**Aztreonam +** (**Levo** or **moxi**) + **linezolid**	Many categories of CAP, *see material beginning at page 39*. Suggestions based on most severe CAP, e.g., MRSA after influenza or Klebsiella pneumonia in an alcoholic.
If illicit use IV drugs	S. aureus	**Vanco if high prevalence of MRSA. Do NOT use empiric vanco + oxacillin pending organism ID.** In vitro nafcillin increased production of toxins by CA-MRSA *(JID 195:202, 2007). Dosages—footnote 33, page 62*		
If suspect intra-abdominal source	Mixture aerobic & anaerobic Gm-neg. bacilli	*See secondary peritonitis, page 47.*		
If petechial rash	Meningococcemia	**Ceftriaxone** 2 gm IV q12h (until sure no meningitis); consider Rocky Mountain spotted fever—*see page 59*		
If suspect urinary source, e.g. pyelonephritis	Aerobic Gm-neg. bacilli & enterococci	*See pyelonephritis, page 34*		
Neutropenia: Child or Adult (absolute PMN count <500 per mm³) in cancer and transplant patients. Guideline: *CID 52:427, 2011 (inpatients); J CLin Oncol 31:794, 2013 (outpatients)*				
Prophylaxis *(J Clin Oncol 31:794, 2013)*				
Post-chemotherapy—impending neutropenia	Pneumocystis (PCP), Viridans strep	In patients expected to have PMN < 100 for > 7 days consider Levo 500-750 mg po Q24. Acute leukemics undergoing intensive induction consider addition of Fluc 400 mg Q24. In patients with AML or MDS who have prolonged neutropenia, consider Posa instead at 200 mg TID *(N Engl J Med 356:348, 2007)*.		
Post allogeneic stem cell transplant	Aerobic Gm-neg bacilli, ↑ risk pneumocystis, herpes viruses, candida aspergillus	**TMP-SMX** (vs. PCP) + **Acyclovir** (vs. HSV/VZV)+ **pre-emptive** monitoring for **CMV** + **Posa** (vs. mold)		In autologous HCT, not active prophylaxis nor CMV screening is recommended. Fluc OK with TMP-SMX and acyclovir.

[33] **P Ceph 3** (**cefotaxime** 2 gm IV q8h, use q4h if life-threatening; **ceftizoxime** 2 gm IV q4h; **ceftriaxone** 2 gm IV q12h), **AP Pen** (**piperacillin** 3 gm IV q4h, **ticarcillin** 3 gm IV q4h), **TC-CL** 3.1 gm IV q4h, **PIP-TZ** 3.375 gm IV q4h or 4-hr infusion of 3.375 gm q8h, **Aminoglycosides** *(see Table 10D, page 109)*, **AMP** 200 mg/kg/day divided q6h, **clinda** 900 mg IV q8h, **IMP** 0.5 gm IV q6h, **MER** 1 gm IV q8h, **ERTA** 1 gm IV q24h, **DORI** 500 mg IV q8h (1-hr infusion), **Nafcillin** or **oxacillin** 2 gm IV q4h, **aztreonam** 2 gm IV q8h, **metro** 1 gm loading dose then 0.5 gm q6h or 1 gm IV q12h, **vanco**: loading dose 25-30 mg/kg IV, then 15-20 mg/kg IV q8-12h (dose in obese pt, *see Table 17C , page 219*), **ceftazidime** 2 gm IV q8h, [**Cefepime** 2 gm IV q12h (q8h if neutropenic), **cefpirome**[NUS] 2 gm IV q12h], **CIP** 400 mg IV q12h, **levo** 750 mg IV q24h, **linezolid** 600 mg IV q12h.

 **NOTE: All dosage recommendations are for adults (unless otherwise indicated) and assume normal renal function. § Alternatives consider allergy, PK, compliance, local resistance, cost*

TABLE 1 (60)

ANATOMIC SITE/DIAGNOSIS/ MODIFYING CIRCUMSTANCES	ETIOLOGIES (usual)	SUGGESTED REGIMENS* PRIMARY	SUGGESTED REGIMENS* ALTERNATIVE§	ADJUNCT DIAGNOSTIC OR THERAPEUTIC MEASURES AND COMMENTS
SYSTEMIC SYNDROMES (FEBRILE/NON-FEBRILE)/Neutropenia *(continued)*				
Empiric therapy—febrile neutropenia (≥38.3°C for > 1 hr or sustained >38°C and absolute neutrophil count <500 cells/μL) (IDSA Guidelines: *CID 52:427, 2012*). *(Outpatients: J CLin Oncol 31:794, 2013)*.				
Low-risk adults Anticipate < 7 days neutropenia, no co-morb, can take po meds	Aerobic Gm-neg bacilli, Viridans strep	**CIP** 750 mg po bid + **AM-CL** 875 /125 mg po bid. Treat until absolute neutrophil count >1000 cells/μL	Treat as outpatients with 24/7 access to inpatient care if: no focal findings, no hypotension, no COPD, no fungal infection, no dehydration, age range 16-60 yrs; motivated and compliant pts & family. If pen allergy: can substitute clinda 300 mg po qid for AM-CL	
High-risk adults and children (Anticipate > 7 days profound neutropenia, active co-morbidities)	**Aerobic Gm-neg. bacilli; to include P. aeruginosa; cephalosporin-resistant viridans strep; MRSA**	**Empiric therapy: CFP, IMP, MERO, DORI**, or **PIP-TAZO**. Consider addition of **Vanco** as below. *Dosages: Footnote[33] and Table 10B* **Include empiric vanco if:** Suspected CLABSI, severe mucositis, SSTI, PNA, or hypotension	**Combination therapy:** If pt has severe sepsis/shock, consider add **Tobra** AND **Vanco** AND **Echinocandin**	Increasing resistance of viridans streptococci to penicillins, cephalosporins & FQs *(CID 34:1469 & 1524, 2002)*. **What if severe IgE-mediated β-lactam allergy?** Aztreonam plus Tobra. Work-up should include blood, urine, CXR with additional testing based on symptoms. Low threshold for CT scan. If cultures remain neg, but pt afebrile, treat until absolute neutrophil count ≥ 500 cells/μL.
Persistent fever and neutropenia after 5 days of empiric antibacterial therapy—*see CID 52:427, 2011.*				
	Candida species, aspergillus, VRE, resistant GNB	Add either (**caspofungin** 70 mg IV day 1, then 50 mg IV q24h or **Micafungin** 100 mg IV q24h or **Anidulafungin** 200 mg IV x 1 dose, then 100 mg IV q24h) **OR voriconazole** 6 mg per kg IV q12h times 2 doses, then 4 mg per kg IV q12h		Conventional **ampho B** causes more fever & nephrotoxicity & lower efficacy than lipid-based ampho B; both **caspofungin** & **voriconazole** better tolerated & perhaps more efficacious than lipid-based ampho B *(NEJM 346:225, 2002 & 351:1391 & 1445, 2005)*.
Shock syndromes				
Septic shock: Fever & hypotension **Bacteremic shock, endotoxin shock** *Surviving Sepsis Campaign: JAMA 305:1469, 2011.* "Bundles": *AJRCCM 1887, 2013. See NEJM 369:840, 2013; CCM 188:77, 2013.*	Bacteremia with aerobic Gm-neg. bacteria or Gm+ cocci	Lower mortality with **sepsis treatment "bundle"** *(AJRCCM 188:77, 2013)* • Blood cultures & serum lactate • Initiate effective antibiotic therapy: o No clear source & MDR GNB are rare: **PIP-TZ** + **Vanco** o No clear source but high prevalence of MDR GNB: **Colistin** + (**MER** or **IMP**) • IV saline/crystalloid: 20-40 mL/kg for hypotension or elevated lactate *(NEJM 369:1243, 2013; JAMA 310:1809, 2013)* • If hypotensive after fluids, nor-epinephrine • Attempt to identify & correct source of bacteremia • Monitor lactate, CVP (target ≥ 8 cm H2O) & central venous O2 sat (target ≥ 70%) • Low tidal volume (6 mL/kg) mechanical ventilation *(NEJM 369:2126, 2013)* • Transfuse if hematocrit < 30% • *See Comment*		"Bundle" substantially reduced mortality. • Hydrocortisone start stress doses: 100 mg IV q8h if BP still low after fluids and one vasopressor *(ARJCCM 185:135, 2012)*. • Insulin Rx: Current target is glucose level of 140-180 mg/dL. Attempts at tight control (80-110 mg/dL) resulted in excessive hypoglycemia *(NEJM 363:2540, 2010)*. • Impact of early effective antibiotic therapy *(CCM 38:1045 & 1211, 2010)*
Septic shock: post-splenectomy or functional asplenia	S. pneumoniae, N. meningitidis, H. influenzae, Capnocytophaga (DF-2)	No dog bite: **Ceftriaxone** 2 gm IV q24h (↑ to 2 gm q12h if meningitis) Post-dog bite: (**Pip-Tazo** 3.375 gm IV q6h OR **MER** 1 gm IV q8h) + **Clinda** 900 mg IV q8h	No dog bite: (**Levo** 750 mg or **Moxi** 400 mg) once IV q24h	Howell-Jolly bodies in peripheral blood smear confirm absence of functional spleen. Often results in **symmetrical peripheral gangrene of digits** due to severe DIC. For prophylaxis, see Table 15A, page 197.

Abbreviations on page 2. **NOTE: All dosage recommendations are for adults (unless otherwise indicated) and assume normal renal function. § Alternatives consider allergy, PK, compliance, local resistance, cost*

TABLE 1 (61)

ANATOMIC SITE/DIAGNOSIS/ MODIFYING CIRCUMSTANCES	ETIOLOGIES (usual)	SUGGESTED REGIMENS*		ADJUNCT DIAGNOSTIC OR THERAPEUTIC MEASURES AND COMMENTS
		PRIMARY	ALTERNATIVE§	
SYSTEMIC SYNDROMES (FEBRILE/NON-FEBRILE)/Neutropenia *(continued)*				
Toxic shock syndrome, Clostridium sordellii				
Clinical picture: shock, capillary leak, hemoconcentration, leukemoid reaction, afebrile Ref: CID 43:1436 & 1447, 2006.	Clostridium sordellii –hemorrhagic & lethal toxins	Fluids, aq. **penicillin G** 18–20 million units per day div. q4–6h + **clindamycin** 900 mg IV q8h. **Surgical debridement is key.**	Occurs in variety of settings that produce anaerobic tissue, e.g., illicit drug use, post-partum. Several deaths reported after use of abortifacient regimen of mifepristone (RU486) & misoprostol. *(NEJM 363:2540, 2010).* 2001-2006 standard medical abortion: po mifepristone & then vaginal misoprostol. Since 2006, switch to buccal, instead of vaginal misoprostol, plus prophylactic Doxy resulted in dramatic decrease in TSS *(NEJM 361:145, 2009).* Mortality nearly 100% if WBC >50,000/μL.	
Toxic shock syndrome, staphylococcal. Review: *LnID 9:281, 1009*				
Colonization by toxin-producing Staph. aureus of: vagina (tampon-assoc.), surgical/traumatic wounds, endometrium, burns	Staph. aureus (toxic shock toxin-mediated)	(**Nafcillin** or **oxacillin** 2 gm IV q4h) or (if MRSA, **vanco** 1 gm IV q12h) + **Clinda** 600-900 mg IV q8h + **IVIG** (Dose in Comment)	(**Cefazolin** 1–2 gm IV q8h) or (if MRSA, **vanco** 1 gm IV q12h OR **dapto** 6 mg/kg IV q24h) **Clinda** 600-900 mg IV q8h+ **IVIG** (Dose in Comment)	**IVIG reasonable** *(see Streptococcal TSS)* — dose 1 gm per kg on day 1, then 0.5 gm per kg days 2 & 3 — antitoxin antibodies present. If suspect TSS, "turn off" toxin production with clinda; report of success with **linezolid** *(JID 195:202, 2007). Exposure of MRSA to nafcillin increased toxin production in vitro: JID 195:202, 2007.*
Toxic shock syndrome, streptococcal. NOTE: For Necrotizing fasciitis without toxic shock, *see page 56.* Ref: *LnID 9:281, 2009.*				
Associated with **invasive disease**, i.e., erysipelas, necrotizing fasciitis; secondary strep infection of varicella. Secondary TSS cases reported *(NEJM 335:547 & 590, 1996; CID 27:150, 1998).*	Group A, B, C, & G Strep. pyogenes, Group B strep ref: *EID 15:223, 2009.*	(**Pen G** 24 million units per day IV in div. doses) + (**clinda** 900 mg IV q8h) **IVIG** associated with ↓ in sepsis-related organ failure *(CID 37:333 & 341, 2003).* IVIG dose: 1 gm per kg day 1, then 0.5 gm per kg days 2 & 3. IVIG preps vary in neutralizing antibody content *(CID 43:743, 2006).* In multicenter retrospect study, no benefit from IVIG-controversial *(CID 1369 & 1377, 2009).*	**Ceftriaxone** 2 gm IV q24h + **clinda** 900 mg IV q8h	**Definition:** Isolation of Group A strep, hypotension and ≥2 of: renal impairment, coagulopathy, liver involvement, ARDS, generalized rash, soft tissue necrosis. Associated with invasive disease. **Surgery usually required.** Mortality with fasciitis 30–50%, myositis 80% even with early rx *(CID 14:2, 1992).* Clinda ↓ toxin production. Use of NSAID may predispose to TSS. For reasons pen G may fail in fulminant S. pyogenes infections *(see JID 167:1401, 1993).*
Toxin-Mediated Syndromes—no fever unless complicated				
Botulism *(CID 41:1167, 2005. As* **biologic weapon:** *JAMA 285:1059, 2001; www.bt.cdc.gov)*				
Food-borne Dyspnea at presentation bad sign *(CID 43:1247, 2006)*	Clostridium botulinum	For all types: Follow vital capacity; other supportive care If no ileus, purge GI tract	Heptavalent equine serum antitoxin—CDC *(see Comment)*	**Equine antitoxin:** Heptavalent currently only antitoxin available (U.S) for non-infant botulism: *CDC (+1 404-639-2206 M-F OR +1 404-639-2888 evenings/weekends).* For infants, *use Baby BIG (human botulism immune globulin): California Infant Botulism Treat & Prevent Program.*
Infant (Adult intestinal botulism is rare variant: EIN 18:1, 2012).		Human botulinum immunoglobulin (BIG) IV, single dose. Call (+1) 510-540-2646. Do not use equine antitoxin.	**No antibiotics;** may lyse C. botulinum in gut and ↑ load of toxin	**Antimicrobials:** May make infant botulism worse. Untested in wound botulism. When used, pen G 10–20 million units per day usual dose. If complications (pneumonia, UTI) occur, avoid antimicrobials with assoc. neuromuscular blockade, i.e., aminoglycosides, tetracycline, polymyxins. **Differential dx:** Guillain-Barré, myasthenia gravis, tick paralysis, organophosphate toxicity, West Nile virus
Wound		Debridement & anaerobic cultures. No proven value of local antitoxin. Role of antibiotics untested.	Trivalent equine antitoxin *(see Comment)*	Wound botulism can result from spore contamination of tar heroin. Ref: *CID 31:1018, 2000.* Mouse bioassay failed to detect toxin in 1/3 of patients *(CID 48:1669, 2009).*

 **NOTE: All dosage recommendations are for adults (unless otherwise indicated) and assume normal renal function. § Alternatives consider allergy, PK, compliance, local resistance, cost*

TABLE 1 (62)

ANATOMIC SITE/DIAGNOSIS/ MODIFYING CIRCUMSTANCES	ETIOLOGIES (usual)	SUGGESTED REGIMENS*		ADJUNCT DIAGNOSTIC OR THERAPEUTIC MEASURES AND COMMENTS
		PRIMARY	ALTERNATIVE§	
SYSTEMIC SYNDROMES/Neutropenia *(continued)*				
Tetanus: Trismus, generalized muscle rigidity, muscle spasm Ref: *AnIM 154:329, 2011.*	C. tetani–production of tetanospasmin toxin	**Six treatment steps:** 1–Urgent endotracheal intubation to protect the airway. Laryngeal spasm is common. Early tracheostomy. 2–Eliminate reflex spasms with diazepam, 20 mg/kg/day IV or midazolam. Reports of benefit combining diazepam with magnesium sulfate *(Ln 368:1436, 2006)*. Worst cases: need neuromuscular blockade with vecuronium. 3–Neutralize toxin: Human hyperimmune globulin IM; start tetanus immunization–no immunity from clinical tetanus. 4–Surgically debride infected source tissue. Start antibiotic: (**Pen G** 3 million units IV q4h or **Doxy** 100 mg IV q12h or **Metro** 1000 mg IV q12h) x 7-10 days. 5–Avoid light as may precipitate muscle spasms. 6–Use beta blockers, e.g., short acting esmolol, to control sympathetic hyperactivity.		
VASCULAR				
IV line infection *(See IDSA Guidelines CID 49:1, 2009).*				
Heparin lock, midline catheter, **non-tunneled** central venous catheter (subclavian, internal jugular), peripherally inserted central catheter (PICC) 2008 study found ↑ infection risk/thrombosis if femoral vein used, esp. if BMI >28.4 *(JAMA 299:2413, 2008). See Comment*	Staph. epidermidis, Staph. aureus (MSSA/MRSA). **Diagnosis:** Fever & either + blood cult from line & peripheral vein **OR** >15 colonies on tip of removed line **OR** culture from catheter positive 2 hrs earlier than peripheral vein culture.	**Vanco** 1 gm IV q12h. **Other alternatives—see Comment.** Other rx and duration: **(1) If S. aureus,** remove catheter. Can use TEE result to determine if 2 or 4 wks of therapy *(JAC 57:1172, 2006)*. **(2) If S. epidermidis,** can try to "save" catheter. 80% cure after 7–10 days of therapy. With only systemic antibiotics, high rate of recurrence *(CID 49:1187, 2009)*. If **leuconostoc** or **lactobacillus** are **Vanco** resistant; need **Pen G**, **Amp** or **Clinda**.		If no response to, or intolerant of, **vanco**: switch to **daptomycin** 6 mg per kg IV q24h. **Quinupristin-dalfopristin** an option: 7.5 mg per kg IV q8h via central line. Culture removed catheter. With "roll" method, >15 colonies *(NEJM 312:1142, 1985)* suggests infection. Lines do not require "routine" changing when not infected. When infected, do not insert new catheter over a wire. Antimicrobial-impregnated catheters may ↓ infection risk; the debate is lively *(CID 37:65, 2003 & 38:1287, 2004 & 39:1829, 2004)*. Are femoral lines more prone to infection than subclavian or internal jugular lines? Meta-analysis found no difference *(CCM 40:2479, 2012)*. However, a number of confounders may influence conclusion *(AnIM 157(10):JC5-8, 2012)*.
Tunnel type indwelling venous catheters and ports (Broviac, Hickman, Groshong, Quinton), dual lumen hemodialysis catheters (Permacath). *For prevention, see below.*	Staph. epidermidis, Staph. aureus, (Candida sp.). Rarely: leuconostoc or lactobacillus—both resistant to vanco *(see Table 2, page 68)* *(Dx, see above)*			If subcutaneous tunnel infected, very low cure rates; need to remove catheter. Beware of silent infection in clotted hemodialysis catheters. Indium scans detect *(Am J Kid Dis 40:832, 2002)*.
Impaired host (burn, neutropenic)	As above + Pseudomonas sp., Enterobacteriaceae, Corynebacterium jeikeium, aspergillus, rhizopus	[**Vanco** + (**Cefepime** or **Ceftaz**) or (**Vanco** + **Pip-Tazo**) or **IMP** or [(**Cefepime** or **Ceftaz**) + **Aminoglycoside**]. *(Dosage in footnotes[27,33], pages 47 and 62).*		Usually have associated septic thrombophlebitis: biopsy of vein to rule out fungi. If fungal, surgical excision + amphotericin B. Surgical drainage, ligation or removal often indicated.
Hyperalimentation	As with tunnel, Candida sp. common *(see Table 11, resistant Candida species)*	If candida, **voriconazole or an echinocandin** (**anidulafungin**, **micafungin**, **caspofungin**) if clinically stable. Dosage: *see Table 11B, page 125.*		Remove venous catheter and discontinue antimicrobial agents if possible. Ophthalmologic consultation recommended. **Rx all patients with + blood cultures.** *See Table 11A, Candidiasis, page 114*
Intravenous lipid emulsion	Staph. epidermidis	**Vanco** 1 gm IV q12h		Discontinue intralipid
	Malassezia furfur	**Fluconazole** 400 mg IV q24h		

 **NOTE: All dosage recommendations are for adults (unless otherwise indicated) and assume normal renal function. § Alternatives consider allergy, PK, compliance, local resistance, cost*

TABLE 1 (63)

ANATOMIC SITE/DIAGNOSIS/ MODIFYING CIRCUMSTANCES	ETIOLOGIES (usual)	SUGGESTED REGIMENS*		ADJUNCT DIAGNOSTIC OR THERAPEUTIC MEASURES AND COMMENTS
		PRIMARY	ALTERNATIVE§	
VASCULAR/IV line infection *(continued)*				
Prevention of Infection of Long-Term IV Lines *CID 52:1087, 2011*	To minimize risk of infection: **Hand washing and** **1.** Maximal sterile barrier precautions during catheter insertion **2.** Use >0.5% chlorhexidine prep with alcohol for skin antisepsis **3.** If infection rate high despite #1 & 2, use either chlorhexidine/silver sulfadiazine or minocycline/rifampin-impregnated catheters or "lock" solutions *(see Comment)*. **4.** If possible, use subclavian vein, avoid femoral vessels. Lower infection risk in jugular vs. femoral vein if BMI >28.4 *(JAMA 299:2413, 2008)*.			**IV line "lock" solutions under study. No FDA-approved product.** Reports of the combination of TMP, EDTA & ethanol *(AAC 55:4430, 2011)*. Trials to begin in Europe. Another report: lock sol'n of sodium citrate, methylene blue, methylparabens *(CCM 39:613, 2011)*. Recent meeting abstracts support 70% ethanol.
Mycotic aneurysm	S. aureus (28-71%), S. epidermidis, Salmonella sp. (15-24%), M.TBc, S. pneumonia, many others	**Vanco** (dose sufficient to achieve trough level of 15-20 µg/mL) + (**ceftriaxone** or **PIP-TZ** or **CIP**) **Treatment is combination of antibiotic + surgical resection with revascularization.**	**Dapto** could be substituted for Vanco. For GNB: **cefepime** or **carbapenems**. For MDR-GNB, **colistin** in combination therapy	No data for ceftaroline or telavancin. Best diagnostic imaging: CT angiogram. Blood cultures positive in 50-85%. **De-escalate to specific therapy when culture results known.** Treatment duration varies but usually 6 wks from date of definitive surgery.
Suppurative (Septic) Thrombophlebitis				
Cranial dural sinus:				
Cavernous Sinus	S. aureus (70%) Streptococcus sp. Anaerobes (rare) Mucormycosis (diabetes)	[**Vanco** (dose for trough conc of 15-20 mcg/mL) + **Ceftriaxone** 2 gm IV q12h], add **Metro** 500 mg IV q8h if dental/sinus source	(**Dapto** 8-12 mg/kg IV q24h OR **Linezolid** 600 mg IV q12h), add **Metro** 500 mg IV q8h if dental/sinus source	• Diagnosis: CT or MRI • Treatment: 1) obtain specimen for culture; 2) empiric antibiotics; 3) may need adjunctive surgery; 4) heparin until afebrile, then coumadin for several weeks
Lateral Sinus: Complication of otitis media/mastoiditis	Polymicrobial (often) Aerobes Anaerobes S. aureus P. aeruginosa B. fragilis Other GNB	**Cefepime** 2 gm IV q8h + **Metro** 500 mg IV q8h + **Vanco** (dose for trough conc of 15-20 mcg/mL)	**Meropenem** 1-2 gm IV q8h + **Linezolid** 600 mg IV q12h	• Diagnosis: CT or MRI • Treatment: 1) consider radical mastoidectomy; 2) obtain cultures; 3) antibiotics; 4) anticoagulation controversial • Prognosis: favorable
Superior Sagittal Sinus: Complication of bacterial meningitis or bacterial frontal sinusitis	S. pneumoniae N. meningitides H. influenzae (rare) S. aureus (very rare)	As for meningitis: **Ceftriaxone** 2 gm IV q12h + **Vanco** (dose for trough conc of 15-20 mcg/mL) + **dexamethasone**	As for meningitis: **Meropenem** 1-2 gm IV q8h + **Vanco** (dose for trough conc of 15-20 mcg/mL) + **dexamethasone**	• Diagnosis: MRI • Prognosis: bad; causes cortical vein thrombosis, hemorrhagic infarcts and brainstem herniation. • Anticoagulants not recommended

 **NOTE: All dosage recommendations are for adults (unless otherwise indicated) and assume normal renal function. § Alternatives consider allergy, PK, compliance, local resistance, cost*

TABLE 1 (64)

ANATOMIC SITE/DIAGNOSIS/ MODIFYING CIRCUMSTANCES	ETIOLOGIES (usual)	SUGGESTED REGIMENS*		ADJUNCT DIAGNOSTIC OR THERAPEUTIC MEASURES AND COMMENTS
		PRIMARY	ALTERNATIVE§	
VASCULAR/Suppurative (Septic) Thrombophlebitis *(continued)*				
Jugular Vein, Lemierre's Syndrome: Complication of pharyngitis, tonsillitis, dental infection, EBV	Fusobacterium necrophorum (anaerobe) Less often: Other Fusobacterium S. pyogenes Bacteroides sp.	(**Pip-Tazo** 3.375 gm IV q6h OR **Amp-Sulb** 3 gm IV q6h) x 4 weeks	[**Imipenem** 500 mg IV q6h OR (**Metro** 500 mg IV q8h + **Ceftriaxone** 2 gm IV once daily)] x 4 weeks. Another option: **Clinda** 600-900 mg IV q8h	• Diagnosis: Preceding pharyngitis and antibiotics therapy, persistent fever and pulmonary emboli • Imaging: Hi-res CT scan • Role of anticoagulants unclear
Pelvic Vein: Includes ovarian vein and deep pelvic vein phlebitis	Aerobic gram-neg bacilli Streptococcus sp. Anaerobes	Antibiotics + anticoagulation (heparin, then coumadin) *Low prevalence of MDR GNB:* **Pip-Tazo** 3.375 gm IV q6h or 4.5 gm IV q8h OR (**Ceftriaxone** 2 gm IV once daily + **Metro** 500 mg IV q8h)	*High prevalence of MDR GNB:* **Meropenem** 1 gm IV q8h. If severe beta-lactam allergy: (**CIP** 400 mg IV q12h + **Metro** 500 mg IV q8h)	• Diagnosis: ovarian vein infection presents 1 week post-partum with fever & local pain; deep pelvic vein presents 3-5 days post-delivery with fever but no local pain. CT or MRI may help. • Treat until afebrile for 48 hrs & WBC normal • Coumadin for 6 weeks
Portal Vein (Pylephlebitis): Complication of diverticulitis, appendicitis and (rarely) other intra-abdominal infection	Aerobic gram-neg bacilli: E. coli, Klebsiella & Proteus most common Other: aerobic/anaerobic streptococci, B. fragilis, Clostridia	*Low prevalence of MDR GNB* (<20%): **Pip-Tazo** 4.5 gm IV q8h OR (**CIP** 400 mg IV q12h + **Metro** 500 mg IV q8h)	*High prevalence of MDR GNB* (≥20%): If ESBL producer: **Meropenem** 1 gm IV q8h. If carbapenemase producer: **Colistin** + **Meropenem** *(See Table 10A for dosing)*	• Diagnosis: Pain, fever, neutrophilia in pt with intra-abdominal infection. Abdominal CT scan • Pyogenic liver abscess is a complication • No anticoagulants unless hypercoagulable disease (neoplasm) • Surgery on vein not indicated

 **NOTE: All dosage recommendations are for adults (unless otherwise indicated) and assume normal renal function. § Alternatives consider allergy, PK, compliance, local resistance, cost*

TABLE 2 – RECOMMENDED ANTIMICROBIAL AGENTS AGAINST SELECTED BACTERIA

BACTERIAL SPECIES	ANTIMICROBIAL AGENT *(See page 2 for abbreviations)*		
	RECOMMENDED	**ALTERNATIVE**	**ALSO EFFECTIVE[1] (COMMENTS)**
Achromobacter xylosoxidans spp xylosoxidans (formerly Alcaligenes)	IMP, MER, DORI (no DORI for pneumonia)	TMP-SMX. Some strains susc. to ceftaz, PIP-TZ	Resistant to aminoglycosides, most cephalosporins & FQs.
Acinetobacter calcoaceticus—baumannii complex	If suscept: IMP or MER or DORI. For MDR strains: Colistin + (IMP or MER) (no DORI for pneumonia)	AM-SB used for activity of sulbactam *(CID 51:79, 2010)*. Perhaps Minocycline IV	Resistant to aminoglycosides, FQs. Minocycline, effective against many strains *(CID 51:79, 2010) (See Table 5A, pg 78)*
Actinomyces israelii	AMP or Pen G	Doxy, ceftriaxone	Clindamycin, erythro
Aeromonas hydrophila & other sp.	CIP or Levo	TMP-SMX or (P Ceph 3, 4)	*See AAC 56:1110, 2012.*
Arcanobacterium (C.) haemolyticum	Erythro; azithro	Benzathine Pen G, Clinda	Sensitive to most drugs, resistant to TMP-SMX *(AAC 38:142, 1994)*
Bacillus anthracis (anthrax): inhalation	*See Table 1, page 43*		
Bacillus cereus, B. subtilis	Vancomycin, clinda	FQ, IMP	
Bacteroides sp., B. fragilis & others	Metronidazole or PIP-TZ	Dori, ERTA, IMP, MER, AM-CL	Increasing resistance to: clinda, cefoxitin, cefotetan.
Bartonella henselae, quintana *See Table 1, pages 30, 45, 52, 57*	Varies with disease entity & immune status. Active: Azithro, clarithro, erythro, doxy & in combination: RIF, gent, ceftriaxone. Not active: CIP, TMP-SMX, Pen, most cephalosporins, aztreonam		
Bordetella pertussis	Azithro or clarithro	TMP-SMX	*See PIDJ 31:78, 2012.*
Borrelia burgdorferi, B. afzelii, B. garinii (Lyme & relapsing fever)	*See specific disease entity*		
Brucella sp.	Drugs & duration vary with localization or non-localization. *See specific disease entities. PLoS One 7:e32090, 2012.*		
Burkholderia (Pseudomonas) cepacia	TMP-SMX or MER or CIP	Minocycline or chloramphenicol	(Usually resist to aminoglycosides, polymyxins) *(AAC 37: 123, 1993 & 43:213, 1999; Inf Med 18:49, 2001)* (Some resist to carbapenems). May need combo rx *(AJRCCM 161:1206, 2000)*.
Burkholderia (Pseudomonas) pseudomallei *Curr Opin Infect Dis 23:554, 2010; CID 41:1105, 2005*	Initially, IV ceftaz or IMP or MER, then po (TMP-SMX + Doxy x 3 mos) ± Chloro *(AAC 49:4010, 2005)*.		(Thai, 12–80% strains resist to TMP-SMX). FQ active in vitro. MER also effective *(AAC 48: 1763, 2004)*
Campylobacter jejuni	Azithro	Erythro or CIP	TMP-SMX, Pen & cephalosporins not active.
Campylobacter fetus	Gentamicin	IMP or ceftriaxone	AMP, chloramphenicol
Capnocytophaga ochracea (DF-1)	Dog bite: Clinda or AM-CL	Septic shock, post-splenectomy: PIP-TZ, Clinda, IMP, DORI, MER	FQ activity variable; aminoglycosides, TMP-SMX & Polymyxins have limited activity. *LN ID 9:439, 2009.*
Capnocytophaga canimorsus (DF-2)	Dog bite: AM-CL		
Chlamydophila pneumoniae	Doxy	Erythro, FQ	Azithro, clarithro
Chlamydia trachomatis	Doxy or azithro	Erythro	
Citrobacter diversus (koseri), C. freundii	Life threatening illness: IMP, MER, DORI	Non-life threatening illness: CIP or Gent	Emergence of resistance: *AAC 52:995, 2007.*
Clostridium difficile	Mild illness: Metronidazole (po)	Moderate/severe illness: Vancomycin (po) or Fidaxomicin *(CID 51:1306, 2010)*.	Bacitracin (po); Nitazoxanide *(CID 43:421, 2006; JAC 59:705, 2007)*. Rifaximin *(CID 44:846, 2007)*. *See also Table 1, page 18 re severity of disease.*
Clostridium perfringens	Pen G ± clindamycin	Doxy	Erythro, chloramphenicol, cefazolin, cefoxitin, AP Pen, carbapenems
Clostridium tetani	Metronidazole or Pen G	Doxy	Role of antibiotics unclear.
Corynebacterium. diphtheriae	Erythro + antitoxin	Pen G + antitoxin	RIF reported effective *(CID 27:845, 1998)*
Corynebacterium jeikeium	Vancomycin + aminoglycoside	Pen G + aminoglycoside	Many strains resistant to Pen *(EJCMID 25:349, 2006)*.
Corynebacterium minutissimum	Clinda 1% lotion	Clarithro or Erythro	Causes erythrasma
Coxiella burnetii (Q fever) acute disease *(CID 52:1431, 2011)*.	Doxy, FQ *(see Table 1, page 31)*	Erythro, Azithro, Clarithro	Endocarditis: doxy + hydroxychloroquine *(JID 188:1322, 2003; LnID 3:709, 2003; LnID 10:527, 2010)*.
chronic disease, e.g., endocarditis	Doxy + hydroxy chloroquine	TMP-SMX, Chloro	

TABLE 2 (2)

BACTERIAL SPECIES	ANTIMICROBIAL AGENT *(See page 2 for abbreviations)*		
	RECOMMENDED	**ALTERNATIVE**	**ALSO EFFECTIVE[1] (COMMENTS)**
Ehrlichia chaffeensis, Ehrlichia ewubguum Anaplasma (Ehrlichia) phagocytophillium	Doxy	RIF *(CID 27:213, 1998)*, Levo *(AAC 47:413, 2003)*.	CIP, oflox, chloramphenicol also active in vitro. Resist to clinda, TMP-SMX, IMP, AMP, erythro, & azithro *(AAC 41:76, 1997)*.
Eikenella corrodens	AM-CL, IV Pen G	TMP-SMX, FQ	Resistant to clinda, cephalexin, erythro, metro, diclox
Elizabethkingae meningosepticum (formerly Chryseobacterium)	Levo or TMP-SMX	CIP, Minocycline	Resistant to Pen, cephalosporins, carbapenems, aminoglycosides, vancomycin *(JCM 44:1181, 2006)*
Enterobacter species	Recommended agents vary with clinical setting and degree and mechanism of resistance.		
Enterococcus faecalis	Highly resistant. *See Table 5A, page 78*		
Enterococcus faecium	Highly resistant. *See Table 5A, page 78*		
Erysipelothrix rhusiopathiae	Penicillin G or amox	P Ceph 3, FQ	IMP, AP Pen (vancomycin, APAG, TMP-SMX resistant)
Escherichia coli	Highly resistant. Treatment varies with degree & mechanism of resistance, *see TABLE 5B.*		
Francisella tularensis (tularemia) *See Table 1, page 45*	Gentamicin, tobramycin, or streptomycin	Mild infection: Doxy or CIP	Chloramphenicol, RIF. Doxy/chloro bacteriostatic → relapses *CID 53:e133, 2011.*
Gardnerella vaginalis (bacterial vaginosis)	Metronidazole or Tinidazole	Clindamycin	*See Table 1, pg 26 for dosage*
Helicobacter pylori	*See Table 1, pg 21*		Drugs effective in vitro often fail in vivo.
Haemophilus aphrophilus (Aggregatibacter aphrophilus)	[(Penicillin or AMP) + gentamicin] or [AM- SB ± gentamicin]	(Ceftriaxone + Gent) or CIP or Levo	Resistant to vancomycin, clindamycin, methicillin
Haemophilus ducreyi (chancroid)	Azithro or ceftriaxone	Erythro, CIP	Most strains resistant to tetracycline, amox, TMP-SMX
Haemophilus influenzae Meningitis, epiglottitis & other life-threatening illness	Cefotaxime, ceftriaxone	AMP if susceptible and ß-lactamase neg, FQs	Chloramphenicol (downgrade from 1st choice due to hematotoxicity).
non-life threatening illness	AM-CL, O Ceph 2/3		Azithro, clarithro, telithro
Klebsiella ozaenae/ rhinoscleromatis	CIP	Levo	*Acta Otolaryngol 131:440, 2010.*
Klebsiella species	Treatment varies with degree & mechanism of resistance, *see TABLE 5B.*		
Lactobacillus species	Pen G or AMP	Clindamycin	**May be resistant to vancomycin**
Legionella sp.	Levo or Moxi	Azithro	Telithro active in vitro.
Leptospira interrogans	Mild: Doxy or amox	Severe: Pen G or ceftriaxone	
Leuconostoc	Pen G or AMP	Clinda	**NOTE: Resistant to vancomycin**
Listeria monocytogenes	AMP + Gent for synergy	TMP-SMX	Erythro, penicillin G (high dose), APAG may be synergistic with β-lactams. Meropenem active in vitro. **Cephalosporin-resistant!**
Moraxella (Branhamella) catarrhalis	AM-CL or O Ceph 2/3, TMP-SMX	Azithro, clarithro, dirithromycin, telithro	Erythro, doxy, FQs
Mycoplasma pneumoniae	Doxy	Azithro	Clindamycin & ß lactams NOT effective. Increasing macrolide resistance *(JAC 68:506, 2013)*.
Neisseria gonorrhoeae (gonococcus)	Ceftriaxone,	Azithro (high dose)	FQs and oral cephalosporins no longer recommended: high levels of resistance.
Neisseria meningitidis (meningococcus)	Ceftriaxone	Chloro, MER	Chloro-resist strains in SE Asia *(NEJM 339:868, 1998) (Prophylaxis: pg 10)*
Nocardia asteroides or **Nocardia brasiliensis**	TMP-SMX + IMP	Linezolid	Amikacin + (IMP or ceftriaxone or cefotaxime)
Pasteurella multocida	Pen G, AMP, amox, cefuroxime, cefpodoxime	Doxy, Levo, Moxi, TMP-SMX	Resistant to cephalexin, oxacillin, clindamycin, erythro, vanco.
Plesiomonas shigelloides	CIP	TMP-SMX	AM-CL, Ceftriaxone & Chloro active. Resistant to: Amp, Tetra, aminoglycosides
Propionibacterium acnes (not acne)	Penicillin, Ceftriaxone	Vanco, Dapto, Linezolid	May be resistant to Metro.
Proteus sp, **Providencia sp**, Morganella sp. (Need in vitro susceptibility)	CIP, PIP-TZ; avoid cephalosporins	May need carbapenem if critically ill	Note: Proteus sp. & Providencia sp. have intrinsic resistance to Polymyxins.
Pseudomonas aeruginosa *(ID Clin No Amer 23:277, 2009)*. Combination therapy? *See Clin Micro Rev 25:450, 2012.*	No in vitro resistance: AP Pen, AP Ceph 3, Dori, IMP, MER, tobramycin, CIP, aztreonam. For serious inf., use AP β-lactam + (tobramycin or CIP)	For UTI, if no in vitro resistance, single drugs effective: AP Pen, AP Ceph 3, cefepime, IMP, MER, aminoglycoside, CIP, aztreonam	If resistant to all beta lactams, FQs, aminoglycosides: Colistin + MER or IMP. Do not use DORI for pneumonia.

TABLE 2 (3)

BACTERIAL SPECIES	ANTIMICROBIAL AGENT *(See page 2 for abbreviations)*		
	RECOMMENDED	**ALTERNATIVE**	**ALSO EFFECTIVE[1] (COMMENTS)**
Rhodococcus (C. equi)	Two drugs: Azithro, Levo or RIF	(Vanco or IMP) + (Azithro, Levo or RIF)	Vancomycin active in vitro; intracellular location may impair efficacy *(CID 34:1379, 2002)*. Avoid Pen, cephalosporins, clinda, tetra, TMP-SMX.
Rickettsia species (includes spotted fevers)	Doxy	Chloramphenicol (in pregnancy), azithro (age < 8 yrs)	*See specific infections (Table 1).*
Salmonella typhi *(CID 50:241, 2010; AAC 54:5201, 2010; BMC ID 51:37, 2005)*	If FQ & nalidixic acid susceptible: CIP	Ceftriaxone, cefixime, azithro, chloro	Concomitant steroids in severely ill. Watch for relapse (1-6%) & ileal perforation. FQ resistance reported with treatment failures *(AAC 52:1278, 2008)*.
Serratia marcescens	If no in vitro resistance: PIP-TZ, CIP, LEVO, Gent	If in vitro resistance: Carbapenem	Avoid extended spectrum Ceph if possible.
Shigella sp.	FQ or azithro	Ceftriaxone is alternative; TMP-SMX depends on susceptibility.	
Staph. aureus, methicillin-susceptible	Oxacillin/nafcillin	P Ceph 1, vanco, teicoplanin[NUS], clinda ceftaroline	ERTA, IMP, MER, BL/BLI, FQ, Pip-Tazo, linezolid, dapto, telavancin.
Staph. aureus, methicillin-resistant (health-care associated) *IDSA Guidelines: CID 52 (Feb 1):1, 2011.*	Vancomycin	Teicoplanin[NUS], TMP-SMX (some strains resistant), linezolid, daptomycin, telavancin, ceftaroline	Fusidic acid[NUS]. >60% CIP-resistant in U.S. (Fosfomycin + RIF). Partially vancomycin-resistant strains (GISA, VISA) & highly resistant strains now described—*see Table 6, pg 79.*
Staph. aureus, methicillin-resistant [community- associated (CA-MRSA)]			CA-MRSA usually not multiply-resistant. Oft resist. to erythro & variably to FQ. Vanco, teico[NUS], telavancin, daptomycin, ceftaroline can be used in pts requiring hospitalization *(see Table 6, pg 79)*. Also, ceftaroline.
Mild-moderate infection	(TMP-SMX or doxy or mino)	Clinda (if D-test neg—*see Table 5A & 6).*	
Severe infection	Vanco or teico[NUS]	Linezolid or daptomycin	
Staph. epidermidis	Vancomycin ± RIF	RIF + (TMP-SMX or FQ), daptomycin *(AAC 51:3420, 2007)*	Cephalothin or nafcillin/oxacillin if sensitive to nafcillin/oxacillin but 75% are resistant. FQs. *(See Table 5A).*
Staph. haemolyticus	TMP-SMX, FQ, nitrofurantoin	Oral cephalosporin	Recommendations apply to UTI only.
Staph. lugdunensis	Oxacillin/nafcillin or penicillin G (if β-lactamase neg.)	P Ceph 1 or vancomycin or teico[NUS]	Approx. 75% are penicillin-susceptible.
Staph. saprophyticus (UTI)	Oral cephalosporin or AM-CL	FQ	Almost always methicillin-susceptible
Stenotrophomonas (Xanthomonas, Pseudomonas) maltophilia	TMP-SMX	TC-CL	Minocycline, tigecycline, CIP, Ceftriaxone, moxifloxacin, ceftaz *(LnID 9:312, 2009; JAC 62:889, 2008)*. [In vitro synergy (TC-CL + TMP-SMX) & (TC-CL + CIP), *JAC 62:889, 2008*].
Streptobacillus moniliformis	Penicillin G	Doxy	Maybe erythro, clinda, ceftriaxone
Streptococcus, anaerobic (Peptostreptococcus)	Penicillin G	Clindamycin	Doxy, vancomycin, linezolid, ERTA *(AAC 51:2205, 2007)*.
Streptococcus anginosus group	Penicillin	Vanco or Ceftriaxone	Avoid FQs; macrolide resistance emerging
Streptococcus pneumoniae penicillin-susceptible	Penicillin G, Amox	Multiple agents effective, e.g., Ceph 2/3, Clinda	If meningitis, higher dose, *see Table 1, page 9.*
penicillin-resistant (MIC ≥2.0)	Vancomycin, Levo, ceftriaxone, Amox (HD), Linezolid		
Streptococcus pyogenes, Groups A, B, C, G: bacteremia	Penicillin G + Clinda	Pen (alone) or Clinda (alone)	*JCM 49:439, 2011.* Pockets of macrolide resistance
Tropheryma whipplei	Doxy + Hydroxychloroquine	None	Clinical failures with TMP-SMX
Vibrio cholerae	Doxy, FQ	Azithro, erythro	Maybe CIP or Levo; some resistance.
Vibrio parahaemolyticus	Doxy	Azithro, CIP	If bacteremic, treat as for V. vulnificus
Vibrio vulnificus, alginolyticus, damsela	Doxy + ceftriaxone	Levo	*CID 52:788, 2011*
Yersinia enterocolitica	CIP or ceftriaxone	TMP-SMX; CIP (if bacteremic)	CIP resistance *(JAC 53:1068, 2004)*, also resistant to Pen, AMP, erythro.
Yersinia pestis (plague)	Streptomycin or Gent	Doxy or CIP	Maybe TMP-SMX (for bubonic, but sub-optimal)

[1] Agents are more variable in effectiveness than "Recommended" or "Alternative." Selection of "Alternative" or "Also Effective" based on in vitro susceptibility testing, pharmacokinetics, host factors such as auditory, renal, hepatic function, & cost.

TABLE 3 – SUGGESTED DURATION OF ANTIBIOTIC THERAPY IN IMMUNOCOMPETENT PATIENTS[1,2]

CLINICAL SITUATION: SITE	CLINICAL SITUATION: CLINICAL DIAGNOSIS	DURATION OF THERAPY (Days)
Bacteremia	Bacteremia with removable focus (no endocarditis)	10–14 *(CID 14:75, 1992) (See Table 1)*
Bone	Osteomyelitis, adult; acute	42
	adult; chronic	Until ESR normal (often > 3 months)
	child; acute; staph. and enterobacteriaceae[3]	21
	child; acute; strep, meningococci, haemophilus[3]	14
Ear	Otitis media with effusion	<2 yrs: 10 (or 1 dose ceftriaxone); ≥2 yrs: 5–7
	Recent meta-analysis suggests 3 days of azithro *(JAC 52:469, 2003)* or 5 days of "short-acting" antibiotics effective for uncomplicated otitis media *(JAMA 279:1736, 1998)*, but may be inadequate for severe disease *(NEJM 347:1169, 2002)*.	
Endo-cardium	Infective endocarditis, native valve	
	Viridans strep	14 or 28 *(See Table 1, page 28)*
	Enterococci	28 or 42 *(See Table 1, page 29)*
	Staph. aureus	14 (R-sided only) or 28 *(See Table 1, page 29)*
GI *Also see Table 1*	Bacillary dysentery (shigellosis)/traveler's diarrhea	3
	Typhoid fever (S. typhi): Azithro	5 (children/adolescents)
	Ceftriaxone	14 [Short course ↑ effective *(AAC 44:450, 2000)*]
	FQ	5–7
	Chloramphenicol	14
	Helicobacter pylori	10–14. For triple-drug regimens, 7 days probably adequate *(AIM 147:553, 2007)*.
	Pseudomembranous enterocolitis (C. difficile)	10
Genital	Non-gonococcal urethritis or mucopurulent cervicitis	7 days doxy or single dose azithro
	Pelvic inflammatory disease	14
Heart	Pericarditis (purulent)	28
Joint	Septic arthritis (non-gonococcal) Adult	14–28 *(Ln 351:197, 1998)*
	Infant/child	Rx as osteomyelitis above. 10-14 days of therapy sufficient *(CID 48:1201, 2009)*, but not complete agreement on this *(CID 48:1211, 2009)*.
	Gonococcal arthritis/disseminated GC infection	7 *(See Table 1, page 23)*
Kidney	Cystitis (bladder bacteriuria)	3 (Single dose extended-release cipro also effective) *(AAC 49:4137, 2005)*
	Pyelonephritis	14 (7 days if CIP used; 5 days if levo 750 mg)
	Recurrent (failure after 14 days rx)	42
Lung	Pneumonia, pneumococcal	Until afebrile 3–5 days (minimum 5 days).
	Community-acquired pneumonia	Minimum 5 days and afebrile for 2-3 days *(CID 44:S55, 2007; AJM 120:783, 2007)*.
	Pneumonia, enterobacteriaceae or pseudomonal	21, often up to 42
	Pneumonia, staphylococcal	21–28
	Pneumocystis carinii, in AIDS;	21
	other immunocompromised	14
	Legionella, mycoplasma, chlamydia	7–14
	Lung abscess	Usually 28–42[4]
Meninges[5] *(CID 39:1267, 2004)*	N. meningitidis	7
	H. influenzae	7
	S. pneumoniae	10–14
	Listeria meningoencephalitis, gp B strep, coliforms	21 (longer in immunocompromised)
Multiple systems	Brucellosis *(See Table 1, page 60)*	42 (add SM or gent for 1st 7–14 days) *(JAC 65:1028, 2010)*
	Tularemia *(See Table 1, pages 45, 59)*	7–14
Muscle	Gas gangrene (clostridial)	10
Pharynx	Group A strep pharyngitis Also see Pharyngitis, *Table 1, page 48*	10 O Ceph 2/3, azithromycin effective at 5 days *(JAC 45, Topic TI 23, 2000; JIC 14:213, 2008)*. 3 days less effective *(Inf Med 18:515, 2001). Single dose extended rel Azithro (2 gm) as effective as 3 days of immediate rel Azithro (CMI 15:1103, 2009). See also 2009 Cochrane Review (www.thecochranelibrary.com).*
	Diphtheria (membranous)	7–14
	Carrier	7
Prostate	Chronic prostatitis (TMP-SMX)	30–90
	(FQ)	28–42
Sinuses	Acute sinusitis	5–14[6]
Skin	Cellulitis	Until 3 days after acute inflamm disappears
Systemic	Lyme disease	*See Table 1, page 58*
	Rocky Mountain spotted fever *(See Table 1, page 59)*	Until afebrile 2 days

1 Early change from IV to po regimens (about 72 hrs) is cost-effective with many infections, i.e., intra-abdominal *(AJM 91:462, 1991)*. There is emerging evidence that normalization of serum procalcitonin level can shorten treatment duration for pneumonia *(JAMA 309:717, 2013)*.
2 The recommended duration is a minimum or average time and should not be construed as absolute.
3 These times are with proviso: sx & signs resolve within 7 days and ESR is normalized *(J.D. Nelson, APID 6:59, 1991)*.
4 After patient afebrile 4-5 days, change to oral therapy.
5 In children relapses seldom occur until 3 days or more after termination of rx. For meningitis in children, *see Table 1, page 8*.
6 Duration of therapy dependent upon agent used and severity of infection. Longer duration (10-14 days) optimal for beta-lactams and patients with severe disease. For sinusitis of mild-moderate severity shorter courses of therapy (5-7 days) effective with "respiratory FQs" (including gemifloxacin, levofloxacin 750 mg), azithromycin. Courses as short as 3 days reported effective for TMP-SMX and azithro and one study reports effectiveness of single dose extended-release azithro. Authors feel such "super-short" courses should be restricted to patients with mild-mod disease *(JAMA 273:1015, 1995; AAC 47:2770, 2003; Otolaryngol-Head Neck Surg 133:194, 2005; Otolaryngol-Head Neck Surg 127:1, 2002; Otolaryngol-Head Neck Surg 134:10, 2006)*.

TABLE 4 – COMPARISON OF ANTIBACTERIAL SPECTRA

Editorial Note: This table is not a source for making treatment decisions. Choice of antibacterial agent must be made in consideration of local/institutional patterns of organism susceptibility and drug resistance, as well as ability of the drug to achieve effective concentrations at the site of infection. Patterns vary considerably based on geography and temporal changes in patterns are continuous. These data are intended to convey a **generalized image** of susceptibility/resistance. These data reflect in vitro susceptibilities, package insert data and/or reports in the published literature. In vitro susceptibility is not a predictor of in vivo efficacy. **Drugs active in vitro, but not used clinically are indicated as: ↕.** ***See specific organism, syndrome or drug for treatment recommendations.***

Organisms	Penicillins		Antistaphylo-coccal Penicillins			Amino-Penicillins			Anti-Pseudomonal Penicillins				Carbapenems					Fluoroquinolones						
	Penicillin G	**Penicillin V**	**Methicillin**	**Nafcillin/Oxacillin**	**Cloxacillin[NUS] /Diclox.**	**AMP/Amox**	**Amox/Clav**	**AMP-Sulb**	**Ticarcillin**	**Ticar-Clav**	**Pip-Tazo**	**Piperacillin**	**Doripenem**	**Ertapenem**	**Imipenem**	**Meropenem**	**Aztreonam**	**Ciprofloxacin**	**Ofloxacin**	**Pefloxacin[NUS]**	**Levofloxacin**	**Moxifloxacin**	**Gemifloxacin**	**Gatifloxacin**
GRAM-POSITIVE:																								
Strep, Group A, B, C, G	+	+	+	+	+	+	+	+	+	+	+	+	+	+	+	+	0	±	±	0	+	+	+	+
Strep. pneumoniae	+	+	+	+	+	+	+	+	+	+	+	+	+	+	+	+	0	±	±	0	+	+	+	+
Viridans strep	±	±	±	±	±	±	±	±	±	±	±	±	+	+	+	+	0	0	0		+	+	+	+
Strep. anginosus gp	+	+	+	+	+	+	+	+	+	+	+	+	+	+	+	+	0	0	0		+	+	+	+
Enterococcus faecalis	+	+	0	0	0	+	+	+	±	±	+	+	±	0	+	±	0	**	**	0	+	+	+	+
Enterococcus faecium	±	±	0	0	0	±	+	+	±	±	±	±	0	0	±	0	0	0	0	0	0	±	±	±
Enterococci, vanco-resistant	0	0	0	0	0	0	0	0	0	0	0	0	0	0	0	0	0	0	0	0	0	0	0	0
Staph. aureus (MSSA)	**0**	**0**	**+**	**+**	**+**	**0**	**+**	**+**	**0**	**+**	**+**	**0**	**+**	**+**	**+**	**+**	**0**	**+**	**+**	**+**	**+**	**+**	**+**	**+**
Staph. aureus (MRSA)	**0**	**0**	**0**	**0**	**0**	**0**	**0**	**0**	**0**	**0**	**0**	**0**	**0**	**0**	**0**	**0**	**0**	**0**	**0**	**0**	**0**	**±**	**±**	**±**
Staph. aureus (CA-MRSA)	**0**	**0**	**0**	**0**	**0**	**0**	**0**	**0**	**0**	**0**	**0**	**0**	**0**	**0**	**0**	**0**	**0**	**±**			**±**	**±**	**±**	**±**
Staph. epidermidis	0	0	+	+	+	0	0	0	±	±	+	0	+	+	+	+	0	+	+	+	+	+	+	+
Corynebacterium jeikeium	0	0	0	0	0	0	0	0	0	0		0		0	0		0	0	0					
Listeria monocytogenes	**+**	**0**	**0**	**0**	**0**	**+**	**↕**	**+**	**+**	**↕**	**↕**	**+**	**+**	**±**	**+**	**+**	**0**	**+**	**0**	**0**	**+**	**+**	**+**	**+**
GRAM-NEGATIVE:																								
Neisseria gonorrhoeae	0	0	0	0	0	0	+	+	↕	↕	↕	↕	↕	↕	↕	↕	+	±	±	±	±	±	±	±
Neisseria meningitidis	**+**	**0**	**0**	**0**	**0**	**+**	**+**	**+**	**+**	**+**	**+**	**+**	**+**	**+**	**+**	**+**	**+**	**+**	**+**	**+**	**+**	**+**		**+**
Moraxella catarrhalis	0	0	0	0	0	0	+	+	0	+	+	±	+	+	+	+	+	+	+	+	+	+	+	+
Haemophilus influenzae	0	0	0	0	0	±	+	+	±	+	+	±	+	+	+	+	+	+	+	+	+	+	+	+
Escherichia coli	**0**	**0**	**0**	**0**	**0**	**±**	**+**	**+**	**±**	**+**	**+**	**+**	**+**	**+**	**+**	**+**	**+**	**+**	**+**	**+**	**+**	**+**	**+**	**+**
Klebsiella sp.	0	0	0	0	0	0	+	+	0	+	+	+	+	+	+	+	+	+	+	+	+	+	+	+
E. coli/ Klebsiella sp, ESBL+	0	0	0	0	0	0	0	0	0	**0**	**0**	0	**+**	**+**	+	+	0	+	+	+	+	+	+	+
E. coli/ Klebsiella sp, KPC+	0	0	0	0	0	0	0	0	0	0	0	0	0	0	0	0	0	0	0	0	0	0	0	0
Enterobacter sp.	0	0	0	0	0	0	0	0	+	+	+	+	+	+	+	+	+	+	+	+	+	+		+

+ = **usually susceptible;** ± = **variably susceptible/resistant;** 0 = **usually resistant;** blank = **no data;** ↕ = **active in vitro, but not used clinically**

** Most strains ±, can be used in UTI, not in systemic infection

TABLE 4 (2)

Organisms	Penicillins		Antistaphylococcal Penicillins			Amino-Penicillins			Anti-Pseudomonal Penicillins				Carbapenems					Fluoroquinolones						
	Penicillin G	**Penicillin V**	**Methicillin**	**Nafcillin/Oxacillin**	**Cloxacillin[NUS] /Diclox.**	**AMP/Amox**	**Amox/Clav**	**AMP-Sulb**	**Ticarcillin**	**Ticar-Clav**	**Pip-Tazo**	**Piperacillin**	**Doripenem**	**Ertapenem**	**Imipenem**	**Meropenem**	**Aztreonam**	**Ciprofloxacin**	**Ofloxacin**	**Pefloxacin[NUS]**	**Levofloxacin**	**Moxifloxacin**	**Gemifloxacin**	**Gatifloxacin**
Serratia sp.	0	0	0	0	0	0	0	0	0	+	+	+	+	+	+	+	+	+	+	+	+	+		+
Salmonella sp.	0	0	0	0	0	±	+	+	+	+	+	+	+	+	+	+		+	+	+	+	+		+
Shigella sp.	0	0	0	0	0	±	+	+	+	+	+	+	+	+	+	+	+	+	+	+	+	+		+
Proteus mirabilis	0	0	0	0	0	+	+	+	+	+	+	+	+	+	+	+	+	+	+	+	+	+		+
Proteus vulgaris	0	0	0	0	0	0	+	+	+	+	+	+	+	+	+	+	+	+	+	+	+	+	+	+
Providencia sp.	0	0	0	0	0	0	+	+	+	+	+	+	+	+	+	+	+	+	+	+	+	+		+
Morganella sp.	0	0	0	0	0	0	±	+	+	+	+	+	+	+	+	+	+	+	+	+	+	+		+
Citrobacter sp.	0	0	0	0	0	0	0	0	+	+	+	+	+	+	+	+	+	+	+	+	+	+		+
Aeromonas sp.	0	0	0	0	0	0	+	+	+	+	+	+	+	+	+	+	+	+	+		+	+		+
Acinetobacter sp.	0	0	0	0	0	0	0	+	0	±	±	0	±	0	±	±	0	±	±		±	±	±	±
Pseudomonas aeruginosa	0	0	0	0	0	0	0	0	+	+	+	+	+	0	+	+	+	+	±		±	±		±
Burkholderia cepacia	0	0	0	0	0	0	0	0	0				±	0	0	+	0	0	0			0		0
Stenotrophomonas maltophilia	0	0	0	0	0	0	0	0		+	±	±	0	0	0	0	0	0	0	0	±	±		±
Yersinia enterocolitica	0	0	0	0	0	0	±	±	±	+		+	+		+		+	+	+	+	+	+		+
Legionella sp.	0	0	0	0	0	0	0	0	0	0	0	0	0	0	0	0	0	+	+	+	+	+	+	+
Pasteurella multocida	+	+	0	0	0	+	+	+	+	+		+	+	+	+		+	+	+	+	+	+		+
Haemophilus ducreyi	+					0	+	+																
MISC.:																								
Chlamydophila sp	0	0	0	0	0	0	0	0	0	0	0	0	0	0	0	0	0	+	+	+	+	+	+	+
M. pneumoniae	0	0	0	0	0	0	0	0	0	0	0	0	0	0	0	0	0	+	+	+	+	+	+	+
ANAEROBES:																								
Actinomyces	+	±	0	0	0	+	+	+				+		+	+		0	0	±			+		+
Bacteroides fragilis	0	±	0	0	0	0	+	+	0	+	+	0	+	+	+	+	0	0	0	0	0	±	0	±
Prevotella melaninogenica	+	0	0	0	0	+	+	+	+	+	+	+	+	+	+	+	0	0	±		+	+		+
Clostridium difficile	↕							↕				↕	↕	↕	↕	↕	0	0			0	0		0
Clostridium (not difficile)	+	+				+	+	+	+	+	+	+	+	+	+	+	0	±	±		+	±		+
Fusobacterium necrophorum	±	±				+	+	+		+	+		+	+	+	+						±		
Peptostreptococcus sp.	+	+	+	+	+	+	+	+	+	+	+	+	+	+	+	+	0	±	±		+	+		+

+ = **usually susceptible;** ± = **variably susceptible/resistant;** 0 = **usually resistant;** blank = **no data;** ↕ = **active in vitro, but not used clinically**

TABLE 4 (3)

	CEPHALOSPORINS																	
											Oral Agents							
	1st Generation	2nd Generation			3rd/4th Generation (including anti-MRSA)						1st Generation		2nd Generation			3rd Generation		
Organisms	**Cefazolin**	**Cefotetan**	**Cefoxitin**	**Cefuroxime**	**Cefotaxime**	**Ceftizoxime**	**Ceftriaxone**	**Ceftaroline**	**Ceftazidime**	**Cefepime**	**Cefadroxil**	**Cephalexin**	**Cefaclor/Loracarbef**	**Cefprozil**	**Cefuroxime axetil**	**Cefixime**	**Ceftibuten**	**Cefpodox/Cefdinir/Cefditoren**
GRAM-POSITIVE:																		
Strep, Group A, B, C, G	+	+	+	+	+	+	+	+	+	+	+	+	+	+	+	+	+	+
Strep. pneumoniae	+	+	+	+	+	+	+	+	+	+	+	+	+	+	+	+	±	+
Viridans strep	+	+	+	+	+	+	+	+	±	+	+	+	+	0	+	+	0	+
Enterococcus faecalis	0	0	0	0	0	0	0	+	0	0	0	0	0	0	0	0	0	0
Staph. aureus (MSSA)	+	+	+	+	+	+	+	+	±	+	+	+	+	+	+	0	0	+
Staph. aureus (MRSA)	0	0	0	0	0	0	0	+	0	0	0	0	0	0	0	0	0	0
Staph. aureus (CA-MRSA)	0	0	0	0	0	0	0	+	0	0	0	0	0	0	0	0	0	0
Staph. epidermidis	±	±	±	±	±	±	±	+	±	±	±	±	±	±	±	0	0	±
Corynebacterium jeikeium	0	0	0	0	0	0	0		0		0	0	0	0	0	0	0	
Listeria monocytogenes	0	0	0	0	0	0	0		0	0	0	0	0	0	0	0	0	0
GRAM-NEGATIVE																		
Neisseria gonorrhoeae	+	±	±	±	±	±	±	±	±	±	0	0	±	±	±	+	±	+
Neisseria meningitidis	0	±	±	+	+	±	+	+	±	+	0	0	±	±	±	±	±	
Moraxella catarrhalis	±	+	+	+	+	+	+	+	+	+	0	0	±	+	+	+	+	+
Haemophilus influenzae	+	+	+	+	+	+	+	+	+	+		0	+	+	+	+	+	+
Escherichia coli	+	+	+	+	+	+	+	+	+	+	+	+	+	+	+	+	+	+
Klebsiella sp.	+	+	+	+	+	+	+	+	+	+	+	+	+	+	+	+	+	+
E. coli/Klebsiella sp, ESBL+	0	0	0	0	0	0	0	0	0	0	0	0	0	0	0	0	0	0
E. coli/Klebsiella sp, KPC+	0	0	0	0	0	0	0	0	0	0	0	0	0	0	0	0	0	0
Enterobacter sp., AmpC neg	0	±	0	±	+	+	+	+	+	+	0	0	0	0	0	0	±	0
Enterobacter sp., AmpC pos	0	0	0	0	0	0	0	0	0	0	0	0	0	0	0	0	0	0
Serratia sp.	0	+	0	0	+	+	+	+	+	+	0	0	0	0	0	±	±	0
Salmonella sp.					+	+	+	+	+	+	0	0				+	+	+
Shigella sp.					+	+	+		+	+	0	0				+	+	+
Proteus mirabilis	+	+	+	+	+	+	+	+	+	+	+	+	+	+	+	+	+	+
Proteus vulgaris	0	+	+	+	+	+	+	+	+	+	0	0	0	0	0	+	+	±
Providencia sp.	0	+	+	0	+	+	+	+	+	+	0	0	0	0	+	+	+	
Morganella sp.	0	+	+	±	+	+	+	+	+	+	0	0	0	0	±	0	0	0
Citrobacter freundii	0	0	0	0	+	0	+		0	+	0	0	0	0	0	0	0	0
Citrobacter diversus	0	±	±	±	+	+	+	+	+	+	0	0	0	0			+	
Citrobacter sp.	0	±	±	±	+	+	+	+	+	+		0	±	0	±	+	+	+
Aeromonas hydrophila	0	+	±	+	+	+	+	+	+	+						+	+	

+ = **usually susceptible;** ± = **variably susceptible/resistant;** 0 = **usually resistant;** blank = **no data;** ‡ = **active in vitro, but not used clinically**

TABLE 4 (4)

Organisms	CEPHALOSPORINS																	
											Oral Agents							
	1st Generation	2nd Generation			3rd/4th Generation (including anti-MRSA)						1st Generation		2nd Generation			3rd Generation		
	Cefazolin	Cefotetan	Cefoxitin	Cefuroxime	Cefotaxime	Ceftizoxime	Ceftriaxone	Ceftaroline	Ceftazidime	Cefepime	Cefadroxil	Cephalexin	Cefaclor/Loracarbef	Cefprozil	Cefuroxime axetil	Cefixime	Ceftibuten	Cefpodox/Cefdinir/Cefditoren
Acinetobacter sp.	0	0	0	0	0	0	0		±	±	0	0	0	0	0	0	0	
Pseudomonas aeruginosa	**0**	**0**	**0**	**0**	**0**	**0**	**0**	**0**	**+**	**+**	**0**	**0**	**0**	**0**	**0**	**0**	**0**	**0**
Burkholderia cepacia	0	0	0	0	±	±	±	0	+	±	0	0	0	0	0	0	+	
Stenotrophomonas maltophilia	0	0	0	0	0	0	0	0	±	0	0	0	0	0	0	0	0	
Yersinia enterocolitica	0	±	±	±	+	+	+		±	+						+	+	
Legionella sp.	**0**	**0**	**0**	**0**	**0**	**0**	**0**	0	**0**	**0**	**0**	**0**	**0**	**0**	**0**	**0**	**0**	**0**
Pasteurella multocida		+		+	+	+	+			+		0				+		+
Haemophilus ducreyi			+		+	+	+		+							+		
ANAEROBES:																		
Actinomyces						+	+											
Bacteroides fragilis	**0**	**±**[1]	**+**	**0**	**0**	**±**	**0**	0	**0**	**0**		**0**	**0**	**0**	**0**	**0**	**0**	
P. melaninogenica		+	+	+	+	+	±		+	0			+	+	+	+		
Clostridium difficile			**0**		**0**	**0**				**0**								
Clostridium (not difficile)		**+**	**+**	**+**	**+**	**+**	**+**		**+**					**+**	**+**	**0**		
Fusobacterium necrophorum			**+**															
Peptostreptococcus sp.		+	+	+	+	+	+		+	+		+	+	+	+	+		

[1] Cefotetan is less active against B. ovatus, B. distasonis, B. thetaiotaomicron.

+ = **usually susceptible;** ± = **variably susceptible/resistant;** 0 = **usually resistant;** blank = **no data;** ↨ = **active in vitro, but not used clinically**

TABLE 4 (5)

Organisms	AMINO-GLYCOSIDES					MACROLIDES			KETOLIDE	TETRA-CYCLINES		GLYCYL-CYCLINE
	Gentamicin	Tobramycin	Amikacin	Chloramphenicol	Clindamycin	Erythro	Azithromycin	Clarithromycin	Telithromycin	Doxycycline	Minocycline	Tigecycline
GRAM-POSITIVE:												
Strep Group A, B, C, G	0	0	0	+	+	±	±	±	+	±	+	+
Strep. pneumoniae	0	0	0	+	+	±	±	±	+	+	+	+
Enterococcus faecalis	S	S	S	±	0	0	0	0	±	0	0	+
Enterococcus faecium	S	0	0	±	0	0	0	0	0	0	0	+
Enterococci, vanco-resistant	0	0	0	0	0	0	0	0	0	0	0	0
Staph. aureus (MSSA)	+	+	+	±	+	±	±	±	+	±	+	+
Staph. aureus (MRSA)	0	0	0	0	0	0	0	0	0	±	±	+
Staph. aureus (CA-MRSA)					±	±	±	±	±	+	+	+
Staph. epidermidis	±	±	±	0	0	±	0	0	0	0	0	+
C. jeikeium	0	0	0	0	0	0	0	0	0	0	0	+
L. monocytogenes	S	S	S	+		+	+	+	+	+	+	+
GRAM-NEGATIVE:												
Neisseria gonorrhoeae	0	0	0	+	0	±	±	±	↕	±	±	↕
Neisseria meningitidis	0	0	0	+	0	↕	↕		↕	+	+	
Moraxella catarrhalis	+	+	+	+	0	+	+	+	+	+	+	+
Haemophilus influenzae	+	+	+	+	0	±	+	+	+	+	+	+
Aeromonas hydrophila	0			+						+	+	+
Escherichia coli	+	+	+	+	0	0	0	0	0	+	+	+
Klebsiella sp.	+	+	+	±	0	0	0	0	0	±	±	+
E. coli/Klebsiella sp, ESBL+	+	+	+	±	0	0	0	0	0	±	±	+
E. coli/Klebsiella sp, KPC+	0	0	0	0	0	0	0	0	0	0	0	+
Enterobacter sp.	+	+	+	0	0	0	0	0	0	0	0	+
Salmonella sp.				+	0	0	±	0	0	±	±	+

Organisms	GLYCO-/LIPOGLYCO-/LIPO-PEPTIDES							MISCELLANEOUS						
	Daptomycin	Vancomycin	Teicoplanin[NUS]	Telavancin	Fusidic Acid[NUS]	Trimethoprim	TMP-SMX	Nitrofurantoin	Fosfomycin	Rifampin	Metronidazole	Quinupristin-dalfopristin	Linezolid	Colistimethate (Colistin)
GRAM-POSITIVE:														
Strep Group A, B, C, G	+	+	+	+	±	+	↕[2]	+		+	0	+	+	0
Strep. pneumoniae	+[3]	+	+	+	±	±	+	+	+	+	0	+	+	0
Enterococcus faecalis	+	+	+	+	+	+	↕[2]	+	+	±	0	0	+	0
Enterococcus faecium	+	±	±	+		0	0	+		0	0	+	+	0
Enterococci, vanco-resistant	+	0	0	0	0	0	0	0	0	0	0	↕	+	0
Staph. aureus (MSSA)	+	+	+	+	+	±	+	+	+	+	0	+	+	0
Staph. aureus (MRSA)	+	+	+	+	+	±	+	+	+	+	0	+	+	0
Staph. aureus (CA-MRSA)	+	+	+	+	+	+	+	+	+	+	0	+	+	0
Staph. epidermidis	+	+	±	+	+	+	±			+	0	+	+	0
C. jeikeium	+	+	+	+	+	0	0	0		+	0	+	+	0
L. monocytogenes	±	+	+	+		+	+		0	+	0	+	+	0
GRAM-NEGATIVE:														
Neisseria gonorrhoeae	0	0	0	0	+	0	±	+		↕	0	↕		0
Neisseria meningitidis	0	0	0	0	+	±	↕			+	0	0	0	0
Moraxella catarrhalis	0						+			+	0	+	±	
Haemophilus influenzae	0					±	±			+	0	±	±	
Aeromonas hydrophila	0	0	0	0			+			0	0			
Escherichia coli	0	0	0	0	0	+	±	+	+	0	0	0	0	+
Klebsiella sp.	0	0	0	0	0	±	±	±	+	0	0	0	0	+
E. coli/Klebsiella sp, ESBL+	0	0	0	0	0	±	±		+	0	0	0	0	+
E. coli/Klebsiella sp, KPC+	0	0	0	0	0	0	0	0	+	±	0	0	0	+
Enterobacter sp.	0	0	0	0	0	±		±	+	0	0	0	0	+
Salmonella sp.	0	0	0	0	0	±	±	+	+	0	0	0	0	

[2] Although active in vitro, TMP-SMX is not clinically effective for Group A strep pharyngitis or for infections due to E. faecalis.
[3] Although active in vitro, daptomycin is not clinically effective for pneumonia caused by strep pneumonia.

+ = **usually susceptible;** ± = **variably susceptible/resistant;** 0 = **usually resistant;** blank = **no data;** ↕ = **active in vitro, but not used clinically**
Antimicrobials such as azithromycin have high tissue penetration & some such as clarithromycin are metabolized to more active compounds, hence in vivo activity may exceed in vitro activity.
****** Vancomycin, metronidazole given po active vs C. difficile; IV vancomycin not effective. **S = Synergistic with cell wall-active antibiotics.**

TABLE 4 (6)

Organisms	AMINO-GLYCOSIDES					MACROLIDES			KETOLIDE	TETRA-CYCLINES		GLYCYL-CYCLINE	GLYCO-/LIPOGLYCO-/LIPO-PEPTIDES							MISCELLANEOUS						
	Gentamicin	Tobramycin	Amikacin	Chloramphenicol	Clindamycin	Erythro	Azithromycin	Clarithromycin	Telithromycin	Doxycycline	Minocycline	Tigecycline	Daptomycin	Vancomycin	Teicoplanin[NUS]	Telavancin	Fusidic Acid[NUS]	Trimethoprim	TMP-SMX	Nitrofurantoin	Fosfomycin	Rifampin	Metronidazole	Quinupristin-dalfopristin	Linezolid	Colistimethate (Colistin)
Shigella sp.	+	+	+	+	0	0	±	0	0	±	±	+		0	0	0	0	±	±	+		0	0	0	0	
Serratia marcescens	+	+	+	0	0	0	0	0	0	0	0	+	0	0	0	0	0	0	±	0	+	0	0		0	0
Proteus vulgaris	+	+	+	±	0	0	0	0	0	0	0	±	0	0	0	0	0	0	0	0	+	0	0		0	0
Acinetobacter sp.	0	0	±	0	0	0	0	0	0	0	+	±	0	0	0	0	0	0	±		0	0	0		0	+
Pseudomonas aeruginosa	**+**	**+**	**+**	**0**	**0**	**0**	**0**	**0**	**0**	**0**	**0**	**0**	**0**	**0**	**0**	**0**	**0**	**0**	**0**	**0**	**0**	**0**	**0**	**0**	**0**	**+**
Burkholderia cepacia	0	0	0	+	0	0	0	0	0	0	±	±	0	0	0	0	0	+	+	0		0	0		0	0
Stenotrophomonas maltophilia	0	0	0	+	0	0	0	0	0	↕	0	+	0	0	0	0	0	0	+	0			0		0	±
Yersinia enterocolitica	+	+	+	+	0	0	0	0	0	0	0		0				0		+				0		0	
Francisella tularensis	+	+	+	+						+			0						+			+	0		0	
Brucella sp.	**S**	**S**	**S**	**+**	**0**	**0**	**0**	**0**	**0**	**+**	**+**		**0**	**0**	**0**	**0**		↕	↕			**S**	**0**		**0**	
Legionella sp.						**+**	**+**	**+**	↕	↕	↕	↕	**0**				**±**	**+**	**+**				**0**			
Haemophilus ducreyi				↕	↕	+	+			0	0		0	0				0	±				0			
Vibrio vulnificus	±	±	±	↕						S	S		0				0						0			
MISC.:																										
Chlamydophila sp.	**0**	**0**	**0**	**+**	**±**	**+**	**+**	**+**	**+**	**+**	**+**	**+**					**0**	**0**		**0**		↕	**0**	↕	↕	
Mycoplasm pneumoniae	**0**	**0**	**0**	**+**	**0**	**+**	**+**	**+**	**+**	**+**	**+**	**+**					**0**						**0**	**+**	**0**	
Rickettsia sp.	**0**	**0**	**0**	**+**		**±**			**+**	**+**	**+**			**0**	**0**	**0**	**0**						**0**			
Mycobacterium avium			**+**				**+**	**+**		**0**	**0**	**0**											**0**	**0**	**0**	
ANAEROBES:																										
Actinomyces	**0**	**0**	**0**	↕	**+**	**+**	**+**	**+**		**+**	**+**			**+**		**+**	**+**						**0**			
Bacteroides fragilis	**0**	**0**	**0**	↕	**±**	**0**	**0**	**0**		**±**	**±**	**+**		**0**		**0**		↕	**0**				**+**		**±**	
Prevotella melaninogenica	0	0	0	+	+		+	+		+	+	+		0		0	+						+	+		
Clostridium difficile	**0**	**0**	**0**	**±**										**+**	**+**	**+**							**+**	**±**	**±**	
Clostridium (not difficile)**				**+**	**±**	**±**	**+**	**+**		**+**	**+**	**+**		**+**	**+**	**+**	**+**						**S**	↕	↕	
Fusobacterium necrophorum	0	0	0	+	+	0	0	0				+											+			
Peptostreptococcus sp.	0	0	0	+	+	±	+	±	+	+	+	+		+	+	+	+						±		+	

+ = **usually susceptible;** ± = **variably susceptible/resistant;** 0 = **usually resistant;** blank = **no data;** ↕ = **active in vitro, but not used clinically**
Antimicrobials such as azithromycin have high tissue penetration & some such as clarithromycin are metabolized to more active compounds, hence in vivo activity may exceed in vitro activity.
** Vancomycin, metronidazole given po active vs C. difficile; IV vancomycin not effective. **S = Synergistic with cell wall-active antibiotics.**

TABLE 5A – TREATMENT OPTIONS FOR SYSTEMIC INFECTION DUE TO MULTI-DRUG RESISTANT GRAM-POSITIVE BACTERIA

ORGANISM	RESISTANT TO	PRIMARY TREATMENT OPTIONS	ALTERNATIVE TREATMENT OPTIONS	COMMENTS
Enterococcus sp.	Vancomycin, Ampicillin, Penicillin, Gentamicin	E. faecium: **Linezolid** 600 mg IV/po q12h x min 8 wks or **Quinu-dalfo** 7.5 mg/kg IV (central line) x min 8 wks. No clearly effective therapy. Can try **Daptomycin** 8-12 mg/kg IV q24h but monitor for emergence of resistance *(NEJM 365:892, 2011; AAC 57:5013, 2013)*.	E. faecalis: (**Imipenem** 500 mg IV q6h + **Ampicillin** 2 gm IV q4h) x min 8 wks or (**Ceftriaxone** 2 gm IV q12h + **Ampicillin** 2 gm IV q4h) x min 8 wks *(CID 56:1261, 2013)*	Daptomycin successful in single pts *(AAC 56:6064, 2012)*; no activity against E. faecalis. Linezolid bacteriostatic with 40% relapse rate in endocarditis *(AnIM 138:133, 2003)*. Role of telavancin unclear.
Staphylococcus aureus *(See also Table 6 for more details)*	Vancomycin (VISA or VRSA) and all beta lactams (except Ceftaroline)	**Daptomycin** 6-12 mg/kg IV q24h or (**Daptomycin** 6-12 mg/kg IV q24h + **Ceftaroline** 600 mg IV q8h *(AAC 56:5296, 2012)*.	**Telavancin** 10 mg/kg IV q24h or **Linezolid** 600 mg IV/po q12h	Confirm dapto susceptibility as VISA strains may be non-susceptible. If prior vanco therapy (or persistent infection on vanco) there is significant chance of developing resistance to dapto *(JAC 66:1696, 2011)*. Addition of an anti-staphylococcal beta-lactam (nafcillin or oxacillin) may restore susceptibility against Dapto-resistant MRSA *(AAC 54:3161, 2010)*. Combination of Dapto + oxacillin has been successful in clearing refractory MRSA bacteremia *(CID 53:158, 2011)*.
Streptococcus pneumoniae	Penicillin G (MIC $\geq$ 4 μg/mL)	If no meningitis: **Ceftriaxone** 2 gm IV once daily OR **Ceftaroline** 600 mg IV q12h OR **Linezolid** 600 mg IV/po q12h	Meningitis: **Vancomycin** 15 mg/kg IV q8h OR **Meropenem** 2 gm IV q8h	Ceftriaxone 2 gm IV q12h should also work for meningitis.

TABLE 5B: TREATMENT OPTIONS FOR SYSTEMIC INFECTION DUE TO SELECTED MULTI-DRUG RESISTANT GRAM-NEGATIVE BACILLI

The suggested treatment options in this Table are usually not FDA-approved. Suggestions are variably based on in vitro data, animal studies, and/or limited clinical experience.

ORGANISM	RESISTANT TO	PRIMARY TREATMENT OPTIONS	ALTERNATIVE TREATMENT OPTIONS	COMMENTS
Acinetobacter baumannii	All Penicillins, All Cephalosporins, Aztreonam, Carbapenems, Aminoglycosides and Fluoroquinolones	Combination therapy: **Polymyxin E (Colistin) + (Imipenem or Meropenem)** *See Table 10A, page 100,* for guidance on Colistin dosing.	**Minocycline** *(IDCP 20:184, 2012)* (in vitro synergy between minocycline and imipenem)	Refs: *Int J Antimicrob Agts 37:244, 2011; BMC Inf Dis 11:109, 2011*. Detergent effect of colistin reconstitutes antibiotic activity of carbapenems and other drugs. Do not use colistin as monotherapy. Colistin + Rifampin failed to influence infection-related mortality *(CID 57:349, 2013)*.
Extended spectrum beta lactamase (ESBL) producing E. coli, Klebsiella pneumoniae, or other Enterobacteriaceae	All Cephalosporins, TMP-SMX, Fluoroquinolones, Aminoglycosides	**Imipenem** 500 mg IV q6h OR **Meropenem** 1 gm IV q8h OR **Doripenem** 500 mg IV q8h *(CID 39:31, 2004)* (Note: **Dori** is **not** FDA approved for treatment of pneumonia).	Perhaps high dose **Cefepime** 2 gm IV q12h *(See Comment)*. **Polymyxin E (Colistin)** + (**MER** or **IMP**). For dosing, see *Table 10A, page 100*.	For UTI: Fosfomycin, nitrofurantoin *(AAC 53:1278, 2009)*. Avoid PIP-TZ even if suscept in vitro *(AAC 57:3402, 2013)*. Cefepime: outcome correlates with MIC. If MIC $\leq$ 1 μg/mL favorable result. If MIV 1-8 μg/mL unfavorable result *(CID 56:488, 2013)*.
Carbapenemase producing aerobic gram-negative bacilli or P. aeruginosa	All Penicillins, Cephalosporins, Aztreonam, Carbapenems, Aminoglycosides, Fluoroquinolones	Combination therapy: **Polymyxin E (Colistin)** + (**MER** or **IMP**). *See Table 10A, page 100,* for guidance on Colistin dosing.	Pneumonia: Inhaled **Colistin**[NAI] 50-75 mg in 3-4 mL saline via nebulizer + **Colistin** + (**MER** or **IMP**)	*See Table 10A, page 100,* for guidance on **Colistin** dosing. For inhalation dosing, *see Table 10F*.
Stenotrophomonas maltophilia	All beta-lactams except Ticar-Clav, Aminoglycosides, Fluoroquinolones	**TMP-SMX** 8-10 mg/kg/day IV divided q6h/q8h/q12h (based on TMP component)	**Ticar-Clav** 3.1 gm IV q4-6h	

TABLE 6 – SUGGESTED MANAGEMENT OF SUSPECTED OR CULTURE-POSITIVE COMMUNITY-ASSOCIATED METHICILLIN-RESISTANT S. AUREUS INFECTIONS

(See footnote[1] for doses)

IDSA Guidelines: *CID 52 (Feb 1):1, 2011*. With the magnitude of the clinical problem and a number of new drugs, it is likely new data will require frequent revisions of the regimens suggested. *(See page 2 for abbreviations)*.
NOTE: Distinction between community and hospital strains of MRSA blurring.

CLINICAL ILLNESS	ABSCESS, NO IMMUNOSUPPRESSION, OUT-PATIENT CARE	PNEUMONIA	BACTEREMIA OR POSSIBLE ENDOCARDITIS OR BACTEREMIC SHOCK	TREATMENT FAILURE *(See footnote[2])*
Management *Drug doses in footnote.*	I&D alone may be sufficient, especially for boil or smaller abscess (e.g., < 5cm). For larger abscesses, multiple lesions, systemic inflammatory response syndrome: I&D PLUS **TMP-SMX** 1 DS (2 DS if BMI > 40) po bid OR **Clinda** 300-450 mg po tid (450 mg dose if BMI > 40) OR **Doxy** 100 mg po bid or **Minocycline** 100 mg po bid	**Vanco** IV or **linezolid** IV	**Vanco** 15-20 mg/kg IV q8-12 h. Confirm adequate vanco troughs of 15-20 µg/mL Switch to alternative regimen if **vanco** MIC > 2 µg/mL. Some reports of failure if **vanco** MIC = 2 µg/mL but whether this is mediated by insensitivity to **vancomycin** per se or to other factor unclear *(JID 204:340, 2011)*. If patient has slow response to vancomycin and isolate has MIC = 2, consider alternative therapy. **Dapto** 6 mg/kg IV q24h (FDA-approved dose but some authorities recommend 8-12 mg/kg for MRSA bacteremia)	**Dapto** 8-12 mg/kg IV q24h; confirm in vitro susceptibility as prior vanco therapy may select for daptomycin non-susceptibility (MIC >1 µg/mL) & some VISA strains are daptomycin non-susceptible. Use combination therapy for bacteremia or endocarditis: dapto + beta-lactam combination therapy [dapto 8-12 mg/kg IV q24h + (Nafcillin 2 gm IV q4h OR Oxacillin 2 gm IV q4h OR Ceftaroline 600 mg IV q8h) appears effective against MRSA strains as salvage therapy even if non-susceptible to dapto *(Int J Antimicrob Agents, 2013 Aug 11, Epub ahead of print, AAC 54:3161, 2010, AAC 56:6192, 2013)*. **Ceftaroline** 600 mg q8h IV *(J Antimicrob Chemother 67:1267, 2012, J Infect Chemother 19:42, 2013, Int J Antimicrob Agents 2013 Aug 11, Epub ahead of print)*. **Linezolid** 600 mg IV/PO q12h (Linezolid is bacteriostatic and should not be used as a single agent in suspected endovascular infection). **Telavancin** 10 mg/kg q24h IV
Comments	**Fusidic acid** 500 mg tid (not available in the US) **+ rifampin** also an option; do not use rifampin alone as resistance rapidly emerges. Patients not responding after 2-3 days should be evaluated for complicated infection and switched to **vancomycin**.	Prospective study of **Linezolid** vs **Vanco** showed slightly higher cure rate with Linezolid, no difference in mortality *(CID 54:621, 2012)*.	Efficacy of IV **TMP-SMX** vs CA-MRSA uncertain. IV **TMP-SMX** was inferior to **vanco** vs bacteremic MSSA *(AnIM 117:390, 1992)*.	

[1] **Clindamycin:** 300 mg po tid. **Daptomycin:** 6 mg/kg IV q24h is the standard, FDA-approved dose for bacteremia and endocarditis but 8-12 mg/kg q24h is recommended by some and for treatment failures. **Doxycycline or minocycline:** 100 mg po bid. **Linezolid:** 600 mg po/IV bid. **Quinupristin-dalfopristin (Q-D):** 7.5 mg per /kg IV q8h via central line. **Rifampin:** Long serum half-life justifies dosing 600 mg po q24h; however, frequency of nausea less with 300 mg po bid. **TMP-SMX-DS:** Standard dose 8–10 mg per kg per day. For 70 kg person = 700 mg TMP component per day. **TMP-SMX** contains 160 mg TMP and 800 mg SMX. The dose for treatment of CA-MRSA skin and soft tissue infections (SSTI) is 1 DS tablet twice daily. **Vancomycin:** 1 gm IV q12h; up to 45-60 mg/kg/day in divided doses may be required to achieve target trough concentrations of 15-20 mcg/mL recommended for serious infections.

[2] The median duration of bacteremia in endocarditis is 7-9 days in patients treated with vancomycin *(AnIM 115:674, 1991)*. Longer duration of bacteremia, greater likelihood of endocarditis *(JID 190:1140, 2004)*. Definition of failure unclear. Clinical response should be factored in. **Unsatisfactory clinical response especially if blood cultures remain positive >2-4 days.**

TABLE 7 – DRUG DESENSITIZATION METHODS

Penicillin. ***Oral route (Pen VK) preferred.*** 1/3 pts develop transient reaction, usually mild. **Perform in ICU setting. Discontinue β-blockers. Have IV line, epinephrine, ECG, spirometer available.** Desensitization works as long as pt is receiving Pen; allergy returns after discontinuance. History of Steven-Johnson, exfoliative dermatitis, erythroderma are contraindications. Skin testing for evaluation of Pen allergy: Testing with major determinant (benzyl Pen polylysine) and minor determinants has negative predictive value (97-99%). Risk of systemic reaction to skin testing <1% *(Ann Allergy Asth Immunol 106:1, 2011)*. General refs: *CID 35:26, 2002; Am J Med 121:572, 2008; Curr Clin Topics ID 13:131, 1993.*

- **Method:** Prepare dilutions using **Pen-VK** oral soln, 250 mg/5mL. Administer each dose @ 15 min intervals in 30 mL water/flavored bev. After Step 14 observe pt for 30 min, then give full therapeutic dose by route of choice. Ref: *Allergy, Prin & Prac, Mosby, 1993, p. 1726.*

Step	Dilution (mg/mL)	mL Administered	Dose/Step		Cumulative Dose Given	
			mg	units	mg	units
1	0.5	0.1	0.05	80	0.05	80
2	0.5	0.2	0.1	160	0.15	240
3	0.5	0.4	0.2	320	0.35	560
4	0.5	0.8	0.4	640	0.75	1,200
5	0.5	1.6	0.8	1,280	1.55	2,480
6	0.5	3.2	1.6	2,560	3.15	5,040
7	0.5	6.4	3.2	5,120	6.35	10,160
8	5	1.2	6	9,600	12.35	19,760
9	5	2.4	12	19,200	24.35	38,960
10	5	4.8	24	38,400	48.35	77,360
11	50	1	50	80,000	98.35	157,360
12	50	2	100	160,000	198.35	317,360
13	50	4	200	320,000	398.35	637,360
14	50	8	400	640,000	798.35	1,277,360

TMP-SMX. Perform in hospital/clinic. Refs: *CID 20:849, 1995; AIDS 5:311, 1991.*

- **Method:** Use **TMP-SMX** oral susp, (40 mg TMP/200 mg SMX)/5 mL. Take with 6 oz water after each dose. Corticosteroids, antihistaminics NOT used.

Hour	Dose (TMP/SMX) (mg)
0	0.004/0.02
1	0.04/0.2
2	0.4/2
3	4/20
4	40/200
5	160/800

Penicillin. *Parenteral (Pen G)* *route*. Follow procedures/notes under Oral (Pen-VK) route. Ref: *Allergy, Prin & Prac, Mosby, 1993, p. 1726.*

- **Method:** Administer **Pen G** IM, IV or sc as follows:

Step	Dilution (units/mL)	mL Administered	Dose/Step (units)	Cumulative Dose Given (units)
1	100	0.2	20	20
2		0.4	40	60
3		0.8	80	140
4	1,000	0.2	200	340
5		0.4	400	740
6		0.8	800	1,540
7	10,000	0.2	2,000	3,540
8		0.4	4,000	7,540
9		0.8	8,000	15,540
10	100,000	0.2	20,000	35,540
11		0.4	40,000	75,540
12		0.8	80,000	155,540
13	1,000,000	0.2	200,000	355,540
14		0.4	400,000	755,540
15		0.8	800,000	1,555,540

Ceftriaxone. Ref: *Allergol Immunopathol (Madr) 37:105, 2009.*

- **Method:** Infuse **Ceftriaxone** IV @ 20 min intervals as follows:

Day	Dose (mg)
1	0.001, then 0.01, then 0.1, then 1
2	1, then 5, then 10, then 50
3	100, then 250, then 500
4	1000

Desensitization Methods for Other Drugs (References)

- **Imipenem-Cilastatin.** *See Ann Pharmacother 37:513, 2003.*
- **Meropenem.** *See Ann Pharmacother 37:1424, 2003.*
- **Daptomycin.** *See Ann All Asthma Immun 100:87, 2008.*
- **Ceftazidime.** *Curr Opin All Clin Immunol 6(6): 476, 2006.*
- **Vancomycin.** *Intern Med 45:317, 2006.*

TABLE 8 – RISK CATEGORIES OF ANTIMICROBICS IN PREGNANCY

DRUG	FDA CATEGORIES*	DRUG	FDA CATEGORIES	DRUG	FDA CATEGORIES	DRUG	FDA CATEGORIES
Antibacterial Agents:		**Antifungal Agents:** *(CID 27:1151, 1998)*		**Antimycobacterial Agents:**		**Antiviral Agents:** *(continued)*	
Aminoglycosides:		Amphotericin B preparations	B	Bedaquiline	B	Fosamprenavir	C
Amikacin, gentamicin, isepamicin^{NUS},		Anidulafungin	C	Quinine	**X**	Foscarnet	C
netilmicin^{NUS}, streptomycin & tobramycin	**D**	Caspofungin	C	Capreomycin	C	Ganciclovir	C
Beta Lactams		Fluconazole (150 mg SD		Clofazimine/cycloserine	"avoid"	Indinavir	C
Penicillins; pens + BLI;		for vaginal candidiasis)	C	Dapsone	C	Interferons	C
cephalosporins; aztreonam	B	Fluconazole (other regimens, uses)	D	Ethambutol	"safe"	Lamivudine	C
Imipenem/cilastatin	C	Itraconazole, ketoconazole, flucytosine	C	Ethionamide	"do not use"	Lopinavir/ritonavir	C
Meropenem, ertapenem, doripenem	B	Micafungin	C	INH, pyrazinamide	C	Maraviroc	B
Chloramphenicol	C	Posaconazole	C	Rifabutin	B	Nelfinavir	B
Ciprofloxacin, oflox, levo, gati,		Terbinafine	B	Rifampin	C	Nevirapine	C
gemi, moxi	C	Voriconazole	**D**	Thalidomide	**X**	Oseltamivir	C
Clindamycin	B	**Antiparasitic Agents:**		**Antiviral Agents:**		Raltegravir	C
Colistin	C	Albendazole/mebendazole	C	Abacavir	C	Ribavirin	**X**
Daptomycin	B	Artemether/lumefantrine	C	Acyclovir	B	Rilpivirine	B
Fosfomycin	B	Atovaquone/proguanil; atovaquone alone	C	Adefovir	C	Rimantadine	C
Fidaxomicin	B	Chloroquine	C	Amantadine	C	Ritonavir	B
Fusidic acid[1]	*See Footnote [1]*	Dapsone	C	Atazanavir	B	Saquinavir	B
Linezolid	C	Eflornithine	C	Cidofovir	C	Simeprevir	C (X w/ribavirin)
Macrolides:		Ivermectin	C	Cobicistat	B	Sofosbuvir	B (X w/ribavirin)
Erythromycins/azithromycin	B	Mefloquine	B	Darunavir	B	Stavudine	C
Clarithromycin	C	Miltefosine	**X**	Delavirdine	C	Telbivudine	B
Metronidazole	B	Nitazoxanide	B	Didanosine (ddI)	B	Tenofovir	B
Nitrofurantoin	B	Pentamidine	C	Dolutegravir	B	Tipranavir	C
Polymyxin B	C	Praziquantel	B	Efavirenz	**D**	Valacyclovir	B
Quinupristin-Dalfopristin	B	Proguanil	C	Elvitegravir/cobicistat/	B	Valganciclovir	C
Rifaximin	C	Pyrimethamine/pyrisulfadoxine	C	emtricitabine/tenofovir		Zalcitabine	C
Sulfonamides/trimethoprim	C	Quinidine	C	Emtricitabine	B	Zanamivir	C
Telavancin	C			Enfuvirtide	B	Zidovudine	C
Telithromycin	C			Entecavir	C		
Tetracyclines, tigecycline	**D**			Etravirine	B		
Tinidazole	C			Famciclovir	B		
Vancomycin	C						

* **FDA Pregnancy Categories: A** = Adequate studies in pregnant women, no risk; **B** = Animal reproduction studies, no fetal risk; no controlled studies in pregnant women; **C** = Animal reproduction studies have shown fetal adverse effect; no controlled studies in humans; potential benefit may warrant use despite potential risk; **D** = Evidence of human fetal risk; potential benefit may warrant use despite potential risk; **X** = Animal and human studies demonstrate fetal abnormalities; risks in pregnant women clearly exceed potential benefits

[1] **Fusidic acid^{NUS}**: potential for neonatal kernicterus

TABLE 9A – SELECTED PHARMACOLOGIC FEATURES OF ANTIMICROBIAL AGENTS

For pharmacodynamics, see Table 9B; for Cytochrome P450 interactions, see Table 9C. Table terminology key at bottom of each page. Additional footnotes at end of Table 9A, page 90.

DRUG	REFERENCE DOSE/ROUTE	PREG RISK	FOOD EFFECT (PO)[1]	ORAL %AB	PEAK SERUM LEVEL (μg/mL)	PROTEIN BINDING (%)	VOL OF DISTRIB (Vd)	AVER SERUM T½, hrs[2]	BILE PEN (%)[3]	CSF[4]/ BLOOD (%)	CSF PEN[5]	AUC (μg*hr/mL)	Tmax (hr)
PENICILLINS: Natural													
Benz Pen G	1.2 million units IM	B			0.15 (SD)								
Penicillin G	2 million units IV	B			20 (SD)	65	0.35 L/kg		500	5-10	Yes: Pen-sens S. pneumo		
Penicillin V	500 mg po	B	Tab/soln no food	60–73	5–6 (SD)	65		0.5					
PEN'ASE-RESISTANT PENICILLINS													
Cloxacillin[NUS]	500 mg po	B	Cap no food	50	7.5–14 (SD)	95	0.1 L/kg	0.5					1–1.5
Dicloxacillin	500 mg po	B	Cap no food	37	10–17 (SD)	98	0.1 L/kg	0.7	5-8				1–1.5
Nafcillin	500 mg	B			30 (SD)	90–94	27.1 L Vss	0.5–1	>100	9–20	Yes	18.1	
Oxacillin	500 mg	B			43 (SD)	90–94	0.4 L/kg	0.5–0.7	25	10-15	Yes		
AMINOPENICILLINS													
Amoxicillin	500 mg po	B	Cap/tab/susp ± food	80	5.5-7.5 (SD)	17	0.36 L/kg	1.2	100–3000	13–14	Yes (IV only)	22	1–2
Amoxicillin ER	775 mg po	B	Tab + food		6.6 (SD)	20		1.2-1.5				29.8	3.1
AM-CL	875/125 mg po	B	Cap/tab/susp ± food	80/30–98	11.6/2.2 (SD)	18/25		1.4/1.1	100–3000			AM: 26.8 - CL: 5.1	
AM-CL-ER	2 tabs [2000/125 mg]	B	Tab + food		17/2.1 (SD)	18/25		1.3/1.0				AM: 71.6 - CL: 5.3	AM: 1.5 CL: 1.03
Ampicillin	2 gm IV	B			100 (SD)	18–22	0.29 L/kg	1.2	100–3000	13–14	Yes		
AM-SB	3 gm IV	B			109-150/48-88 (SD)	28/38		1.2				AM: 120- SB: 71	
ANTIPSEUDOMONAL PENICILLINS													
PIP-TZ	3/.375 gm IV	B			242/24 (SD)	16–48	PIP: 0.24 L/kg	1.0	>100			PIP: 242 - TZ: 25	
TC-CL	3.1 gm IV	B			330/8 (SD)	45/25	TC: 9.7 Vss	1.2/1.0				TC: 485 - CL: 8.2	
CEPHALOSPORINS—1st Generation													
Cefadroxil	500 mg po	B	Cap/tab/susp ± food	90	16 (SD)	20	0.31 L/kg V/F	1.5	22			47.4	
Cefazolin	1 gm IV	B			188 (SD)	73–87	0.19 L/kg	1.9	29–300	1–4	No	236	
Cephalexin	500 mg po	B	Cap/tab/susp ±	90	18 (SD)	5–15	0.38 L/ kg V/F	1.0	216			29	1

Preg Risk: FDA risk categories: A = no risk in adequate human studies, **B** = animal studies suggest no fetal risk, but no adequate human studies, **C** = adverse fetal effects in animals, but no adequate studies in humans; potential benefit may warrant use despite potential risk, **D** = evidence of human risk, but potential benefit may warrant use despite potential risk **X** = evidence of human risk that clearly exceeds potential benefits; **Food Effect (PO dosing): + food** = take with food, **no food** = take without food, **± food** = take with or without food; **Oral % AB** = % absorbed; **Peak Serum Level: SD** = after single dose, **SS** = steady state after multiple doses; **Volume of Distribution (Vd): V/F** = Vd/oral bioavailability, **Vss** = Vd at steady state, **Vss/F** = Vd at steady state/oral bioavailability; **CSF Penetration:** therapeutic efficacy comment based on dose, usual susceptibility or target organism & penetration into CSF; **AUC** = area under drug concentration curve; **24hr** = AUC 0-24; **Tmax** = time to max plasma concentration.

TABLE 9A (2) *(Footnotes at the end of table)*

DRUG	REFERENCE DOSE/ROUTE	PREG RISK	FOOD EFFECT (PO)[1]	ORAL %AB	PEAK SERUM LEVEL (μg/mL)	PROTEIN BINDING (%)	VOL OF DISTRIB (Vd)	AVER SERUM T½, hrs[2]	BILE PEN (%)[3]	CSF[4]/ BLOOD (%)	CSF PEN[5]	AUC (μg*hr/mL)	Tmax (hr)
CEPHALOSPORINS—2nd Generation													
Cefaclor	500 mg po	B	Cap/susp ± food	93	13 (SD)	22–25	0.33 L/kg V/F	0.8	≥60			20.5	0.5–1.0
Cefaclor–ER	500 mg po	B	Tab + food		8.4 (SD)	22–25		0.8	≥60			18.1	2.5
Cefotetan	1 gm IV	B			158 (SD)	78–91	10.3 L	4.2	2–21			504	
Cefoxitin	1 gm IV	B			110 (SD)	65–79	16.1 L Vss	0.8	280	3	No		
Cefprozil	500 mg po	B	Tab/susp ± food	95	10.5 (SD)	36	0.23 L/kg Vss/F	1.5				25.7	
Cefuroxime	1.5 gm IV	B			100 (SD)	33–50	0.19 L/kg Vss	1.5	35–80	17–88	Marginal	150	
Cefuroxime axetil	250 mg tabs po	B	Susp + food; Tab ± food	52	4.1 (SD)	50	0.66 L/kg V/F	1.5				12.9	2.5
CEPHALOSPORINS—3rd Generation													
Cefdinir	300 mg po	B	Cap/susp ± food	25	1.6 (SD)	60–70	0.35 L/kg V/F	1.7				7.1	2.9
Cefditoren pivoxil	400 mg po	B	Tab + food	16	4 (SD)	88	9.3 L Vss/F	1.6				20	1.5–3.0
Cefixime	400 mg tabs po	B	Tab/susp ± food	50	3–5 (SD)	65	0.93 L/kg V/F	3.1	800			25.8	4
Cefotaxime	1 gm IV	B			100	30–51	0.28 L/kg	1.5	15–75	10	Yes	70	
Cefpodoxime proxetil	200 mg po	B	Tab + food Susp ± food	46	2.3 (SD)	40	0.7 L/kg V/F	2.3	115			14.5	2-3
Ceftazidime	1 gm IV	B			69 (SD)	<10	0.24 L/kg Vss	1.9	13–54	20–40	Yes	127	
Ceftibuten	400 mg po	B	Cap/susp no food	80	15 (SD)	65	0.21 L/kg V/F	2.4				73.7	2.6
Ceftizoxime	1 gm IV	B			60 (SD)	30	0.34 L/kg	1.7	34–82			85	
Ceftriaxone	1 gm IV	B			150 (SD), 172-204 (SS)	85–95	5.8-13.5 L	8	200–500	8–16	Yes	1006	
CEPHALOSPORIN—4th Generation and Anti-MRSA													
Cefepime	2 gm IV	B			164 (SD)	20	18 L Vss	2.0	10-20	10	Yes	284.8	
Ceftaroline	600 mg IV	B			21.3	20	20.3 Vss	2.7				56.3	
Ceftobiprole[NUS]	500 mg IV	B			33–34.2 (SD)	16	18 L Vss	2.9–3.3				116	
CARBAPENEMS													
Doripenem	500 mg IV	B			23	8.1	16.8 L Vss	1	117 (0–611)			36.3	
Ertapenem	1 gm IV	B			154	95	0.12 L/kg Vss	4	10			572.1	
Imipenem	500 mg IV	C			40	15–25	0.27 L/kg	1	minimal	8.5	+[6]	42.2	
Meropenem	1 gm IV	B			49	2	0.29 L/kg	1	3–300	Approx. 2	+	72.5	

Preg Risk: FDA risk categories: A = no risk, **B** = No risk – human studies, **C** = toxicity in animals - inadequate human studies, **D** = human risk, but benefit may outweigh risk, **X** = fetal abnormalities – risk > benefit; **Food Effect (PO dosing): + food** = take with food, **no food** = take without food, **± food** = take with or without food; **Oral % AB** = % absorbed; **Peak Serum Level: SD** = after single dose, **SS** = steady state after multiple doses; **Volume of Distribution (Vd): V/F** = Vd/oral bioavailability, **Vss** = Vd at steady state, **Vss/F** = Vd at steady state/oral bioavailability; **CSF Penetration:** therapeutic efficacy comment based on dose, usual susceptibility or target organism & penetration into CSF; **AUC** = area under drug concentration curve; **24hr** = AUC 0-24; **Tmax** = time to max plasma concentration.

TABLE 9A (3) *(Footnotes at the end of table)*

DRUG	REFERENCE DOSE/ROUTE	PREG RISK	FOOD EFFECT (PO)[1]	ORAL %AB	PEAK SERUM LEVEL (μg/mL)	PROTEIN BINDING (%)	VOL OF DISTRIB (Vd)	AVER SERUM T½, hrs[2]	BILE PEN (%)[3]	CSF[4]/ BLOOD (%)	CSF PEN[5]	AUC (μg*hr/mL)	Tmax (hr)
MONOBACTAM													
Aztreonam	1 gm IV	B			90 (SD)	56	12.6 L Vss	2	115–405	3–52	±	271	
AMINOGLYCOSIDES													
Amikacin, gentamicin, kanamycin, tobramycin—*see Table 10D, page 109, for dose & serum levels*		D				0–10	0.26 L/kg	2.5	10–60	0–30	No; intrathecal dose: 5–10 mg		
Neomycin	po	D	Tab/soln ± food	<3	0								
FLUOROQUINOLONES[7]													
Ciprofloxacin	750 mg po q12h	C	± food	70	3.6 (SS)	20–40	2.4 L/kg	4	2800–4500			31.6 (24 hr)	1-2
	400 mg IV q12h	C	± food		4.6 (SS)	20–40		4	2800–4500	26	1 μg/mL: Inadequate for Strep. sp. *(CID 31:1131, 2000)*.	25.4 (24 hr)	
	500 mg ER po q24h	C	± food		1.6 (SS)	20–40		6.6				8 (24 hr)	1.5
	1000 mg ER po q24h	C	± food		3.1 (SS)	20–40		6.3				16 (24 hr)	2.0
Gemifloxacin	320 mg po q24h	C	Tab ± food	71	1.6 (SS)	55–73	2-12 L/kg Vss/F	7				9.9 (24 hr)	0.5-2.0
Levofloxacin	500 mg po/IV q24h	C	Tab ± food	99	5.7/6.4 (SS)	24–38	74-112 L Vss	7		30–50		PO:47.5, IV 54.6 (24 hr)	PO: 1.3
	750 mg po/IV q24h	C	Tab ± food Oral soln: no food	99	8.6/12.1 (SS)	24–38	244 L Vss	7				PO 90.7, IV 108 (24 hr)	PO: 1.6
Moxifloxacin	400 mg po/IV q24h	C	Tab ± food	89	4.2-4.6/4.5 (SS)	30–50	2.2 L/kg	10–14		>50	Yes *(CID 49:1080, 2009)*	PO 48, IV 38 (24 hr)	PO: 1-3
Ofloxacin	400 mg po/IV q12h	C	Tab ± food	98	4.6/6.2 (SS)	32	1-2.5 L/kg	7				PO 82.4, IV 87 (24 hr)	PO: 1-2
Prulifloxacin[NUS]	600 mg po		± food		1.6 (SD)	45	1231L	10.6–12.1		negligible	no	7.3	1
MACROLIDES, AZALIDES, LINCOSAMIDES, KETOLIDES													
Azithromycin	500 mg po	B	Tab/Susp ± food	37	0.4 (SD)	7–51	31.1 L/kg	68	High			4.3	2.5
	500 mg IV	B			3.6 (SD)	7–51	33.3 L/kg	12/68				9.6 (24 hr, pre SS)	
Azithromycin-ER	2 gm po	B	Susp no food	∝ 30	0.8 (SD)	7–50	31.1 L/kg	59	High			20	5.0
Clarithromycin	500 mg po q12h	C	Tab/Susp ± food	50	3–4 (SS)	65–70	4 L/kg	5–7	7000			20 (24 hr)	2.0-2.5
	1000 mg ER po q24h	C	Tab + food	∝ 50	2–3 (SS)	65–70							5-8

Preg Risk: FDA risk categories: A = no risk, **B** = No risk – human studies, **C** = toxicity in animals - inadequate human studies, **D** = human risk, but benefit may outweigh risk, **X** = fetal abnormalities – risk > benefit; **Food Effect (PO dosing): + food** = take with food, **no food** = take without food, **± food** = take with or without food; **Oral % AB** = % absorbed; **Peak Serum Level: SD** = after single dose, **SS** = steady state after multiple doses; **Volume of Distribution (Vd): V/F** = Vd/oral bioavailability, **Vss** = Vd at steady state, **Vss/F** = Vd at steady state/oral bioavailability; **CSF Penetration:** therapeutic efficacy comment based on dose, usual susceptibility or target organism & penetration into CSF; **AUC** = area under drug concentration curve; **24hr** = AUC 0-24; **Tmax** = time to max plasma concentration.

TABLE 9A (4) *(Footnotes at the end of table)*

DRUG	REFERENCE DOSE/ROUTE	PREG RISK	FOOD EFFECT (PO)[1]	ORAL %AB	PEAK SERUM LEVEL (µg/mL)	PROTEIN BINDING (%)	VOL OF DISTRIB (Vd)	AVER SERUM T½, hrs[2]	BILE PEN (%)[3]	CSF[4]/ BLOOD (%)	CSF PEN[5]	AUC (µg*hr/mL)	Tmax (hr)
MACROLIDES, AZALIDES, LINCOSAMIDES, KETOLIDES *(continued)*													
Erythromycin													
Oral (various)	500 mg po	B	Tab/Susp no food DR Caps ± food	18–45	0.1–2 (SD)	70–74	0.6 L/kg	2–4		2–13	No		Delayed Rel: 3
Lacto/glucep	500 mg IV	B			3–4 (SD)	70–74		2–4					
Telithromycin	800 mg po q24h	C	Tab ± food	57	2.3 (SS)	60–70	2.9 L/kg	10	7			12.5 (24 hr)	1
Clindamycin	150 mg po	B	Cap ± food	90	2.5 (SD)	85–94	1.1 L/kg	2.4	250–300		No		0.75
	900 mg IV	B			14.1 (SS)	85–94		2.4	250–300		No		
MISCELLANEOUS ANTIBACTERIALS													
Chloramphenicol	1 gm po q6h	C	Cap ± food	High	18 (SS)	25–50	0.8 L/kg	4.1		45–89	Yes		
Colistin (Polymyxin E)	150 mg IV	C			5–7.5 (SD)	approx 50	0.34 L/kg	2–3	0		No *(AAC 53:4907, 2009)*		
Daptomycin	4–6 mg/kg IV q24h	B			58–99 (SS)	92	0.1 L/kg Vss	8–9		0-8		494-632 (24 hr)	
Doxycycline	100 mg po	B	Tab/cap/susp + food		1.5–2.1 (SD)	93	53–134 L Vss	18	200–3200		No (26%)	31.7	2
Fosfomycin	3 gm po	-	Sachet ± food		26 (SD)	<10	136.1 L Vss/F	5.7				150	
Fusidic acid[NUS]	500 mg po	C	Tab + food	91	30 (SD)	95-99	0.3 L/kg	5-15	100–200			315	2–4
Linezolid	600 mg po/IV q12h	C	Tab/susp ± food	100	15–20 (SS)	31	40–50 L Vss	5		60–70	Yes *(AAC 50:3971, 2006)*	PO: 276/IV: 179 (24 hr)	PO: 1.3
Metronidazole	500 mg po/IV q6h	B	ER tab no food, Tab/cap ± food		20–25 (SS)	20	0.6–0.85 L/kg	6–14	100	45–89		560 (24 hr)	Immed Rel: 1.6 ER: 6.8
Minocycline	200 mg po	D	Cap/tab ± food		2.0–3.5 (SD)	76	80–114 L Vss	16	200–3200			48.3	2.1
Polymyxin B	0.45-3.4 mg/kg/day IV	C			2.8 (SS, not peak)	60		4.5-6 (old data)			No	66.9 (24 hr)	
Quinu-Dalfo	7.5 mg/kg IV q8h	B			3.2/8 (SS)		0.45/0.24 L/kg Vss	1.5				Quinu: 21.6 Dal: 31.8	
Rifampin	600 mg po	C	Cap no food	70-90	4–32 (SD)	80	0.65 L/kg Vss	2–5	10,000	7–56	Yes	58	1.5–2
Rifaximin	200 mg po	C	Tab ± food	<0.4	0.004–0.01 (SD)	67.5		2–5			No	0.008	1
Tetracycline	250 mg po	D	Cap no food		1.5–2.2 (SD)		1.3 L/kg	6–12	200–3200		No (7%)	30	2–4
Telavancin	10 mg/kg q24h	C			108 (SS)	90	0.13 L/kg	8.1	Low			780 (24 hr)	

Preg Risk: FDA risk categories: A = no risk, **B** = No risk – human studies, **C** = toxicity in animals - inadequate human studies, **D** = human risk, but benefit may outweigh risk, **X** = fetal abnormalities – risk > benefit; **Food Effect (PO dosing): + food** = take with food, **no food** = take without food, **± food** = take with or without food; **Oral % AB** = % absorbed; **Peak Serum Level: SD** = after single dose, **SS** = steady state after multiple doses; **Volume of Distribution (Vd): V/F** = Vd/oral bioavailability, **Vss** = Vd at steady state, **Vss/F** = Vd at steady state/oral bioavailability; **CSF Penetration:** therapeutic efficacy comment based on dose, usual susceptibility or target organism & penetration into CSF; **AUC** = area under drug concentration curve; **24hr** = AUC 0-24; **Tmax** = time to max plasma concentration.

TABLE 9A (5) *(Footnotes at the end of table)*

DRUG	REFERENCE DOSE/ROUTE	PREG RISK	FOOD EFFECT (PO)[1]	ORAL %AB	PEAK SERUM LEVEL (µg/mL)	PROTEIN BINDING (%)	VOL OF DISTRIB (Vd)	AVER SERUM T½, hrs[2]	BILE PEN (%)[3]	CSF[4]/ BLOOD (%)	CSF PEN[5]	AUC (µg*hr/mL)	Tmax (hr)
MISCELLANEOUS ANTIBACTERIALS *(continued)*													
Tigecycline	50 mg IV q12h	D			0.63 (SS)	71–89	7–9 L/kg	42	138		No	4.7 (24 hr)	
Trimethoprim (TMP)	100 mg po	C	Tab ± food	80	1 (SD)	44	100-120 V/F	8–15					1–4
TMP-SMX-DS	160/800 mg po q12h	C	Tab/susp ± food	85	1–2/40–60 (SS)	TMP: 44 SMX: 70	TMP: 100-120 L SMX: 12-18 L	TMP: 11 SMX: 9	100–200	50/40			TMP PO: 1–4 SMX IV: 1–4
	160/800 mg IV q8h	C			9/105 (SS)				40–70				
Vancomycin	1 gm IV q12h	C			20–50 (SS)	<10–55	0.7 L/kg	4–6	50	7–14			
ANTIFUNGALS													
Amphotericin B:													
Standard	0.4–0.7 mg/kg IV	B			0.5–3.5 (SS)		4 L/kg	24		0		17	
Lipid (ABLC)	5 mg/kg IV	B			1–2.5 (SS)		131 L/kg	173				14 (24 hr)	
Cholesteryl complex	4 mg/kg IV	B			2.9 (SS)		4.3 L/kg	39				36 (24 hr)	
Liposomal	5 mg/kg IV	B			83 (SS)		0.1-0.4 L/kg Vss	6.8 ± 2.1				555 (24 hr)	
Fluconazole	400 mg po/IV	D	Tab/susp ± food	90	6.7 (SD)	10	50 L V/F	20–50		50–94	Yes		PO: 1–2
	800 mg po/IV	D	Tab/susp ± food	90	Approx. 14 (SD)			20–50					
Itraconazole	200 mg po soln	C	Soln no food	Low	0.3–0.7 (SD)	99.8	796 L	35		0		29.3 (24 hr)	2.5 Hydroxy: 5.3
Ketoconazole	200 mg po	C	Tab ± food	75	1-4 (SD)	99	1.2 L/kg	6-9	ND	<10	No	12	1–2
Posaconazole	200 mg po (susp) 300 mg po q24h (tab)	C	All preps + food	54 (tab)	Susp 0.2-1.0 (SD) Tab 2.1-2.9 (SS)	98-99	287L	20-66			Yes (*JAC 56:745, 2005*)	Susp 15.1 Tab 37.9-51.6	All preps 3–5
Voriconazole	200 mg po q12h	D	Tab/susp no food	96	3 (SS)	58	4.6 L/kg Vss	6		22–100	Yes (*CID 37:728, 2003*)	39.8 (24 hr)	1–2
Anidulafungin	200 mg IV x 1, then 100 mg IV q24h	C			7.2 (SS)	>99	30-50 L	26.5			No	112 (24 hr)	
Caspofungin	70 mg IV x 1, then 50 mg IV qd	C			9.9 (SD)	97	9.7 L Vss	9–11			No	87.3 (24 hr)	
Flucytosine	2.5 gm po	C	Cap ± food	78-90	30–40 (SD)		0.6 L/kg	3–6		60–100	Yes		2
Micafungin	150 mg IV q24h	C			16.4 (SS)	>99	0.39 L/kg	15–17			No	167 (24 hr)	
ANTIMYCOBACTERIALS													
Bedaquiline	400 mg po qd	B	Tab + food	ND	3.3 (Wk 2)	>99	~ 60x total body water Vss	24–30	ND	ND	ND	22 (24hr)	5
Capreomycin	15 mg/kg IM	C			25–35 (SD)	ND	0.4 L/kg	2–5	ND	<10	No	ND	1–2
Cycloserine	250 mg po	C	Cap, no food	70-90	4–8 (SD)	<20	0.47 L/kg	10	ND	54–79	Yes	110	1–2
Ethambutol	25 mg/kg po	C	Tab + food	80	2–6 (SD)	10–30	6 L/kg Vss/F	4		10–50	No	29.6	2–4

Preg Risk: FDA risk categories: A = no risk, **B** = No risk – human studies, **C** = toxicity in animals - inadequate human studies, **D** = human risk, but benefit may outweigh risk, **X** = fetal abnormalities – risk > benefit; **Food Effect (PO dosing): + food** = take with food, **no food** = take without food, **± food** = take with or without food; **Oral % AB** = % absorbed; **Peak Serum Level: SD** = after single dose, **SS** = steady state after multiple doses; **Volume of Distribution (Vd): V/F** = Vd/oral bioavailability, **Vss** = Vd at steady state, **Vss/F** = Vd at steady state/oral bioavailability; **CSF Penetration:** therapeutic efficacy comment based on dose, usual susceptibility or target organism & penetration into CSF; **AUC** = area under drug concentration curve; **24hr** = AUC 0-24; **Tmax** = time to max plasma concentration.

TABLE 9A (6) *(Footnotes at the end of table)*

DRUG	REFERENCE DOSE/ROUTE	PREG RISK	FOOD EFFECT (PO)[1]	ORAL %AB	PEAK SERUM LEVEL (μg/mL)	PROTEIN BINDING (%)	VOL OF DISTRIB (Vd)	AVER SERUM T½, hrs[2]	BILE PEN (%)[3]	CSF[4]/BLOOD (%)	CSF PEN[5]	AUC (μg*hr/mL)	Tmax (hr)
ANTIMYCOBACTERIALS *(continued)*													
Ethionamide	500 mg po	C	Tab ± food	90	2.2 (SD)	10-30	80 L	1.9	ND	∞100	Yes	10.3	1.5
Isoniazid	300 mg po	C	Tab/syrup no food	100	3–5 (SD)		0.6-1.2 L/kg	0.7–4		Up to 90	Yes	20.1	1-2
Para-aminosalicylic acid (PAS)	4 gm po	C	Gran + food	ND	20 (SD)	50-73	0.9-1.4 L/kg (V/F)	0.75–1.0	ND	10–50	Marg	108	8
Pyrazinamide	20–25 mg/kg po	C	Tab ± food	95	30–50 (SD)	5–10		10–16		100	Yes	500	2
Rifabutin	300 mg po	B	Cap + food	20	0.2-0.6 (SD)	85	9.3 L/kg (Vss)	32–67	300–500	30–70	ND	8.6	2.5–4.0
Rifampin	600 mg po	C	Cap no food	70–90	4–32 (SD)	80	0.65 L/kg Vss	2–5	10,000	7–56	Yes	58	1.5–2
Rifapentine	600 mg po q72h	C	Tab + food	ND	15 (SS)	98	70 L	13-14	ND	ND	ND	320 over 72hrs	4.8
Streptomycin	1 gm IV	D			25–50 (SD)	0–10	0.26 L/kg	2.5	10–60	0–30	No; Intrathecal: 5–10 mg		
ANTIPARASITICS													
Albendazole	400 mg po	C	Tab + food		0.5–1.6	70							Sulfoxide: 2–5
Artemether/ Lumefantrine	4 tabs po: 80/480 mg	C	Tab + food		Art: 9 (SS), D-Art: 1, Lum: 5.6-9 (not SS)			Art: 1.6, D-Art: 1.6, Lum: 101					Art: 1.5–2.0 Lum: 6-8
Atovaquone	750 mg po bid	C	Susp + food	47	24 (SS)	99.9	0.6 L/kg Vss	67		<1	No	801 (750 mg x 1)	
Dapsone	100 mg po q24h	C	Tab ± food	70–100	1.1 (SS)	70	1.5 L/kg	10–50					2-6
Ivermectin	12 mg po	C	Tab no food		0.05–0.08 (SD)		9.9 L/kg						4
Mefloquine	1.25 gm po	B	Tab + food		0.5–1.2 (SD)	98	20 L/kg	13–24 days					17
Miltefosine	50 mg po tid	X	Cap + food		31 (SD)	95		7–31 (long) *AAC 52:2855, 2008*					
Nitazoxanide	500 mg po tab	B	Tab/susp + food		9–10 (SD)	99						41.9 Tizoxanide	Tizoxanide: 1-4
Proguanil[8]	100 mg	C	Tab + food		No data	75	1600-2000 L V/F						
Pyrimethamine	25 mg po	C	Tab ± food	"High"	0.1–0.3 (SD)	87	3 L/kg	96					2-6
Praziquantel	20 mg per kg po	B	Tab + food	80	0.2–2.0 (SD)		8000 L V/F	0.8–1.5				1.51	1-3
Tinidazole	2 gm po	B	Tab + food	48	48 (SD)	12	50 L	13				902	1.6

Preg Risk: FDA risk categories: A = no risk, **B** = No risk – human studies, **C** = toxicity in animals - inadequate human studies, **D** = human risk, but benefit may outweigh risk, **X** = fetal abnormalities – risk > benefit; **Food Effect (PO dosing): + food** = take with food, **no food** = take without food, **± food** = take with or without food; **Oral % AB** = % absorbed; **Peak Serum Level: SD** = after single dose, **SS** = steady state after multiple doses; **Volume of Distribution (Vd): V/F** = Vd/oral bioavailability, **Vss** = Vd at steady state, **Vss/F** = Vd at steady state/oral bioavailability; **CSF Penetration:** therapeutic efficacy comment based on dose, usual susceptibility or target organism & penetration into CSF; **AUC** = area under drug concentration curve; **24hr** = AUC 0-24; **Tmax** = time to max plasma concentration.

TABLE 9A (7) *(Footnotes at the end of table)*

DRUG	REFERENCE DOSE/ROUTE	PREG RISK	FOOD EFFECT (PO)[1]	ORAL %AB	PEAK SERUM LEVEL (μg/mL)	PROTEIN BINDING (%)	VOL OF DISTRIB (Vd)	AVER SERUM T½, hrs[2]	BILE PEN (%)[3]	CSF[4]/ BLOOD (%)	CSF PEN[5]	AUC (μg*hr/mL)	Tmax (hr)
ANTIVIRAL DRUGS—NOT HIV													
Acyclovir	400 mg po bid	B	Tab/cap/susp ± food	10–20	1.21 (SS)	9–33	0.7 L/kg	2.5–3.5				7.4 (24 hr)	
Adefovir	10 mg po	C	Tab ± food	59	0.02 (SD)	≤4	0.37 L/kg Vss	7.5				0.22	1.75
Boceprevir	800 mg po q8h	B	Cap + food		1.7 (SS)	75	772L (Vss/F)	3.4	ND	ND	ND	5.41 (8 hr)	
Cidofovir w/Probenecid	5 mg/kg IV	C			19.6 (SD)	<6	0.41 L/kg (VSS)	2.2	ND	0	No	40.8	1.1
Entecavir	0.5 mg po q24h	C	Tab/soln no food	100	4.2 ng/mL (SS)	13	>0.6 L/kg V/F	128–149				0.14	0.5–1.5
Famciclovir	500 mg po	B	Tab ± food	77	3–4 (SD)	<20	1.1 L/kg*	2–3				8.9 Penciclovir	Penciclovir: 0.9
Foscarnet	60 mg/kg IV	C			155 (SD)	4	0.46 L/kg	<1	No			2195 μM*hr	
Ganciclovir	5 mg/kg IV	C			8.3 (SD)	1–2	0.7 L/kg Vss	3.5				24.5	
Oseltamivir	75 mg po bid	C	Cap/susp ± food	75	0.065/0.35[9] **(SS)**	3	23-26 L/kg Vss*	1–3				5.4 (24 hr) Carboxylate	
Peramivir	600 mg IV	?			35-45 (SD)	<30	ND	7.7–20.8	ND	ND	ND	90-95	ND
Ribavirin	600 mg po	X	Tab/cap/soln + food	64	0.8 (SD)		2825 L V/F	44				25.4	2
Rimantadine	100 mg po	C	Tab ± food		0.05–0.1 (SD)		17-19 L/kg	25				3.5	6
Simeprevir	400 mg po	B	Tab +/- food	ND	0.6	61–65	ND	0.5-0.75	ND	ND	ND	0.9	0.5–2
Sofosbuvir	150 mg po	C	Cap + food	ND	ND	>99.9	ND	41	ND	ND	ND	57.5 (24 hr)	4–6
Telaprevir	750 mg po q8h	B	Tab+ food (high fat)		3.51 (SS)	59-76	252L (V/F)	4.0-4.7 (SD)	ND	ND	ND	22.3 (8 hr)	
Telbivudine	600 mg po q24h	B	Tab/soln ± food		3.7 (SS)	3.3	>0.6 L/kg V/F	40–49				26.1 (24 hr)	2
Valacyclovir	1000 mg po	B	Tab ± food	55	5.6 (SD)	13–18	0.7 L/kg	3				19.5 Acyclovir	
Valganciclovir	900 mg po q24h	C	Tab/soln + food	59	5.6 (SS)	1–2	0.7 L/kg	4				29.1 Ganciclovir	Ganciclovir: 1–3

Preg Risk: FDA risk categories: A = no risk, **B** = No risk – human studies, **C** = toxicity in animals - inadequate human studies, **D** = human risk, but benefit may outweigh risk, **X** = fetal abnormalities – risk > benefit; **Food Effect (PO dosing): + food** = take with food, **no food** = take without food, **± food** = take with or without food; **Oral % AB** = % absorbed; **Peak Serum Level: SD** = after single dose, **SS** = steady state after multiple doses; **Volume of Distribution (Vd): V/F** = Vd/oral bioavailability, **Vss** = Vd at steady state, **Vss/F** = Vd at steady state/oral bioavailability; **CSF Penetration:** therapeutic efficacy comment based on dose, usual susceptibility or target organism & penetration into CSF; **AUC** = area under drug concentration curve; **24hr** = AUC 0-24; **Tmax** = time to max plasma concentration.

TABLE 9A (8) *(Footnotes at the end of table)*

DRUG	REFERENCE DOSE/ROUTE	PREG RISK	FOOD EFFECT (PO Prep)	ORAL %AB	PEAK SERUM LEVEL (μg/mL)	PROT BIND (%)	VOL DISTRIB (Vd)	AVER SERUM T½, hrs[2]	INTRA CELL T½, HOURS	CSF[4]/ BLOOD (%)	CSF PEN[5]	AUC (μg*hr/mL)	Tmax (hr)
ANTI RETROVIRAL DRUGS													
Abacavir (ABC)	600 mg po q24h	C	Tab/soln ± food	83	4.3 (SS)	50	0.86 L/kg	1.5	12–26	Low	No	12 (24 hr)	
Atazanavir (ATV)	400 mg po q24h	B	Cap + food	Good	2.3 (SS)	86	88.3 L V/F	7		Intermed	?	22.3 (24 hr)	2.5
Darunavir (DRV)	(600 mg+ 100 mg RTV) bid	B	Tab + food	82	3.5 (SS)	95	2 L/kg	15		Intermed	?	116.8 (24 hr)	2.5–4.0
Delavirdine (DLV)	400 mg po tid	C	Tab ± food	85	19 ± 11(SS)	98		5.8	3			180 μM*hr	1
Didanosine (ddI)	400 mg EC[10] po	B	Cap no food	30–40	?	<5	308-363 L	1.4	25–40	Intermed	?	2.6	2
Dolutegravir	50 mg po	B	± food		3.67 (SS)	>99	17.4 (V/F)	14				53.6	2-3
Efavirenz (EFV)	600 mg po q24h	D	Cap/tab no food	42	4.1 (SS)	99	252 L V/F	52–76	3			184 μM*hr (24 hr)	3-5
Elvitegravir (with cobicistat, TDF and FTC, as Stribild)	150 mg (EVG) 150 mg (Cobi) 200 mg (FTC) 300 mg (TDF)	B	Tab + Food	No data	EVG: 1.7 Cobi: 1.1	98-99 (EVG, cobi)		EVG: 12.9 Cobi: 3.5				EVG: 23 Cobi: 8.3	EVG: 4 Cobi: 3
Emtricitabine (FTC)	200 mg po q24h	B	Cap/soln ± food	93	1.8 (SS)	<4		10	39	Intermed	?	10 (24 hr)	1–2
Enfuvirtide (ENF)	90 mg sc bid	B		84	5 (SS)	92	5.5 L	4				97.4 (24 hr)	
Etravirine (ETR)	200 mg po bid	B	Tab + food		0.3 (SS)	99.9		41	2			9 (24 hr)	2.5–4.0
Fosamprenavir (FPV)	(700 mg po+ 100 mg RTV) bid	C	Boosted ped susp + food Adult susp no food Tab ± food	No data	6 (SS)	90		7.7	No data	Intermed	?	79.2 (24 hr)	2.5
Indinavir (IDV)	800 mg po tid	C	Boosted cap + food, Cap alone no food	65	9 (SS)	60		1.2–2		High	Yes	92.1 μM*hr (24 hr)	0.8
Lamivudine (3TC)	300 mg po	C	Tab/soln ± food	86	2.6 (SS)	<36	1.3 L/kg	5–7	18–22	Intermed	?	11	
Lopinavir/RTV (LPV/r)	400 mg po bid	C	Soln + food	No data	9.6 (SS)	98–99		5–6 (LPV)		Intermed	?	186 LPV	LPV: 4
Maraviroc (MVC)	300 mg po bid	B	Tab ± food	33	0.3–0.9 (SS)	76	194 L	14–18		Intermed	?	3 (24 hr)	0.5-4.0
Nelfinavir (NFV)	1250 mg po bid	B	Tab/powd + food	20–80	3–4 (SS)	98	2-7 L/kg V/F	3.5–5		Low	No	53 (24 hr)	
Nevirapine (NVP)	200 mg po	C	Tab/susp ± food	>90	2 (SD)	60	1.2 L/kg Vss	25–30	4	High	Yes	110 (24 hr)	
Raltegravir (RAL)	400 mg po bid	C	Tab ± food	No data	5.4 (SS)	83	287 L Vss/F	9		Intermed	?	28.6 μM*hr (24 hr)	3
Rilpivirine	25 mg po	B	Tab + food	No data	0.1–0.2 (SD)	99.7	152L	45–50	ND	-	-	2.4 (24 hr)	-
Ritonavir (RTV)	600 mg po bid	B	Cap/soln + food	65	11.2 (SS)	98–99	0.41 L/kg V/F	3–5		Low	No		Soln: 2-4

Preg Risk: FDA risk categories: A = no risk, **B** = No risk – human studies, **C** = toxicity in animals - inadequate human studies, **D** = human risk, but benefit may outweigh risk, **X** = fetal abnormalities – risk > benefit; **Food Effect (PO dosing): + food** = take with food, **no food** = take without food, **± food** = take with or without food; **Oral % AB** = % absorbed; **Peak Serum Level: SD** = after single dose, **SS** = steady state after multiple doses; **Volume of Distribution (Vd): V/F** = Vd/oral bioavailability, **Vss** = Vd at steady state, **Vss/F** = Vd at steady state/oral bioavailability; **CSF Penetration:** therapeutic efficacy comment based on dose, usual susceptibility or target organism & penetration into CSF; **AUC** = area under drug concentration curve; **24hr** = AUC 0-24; **Tmax** = time to max plasma concentration.

TABLE 9A (9) *(Footnotes at the end of table)*

DRUG	REFERENCE DOSE/ROUTE	PREG RISK	FOOD EFFECT (PO Prep)	ORAL %AB	PEAK SERUM LEVEL (µg/mL)	PROT BIND (%)	VOL DISTRIB (Vd)	AVER SERUM T½, hrs[2]	INTRA CELL T½, HOURS	CSF[4]/ BLOOD (%)	CSF PEN[5]	AUC (µg*hr/mL)	Tmax (hr)
ANTI RETROVIRAL DRUGS *(continued)*													
Saquinavir (SQV)	(1000 + 100 RTV) mg po bid	B	Tab/cap + food	4	0.37 min (SS conc)	97	700 L Vss	1–2		Low	No	29.2 (24 hr)	
Stavudine (d4T)	40 mg bid	C	Cap/soln ± food	86	0.54 (SS)	<5	46L	1	3-5			2.6 (24 hr)	1
Tenofovir (TDF)	300 mg po	B	Tab ± food	25 fasted 39 w/food	0.3 (SD)	<1–7	1.3 L/kg Vss	17	>60	Low	No	2.3	1
Tipranavir (TPV)	(500 + 200 RTV) mg po bid	C	Cap/soln + food		47–57 (SS)	99.9	7.7–10 L	5.5–6		Low	No	1600 µM*hr (24 hr)	3
Zidovudine (ZDV)	300 mg po	C	Tab/cap/syrup ± food	60	1–2	<38	1.6 L/kg	0.5–3	11	High	Yes	2.1	0.5-1.5

1 Refers to adult oral preparations unless otherwise noted.
2 Assumes CrCl >80 mL per min.
3 Peak concentration in bile/peak concentration in serum x 100. If blank, no data.
4 CSF levels with inflammation
5 Judgment based on drug dose & organism susceptibility. CSF concentration ideally ≥10 above MIC.
6 Concern over seizure potential; *see Table 10B*.
7 Take all po FQs 2–4 hours before sucralfate or any multivalent cations: Ca^{++}, Fe^{++}, Zn^{++}.
8 Given with atovaquone as Malarone for malaria prophylaxis.
9 Oseltamivir/oseltamivir carboxylate.
10 EC = enteric coated.

Preg Risk: FDA risk categories: A = no risk, **B** = No risk – human studies, **C** = toxicity in animals - inadequate human studies, **D** = human risk, but benefit may outweigh risk, **X** = fetal abnormalities – risk > benefit; **Food Effect (PO dosing): + food** = take with food, **no food** = take without food, **± food** = take with or without food; **Oral % AB** = % absorbed; **Peak Serum Level: SD** = after single dose, **SS** = steady state after multiple doses; **Volume of Distribution (Vd): V/F** = Vd/oral bioavailability, **Vss** = Vd at steady state, **Vss/F** = Vd at steady state/oral bioavailability; **CSF Penetration:** therapeutic efficacy comment based on dose, usual susceptibility or target organism & penetration into CSF; **AUC** = area under drug concentration curve; **24hr** = AUC 0-24; **Tmax** = time to max plasma concentration.

TABLE 9B – PHARMACODYNAMICS OF ANTIBACTERIALS*

BACTERIAL KILLING/PERSISTENT EFFECT	DRUGS	THERAPY GOAL	PK/PD MEASUREMENT
Concentration-dependent/Prolonged persistent effect	Aminoglycosides; daptomycin; ketolides; quinolones; metro	High peak serum concentration	24-hr AUC[1]/MIC
Time-dependent/No persistent effect	Penicillins; cephalosporins; carbapenems; monobactams	Long duration of exposure	Time above MIC
Time-dependent/Moderate to long persistent effect	Clindamycin; erythro/azithro/clarithro; linezolid; tetracyclines; vancomycin	Enhanced amount of drug	24-hr AUC[1]/MIC

* Adapted from *Craig, WA: IDC No. Amer 17:479, 2003* & *Drusano, G.L.: CID 44:79, 2007*

TABLE 9C– ENZYME -AND TRANSPORTER- MEDIATED INTERACTIONS OF ANTIMICROBIALS

Cytochrome P450 isoenzyme terminology:
e.g., 3A4: **3** = family, **A** = subfamily, **4** = gene; **PGP** = P-glycoprotein; **UGT** = uridine diphosphate glucuronosyltransferase; **OATP** = organic anion transporter polypeptide; **OCT** = organic cation transporter; **BCRP** = breast cancer resistance protein

DRUG	Substrate	Inhibits	Induces
Antibacterials			
Azithromycin (all)	PGP	PGP (weak)	
Chloramphenicol		2C19, 3A4	
Ciprofloxacin (all)		1A2, 3A4 (minor)	
Clarithromycin (all)	3A4	3A4, PGP	
Erythromycin (all)	3A4, PGP	3A4, PGP	
Metronidazole		2C9	
Nafcillin			2C9 (?), 3A4
Quinu-Dalfo		3A4	
Rifampin	PGP		1A2, 2C9, 2C19, 2D6 (Weak), 3A4, PGP
Telithromycin		3A4, PGP	
TMP-SMX	SMX: 2C9 (major), 3A4	SMX: 2C9 TMP: 2C8	
Trimethoprim		2C8	
Antifungals			
Fluconazole (400 mg)	3A4 (minor), PGP	2C9, 2C19, 3A4, UGT	
Itraconazole	3A4, PGP	3A4, PGP	
Ketoconazole	3A4	3A4, PGP	
Posaconazole	PGP, UGT	3A4, PGP	
Terbinafine	2D6		
Voriconazole	2C9, 2C19, 3A4	2C9, 2C19 (major), 3A4	
Antimycobacterials (Also Rifampin, above)			
Bedaquiline	3A4		
Ethionamide	3A4 (?)		
Isoniazid	2E1	2C19, 3A4	
Rifabutin	3A4		
Rifapentine		2C9, 3A4	3A4, UGT
Dapsone	3A4		

DRUG	Substrate	Inhibits	Induces
Antiparasitics			
Mefloquine	3A4, PGP	PGP	
Praziquantel	3A4		
Proguanil	2C19 (conversion to cycloguanil)		
Tinidazole	3A4		
Antiretrovirals			
Atazanavir	3A4	1A2, 2C9, 3A4	
Cobicistat	3A4, 2D6	3A4, 2D6, PGP, BCRP, OATP1B1, OATP1B3	
Darunavir	3A4	3A4	
Delavirdine	2D6, 3A4	2C9, 2C19, 3A4	
Efavirenz	2B6, 3A4	2B6, 2C9, 2C19	2C19, 3A4
Elvitegravir	CYP3A, UGT		2C9
Etravirine	2C9, 2C19, 3A4	2C9, 2C19 (weak)	3A4
Fosamprenavir	3A4	2C19, 3A4	
Indinavir	3A4, PGP	3A4, PGP	
Lopinavir	3A4	3A4	
Maraviroc	3A4, PGP	2D6	
Nelfinavir	2C9, 2C19, 3A4, PGP	3A4, PGP	3A4
Nevirapine	2B6, 3A4		3A4
Raltegravir	UGT		
Ritonavir	2D6, 3A4, PGP	2B6, 2C9, 2C19, 2D6, 3A4, PGP	3A4, 1A2 (?), 2C9 (?), PGP (?)
Saquinavir	3A4, PGP	3A4, PGP	
Tipranavir	3A4, PGP	1A2, 2C9, 2C19, 2D6	3A4, PGP (weak)

Refs: Hansten PD, Horn JR. The top 100 drug interactions: a guide to patient management 2012; E. Freeland (WA): H&H Publications; 2010; and package inserts.

TABLE 10A – ANTIBIOTIC DOSAGE* AND SIDE-EFFECTS

CLASS, AGENT, GENERIC NAME (TRADE NAME)	USUAL ADULT DOSAGE*	ADVERSE REACTIONS, COMMENTS *(See Table 10B for Summary)*
NATURAL PENICILLINS		
Benzathine penicillin G (Bicillin L-A)	**600,000–1.2 million units IM q2–4 wks**	**Allergic reactions a major issue.** 10% of all hospital admissions give history of pen allergy; but only 10% have allergic reaction if given penicillin. Why? Possible reasons: inaccurate history, waning immunity with age, aberrant response during viral illness, if given **Bicillin C-R IM (procaine Pen + benzathine Pen)** could be reaction to procaine. **Most serious reaction is immediate IgE-mediated anaphylaxis;** incidence only 0.05% but 5-10% fatal. Other IgE-mediated reactions: urticaria, angioedema, laryngeal edema, bronchospasm, abdominal pain with emesis, or hypotension. All appear within 4 hrs. Can form IgE antibody against either the beta-lactam ring or the R-group side chain. **Morbilliform rash after 72 hrs is not IgE-mediated and not serious.** **Serious late allergic reactions:** Coombs-positive hemolytic anemia, neutropenia, thrombocytopenia, serum sickness, interstitial nephritis, hepatitis, eosinophilia, drug fever. **Cross-allergy to cephalosporins and carbapenems** varies from 0-11%. One factor is similarity, or lack of similarity, of side chains. **For pen desensitization,** *see Table 7.* For skin testing, suggest referral to allergist. High **CSF** concentrations cause seizures. Reduce dosage with renal impairment, *see Table 17A.* Allergy refs: *AJM 121:572, 2008; NEJM 354:601, 2006.*
Penicillin G	**Low: 600,000–1.2 million units IM per day** **High: ≥20 million units IV q24h(=12 gm) div q4h**	
Penicillin V (250 & 500 mg caps)	**0.25–0.5 gm po bid, tid, qid before meals & at bedtime.** Pen V preferred over Pen G for oral therapy due to greater acid stability.	
PENICILLINASE-RESISTANT PENICILLINS		
Dicloxacillin (Dynapen) (250 & 500 mg caps)	**0.125–0.5 gm po q6h before meals**	Blood levels ~2 times greater than cloxacillin so preferred for po therapy. Acute hemorrhagic cystitis reported. Acute abdominal pain with GI bleeding without antibiotic-associated colitis also reported.
Flucloxacillin[NUS] (Floxapen, Lutropin, Staphcil)	**0.25–0.5 gm po q6h** **1–2 gm IV q4h**	Cholestatic hepatitis occurs in 1:15,000 exposures: more frequently in age > 55yrs, females and therapy > 2wks duration. Can appear wks after end of therapy and take wks to resolve *(JAC 66:1431, 2011)*. **Recommendation: use only in severe infection.**
Nafcillin (Unipen, Nafcil)	**1–2 gm IV/IM q4h.** Due to > 90% protein binding, need 12gm/day for bacteremia.	Extravasation can result in tissue necrosis. With dosages of 200–300 mg per kg per day hypokalemia may occur. **Reversible neutropenia (over 10% with ≥21-day rx, occasionally WBC <1000 per mm³).**
Oxacillin (Prostaphlin)	**1–2 gm IV/IM q4h.** Due to > 90% protein binding, need 12gm/day for bacteremia.	**Hepatic dysfunction with ≥12 gm per day.** LFTs usually ↑ 2–24 days after start of rx, reversible. In children, more rash and liver toxicity with oxacillin as compared to nafcillin *(CID 34:50, 2002)*.
AMINOPENICILLINS		
Amoxicillin (Amoxil, Polymox)	**250 mg–1 gm po tid**	IV available in UK & Europe. IV amoxicillin rapidly converted to ampicillin. Rash with infectious mono– *see Ampicillin*. Increased risk of cross-allergenicity with oral cephalosporins with identical side-chains: cefadroxil, cefprozil.
Amoxicillin extended release (Moxatag)	**One 775 mg tab po once daily**	Allergic reactions, C. difficile associated diarrhea, false positive test for urine glucose with clinitest.
Amoxicillin-clavulanate (Augmentin) **AM-CL extra-strength peds suspension (ES-600)** **AM-CL-ER—extended release adult tabs**	*See Comment for adult products* **Peds Extra-Strength susp.: 600/42.9 per 5 mL. Dose: 90/6.4 mg/kg div bid.** For adult formulations, *see Comments* IV amox-clav available in Europe	With bid regimen, less clavulanate & less diarrhea. In pts with immediate allergic reaction to AM-CL, ⅓ due to Clav component *(J Allergy Clin Immunol 125:502, 2010)*. Positive blood tests for 1,3-beta D-glucan with IV AM-CL *(NEJM 354:2834, 2006)*. Hepatotoxicity linked to clavulanic acid; AM-CL causes 13-23% of drug-induced liver injury. Onset delayed. Usually mild; rare liver failure *(JAC 66:1431, 2011)*. **Comparison adult Augmentin dosage regimens:** Augmentin 500/125 1 tab po tid Augmentin 875/125 1 tab po bid Augmentin-XR 1000/62.5 2 tabs po bid
Ampicillin (Principen) (250 & 500 mg caps)	**0.25–0.5 gm po q6h.** **50–200 mg/kg IV/day.**	A maculopapular rash occurs (not urticarial), **not true penicillin allergy,** in 65–100% pts with infectious mono, 90% with chronic lymphocytic leukemia, and 15–20% in pts taking allopurinol. EBV-associated rash does not indicate permanent allergy; post-EBV no rash when challenged. Increased risk of true cross-allergenicity with oral cephalosporins with identical side chains: cefaclor, cephalexin, loracarbef.

*NOTE: all dosage recommendations are for adults (unless otherwise indicated) & assume normal renal function.
(See page 2 for abbreviations)

TABLE 10A (2)

CLASS, AGENT, GENERIC NAME (TRADE NAME)	USUAL ADULT DOSAGE*	ADVERSE REACTIONS, COMMENTS *(See Table 10B for Summary)*
AMINOPENICILLINS *(continued)*		
Ampicillin-sulbactam (Unasyn)	**1.5–3 gm IV q6h; for Acinetobacter: 3 gm (Amp 2 gm/Sulb 1 gm) IV q4h**	Supplied in vials: ampicillin 1 gm, sulbactam 0.5 gm or amp 2 gm, sulbactam 1 gm. AM-SB is not active vs pseudomonas. Total daily dose sulbactam ≤4 gm. Increasing resistance of aerobic gram-negative bacilli. Sulbactam doses up to 9-12 gm/day evaluated *(J Infect 56:432, 2008). See also CID 50:133, 2010.*
EXTENDED SPECTRUM PENICILLINS. NOTE: Platelet dysfunction may occur with any of the antipseudomonal penicillins, esp. in renal failure patients.		
Piperacillin (Pipracil) (Hard to find PIP alone; usually PIP-TZ)	**3–4 gm IV q4–6h (max 24 gm/day). For urinary tract infection: 2 gm IV q6h.** *See Comment*	1.85 mEq Na^+ per gm. *See PIP-TZ comment on extended infusion.* For P. aeruginosa infections: 3 gm IV q4h. Associated with bleeding due to impaired platelet aggregation *(JID 155:1242, 1987; J Lab Clin Med 108:217, 1986).*
ANTIPSEUDOMONAL PENICILLINS		
Piperacillin-tazobactam (PIP-TZ) (Zosyn) Prolonged infusion dosing, *see Comment and Table 10E.* Obesity dosing, *see Table 17C .*	**Formulations:** PIP/TZ: **2/0.25 gm (2.25 gm)** PIP/TZ: **3/0.375 gm (3.375 gm)** PIP/TZ: **4/0.5 gm (4.5 gm)** **Standard Dose (no P. aeruginosa): 3.375 gm IV q6h or 4.5 gm IV q8h** **Standard Dose for P. aeruginosa: 3.375 gm IV q4h or 4.5 gm IV q6h**	Based on PK/PD studies, there is emerging evidence in support of **prolonged infusion** of PIP-TZ: Initial "loading" dose of 4.5 gm over 30 min, then ,4 hrs later, start 3.375 gm IV over 4 hrs q 8h (CrCl≥20) or 3.375 gm IV over 4 hrs q12h (CrCl<20) *(CID 44:357, 2007; AAC 54:460, 2010).* • Cystic fibrosis + P. aeruginosa infection: 350-450 mg/kg/day div q4-6h • P. aeruginosa pneumonia: Combine PIP-TZ with CIP or Tobra. Misc: Assoc false-pos galactomannan test for aspergillus, thrombocytopenia 2.79 mEq Na^+ per gram of PIP. For obesity dosing adjustment *see Table 17C , page 219.* In critically ill pts, may contribute to thrombocytopenia *(PLoS One 8(11):e81477).*
Temocillin[NUS]	**2 gm IV q12h.**	Semi-synthetic penicillin stable in presence of classical & ESBLs plus AmpC beta-lactamases. Source: *www.eumedica.be*
Ticarcillin disodium (Ticar)	**3 gm IV q4–6h.**	Coagulation abnormalities common with large doses, interferes with platelet function, ↑ bleeding times; may be clinically significant in pts with renal failure. (4.5 mEq Na^+ per gm)
Ticarcillin-clavulanate (Timentin)	**3.1 gm IV q4–6h.**	Supplied in vials: ticarcillin 3 gm, clavulanate 0.1 gm per vial. 4.5–5 mEq Na^+ per gm. Diarrhea due to clavulanate. Rare reversible cholestatic hepatitis secondary to clavulanate *(ArIM 156:1327, 1996).* In vitro activity vs. Stenotrophomonas maltophilia.
CARBAPENEMS. Review: *AAC 55:4943, 2011.* **NOTE: Cross allergenicity: In studies of pts with history of Pen-allergy but no confirmatory skin testing, 0-11% had allergic reactions with cephalosporin therapy** *(JAC 54:1155, 2004).* **In better studies, pts with positive skin tests for Pen allergy were given Carbapenem: no reaction in 99%** *(Allergy 63:237, 2008; NEJM 354:2835, 2006; J Allergy Clin Immunol 124:167, 2009).* **Increasing reports of carbapenemase-producing aerobic gram-negative bacilli** *(JCM 48:1019, 2010; Ln ID 11:381, 2011; CID 53:49 & 60, 2011).*		
Doripenem (Doribax) Ref: *CID 49:291, 2009. For prolonged infusion dosing, see Table 10E*	Intra-abdominal & complicated UTI: **500 mg IV q8h (1-hr infusion).** For prolonged infusion, *see Table 10E, page 110 .* Do not use for pneumonia	Most common adverse reactions (≥5%): Headache, nausea, diarrhea, rash & phlebitis. Seizure reported in post-marketing surveillance. Can lower serum valproic acid levels. Adjust dose if renal impairment. Somewhat more stable in solution than **IMP** or **MER** *(JAC 65:1023, 2010; CID 49:291, 2009).* FDA safety announcement (01/05/12): Trial of Dori for the treatment of VAP stopped early due to safety concerns. Compared to IMP, patients treated with Dori were observed to have excess mortality and poorer cure rate. **NOTE: Dori is not approved to treat any type of pneumonia; Dori is not approved for doses greater than 500 mg q8h.**
Ertapenem (Invanz)	**1 gm IV/IM q24h.**	**Lidocaine** diluent for IM use; ask about lidocaine allergy. Standard dosage may be inadequate in obesity (BMI ≥40). Reports of DRESS (drug rash eosinophilia systemic symptoms) Syndrome. Visual hallucinations reported *(NZ Med J 122:76, 2009).* No predictable activity vs. P. aeruginosa.
Imipenem + cilastatin (Primaxin) Ref: *JAC 58:916, 2006*	**0.5 gm IV q6h**; for P. aeruginosa: 1 gm q6–8h *(see Comment).*	For infection due to P. aeruginosa, increase dosage to 3 or 4 gm per day div. q8h or q6h. Continuous infusion of carbapenems may be more efficacious & safer *(AAC 49:1881, 2005).* Seizure comment, *see footnote[2], Table 10B, page 104.* Cilastatin blocks enzymatic degradation of Imipenem in lumen of renal proximal tubule & also prevents tubular toxicity.

(See page 2 for abbreviations)

*NOTE: all dosage recommendations are for adults (unless otherwise indicated) & assume normal renal function.

TABLE 10A (3)

CLASS, AGENT, GENERIC NAME (TRADE NAME)	USUAL ADULT DOSAGE*	ADVERSE REACTIONS, COMMENTS *(See Table 10B for Summary)*
CARBAPENEMS *(continued)*		
Meropenem (Merrem)	**0.5–1 gm IV q8h. Up to 2 gm IV q8h for meningitis. Prolonged infusion** in critically ill: If CrCl ≥ 50: 2gm (over 3hr) q8h If CrCl 30-49: 1gm (over 3hr) q8h If CrCl 10-29: 1gm (over 3hr) q12h *(Inten Care Med 37:632, 2011)*.	For seizure incidence comment, *see Table 10B, page 104*. Comments: Does not require a dehydropeptidase inhibitor (cilastatin). Activity vs aerobic gm-neg. slightly ↑ over IMP, activity vs staph & strep slightly ↓; anaerobes: B. ovatus, B. distasonis more resistant to meropenem.
MONOBACTAMS		
Aztreonam (Azactam)	**1 gm q8h–2 gm IV q6h.**	Can be used in pts with allergy to penicillins/cephalosporins. Animal data and a letter raise concern about cross-reactivity with ceftazidime *(Rev Infect Dis 7(Suppl4):S613, 1985; Allergy 53:624, 1998)*; **side-chains of aztreonam and ceftazidime are identical.**
Aztreonam for Inhalation (Cayston)	**75 mg inhaled tid x 28 days.** Use bronchodilator before each inhalation.	Improves respiratory symptoms in CF pts colonized with P. aeruginosa. Alternative to inhaled Tobra. AEs: bronchospasm, cough, wheezing. So far, no emergence of other resistant pathogens. Ref: *Chest 135:1223, 2009.*
CEPHALOSPORINS (1st parenteral, then oral drugs). NOTE: Prospective data demonstrate correlation between use of cephalosporins (esp. 3rd generation) and ↑ risk of C. difficile toxin-induced diarrhea. May also ↑ risk of colonization with vancomycin-resistant enterococci. *See Oral Cephalosporins, page 95*, **for important note on cross-allergenicity.**		
1st Generation, Parenteral		
Cefazolin (Ancef, Kefzol)	**1-1.5 gm IV/IM q8h, occasionally 2 gm IV q8h for serious infections, e.g., MSSA bacteremia (max. 12 gm/day)**	Do not give into lateral ventricles—seizures! No activity vs. community-associated MRSA. Rare failures if cefazolin treatment of MSSA bacteremia due to hyperproduction of type A beta lactamase *(AAC 53:3437, 2009)*.
2nd Generation, Parenteral (Cephamycins): May be active in vitro vs. ESBL-producing aerobic gram-negative bacilli. Do not use as there are no clinical data for efficacy.		
Cefotetan (Cefotan)	**1–3 gm IV/IM q12h. (max. dose not >6 gm q24h).**	Increasing resistance of B. fragilis, Prevotella bivia, Prevotella disiens (most common in pelvic infections); do not use for intra-abdominal infections. Methylthiotetrazole (MTT) side chain can inhibit vitamin K activation. Avoid alcohol-disulfiram reaction.
Cefoxitin (Mefoxin)	**1 gm q8h–2 gm IV/IM q6-8h.**	Increasing resistance of B. fragilis isolates.
Cefuroxime (Kefurox, Ceftin, Zinacef)	**0.75–1.5 gm IV/IM q8h.**	Improved activity against H. influenzae compared with 1st generation cephalosporins. *See Cefuroxime axetil for oral preparation.*
3rd Generation, Parenteral—Use correlates with incidence of C. difficile toxin diarrhea; all are inactivated by ESBLs and amp C cephalosporinase from aerobic gram-negative bacilli.		
Cefoperazone-sulbactam[NUS] (Sulperazon)	**Usual dose (Cefoperazone comp) 1–2 gm IV q12h;** if larger doses, do not exceed 4 gm/day of sulbactam.	In SE Asia & elsewhere, used to treat intra-abdominal, biliary, & gyn. infections. Other uses due to broad spectrum of activity. Possible clotting problem due to side-chain.
Cefotaxime (Claforan)	**1 gm q8–12h to 2 gm IV q4h.**	Maximum daily dose: 12 gm; give as 4 gm IV q8h. Similar to ceftriaxone but requires multiple daily doses.
Ceftazidime (Fortaz, Tazicef)	**Usual dose: 1–2 gm IV/IM q8–12h.** **Prolonged infusion dosing:** Initial dose: 15 mg/kg over 30 min, then immediately begin: If CrCl > 50: 6 gm (over 24 hr) daily If CrCl 31-50: 4 gm (over 24 hr) daily If CrCl 10-30: 2 gm (over 24 hr) daily *(AAC 49:3550, 2005; Infect 37:418, 2009)*.	Often used in healthcare-associated infections, where P. aeruginosa is a consideration. Use may result in ↑ incidence of C. difficile-assoc. diarrhea and/or selection of vancomycin-resistant E. faecium. Risk of cross-allergenicity with aztreonam (same side chain).
Ceftizoxime (Cefizox)	From **1-2 gm IV q8-12h** up to **2 gm IV q4h**.	Maximum daily dose: 12 gm; can give as 4 gm IV q8h
Ceftriaxone (Rocephin)	Commonly used IV dosage in adults: **1-2 gm once daily** Purulent meningitis: **2 gm q12h.** Can give **IM** in 1% lidocaine.	**"Pseudocholelithiasis"** 2° to sludge in gallbladder by ultrasound (50%), symptomatic (9%) *(NEJM 322:1821, 1990)*. More likely with ≥2 gm per day with pt on total parenteral nutrition and not eating *(AnIM 115:712, 1991)*. Clinical significance still unclear but has led to cholecystectomy *(JID 17:356, 1995)* and gallstone pancreatitis *(Ln 17:662, 1998)*. In pilot study: 2 gm once daily by continuous infusion superior to 2 gm bolus once daily *(JAC 59:285, 2007)*. For Ceftriaxone Desensitization, *see Table 7, page 80.*

(See page 2 for abbreviations)

*NOTE: all dosage recommendations are for adults (unless otherwise indicated) & assume normal renal function.

TABLE 10A (4)

CLASS, AGENT, GENERIC NAME (TRADE NAME)	USUAL ADULT DOSAGE*	ADVERSE REACTIONS, COMMENTS *(See Table 10B for Summary)*
CEPHALOSPORINS (1st parenteral, then oral drugs) *(continued)*		
Other Generation, Parenteral: All are substrates for ESBLs & amp C cephalosporinase for aerobic gram-negative bacilli. Cefepime penetrates to target faster than other cephalosporins.		
Cefepime (Maxipime) Obesity dosing, *see Table 17C*	**Usual dose: 1–2 gm IV q8-12h.** **Prolonged infusion dosing:** Initial dose: 15 mg/kg over 30 min, then immediately begin: If CrCl > 60: 6 gm (over 24 hr) daily If CrCl 30-60: 4 gm (over 24 hr) daily If CrCl 11-29: 2 gm (over 24 hr) daily	Active vs P. aeruginosa and many strains of Enterobacter, Serratia, C. freundii resistant to ceftazidime, cefotaxime, aztreonam *(LnID 7:338, 2007)*. More active vs MSSA than 3rd generation cephalosporins. Neutropenia after 14 days rx *(Scand J Infect Dis 42:156, 2010)*. Prolonged or extended infusion: *AAC 57:2907, 2013* Case of red man syndrome reported *(AAC 56:6387,* 2012). FDA Safety warning (June 2012): risk of non-convulsive status epilepticus, especially in pts with renal insufficiency when doses not adjusted. Seizure activity resolved after drug discontinuation and/or hemodialysis in the majority of pts.
Cefpirome[NUS] (HR 810)	**1–2 gm IV q12h**	Similar to cefepime; ↑ activity vs enterobacteriaceae, P. aeruginosa, Gm + organisms. Anaerobes: less active than cefoxitin, more active than cefotax or ceftaz.
Ceftaroline fosamil (Teflaro)	**600 mg IV q12h (1-hr infusion)** Pneumonia/bacteremia 600 mg IV q8h[NAI]. *See Comment*	Avid binding to PBP 2a; active vs. MRSA. Inactivated by Amp C & ESBL enzymes. Approved for MRSA skin and skin structure infections and CAP not due to MRSA. Active in vitro vs. VISA, VRSA. Refs: *CID 52:1156, 2011; Med Lett 53:5, 2011*. Used (NAI) for MRSA pneumonia and bacteremia *(J Infect Chemother 19:42, 2013)*.
Ceftobiprole[NUS]	**0.5 gm IV q8h for mixed gm- neg & gm-pos infections. 0.5 gm IV q12h for gm-pos infections**	Infuse over 2 hrs for q8h dosing, over 1 hr for q12h dosing. Associated with caramel-like taste disturbance. Ref.: *Clin Microbiol Infections 13(Suppl 2):17 & 25, 2007*. Active vs. MRSA.
Oral Cephalosporins		**Cross-Allergenicity: Patients with a history of IgE-mediated allergic reactions to penicillin (e.g., bronchospasm anaphylaxis, angioneurotic edema, immediate urticaria) should not receive a cephalosporin.** If the history is a "measles-like" rash to penicillin, available data suggest a 5–10% risk of rash in such patients; there is no enhanced risk of anaphylaxis. • In pts with history of Pen "reaction" and no skin testing, 0.2-8.4% react to a cephalosporin *(Aller Asthma Proc 26:135, 2006)*. If positive Pen G skin test, only 2% given a cephalosporin will react. Can predict with cephalosporin skin testing, but not easily available *(An IM 141:16, 2004; AJM 125:572, 2008)*. • IgE antibodies against either ring structure or side chains; 80% pts lose IgE over 10 yrs post-reaction *(J Aller Clin Immunol 103:918, 1999)*. Amox, Cefadroxil, Cefprozil have similar side chains; Amp, Cefaclor, Cephalexin, Cephedrine have similar side chains. • If Pen/Ceph skin testing not available or clinically no time, proceed with cephalosporin if history does not suggest IgE-mediated reaction, prior reaction more than 10 yrs ago or cephalosporin side chain differs from implicated Pen. Any of the cephalosporins can result in **C. difficile toxin**-mediated diarrhea/enterocolitis. The reported frequency of nausea/vomiting and non-C. difficile toxin diarrhea is summarized in *Table 10B*. There are **few drug-specific adverse effects, e.g.:** **Cefaclor:** Serum sickness-like reaction 0.1–0.5%—arthralgia, rash, erythema multiforme but no adenopathy, proteinuria or demonstrable immune complexes. Appear due to mixture of drug biotransformation and genetic susceptibility *(Ped Pharm & Therap 125:805, 1994)*. **Cefdinir:** Drug-iron complex causes red stools in roughly 1% of pts. **Cefditoren pivoxil:** Hydrolysis yields pivalate. Pivalate absorbed (70%) & becomes pivaloylcarnitine which is renally excreted; 39–63% ↓ **in serum carnitine concentrations.** Carnitine involved in fatty acid (FA) metabolism & FA transport into mitochondria. Effect transient & reversible. Contraindicated in patients with carnitine deficiency or those in whom inborn errors of metabolism might result in clinically significant carnitine deficiency. Also contains caseinate (milk protein); **avoid if milk allergy** (not same as lactose intolerance). Need gastric acid for optimal absorption. **Cefpodoxime:** There are rare reports of acute liver injury, bloody diarrhea, pulmonary infiltrates with eosinophilia. **Cephalexin:** Can cause false-neg. urine dipstick test for leukocytes.
1st Generation, Oral		
Cefadroxil (Duricef) (500 mg caps, 1 gm tabs)	**0.5–1 gm po q12h.**	
Cephalexin (Keflex) (250 & 500 mg tabs)	**0.25–1 gm po q6h (max 4 gm/day).**	
2nd Generation, Oral		
Cefaclor (Ceclor, Raniclor) (250 & 500 mg caps)	**0.25–0.5 gm po q8h.**	
Cefprozil (Cefzil) (250 & 500 mg tabs)	**0.25–0.5 gm po q12h.**	
Cefuroxime axetil po (Ceftin)	**0.125–0.5 gm po q12h.**	
3rd Generation, Oral		
Cefdinir (Omnicef) (300 mg cap)	**300 mg po q12h or 600 mg q24h.**	
Cefditoren pivoxil (Spectracef)	**400 mg po bid.**	
Cefixime (Suprax) (400 mg tab)	**0.4 gm po q12–24h.**	
Cefpodoxime proxetil (Vantin)	**0.1–0.2 gm po q12h.**	
Ceftibuten (Cedax) (400 mg tab)	**0.4 gm po q24h.**	

(See page 2 for abbreviations)

*NOTE: all dosage recommendations are for adults (unless otherwise indicated) & assume normal renal function.

TABLE 10A (5)

CLASS, AGENT, GENERIC NAME (TRADE NAME)	USUAL ADULT DOSAGE*	ADVERSE REACTIONS, COMMENTS *(See Table 10B for Summary)*
AMINOGLYCOSIDES AND RELATED ANTIBIOTICS—*See Table 10D, page 109, and Table 17A, page 211*		
GLYCOPEPTIDES, LIPOGLYCOPEPTIDES, LIPOPEPTIDES		
Teicoplanin[NUS] (Targocid)	**For septic arthritis—maintenance dose 12 mg/kg per day; S. aureus endocarditis—trough serum levels >20 mcg/mL required (12 mg/kg q12h times 3 loading dose, then 12 mg/kg q24h)**	Hypersensitivity: fever (at 3 mg/kg 2.2%, at 24 mg per kg 8.2%), skin reactions 2.4%. Marked ↓ platelets (high dose ≥15 mg per kg per day). Red neck syndrome less common than with vancomycin.
Telavancin (Vibativ) Lipoglycopeptide Ref: *CID 49:1908, 2009. Med Lett 52:1, 2010.*	10 mg/kg IV q24h if CrCl >50 mL/min. Infuse each dose over 1 hr. Adjust dose if wt ≥30% over IBW, *see Table 10D.*	**Avoid during pregnancy: teratogenic in animals.** Do pregnancy test before therapy. Adverse events: **dysgeusia (taste) 33%;** nausea 27%; vomiting 14%; headache 14%; ↑ creatinine (3.1%); foamy urine; flushing if infused rapidly. In clin trials, **evidence of renal injury** in 3% telavancin vs. 1% vanco. In practice, renal injury reported in 1/3 of 21 complicated pts *(JAC 67:723, 2012).*
Vancomycin (Vancocin) Guidelines Ref: *CID 49:325, 2009.* *See Comments for po dose.* Continuous infusion dosing, *see Table 10E*	**Initial doses based on actual wt, including for obese pts.** Subsequent doses adjusted based on measured trough serum levels. **For critically ill pts, give loading dose of 25-30 mg/kg IV then 15-20 mg/kg IV q8-12h.** Target trough level is 15-20 µg/mL. For individual doses over 1 gm, infuse over 1.5-2 hrs. **Dosing for morbid obesity (BMI ≥40 kg/m²): If CrCl ≥50 mL/min & pt not critically ill:** 30 mg/kg/day divided q8-12h—no dose over 2 gm. Infuse doses of 1 gm or more over 1.5-2 hrs. Check trough levels. **Morbid obesity & critically ill:** Loading dose of 25-30 mg/kg (based on actual wt), then 15-20 mg/kg (actual wt) IV q8-12h. Infuse over 1.5-2 hrs. **Limit maximal single dose to 2 gm.** Oral tabs for C. difficile: 125 mg po q6h Generic drug now available	Vanco treatment failure of MRSA bacteremia associated with Vanco trough concentration <15 µg/mL & MIC > 1 µg/mL *(CID 52:975, 2011)*. IDSA Guideline supports target trough of 15-20 µg/mL *(CID 52:e18, 2011)*. Pertinent issues: • Max Vanco effect vs. MRSA when ratio of AUC/MIC > 400 *(CID 52:975, 2011)*. • MIC values vary with method used, so hard to be sure/compare *(JCM 49:269, 2011)*. • With MRSA Vanco MIC = 1 & Vanco dose >3 gm/day IV, AUC/MIC > 400 in 80% with est. risk of nephrotoxicity of 25%. With MIC = 2 & 4 gm/day IV, AUC/MIC > 400 in only 57% (nephrotoxicity risk 35%) *(CID 52:969, 2011)*. • Higher Vanco doses assoc with nephrotoxicity; causal relation unproven; other factors: renal disease, other nephrotoxic drugs, shock/vasopressors, radiographic contrast *(AAC 52:1330, 2008; AAC 55:3278, 2011; AJM 123:182e1, 2010)*. • If pt clinically failing Vanco (regardless of MIC or AUC/MIC), consider other drugs active vs. MRSA: ceftaroline, daptomycin, linezolid, telavancin. *(see Table 5A for MDR options)*. **PO vanco for C. difficile colitis: 125 mg po q6h.** Commercial po formulation very expensive. Can compound po vanco from IV formulation: 5 g, IV vanco powder + 47.5 mL sterile H_2O, 0.2 gm saccharin, 0.05 gm stevia powder, 40 mL glycerin and then enough cherry syrup to yield 100 mL = 50 mg vanco/mL. Oral dose = 2.5 mL q6h po. **Intrathecal dose:** 5-10 mg/day (infants); 10-20 mg/day (children & adults) to target CSF concentration of 10-20 µg/mL. **Nephrotoxicity:** Risk increases with dose and duration; reversible *(AAC 57:734, 2013)*. **Red Neck Syndrome:** consequence of rapid infusion with non-specific histamine release. **Other adverse effects:** rash, immune thrombocytopenia *(NEJM 356:904, 2007)*, fever, neutropenia, initial report of dose-dependent decrease in platelet count *(JAC 67:727, 2012)*, **IgA bullous dermatitis** *(CID 38:442, 2004)*. **Obesity dosing:** Frequent under dosing *(AJM 121:515, 2008)*. For obesity dosing adjustments, *see Table 17C , page 219.* For CrCl calculation for morbidly obese patient *see Table 10D or Am J Health Sys Pharm 66:642, 2009.*
Daptomycin (Cubicin) (Ref on resistance: *CID 50:S10, 2010*). Case series success in treating right- & left-sided endocarditis with higher dose of 8-10 mg/kg/day *(JAC 68:936 & 2921, 2013)*.	**Skin/soft tissue: 4 mg per kg IV over 2 or 30 minutes q24h** **Bacteremia/right-sided endocarditis: 6 mg per kg IV over 2 or 30 minutes q24h; up to 12 mg/kg IV q24h under study** **Morbid obesity:** base dose on total body weight *(AAC 51:2741, 2007)*, for other dosing recommendations, *see Table 17C , page 219.* Dapto + ceftaroline may work as salvage therapy in pts with refractory MRSA bacteremia *(AAC 57:66, 2013; AAC 56:5296, 2012)*.	**Pneumonia:** Dapto failed to eradicate *S. pneumo* with a trend toward failure to eradicate *S. aureus* in trials of CAP *(CID 46:1142, 2008)*. In animal models Dapto failed vs. *S. pneumo* but efficacious vs. *S. aureus*. Perhaps difference due to Dapto inactivation by surfactant *(JID 191:2149, 2005)*. In theory, less functional surfactant with necrotizing *S. aureus* pneumonia; *S. pneumo* rarely necrotizing. Dapto efficacious in pts with right-sided endocarditis & hematogenous pneumonia; *(NEJM 355:653, 2006)*. Disturbing case report: pt developed *S. aureus* pneumonia while on dapto *(CID 49:1286, 2009)*. **Dapto Resistance:** Can occur de novo, after or during Vanco therapy, or after or during Dapto therapy *(CID 50(Suppl 1):S10, 2010)*. As Dapto MIC increases, MRSA more susceptible to TMP-SMX, nafcillin, oxacillin *(AAC 54:5187, 2010; CID 53:158, 2011)*. **Potential muscle toxicity:** At 4 mg per kg per day, ↑ CPK in 2.8% dapto pts & 1.8% comparator-treated pts. Risk increases if min conc ≥24.3 mg/L *(CID 50:1568, 2010)*. Suggest weekly CPK; DC dapto if CPK exceeds 10x normal level or if symptoms of myopathy and CPK > 1,000. Package insert: stop statins during dapto rx. Dapto interferes with protime reagents & artificially prolongs the PT. *(Blood Coag & Fibrinolysis 19:32, 2008)*. **NOTE:** Dapto well-tolerated in healthy volunteers at doses up to 12 mg/kg q24h x 14d *(AAC 50:3245, 2006)* and in pts given mean dose of 8 mg/kg/day *(CID 49:177, 2009)*. **Immune thrombocytopenia** reported *(AAC 56:6430, 2012)*. Reversible neutropenia with long-term use reported *(CID 56:1353, 2013)*. **Eosinophilic pneumonia**/chronic steroid-dep pneumonia reported *(CID 50:737, 2010; CID 50:e63, 2010)*.

(See page 2 for abbreviations) *NOTE: all dosage recommendations are for adults (unless otherwise indicated) & assume normal renal function.

TABLE 10A (6)

CLASS, AGENT, GENERIC NAME (TRADE NAME)	USUAL ADULT DOSAGE*	ADVERSE REACTIONS, COMMENTS *(See Table 10B for Summary)*
CHLORAMPHENICOL, CLINDAMYCIN(S), ERYTHROMYCIN GROUP, KETOLIDES, OXAZOLIDINONES, QUINUPRISTIN-DALFOPRISTIN		
Chloramphenicol (Chloromycetin)	**50-100 mg/kg/day po/IV div q6h (max 4 gm/day)**	No oral drug distrib in U.S. Hematologic (↓ RBC ~1/3 pts, aplastic anemia 1:21,600 courses). Gray baby syndrome in premature infants, anaphylactoid reactions, optic atrophy or neuropathy (very rare), digital paresthesias, minor disulfiram-like reactions.
Clindamycin (Cleocin)	**0.15–0.45 gm po q6h. 600–900 mg IV/IM q8h**.	Based on number of exposed pts, these drugs are the most frequent cause of **C. difficile toxin-mediated diarrhea**. In most severe form can cause pseudomembranous colitis/toxic megacolon. Available as caps, IV soln, topical (for acne) & intravaginal suppositories & cream. **Used to inhibit synthesis of toxic shock syndrome toxins.**
Lincomycin (Lincocin)	**0.6 gm IV/IM q8h.**	Risk of C. difficile colitis. Rarely used.
Erythromycin Group (Review drug interactions before use)		
Azithromycin (Zithromax) **Azithromycin ER** (Zmax)	**po preps:** Tabs 250 & 600 mg. Peds suspension: 100 & 200 mg per 5 mL. Adult ER suspension: 2 gm. Dose varies with indication, *see Table 1*, Acute otitis media *(page 11)*, acute exac. chronic bronchitis *(page 37)*, Comm.-acq. pneumonia *(pages 39–40)*, & sinusitis *(page 50)*. **IV:** 0.5 gm per day.	**Motilin:** activates duodenal/jejunal receptors that initiate peristalsis. Erythro (E) and E esters activate motilin receptors and cause uncoordinated peristalsis with resultant anorexia, nausea or vomiting. Less binding and GI distress with azithromycin/clarithromycin. No peristalsis benefit *(JAC 59:347, 2007)*. Systemic erythro in 1st 2 wks of life associated with **infantile hypertrophic pyloric stenosis** *(J Ped 139:380, 2001)*. **Frequent drug-drug interactions:** *see Table 22, page 224*. Major concern is prolonged QT_c interval on EKG. **Prolonged QTc:** Erythro, clarithro & azithro all increase risk of ventricular tachycardia via increase in QTc interval. Can be congenital or acquired *(NEJM 358:169, 2008)*. Two studies show variable degree of increased risk of CV death among azithro recipients: presumably from prolonged QTc *(NEJM 366:1881, 2012; NEJM 366:1665 & 1704, 2013)*. Caution if positive family history of sudden cardiac death, electrolyte abnormalities or concomitant drugs that prolong QTc. Refs on risk of CV death with azithro use: *NEJM 366:1881, 2012; NEJM 368:1704, 2013.* ↑ **risk QTc >500 msec! Risk amplified by other drugs** [macrolides, antiarrhythmics, & drug-drug interactions *(see FQs page 99 for list)*]. *www.qtdrugs.org* & *www.torsades.org*. Cholestatic hepatitis in approx. 1:1000 adults (not children) given E estolate. **Drug-drug interactions of note:** Erythro or clarithro with statins: high statin levels, rhabdomyolysis *(Ann Int Med 158:869, 2013)*; concomitant clarithro & colchicine (gout) can cause fatal colchicine toxicity (pancytopenia, renal failure) *(CID 41:291, 2005)*. Concomitant clarithro & Ca++ channel blockers increase risk of hypotension, kidney injury *(JAMA 310:2544, 2013)*. **Transient reversible tinnitus or deafness** with ≥4 gm per day of erythro IV in pts with renal or hepatic impairment. Reversible sensorineural hearing loss with Azithro *(J Otolaryngol 36:257, 2007)*. Dosages of oral erythro preparations expressed as base equivalents. Variable amounts of erythro esters required to achieve same free erythro serum level. **Azithromycin** reported to exacerbate symptoms of myasthenia gravis.
Erythromycin Base and esters (Erythrocin) IV name: E. lactobionate	**0.25 gm q6h–0.5 gm po/IV q6h: 15–20 mg/kg up to 4 gm q24h. Infuse over 30+ min.**	
Clarithromycin (Biaxin) or clarithro extended release (Biaxin XL)	**0.5 gm po q12h**. **Extended release: Two 0.5 gm tabs po per day.**	
Fidaxomicin (Dificid) (200 mg tab)	**One 200 mg tab po bid x 10 days with or without food**	Approved for treatment of C. difficile toxin-mediated diarrhea. Potent activity vs. C. diff., including hypervirulent NAP1/B1/027 strains. Minimal GI absorption; high fecal concentrations. Limited activity vs. normal bowel flora. In trial vs. po Vanco, lower relapse rate vs. non NAP1 strains than Vanco *(NEJM 364:422, 2011)*. Cohort study reported slight in cardiovascular mortality during 5 days of therapy with azithromycin *(NEJM 366: 1881, 2012)*, leading to a drug safety statement by FDA *(http://www.fda.gov/Drugs/DrugSafety/ucm304372.htm)*. Mortality difference did not persist after therapy.
Ketolide: **Telithromycin** (Ketek) *(Med Lett 46:66, 2004; Drug Safety 31:561, 2008)*	**Two 400 mg tabs po q24h.** 300 mg tabs available.	Drug warnings: acute liver failure & serious liver injury post treatment. *(AnIM 144:415, 447, 2006)*. **Uncommon: blurred vision** 2° slow accommodation; may cause exacerbation of **myasthenia gravis (Black Box Warning: Contraindicated in this disorder)**. Liver, eye and myasthenia complications may be due to inhibition of nicotinic acetylcholine receptor at neuromuscular junction *(AAC 54:5399, 2010)*. Potential QT_c prolongation. Several **drug-drug interactions** *(Table 22, pages 224–225)* *(NEJM 355:2260, 2006)*.

(See page 2 for abbreviations)

*NOTE: all dosage recommendations are for adults (unless otherwise indicated) & assume normal renal function.

TABLE 10A (7)

CLASS, AGENT, GENERIC NAME (TRADE NAME)	USUAL ADULT DOSAGE*	ADVERSE REACTIONS, COMMENTS *(See Table 10B for Summary)*
CHLORAMPHENICOL, CLINDAMYCIN(S), ERYTHROMYCIN GROUP, KETOLIDES, OXAZOLIDINONES, QUINUPRISTIN-DALFOPRISTIN *(continued)*		
Linezolid (Zyvox) (600 mg tab) Review: *JAC 66(Suppl4):3, 2011*	**PO or IV dose: 600 mg q12h.** Available as 600 mg tabs, oral suspension (100 mg per 5 mL), & IV solution. Special populations Refs: Renal insufficiency *(J Infect Chemother 17:70, 2011)*; Liver transplant *(CID 42:434, 2006)*; Cystic fibrosis *(AAC 48:281, 2004)*; Burns *(J Burn Care Res 31:207, 2010)*. Obesity: clinical failure with standard dose in 265 kg patient *(Ann Pharmacother 47:e25, 2013)*.	**Reversible myelosuppression:** thrombocytopenia, anemia, & neutropenia reported. Most often after >2 wks of therapy. Incidence of thrombocytopenia after 2 wks of rx: 7/20 osteomyelitic pts; 5/7 pts treated with vanco & then linezolid. Refs.: *CID 37:1609, 2003 & 38:1058 & 1065, 2004*. 6-fold increased risk in pts with ESRD *(CID 42:66, 2006)*. **Lactic acidosis; peripheral neuropathy, optic neuropathy:** After 4 or more wks of therapy. Data consistent with time and dose-dependent inhibition of intramitochondrial protein synthesis *(CID 42:1111, 2006; AAC 50:2042, 2006; Pharmacotherapy 27:771, 2007)*. Neuropathy, not reversible. **Inhibitor of monoamine oxidase;** risk of severe hypertension if taken with foods rich in tyramine. Avoid concomitant pseudoephedrine, phenylpropanolamine, and caution with SSRIs[1]. **Serotonin syndrome** (fever, agitation, mental status changes, tremors). Risk with concomitant SSRIs: *(CID 42:1578 and 43:180, 2006)*. Actual incidence seems low *(JAC 67:494, 2012; AAC 57:5901, 2013)*. Other adverse effects: black hairy tongue and acute interstitial nephritis *(IDCP 17:61, 2009)*. **Rhabdomyolysis:** a case of this entity, probably related to linezolid, was reported in a patient receiving linezolid as a component of multi-drug therapy for XDR tuberculosis *(CID 54:1624, 2012)*. **Resistance:** Linezolid resistant S. epidermidis and MRSA due to other mobil gene that methylates ribosomal target of Linezolid or primarily, to mutation of the 23S rRNA binding site *(JAC 68:4, 2013)*.
Quinupristin + dalfopristin (Synercid) *(CID 36:473, 2003)*	**7.5 mg per kg IV q8h via central line**	Venous irritation (5%); none with central venous line. Asymptomatic ↑ in unconjugated bilirubin. **Arthralgia** 2%–50% *(CID 36:476, 2003)*. **Note:** E. faecium susceptible; E. faecalis resistant. **Drug-drug interactions:** Cyclosporine, nifedipine, midazolam, many more—*see Table 22*.
TETRACYCLINES		
Doxycycline (Vibramycin, Doryx, Monodox, Adoxa, Periostat) (20, 50, 75, 100 mg tab)	**0.1 gm po/IV q12h**	Similar to other tetracyclines. ↑ nausea on empty stomach. Erosive esophagitis, esp. if taken at bedtime; **take with lots of water.** Phototoxicity & photo-onycholysis occur but less than with tetracycline. Deposition in teeth less. Can be used in patients with renal failure. *Comments:* Effective in treatment and prophylaxis for malaria, leptospirosis, typhus fevers.
Minocycline (Minocin, Dynacin) (50, 75, 100 mg cap; 45, 90, 135 mg ext rel tab; IV prep)	**200 mg po/IV loading dose, then 100 mg po/IV q12h** IV minocycline no longer available.	**Vestibular symptoms** (30–90% in some groups, none in others): vertigo 33%, ataxia 43%, nausea 50%, vomiting 3%, women more frequently than men. Hypersensitivity pneumonitis, reversible, ~34 cases reported *(BMJ 310:1520, 1995)*. Can increase **pigmentation** of the skin with long-term use. *Comments:* More effective than other tetracyclines vs staph and in prophylaxis of meningococcal disease. P. acnes: many resistant to other tetracyclines, not to mino. Induced autoimmunity reported in children treated for acne *(J Ped 153:314, 2008)*. Active vs Nocardia asteroides, Mycobacterium marinum and many acinetobacter isolates.
Tetracycline, Oxytetracycline (Sumycin) (250, 500 mg cap) *(CID 36:462, 2003)*	**0.25–0.5 gm po q6h, 0.5–1 gm IV q12h**	GI (oxy 19%, tetra 4), anaphylactoid reaction (rare), deposition in teeth, negative N balance, hepatotoxicity, enamel agenesis, pseudotumor cerebri/encephalopathy. Outdated drug: Fanconi syndrome. *See drug-drug interactions, Table 22*. **Contraindicated in pregnancy, hepatotoxicity in mother, transplacental to fetus.** *Comments:* **Pregnancy:** IV dosage over 2 gm per day may be associated with fatal hepatotoxicity. (Ref: *JAC 66:1431, 2011*).
Tigecycline (Tygacil) Meta-analysis & editorial: *Ln ID 11:804 & 834, 2011*. Also *CID 54:1699 & 1710, 2012*.	**100 mg IV initially, then 50 mg IV q12h with po food, if possible to decrease risk of nausea.** **If severe liver dis. (Child Pugh C):** 100 mg IV initially, then 25 mg IV q12h	**Warning:** excess deaths & non-cure: in 7 pts, 0.7% increase in mortality & 2.9% increase in non-cure rates *(CID 54:1699 & 1710, 2012)*. Derivative of tetracycline. High incidence of nausea (25%) & vomiting (20%) but only 1% of pts discontinued therapy due to an adverse event. Pregnancy Category D. Do not use in children under age 18. Like other tetracyclines, may cause photosensitivity, pseudotumor cerebri, pancreatitis, a catabolic state (elevated BUN) and maybe hyperpigmentation *(CID 45:136, 2007)*. **Tetracycline, minocycline & tigecycline** associated with acute pancreatitis *(Int J Antimicrob Agents, 34:486, 2009)*. **Dear Doctor Letter (4/27/09):** lower cure rate and higher mortality in pts with VAP treated with tigecycline. Ref: *Diag Micro Infect Dis 68:140, 2010*. **Black Box Warning:** All cause mortality higher in pts treated with tigecycline (2.5%) than comparators (1.8%) in meta-analysis of clinical trials. Cause of mortality risk difference of 0.6% (95% CI 0.1, 1.2) not established. Tigecycline should be reserved for use in situations when alternative treatments are not suitable *(FDA MedWatch Sep 27, 2013)*. Poor result probably due to low serum levels *(AAC 56:1065 & 1466, 2012)*; high doses superior to low doses for HAP *(AAC 57:1756, 2013)*.

[1] **SSRI** = selective serotonin reuptake inhibitors, e.g., fluoxetine (Prozac).

(See page 2 for abbreviations) *NOTE: all dosage recommendations are for adults (unless otherwise indicated) & assume normal renal function.

TABLE 10A (8)

CLASS, AGENT, GENERIC NAME (TRADE NAME)	USUAL ADULT DOSAGE*	ADVERSE REACTIONS, COMMENTS *(See Table 10B for Summary)*
FLUOROQUINOLONES (FQs): All can cause false-positive urine drug screen for opiates *(Pharmacother 26:435, 2006)*. Toxicity review: *Drugs Aging 27:193, 2010.*		
Ciprofloxacin (Cipro) and **Ciprofloxacin-extended release** (Cipro XR, Proquin XR) (100, 250, 500, 750 mg tab; 500 mg ext rel tab)	Usual Parenteral Dose: **400 mg IV q12h** For P. aeruginosa: **400 mg IV q8h** Uncomplicated Urethritis/cystitis (Oral) Dose: **250 mg po bid or CIP XR 500 mg po once daily** Other Indications (Oral): **500-750 mg po bid**	FQs are a common precipitant of **C. difficile toxin-mediated diarrhea.** **Children:** No FQ approved for use under age 16 based on joint cartilage injury in immature animals. Articular SEs in children est. at 2–3% *(LnID 3:537, 2003)*. The exception is anthrax. Pathogenesis believed to involve FQ chelation of Mg++ and damaging chondrites *(AAC 51:1022, 2007; Int J Antimicrob Agents 33:194, 2009)*. **CNS toxicity:** Poorly understood. Varies: lightheadedness, confusion, seizures. May be aggravated by NSAIDs. Peripheral neuropathy occurs: rapid onset, potentially permanent injury. **Gemi skin rash:** Macular rash after 8–10 days of rx. Incidence of rash with ≤5 days of therapy only 1.5%. Frequency highest females, < age 40, treated 14 days (22.6%). In men, < age 40, treated 14 days, frequency 7.7%. Mechanism unclear. Indication to DC therapy. Ref: Diag Micro Infect Dis 68:140, 2010. **Hypoglycemia/hyperglycemia (Dysglycemia):** Increased risk, esp. of hypoglycemia in diabetic pts from any of the marketed FQs *(CID 57:971, 2013)*. **Thrombocytopenia** in critically ill *(PLoS One 8(11):e81477)*. **Opiate screen false-positives:** FQs can cause false-positive urine assay for opiates *(Ann Pharmacotherapy 38:1525, 2004)*. **Photosensitivity:** *See Table 10C, page 108.* Rarely, retinal detachment *(JAMA 307:1414, 2012)*. **QT_c (corrected QT) interval prolongation:** ↑ QT_c (>500 msec or >60 msec from baseline) is considered possible with any FQ. ↑ QT_c can lead to torsades de pointes and ventricular fibrillation. Overall risk is 4.7/10,000 person yrs *(CID 55:1457, 2012)*. Risk low with current marketed drugs. Risk ↑ in women, ↓ K^+, ↓ mg^{++}, bradycardia. (Refs.: *CID 43:1603, 2006)*. Major problem is ↑ risk with concomitant drugs.
Gatifloxacin (Tequin)[NUS] *See comments*	**200–400 mg IV/po q24h.** *(See comment)* Ophthalmic solution (Zymar)	
Gemifloxacin (Factive) (320 mg tab)	**320 mg po q24h.**	
Levofloxacin (Levaquin) (250, 500, 750 mg tab)	**250–750 mg po/IV q24h.** For most indications, 750 mg is preferred dose. PO therapy: avoid concomitant dairy products, multivitamins, iron, antacids due to chelation by multivalent cations & interference with absorption. No dose adjustment for morbid obesity.	**Avoid concomitant drugs with potential to prolong QTc such as:** **Antiarrhythmics:** Amiodarone, Disopyramide, Dofetilide, Flecainide, Ibutilide, Procainamide, Quinidine, quinine, Sotalol **Anti-Infectives:** Azoles (not posa), Clarithro/erythro, FQs (not CIP), Halofantrine, NNRTIs, Protease Inhibitors, Pentamidine, Telavancin, Telithromycin **Anti-Hypertensives:** Bepridil, Isradipine, Nicardipine, Moexipril **CNS Drugs:** Fluoxetine, Haloperidol, Phenothiazines, Pimozide, Quetiapine, Risperidone, Sertraline, Tricyclics, Venlafaxine, Ziprasidone **Misc:** Dolasetron, Droperidol, Fosphenytoin, Indapamide, Methadone, Naratriptan, Salmeterol, Sumatriptan, Tamoxifen, Tizanidine **Updates online: www.qtdrugs.org; www.torsades.org**
Moxifloxacin (Avelox)	**400 mg po/IV q24h.** Note: no need to increase dose for morbid obesity *(JAC 66:2330, 2011)*. Ophthalmic solution (Vigamox)	**Tendinopathy:** Over age 60, approx. 2–6% of all Achilles tendon ruptures attributable to use of FQ *(ArIM 163:1801, 2003)*. ↑ risk with concomitant steroid, renal disease or post-transplant (heart, lung, kidney) *(CID 36:1404, 2003)*. Overall incidence is low *(Eur J Clin Pharm 63:499, 2007)*. **Chelation:** Risk of chelation of oral FQs by multivalent cations **(Ca++, Mg++, Fe++, Zn++)**. Avoid dairy products, multivitamins *Clin Pharmacokinet 40 (Suppl1) 33:2001)*. **Allergic Reactions:** Rare (1:50,000). IgE-mediated: urticaria, anaphylaxis. 3 pts with Moxi immediate reactions tolerated CIP *(Ann Pharmacother 44:740, 2010)*. **Myasthenia gravis:** Any of the FQs may exacerbate muscle weakness in pts. with myasthenia gravis. **Retinal detachment:** One study found an association with FQs *(JAMA 307:1414, 2012)* another did not *(JAMA 310:2151 & 2184, 2013)*
Ofloxacin (Floxin)	**200–400 mg po bid.** Ophthalmic solution (Ocuflox)	

(See page 2 for abbreviations)

*NOTE: all dosage recommendations are for adults (unless otherwise indicated) & assume normal renal function.

TABLE 10A (9)

CLASS, AGENT, GENERIC NAME (TRADE NAME)	USUAL ADULT DOSAGE*	ADVERSE REACTIONS, COMMENTS (*See Table 10B for Summary*)
POLYMYXINS (POLYPEPTIDES) Note: Proteus sp., Providencia sp, Serratia sp., B. cepacia are intrinsically resistant to polymyxins.		
Polymyxin B (Poly-Rx) 1 mg = 10,000 international units Avoid monotherapy, see *Colistin*.	Doses based on actual body weight. ***LOADING DOSE:*** 2.5 mg/kg IV over 2 hrs. ***MAINTENANCE DOSE:*** 12 hrs later 1.5 mg/kg over 1 hr, then repeat q12h. Combination therapy with carbapenem suggested to increase efficacy and reduce risk of resistance. No dose reduction for renal insufficiency. **Intrathecal therapy for meningitis:** 5 mg/day into CSF x 3-4 days, then 5 mg every other day x 2 or more weeks.	**Adverse effects: Neurologic:** rare but serious is neuromuscular blockade; other, circumoral paresthesias, extremity numbness, blurred vision, drowsy, irritable, ataxia; can manifest as respiratory arrest (*Chest 141:515, 2012*). **Renal:** reversible acute tubular necrosis. Renal injury in 42% (Polymyxin B) vs. 60% (Colistin) (*CID 57:1300, 2013*). PK study showed no need to reduce dose for renal insufficiency (*CID 57:524, 2013*).
Colistin, Polymyxin E (Colymycin) **All doses are based on mg of Colistin base.** **Calculated doses are higher than the package insert dosing; need to avoid underdosage in the critically ill.** **Do not use as monotherapy (combine with carbapenem or rifampin)** Dosing formula based on PK study of 105 pts (*AAC 55:3284, 2011*). Loading dose (*AAC 53:3430, 2009*). PK/PD studies (*AAC 54:3783, 2010 (in vitro), JAC 65:1984, 2010 (in vivo)*). **Recommendations are evolving: see Sanford Guide digital editions for most current information and dosing calculator.**	• ***Severe Systemic Infection:*** ***LOADING DOSE:*** 3.5 (targeted average serum steady state level) x 2 x body weight in kg (lower of ideal or actual weight) IV. This will often result in a loading dose of over 300 mg of colistin base. First maintenance dose is given 12 hrs. later. ***MAINTENANCE DOSE:*** Formula for calculating the daily maintenance dosage: ▪ 3.5 (the desired serum steady state concentration) x [(1.5 x CrCln) +30] = total daily dose. Divide and give q8h or maybe q12h. The maximum suggested daily dose is 475 mg. ▪ **NOTE:** CrCln is the Creatinine Clearance (CrCl) normalized (n) for Body Surface Area (BSA) such that the CrCln = CrCl x BSA in m^2/1.73 m^2. • *Combination therapy is recommended for all pts:* **Colistin** (as above) + [(**IMP** or **MER**) or **RIF**] • ***Cystic fibrosis:*** 3-8 mg/kg/day q8h (based on IBW) • **Intrathecal or intraventricular for meningitis:** 10 mg/day • ***Inhalation therapy:*** 50-75 mg in 3-4 mL of Saline via nebulizer 2-3x/day	• **GNB Resistance**: Some sp. are intrinsically resistant: Serratia sp, Proteus sp, Providencia sp., B. cepacia. In vitro and in animal models, gram-negative bacilli quickly become resistant; concomitant Tigecycline or Minocycline may attenuate risk of resistance (*JAC 60:421, 2007*). Synergy with Rifampin or Tigecycline unpredictable. The greater the resistance of GNB to Colistin, the greater the susceptibility to beta-lactams (AM-SB, PIP-TZ, extended spectrum Ceph, maybe carbapenems). • **Caveat**: higher doses of colistin (> 5 mg/kg of ideal body weight per day) are associated with increased risk of nephrotoxicity and should be reserved for critically ill patients (Clin Infect Dis 53:879, 2011). • **Bactericidal activity concentration dependent** but no post-antibiotic effect; do not dose once daily. • **Nephrotoxic:** exact risk unclear, but increased by concomitant nephrotoxins (IV contrast), hypotension, maybe Rifampin. Reversible. • **Neurotoxicity.** Frequent: circumoral paresthesia, vertigo, abnormal vision, confusion, ataxia. Rare: neuromuscular blockade with respiratory failure. • **Caution:** Some colistimethate products are expressed in IUs. To convert IUs to mg of colistin base: 1,000,000 IUs colistimethate = 80 mg colistimethate base = 30 mg colistin base. *See CID 58:139, 2014.*
MISCELLANEOUS AGENTS		
Fosfomycin (Monurol) (3 gm packet)	**3 gm with water po times 1 dose.** For emergency use: single patient IND for IV use. From FDA: 1-888-463-6332.	Diarrhea in 9% compared to 6% of pts given nitrofurantoin and 2.3% given TMP-SMX. Available outside U.S., IV & PO, for treatment of multi-drug resistant bacteria. For MDR-GNB: 6-12 gm/day IV divided q6-8h. Ref: *Int J Antimicrob Ag 37:415, 2011*.
Fusidic acid[NUS] (Fucidin, Taksta)	**500 mg po/IV tid (Denmark & Canada)** **US: loading dose of 1500 mg po bid x 1 day, then 60 mg po bid**	Activity vs. MRSA of importance. Approved outside the U.S.; currently in U.S. clinical trials. Ref for proposed US regimen: *CID 52 (Suppl 7):S520, 2011*.

(*See page 2 for abbreviations*)

*NOTE: all dosage recommendations are for adults (unless otherwise indicated) & assume normal renal function.

TABLE 10A (10)

CLASS, AGENT, GENERIC NAME (TRADE NAME)	USUAL ADULT DOSAGE*	ADVERSE REACTIONS, COMMENTS *(See Table 10B for Summary)*
MISCELLANEOUS AGENTS *(continued)*		
Methenamine hippurate (Hiprex, Urex)	**1 gm po bid**	Nausea and vomiting, skin rash or dysuria. Overall ~3%. Methenamine requires (pH ≤5) urine to liberate formaldehyde. Useful in suppressive therapy after infecting organisms cleared; do not use for pyelonephritis. *Comment:* Do not force fluids; may dilute formaldehyde. Of no value in pts with chronic Foley. If urine pH >5.0, co-administer ascorbic acid (1–2 gm q4h) to acidify the urine; cranberry juice (1200–4000 mL per day) has been used, results ±. Do not use concomitantly with sulfonamides (precipitate), or in presence of renal or severe hepatic dysfunction.
Methenamine mandelate (Mandelamine)	**1 gm po qid**	
Metronidazole (Flagyl) (250, 375, 500 mg tab/cap) Ref.: *Activity vs. B. fragilis* Still drug of choice *(CID 50 (Suppl 1):S16, 2010).*	Anaerobic infections: **usually IV, 7.5 mg per kg (~500 mg) q6h (not to exceed 4 gm q24h).** With long T½, **can use IV at 15 mg per kg q12h.** If life-threatening, use loading dose of **IV 15 mg per kg. Oral dose: 500 mg qid; extended release tabs** available 750 mg	**Common AEs:** nausea (12%), metallic taste, "furry" tongue. Avoid alcohol during 48 hrs after last dose to avoid disulfiram reaction (N/V, flushing, tachycardia, dyspnea). Neurologic AEs with high dose/long Rx: peripheral, autonomic and optic neuropathy *(J Child Neurol 21:429, 2006).* Aseptic meningitis, encephalopathy, seizures & reversible cerebellar lesion reported *(NEJM 346:68, 2002).* Also: topical & vaginal gels. Can use IV soln as enema for *C. diff colitis.* Resistant anaerobic organisms: Actinomycetes, Peptostreptococci. Once-daily IV dosing of 1,500 mg: rational based on long serum T1/2; standard in Europe; supportive retrospective studies in adults with intra-abdominal infections *(JAC 19:410, 2007).*
Nitazoxanide	*See Table 13B, page 154*	
Nitrofurantoin macrocrystals (Macrobid, Macrodantin, Furadantin) (25, 50, 100 mg caps)	Active UTI: **Furadantin/Macrodantin 50-100 mg po qid x 5-7 days OR Macrobid 100 mg po bid x 5-7 days** Dose for long-term UTI suppression: **50–100 mg at bedtime**	Absorption ↑ with meals. Increased activity in acid urine, much reduced at pH 8 or over. Nausea and vomiting, **peripheral neuropathy,** pancreatitis. **Pulmonary reactions** (with chronic rx): acute ARDS type, **chronic desquamative interstitial pneumonia with fibrosis**. Intrahepatic cholestasis & **hepatitis** similar to chronic active hepatitis. Hemolytic anemia in G6PD deficiency. Drug rash, eosinophilia, systemic symptoms (DRESS) hypersensitivity syndrome reported *(Neth J Med 67:147, 2009).* Concern that efficacy may be reduced and AEs increased with CrCl under 40mL/min. Should not be used in infants <1 month of age. Birth defects: increased risk reported *(Arch Ped Adolesc Med 163:978, 2009).*
Rifampin (Rimactane, Rifadin) (150, 300 mg cap)	**300 mg po/IV bid or 600 mg po/IV qd.** Rapid selection of resistant bacteria if used as monotherapy	Causes orange-brown discoloration of sweat, urine, tears, contact lens. **Many important drug-drug interactions,** *see Table 22.* Immune complex flu-like syndrome: fever, headache, myalgias, arthralgia--especially with intermittent rx. Thrombocytopenia, vasculitis reported *(C Ann Pharmacother 42: 727, 2008).* Can cause interstitial nephritis. Risk-benefit of adding RIF to standard therapies for S. aureus endocarditis *(AAC 52:2463, 2008). See also, Antimycobacterial Agents, Table 12B, page 140.*
Rifaximin (Xifaxan) (200, 550 mg tab)	Traveler's diarrhea: **200 mg tab po tid** times 3 days. Hepatic encephalopathy: **550 mg tab po bid.** C. diff diarrhea as "chaser": **400 mg po bid**	For traveler's diarrhea and hepatic encephalopathy *(AAC 54:3618, 2010; NEJM 362:1071, 2010).* In general, adverse events equal to or less than placebo.
Sulfonamides [e.g., sulfisoxazole (Gantrisin), sulfamethoxazole (Gantanol), (Truxazole), sulfadiazine]	Dose varies with indications. *See Nocardia & Toxoplasmosis*	**CNS:** fever, headache, dizziness; **Derm:** mild rash to life threatening Stevens-Johnson syndrome, toxic epidermal necrolysis, photosensitivity; **Hem:** agranulocytosis, aplastic anemia; **Cross-allergenicity:** other sulfa drugs, sulfonylureas, diuretics, crystalluria (esp. sulfadiazine-need ≥ 1500 mL po fluid/day); **Other:** serum sickness, hemolysis if G6PD def, polyarteritis, SLE reported.
Tinidazole (Tindamax)	**Tabs 250, 500 mg.** Dose for giardiasis: 2 gm po times 1 with food.	**Adverse reactions:** metallic taste 3.7%, nausea 3.2%, anorexia/vomiting 1.5%. All higher with multi-day dosing. Avoid alcohol during & for 3 days after last dose; cause disulfiram reaction, flushing, N/V, tachycardia.
Trimethoprim (Trimpex, Proloprim, and others) (100, 200 mg tab)	**100 mg po q12h or 200 mg po q24h.**	**CNS:** drug fever, aseptic meningitis; **Derm:** rash (3-7% at 200 mg/day), phototoxicity, Stevens-Johnson syndrome (rare), toxic epidermal necrolysis (rare); **Renal:** ↑ K+, ↓ Na+, ↑ Cr; **Hem:** neutropenia, thrombocytopenia, methemoglobinemia.

*NOTE: all dosage recommendations are for adults (unless otherwise indicated) & assume normal renal function.

TABLE 10A (11)

CLASS, AGENT, GENERIC NAME (TRADE NAME)	USUAL ADULT DOSAGE*	ADVERSE REACTIONS, COMMENTS *(See Table 10B for Summary)*
MISCELLANEOUS AGENTS *(continued)*		
Trimethoprim (TMP)-Sulfamethoxazole (SMX) (Bactrim, Septra, Sulfatrim, Cotrimoxazole) Single-strength (SS) is 80 TMP/400 SMX, double-strength (DS) 160 TMP/800 SMX	**Standard po rx: 1 DS tab bid.** **P. carinii:** *see Table 11A, page 123.* **IV rx (base on TMP component): standard 8–10 mg per kg IV per day divided q6h, q8h, or q12h.** **For shigellosis: 2.5 mg per kg IV q6h**.	Adverse reactions in 10%: GI: nausea, vomiting, anorexia. Skin: Rash, urticaria, photosensitivity. More serious (1–10%): **Stevens-Johnson syndrome & toxic epidermal necrolysis.** Skin reactions may represent toxic metabolites of SMX rather than allergy *(Ann Pharmacotherapy 32:381, 1998)*. Daily ascorbic acid 0.5–1.0 gm may promote detoxification *(JAIDS 36:1041, 2004)*. Rare hypoglycemia, esp. AIDS pts: *(LnID 6:178, 2006)*. **Sweet's Syndrome** can occur. TMP competes with creatinine for tubular secretion; serum creatinine can ↑; TMP also blocks distal renal tubule secretion of K^+. ↑ serum K^+ in 21% of pts *(AnIM 124:316, 1996)*. Risk of hyperkalemia increased 7x if concomitant ACE inhibitor *(Arch Int Med 170:1045, 2010)*. Discussion of renal injury *(JAC 67:1271, 2012)*. TMP one etiology of **aseptic meningitis.** Report of psychosis during treatment of PCP *(JAC 66:1117, 2011)*. TMP-SMX contains sulfites and may trigger asthma in sulfite-sensitive pts. Frequent drug cause of thrombocytopenia. No cross allergenicity with other sulfonamide non-antibiotic drugs *(NEJM 349:1628, 2003)*. **For TMP-SMX desensitization,** *see Table 7, page 80.*
Topical Antimicrobial Agents Active vs. S. aureus & Strep. pyogenes *(CID 49:1541, 2009)*. **Review of topical antiseptics, antibiotics** *(CID 49:1541, 2009)*.		
Bacitracin (Baciguent)	20% bacitracin zinc ointment, apply 1-5 x/day.	Active vs. staph, strep & clostridium. Contact dermatitis occurs. Available without prescription.
Fusidic acid[NUS] ointment	**2% ointment, apply tid**	Available in Canada and Europe *(Leo Laboratories)*. Active vs. S. aureus & S. pyogenes.
Mupirocin (Bactroban)	**Skin cream or ointment 2%: Apply tid times 10 days. Nasal ointment 2%: apply bid times 5 days.**	Skin cream: itch, burning, stinging 1–1.5%; Nasal: headache 9%, rhinitis 6%, respiratory congestion 5%. Not active vs. enterococci or gm-neg bacteria. Summary of resistance: *CID 49:935, 2009.* If large amounts used in azotemic pts, can accumulate polyethylene glycol *(CID 49:1541, 2009)*.
Polymyxin B—Bacitracin (Polysporin)	5000 units/gm; 400 units/gm. Apply 1-4x/day	Polymyxin active vs. some gm-neg bacteria but not Proteus sp., Serratia sp. or gm-pos bacteria. *See Bacitracin comment above.* Available without prescription.
Polymyxin B—Bacitracin—Neomycin (Neosporin, triple antibiotic ointment (TAO))	5000 units/gm; 400 units/gm; 3.5 mg/gm. Apply 1-3x/day.	*See Bacitracin and polymyxin B comments above.* Neomycin active vs. gm-neg bacteria and staphylococci; not active vs. streptococci. Contact dermatitis incidence 1%; risk of nephro- & oto-toxicity if absorbed. TAO spectrum broader than mupirocin and active mupirocin-resistant strains *(DMID 54:63, 2006)*. Available without prescription.
Retapamulin (Altabax)	1% ointment; apply bid. 5, 10 & 15 gm tubes.	Microbiologic success in 90% S. aureus infections and 97% of S. pyogenes infections *(J Am Acd Derm 55:1003, 2006)*. Package insert says **do not use for MRSA** (not enough pts in clinical trials). Active vs. some mupirocin-resistant S. aureus strains.
Silver sulfadiazine	1% cream, apply once or twice daily.	A sulfonamide but the active ingredient is released silver ions. Activity vs. gram-pos & gram-neg bacteria (including P. aeruginosa). Often used to prevent infection in pts with 2nd/3rd degree burns. Rarely, may stain into the skin.

(See page 2 for abbreviations)

*NOTE: all dosage recommendations are for adults (unless otherwise indicated) & assume normal renal function.

TABLE 10B – SELECTED ANTIBACTERIAL AGENTS—ADVERSE REACTIONS—OVERVIEW

Adverse reactions in individual patients represent all-or-none occurrences, even if rare. After selection of an agent, the physician should read the manufacturer's package insert [statements in the product labeling (package insert) must be approved by the FDA].

Numbers = frequency of occurrence (%); + = occurs, incidence not available; ++ = significant adverse reaction; 0 = not reported; R = rare, defined as <1%.

NOTE: Important reactions in bold print. A blank means no data found.

	PENICILLINS, CARBAPENEMS, MONOBACTAMS, AMINOGLYCOSIDES																		MISC.	
		PENICILLINASE-RESISTANT ANTI-STAPH. PENICILLINS			AMINOPENICILLINS				AP PENS				CARBAPENEMS					AMINOGLYCO-SIDES		
ADVERSE REACTIONS	Penicillin G, V	Dicloxacillin	Nafcillin	Oxacillin	Amoxicillin	Amox-Clav	Ampicillin	Amp-Sulb	Piperacillin	Pip-Taz	Ticarcillin	Ticar-Clav	Doripenem	Ertapenem	Imipenem	Meropenem	Aztreonam	Amikacin Gentamicin Kanamycin Netilmicin[NUS] Tobramycin	Linezolid	Telithromycin
Rx stopped due to AE						2-4.4			3.2	3.2			3.4			1.2	<1			
Local, phlebitis	+		++	+				3	4	1	3		4-8	4	3	1	4			
Hypersensitivity	+												R		3	3				
Fever	+	+	+	+	+	+	+	+	+	2	+	+	+	+	+		2	+	+	
Rash	**3**	**4**	**4**	**4**	**5**	**3**	**5**	**2**	**1**	**4**	**3**	**2**	**1-5**	**+**	**+**	**+**	**2**			
Photosensitivity	0	0	0	0	0	0	0	0	0	0	0	0			0		+			
Anaphylaxis	R	0	R	R	R	R	R	+	R	R	+	+	R	+	+	+	+			
Serum sickness	4								+	+	+	+			+		+			
Hematologic																				
+ Coombs	3	0	R	R	+	0	+	0	+	+	0	+		1	2	+	R			
Neutropenia	R	0	+	R	+	+	+	+	6	+	0	+	R	+	+	+	+		1.1	
Eosinophilia	+	+	22	22	2	+	22	22	+	+	+	+		+	+	+	8			
Thrombocytopenia	R	0	R	R	R	R	R	R	+	+	R	R	+		+	+	+		3–10 *(see 10C)*	
↑ PT/PTT	R	0	+[1]	0	+	+	+	0	+	+	+	+			R		R			
GI																				
Nausea/vomiting		+	0	0	2	3	2	+	+	7	+	1	4-12	3	2	4	R		3/1	7/2
Diarrhea		+	0	0	**5**	**9**	**10**	**2**	2	11	3	1	6-11	6	2	5	R		4	10
C. difficile colitis		R	R	R	R	+	R	+	+	+	+	+	R		+		+		+	+
Hepatic, ↑ LFTs	R	R	0	+	R	+	R	6	+	+	0	+	+	6	4	4	2		1.3	
Hepatic failure	0	0	0	0	0	0	0	0	0	0	0	0			0					+
Renal: ↑ BUN, Cr	R	0	0	0	R	R	R	R	+	+	R	R			+	0	0	**5–25[2]**		
CNS																				
Headache	R	0	R	R	0	+	R	R	R	8	R	R	4-16	2	+	3	+		2	2
Confusion	R	0	R	R	0	0	R	R	R	R	R	R			+		+		+	

[1] A case of antagonism of warfarin effect has been reported *(Pharmacother 27:1467, 2007)*.

[2] Varies with criteria used.

TABLE 10B (2)

ADVERSE REACTIONS	PENICILLINS, CARBAPENEMS, MONOBACTAMS, AMINOGLYCOSIDES																			
		PENICILLINASE-RESISTANT ANTI-STAPH. PENICILLINS			AMINOPENICILLINS				AP PENS				CARBAPENEMS					AMINOGLYCOSIDES	MISC.	
	Penicillin G, V	Dicloxacillin	Nafcillin	Oxacillin	Amoxicillin	Amox-Clav	Ampicillin	Amp-Sulb	Piperacillin	Pip-Taz	Ticarcillin	Ticar-Clav	Doripenem	Ertapenem	Imipenem	Meropenem	Aztreonam	Amikacin Gentamicin Kanamycin Netilmicin[NUS] Tobramycin	Linezolid	Telithromycin
CNS *(continued)*																				
Seizures	R	0	0	+	0	R	R	0	0	R	R	+	*See footnote*[3]				+			
Special Senses																				
Ototoxicity	0	0	0	0	0	0	0	0	0	0	0	0			R		0	3–14[4]		
Vestibular	0	0	0	0	0	0	0	0	0	0	0	0			0		0	4–6[4]		
Cardiac																				
Dysrhythmias	R	0		0	0	0	0	0	0	0	0	0			0		+			
Miscellaneous, Unique *(Table 10A)*	+	+	+	+	+	+	+	+		+				+	+		+		+	++
Drug/drug interactions, common *(Table 22)*	0	0	0	0	0	0	0	0	0	0	0	0	+		0		0	+	+	+

ADVERSE REACTIONS	CEPHALOSPORINS/CEPHAMYCINS																				
	Cefazolin	Cefotetan	Cefoxitin	Cefuroxime	Cefotaxime	Ceftazidime	Ceftizoxime	Ceftriaxone	Cefepime	Ceftaroline	Ceftobiprole[NUS]	Cefaclor/Cef.ER[5] /Loracarbef[NUS]	Cefadroxil	Cefdinir	Cefixime	Cefpodoxime	Cefprozil	Ceftibuten	Cefditoren pivoxil	Cefuroxime axetil	Cephalexin
Rx stopped due to AE									1.5	2.7	4			3		2.7	2	2	2	2.2	
Local, phlebitis	+	R	R	2	5	1	4	2	1	2	1.9										
Hypersensitivity	5	1				2			+		R	2									
Fever	+	+	+			R	+	R			1.3	+				R	+		R	R	
Rash	+		2	R	2	2	2	2	2	3	2.7	1	+	R	1	1	1	R	R	R	1
Photosensitivity	0	0	0	0	0	R	0	0													

[3] **All β-lactams in high concentration can cause seizures** *(JAC 45:5, 2000)*. In rabbit, IMP 10x more neurotoxic than benzyl penicillin *(JAC 22:687, 1988)*. In clinical trial of IMP for pediatric meningitis, trial stopped due to seizures in 7/25 IMP recipients; hard to interpret as purulent meningitis causes seizures *(PIDJ 10:122, 1991)*. Risk with IMP ↓ with careful attention to dosage *(Epilepsia 42:1590, 2001)*.
Postulated mechanism: Drug binding to $GABA_A$ receptor. IMP binds with greater affinity than MER.
Package insert, percent seizures: ERTA 0.5, IMP 0.4, MER 0.7. However, in 3 clinical trials of MER for bacterial meningitis, no drug-related seizures *(Scand J Inf Dis 31:3, 1999; Drug Safety 22:191, 2000)*. In febrile neutropenic cancer pts, IMP-related seizures reported at 2% *(CID 32:381, 2001; Peds Hem Onc 17:585, 2000)*. Also reported for DORI.

[4] Varies with criteria used.

[5] Cefaclor extended release tablets.

TABLE 10B (3)

ADVERSE REACTIONS	CEPHALOSPORINS/CEPHAMYCINS																				
	Cefazolin	**Cefotetan**	**Cefoxitin**	**Cefuroxime**	**Cefotaxime**	**Ceftazidime**	**Ceftizoxime**	**Ceftriaxone**	**Cefepime**	**Ceftaroline**	**Ceftobiprole**[NUS]	**Cefaclor/Cef.ER**[5] **/Loracarbef**[NUS]	**Cefadroxil**	**Cefdinir**	**Cefixime**	**Cefpodoxime**	**Cefprozil**	**Ceftibuten**	**Cefditoren pivoxil**	**Cefuroxime axetil**	**Cephalexin**
Hypersensitivity *(continued)*																					
Anaphylaxis	R	+				R					R	R				R				R	
Serum sickness												≤0.5[6]	+								+
Hematologic																					
+ Coombs	3	+	2	R	6	4			14	9.8		R							R	R	+
Neutropenia	+		2	R	+	1	+	2	1		+	+	+	R	R	R	R		R		3
Eosinophilia		+	3	7	1	8	4	6	1		+			R	R	3	2	5	R	1	9
Thrombocytopenia	+					+	+		+		+	2			R	R	+	R			
↑ PT/PTT		++	+		+	+	+	+	+												
GI			2									3		3	13			6			2
Nausea/vomiting		1		R	R	R		R	1	4/2	+	2			7	4	4	2	6/1	3	
Diarrhea		4		R	1	1		3	1	5	9.1/4.8	1–4		15	16	7	3	3	1.4	4	
C. difficile colitis	+	+	+	+	+	+	+	+	+	+	<1	+	+	+	+	+	+	+	+	+	+
Hepatic, ↑ LFTs	+	1	3	4	1	6	4	3	+	2	<2	3	+	1	R	4	2	R	R	2	+
Hepatic failure	0	0	0	0	0	0	0	0	0												
Renal: ↑ BUN, Cr	+		3			R		1	+		R	+		R	+	4	R	R	R		+
CNS																					
Headache	0					1		R	2		4.5	3		2		1	R	R	2	R	+
Confusion	0											+					R				+
Seizures	0								+[7]		R										
Special Senses																					
Ototoxicity	0	0	0		0	0	0	0				0	0	0	0	0	0	0		0	0
Vestibular	0	0	0		0	0	0	0				0	0	0	0	0	0	0		0	0
Cardiac																					
Dysrhythmias	0	0	0		0	0	0	0				0	0	0	0	0	0	0		0	0
Miscellaneous, Unique *(Table 10A)*								+			+	+							+		
Drug/drug interactions, common *(Table 22)*	0	0	0	0	0	0	0	0				0	0		0	0	0	0		0	0

[6] Serum sickness requires biotransformation of parent drug plus inherited defect in metabolism of reactive intermediates *(Ped Pharm & Therap 125:805, 1994)*.
[7] FDA warning of seizure risk when dose not adjusted for renal insufficiency.

TABLE 10B (4)

ADVERSE REACTIONS	MACROLIDES			QUINOLONES						OTHER AGENTS											
	Azithromycin, Reg. & ER[8]	Clarithromycin, Reg. & ER[8]	Erythromycin	Ciprofloxacin/Cipro XR	Gatifloxacin[NUS]	Gemifloxacin	Levofloxacin	Moxifloxacin	Ofloxacin	Chloramphenicol	Clindamycin	Colistimethate (Colistin)	Daptomycin	Metronidazole	Quinupristin-dalfopristin	Rifampin	Telavancin	Tetracycline/Doxy/Mino	Tigecycline	TMP-SMX	Vancomycin
Rx stopped due to AE	1	3		3.5	2.9	2.2	4.3	3.8	4				2.8						5		
Local, phlebitis					5		0.1–1				+		6		++			+	2		13
Hypersensitivity																1		R		++	**8**
Fever				R	R		R			+	+	+	2			+		+	7	+	1
Rash	R		+	3	R	1–22[9]	2	R	2	+	+	+	4	+	R		4	+	2.4	+	3
Photosensitivity	R			R	R	R	+	R	R		4							+	+	+	0
Anaphylaxis			+	R		R	+		R					R							R
Serum sickness							+				+										
Hematologic				R														R			
Neutropenia	R	1		R	R				1	+	+			+				+		+	2
Eosinophilia				R			+		1		+							+		+	+
Thrombocytopenia	R	R		R			0.1–1			+	+			R				+		+	+
↑ PT/PTT		1																	4		0
GI			++																	3	
Nausea/vomiting	3	3[10]	**25**	**5**	**8/<3**	**2.7**	**7/2**	**7/2**	**7**		+	+	6.3	**12**		+	27/14	+	30/20	+	+
Diarrhea	5	3–6	**8**	2	4	3.6	5	5	4	+	**7**		5	+		+	7	+	13	3	
C. difficile colitis		+	+	**R**	**R**	**R**	**R**	**R**	**R**		++		+			R		+			+
Hepatic, ↑ LFTs	R	R	+	2	R	1.5	0.1–1		2		+				2	+		+	4		0
Hepatic failure	0	R	R				+									+		+			0
Renal																					
↑ BUN, Cr	+	4		1					R		0	++	R			+	3	+	2	+	5
CNS														++							
Dizziness, light headedness				R	3	0.8	**3**	**2**	**3**								3.1		3.5		
Headache	R	2		1	4	1.2	6	2		+	+		5	+				+		+	
Confusion			+	+	+		0.1–1	R	2	+				+		+				+	
Seizures			+	+	+		0.1–1		R					+							

[8] Regular and extended-release formulations.
[9] **Highest frequency:** females <40 years of age after 14 days of rx; with 5 days or less of Gemi, incidence of rash <1.5%.
[10] Less GI upset/abnormal taste with ER formulation.

TABLE 10B (5)

ADVERSE REACTIONS	MACROLIDES			QUINOLONES						OTHER AGENTS											
	Azithromycin, Reg. & ER[8]	Clarithromycin, Reg. & ER[8]	Erythromycin	Ciprofloxacin/Cipro XR	Gatifloxacin[NUS]	Gemifloxacin	Levofloxacin	Moxifloxacin	Ofloxacin	Chloramphenicol	Clindamycin	Colistimethate (Colistin)	Daptomycin	Metronidazole	Quinupristin-dalfopristin	Rifampin	Telavancin	Tetracycline/Doxy/Mino	Tigecycline	TMP-SMX	Vancomycin
Special senses																					
Ototoxicity	+		+	0					0												R
Vestibular																		21[11]			
Cardiac																					
Dysrhythmias	+	+	+	R	+[12]	+[12]	R[12]	+[12]	+[12]		R										0
Miscellaneous, Unique *(Table 10A)*	+		+	+	+	+	+	+	+	+	+	+	+	+	+	+	+	+	+	+	+
Drug/drug interactions, common *(Table 22)*	+	+	+	+	+	+	+	+	+						++	++		+	+	+	

[11] Minocycline has 21% vestibular toxicity.
[12] Fluoroquinolones as class are associated **with QT_c prolongation**. Ref.: *CID 34:861, 2002*.

TABLE 10C – ANTIMICROBIAL AGENTS ASSOCIATED WITH PHOTOSENSITIVITY

The following drugs (listed alphabetically) are known to cause photosensitivity in some individuals. Note that photosensitivity lasts for several days after the last dose of the drug, at least for tetracyclines. There is no intent to indicate relative frequency or severity of reactions. *Ref: Drug Saf 34:821, 2011.*

DRUG OR CLASS	COMMENT
Azole antifungals	Voriconazole, Itraconazole, Ketoconazole, but not Fluconazole
Cefotaxime	Manifested as photodistributed telangiectasia
Ceftazidime	Increased susceptibility to sunburn observed
Dapsone	Confirmed by rechallenge
Efavirenz	Three reports
Flucytosine	Two reports
Fluoroquinolones	Worst offenders have halogen atom at position 8 (Lomefloxacin, Sparfloxacin)
Griseofulvin	Not thought to be a potent photosensitizer
Isoniazid	Confirmed by rechallenge
Pyrazinamide	Confirmed by rechallenge
Quinine	May cross-react with quinidine
Saquinavir	One report
Tetracyclines	Least common with Minocycline
Trimethoprim	Alone and in combination with Sulfamethoxazole

TABLE 10D – AMINOGLYCOSIDE ONCE-DAILY AND MULTIPLE DAILY DOSING REGIMENS

(See Table 17A, page 211, if estimated creatinine clearance <90 mL per min.)

- General Note: dosages are given as **once daily dose (OD)** and **multiple daily doses (MDD).**
- For **calculation of dosing weight in non-obese patients** use **Ideal Body Weight (IBW):**
  - **Female:** 45.5 kg + 2.3 kg per inch over 60 inch height = dosing weight in kg;
  - **Male:** 50 kg + 2.3 kg per inch over 60 inch height = dosing weight in kg.
- **Adjustment for calculation of dosing weight in obese patients** (actual body weight (ABW) is ≥ 30% above IBW): IBW + 0.4 (ABW minus IBW) = adjusted weight (*Pharmacotherapy 27:1081, 2007; CID 25:112, 1997*).
- If CrCl >90 mL/min, use doses in this table. If CrCl <90, *use doses in Table 17A, page 211.*
- **For non-obese patients, calculate estimated creatinine clearance (CrCl) as follows:**

$$\frac{(140 \text{ minus age})(\text{IBW in kg})}{72 \times \text{serum creatinine}} = \text{CrCl in mL/min for men. Multiply answer by 0.85 for women (estimated)}$$

- **For morbidly obese patients, calculate estimated creatinine clearance (CrCl) as follows** (*AJM 84:1053, 1988*):

$$\frac{(137 \text{ minus age}) \times [(0.285 \times \text{wt in kg}) + (12.1 \times \text{ht in meters}^2)]}{51 \times \text{serum creatinine}} = \text{CrCl (obese male)}$$

$$\frac{(146 \text{ minus age}) \times [(0.287 \times \text{wt in kg}) + (9.74 \times \text{ht in meters}^2)]}{60 \times \text{serum creatinine}} = \text{CrCl (obese female)}$$

DRUG	MDD AND OD IV REGIMENS/ TARGETED PEAK (P) AND TROUGH (T) SERUM LEVELS	COMMENTS For more data on once-daily dosing, *see AAC 55:2528, 2011 and Table 17A, page 210*
Gentamicin (Garamycin), **Tobramycin** (Nebcin)	MDD: 2 mg per kg load, then 1.7 mg per kg q8h P 4–10 mcg/mL, T 1–2 mcg per mL OD: 5.1 (7 if critically ill) mg per kg q24h P 16–24 mcg per mL, T <1 mcg per mL	**All aminoglycosides have potential to cause tubular necrosis and renal failure, deafness due to cochlear toxicity, vertigo due to damage to vestibular organs, and rarely neuromuscular blockade.** Risk minimal with oral or topical application due to small % absorption unless tissues altered by disease. Risk of nephrotoxicity ↑ with concomitant administration of cyclosporine, vancomycin, ampho B, radiocontrast. Risk of nephrotoxicity ↓ by concomitant AP Pen and perhaps by once-daily dosing method (especially if baseline renal function normal). In general, same factors influence risk of ototoxicity. **NOTE: There is no known method to eliminate risk of aminoglycoside nephro/ototoxicity. Proper rx attempts to ↓ the % risk.** The clinical trial data of OD aminoglycosides have been reviewed extensively by meta-analysis *(CID 24:816, 1997)*. **Serum levels:** Collect peak serum level (PSL) exactly 1 hr after the start of the infusion of the 3rd dose. In critically ill pts, PSL after the 1st dose as volume of distribution and renal function may change rapidly. Other dosing methods and references: For once-daily 7 mg per kg per day of gentamicin—Hartford Hospital method (may under dose if <7 mg/kg/day dose), *see AAC 39:650, 1995.* One in 500 patients (Europe) have mitochondrial mutation that predicts cochlear toxicity *(NEJM 360:640 & 642, 2009)*. Aspirin supplement (3 gm/day) attenuated risk of cochlear injury from gentamicin *(NEJM 354:1856, 2006)*. Vestibular injury usually bilateral & hence no vertigo but imbalance & oscillopsia *(Med J Aust 196:701, 2012)*.
Kanamycin (Kantrex), **Amikacin** (Amikin), Streptomycin	MDD: 7.5 mg per kg q12h P 15–30 mcg per mL, T 5–10 mcg per mL OD: 15 mg per kg q24h P 56–64 mcg per mL, T <1 mcg per mL	
Netilmicin[NUS]	MDD: 2 mg per kg q8h P 4–10 mcg per mL, T 1–2 mcg per mL OD: 6.5 mg per kg q24h P 22–30 mcg per mL, T <1 mcg per mL	
Isepamicin[NUS]	Only OD: Severe infections 15 mg per kg q24h, less severe 8 mg per kg q24h	
Spectinomycin (Trobicin)[NUS]	2 gm IM times 1–gonococcal infections	
Neomycin–oral	Prophylaxis GI surgery: 1 gm po times 3 with erythro, *see Table 15B, page 198* For hepatic coma: 4–12 gm per day po	
Tobramycin—inhaled (Tobi): *See Cystic fibrosis, Table 1, page 43*. Adverse effects few: transient voice alteration (13%) and transient tinnitus (3%).		
Paromomycin—oral: *See Entamoeba and Cryptosporidia, Table 13A, page 143.*		

TABLE 10E: PROLONGED OR CONTINUOUS INFUSION DOSING OF SELECTED BETA LACTAMS

Based on current and rapidly changing data, it appears that prolonged or continuous infusion of beta-lactams is at least as successful as intermittent dosing. Hence, this approach can be part of stewardship programs as supported by recent publications.

Antibiotic stability is a concern. Factors influencing stability include drug concentration, IV infusion diluent *(e.g. NS vs. D5W)*, type of infusion device, and storage temperature *(Ref: P&T 36:723, 2011)*. Portable pumps worn close to the body expose antibiotics to temperatures closer to body temperature (37°C) than to room temperature (around 25°C). Carbapenems are particularly unstable and may require wrapping of infusion pumps in cold packs or frequent changes of infusion bags or cartridges.

A meta-analysis of observational studies found reduced mortality among patients treated with extended or continuous infusion of carbapenems or piperacillin-tazobactam (pooled data) as compared to standard intermittent regimens. The results were similar for extended and continuous regimens when considered separately. There was a mortality benefit with piperacillin-tazobactam but not carbapenems *(CID 56:272, 2013)*. The lower mortality could, at least in part, be due to closer professional supervision engendered by a study environment. On the other hand, a small prospective randomized controlled study of continuous vs. intermittent pip-tazo, ticar-clav, and meropenem found a higher clinical cure rate and a trend toward lower mortality in the continuous infusion patients *(CID 56:236, 2013)*.

DRUG/METHOD	MINIMUM STABILITY	RECOMMENDED DOSE	COMMENTS
Cefepime (Continuous)	@ 37°C: 8 hours @ 25°C: 24 hours @ 4°C: ≥24 hours	Initial dose: 15 mg/kg over 30 min, then immediately begin: • If CrCl > 60: 6 gm (over 24 hr) daily • If CrCl 30-60: 4 gm (over 24 hr) daily • If CrCl 11-29: 2 gm (over 24 hr) daily	CrCl adjustments extrapolated from prescribing information, not clinical data. Refs: *JAC 57:1017, 2006; Am. J. Health Syst. Pharm. 68:319, 2011.*
Ceftazidime (Continuous)	@ 37°C: 8 hours @ 25°C: 24 hours @ 4°C: ≥24 hours	Initial dose: 15 mg/kg over 30 min, then immediately begin: • If CrCl > 50: 6 gm (over 24 hr) daily • If CrCl 31-50: 4 gm (over 24 hr) daily • If CrCl 10-30: 2 gm (over 24 hr) daily	CrCl adjustments extrapolated from prescribing information, not clinical data. Refs: *Br J Clin Pharmacol 50:184, 2000; IJAA 17:497, 2001; AAC 49:3550, 2005; Infect 37: 418, 2009; JAC 68:900, 2013.*
Doripenem (Prolonged)	@ 37°C: 8 hours (in NS) @ 25°C: 24 hours (in NS) @ 4°C: 24 hours (in NS)	• If CrCl ≥ 50: 500 mg (over 4 hr) q8h • If CrCl 30-49: 250 mg (over 4 hr) q8h • If CrCl 10-29: 250 mg (over 4 hr) q12h	Based on a single study *(Crit Care Med 36:1089, 2008)*.
Meropenem (Prolonged)	@ 37°C: <4 hours @ 25°C: 4 hours @ 4°C: 24 hours	• If CrCl ≥ 50: 2 gm (over 3 hr) q8h • If CrCl 30-49: 1 gm (over 3 hr) q8h • If CrCl 10-29: 1 gm (over 3 hr) q12h	Initial 1 gm dose reasonable but not used by most investigators. Ref: *Intens Care Med 37:632, 2011.*
Pip-Tazo (Prolonged)	@ 37°C: 24 hours @ 25°C: 24 hours @ 4°C: no data	Initial dose: 4.5 gm over 30 min, then 4 hrs later start: • If CrCl ≥ 20: 3.375 gm (over 4 hr) q8h • If CrCl < 20: 3.375 gm (over 4 hr) q12h	Reasonable to begin first infusion 4 hrs after initial dose. Refs: *CID 44:357, 2007; AAC 54:460, 2010. See CID 56:236, 245 & 272, 2013.* In obese patients (> 120 kg), may need higher doses: 6.75 gm or even 9 gm (over 4 hrs) q8h to achieve adequate serum levels of tazobactam *(Int J Antimicrob Agts 41:52, 2013)*.
Vancomycin (Continuous)	@ 37°C: 48 hours @ 25°C: 48 hours @ 4°C: 58 days (at conc 10 μg/mL)	Loading dose of 15-20 mg/kg over 30-60 minutes, then 30 mg/kg by continuous infusion over 24 hrs. No data on pts with renal impairment.	Adjust dose to target plateau concentration of 20-25 μg/mL. Higher plateau concentrations (30-40 μg/mL) achieved with more aggressive dosing increase the risk of nephrotoxicity *(Ref: Clin Micro Inf 19:E98, 2013)*.

TABLE 10F: INHALATION ANTIBIOTICS

Introductory remarks: There is interest in inhaled antimicrobials for several patient populations, such as those with bronchiectasis due to cystic fibrosis or as a result of other conditions. Interest is heightened by growing incidence of infection due to multi-drug resistant Gram-negative bacilli. Isolates of *P. aeruginosa, A. baumannii,* or *Klebsiella* species susceptible only to colistin are of special concern.

There are a variety of ways to generate aerosols for inhalation: inhalation of dry powder, jet nebulizers, ultrasonic nebulizers, and most recently, vibrating mesh nebulizers. The vibrating mesh inhalers generate fine particle aerosols with enhanced delivery of drug to small airways *(Cochrane Database of Systematic Reviews 4:CD007639, 2013).*

Inhaled DRUG	DELIVERY SYSTEM	DOSE	COMMENT
Amikacin + Ceftazidime	Vibrating plate nebulizer	AMK: 25 mg/kg once daily x 3 days Ceftaz: 15 mg/kg q3h x 8 days	Radiographic and clinical cure of *P. aeruginosa* ventilator-associated pneumonia (VAP) similar to IV AMK/Ceftaz, including strains with intermediate resistance *(AJRCCM 184:106. 2011).*
Aztreonam (Cayston)	Altera vibrating mesh nebulizer	75 mg tid x 28 days (every other month)	Improves pulmonary function, reduces bacterial load, reduces frequency of exacerbations, and improves symptoms in cystic fibrosis (CF) pts *(Exp Opin Pharmacother 14:2115, 2013).*
Colistin	Various *(see comment)*	Various (see comment)	Much variability and confusion in dosing. Nebulized colistimethate (CMS) 1-2 million U (33-66 mg colistin base) effective for CF *(Exp Opin Drug Deliv 9:333, 2012).* Adjunctive role for VAP still unclear *(CID 43:S89, 2006; CID 51:1238, 2010).* "High-dose" nebulized CMS (400 mg q8h) via **vibrating-mesh nebulizer effective for VAP due to multidrug-resistant P. aeruginosa and A. baumannii** *(Anesth 117:1335, 2012).* Efficacy of adding inhaled colistin to IV colistin for VAP due to GNB susceptible only to colistin was studied. Colistin: 1 million IU q8h (as CMS) nebulized with either jet or ultrasonic nebulizer. Higher cure rate with combined inhaled plus IV colistin as compared to IV colistin alone *(Chest 144: 1768, 2013).*
Fosfomycin + Tobramycin (FTI) 4:1 wt/wt	eFlow vibrating mesh nebulizer	FTI 160/40 or 80/20 bid x 28 days	Both doses maintained improvements in FEV_1 following a 28-day inhaled aztreonam run-in (vs. placebo) in CF patients with *P. aeruginosa*; FTI 80/20 better tolerated than 160/40 *(AJRCCM 185:171, 2012).*
Levofloxacin	eFlow vibrating mesh nebulizer	240 mg bid x 28 days	Reduced sputum density of *P. aeruginosa*, need for other antibiotics, and improved pulmonary function compared to placebo in CF pts (AJRCCM 183:1510, 2011).
Liposomal Amikacin	PARI LC STAR jet nebulizer	500 mg qd x 28 days (every other month)	Company reports Phase 3 study in CF pts with *P. aeruginosa* has met primary endpoint of non-inferiority compared to TOBI for FEV_1 improvement. Insmed website: *http://investor.insmed.com/releasedetail.cfm?ReleaseID=774638.* Accessed November 30, 2013.
Tobramycin (TOBI)	PARI LC PLUS jet nebulizer	300 mg bid x 28 days (every other month)	Cost: about $6700 for one treatment cycle *(Med Lett 55:51, 2013)*
Tobramycin (TOBI Podhaler)	28 mg dry powder caps	4 caps (112 mg) bid x 28 days (every other month)	Improvement in FEV_1 similar to Tobra inhaled solution in CF patients with chronic *P. aeruginosa* but more airway irritation with the powder. Cost of one month treatment cycle about $6700 *(Med Lett 55:51, 2013).*

TABLE 11A – TREATMENT OF FUNGAL INFECTIONS—ANTIMICROBIAL AGENTS OF CHOICE*

TYPE OF INFECTION/ORGANISM/ SITE OF INFECTION	ANTIMICROBIAL AGENTS OF CHOICE		COMMENTS
	PRIMARY	ALTERNATIVE	
Aspergillosis (A. fumigatus most common, also A. flavus and others) *(See NEJM 360:1870, 2009 for excellent review).*			
Allergic bronchopulmonary aspergillosis (ABPA) Clinical manifestations: wheezing, pulmonary infiltrates, bronchiectasis & fibrosis. Airway colonization assoc. with ↑ blood eosinophils, ↑ serum IgE, ↑ specific serum antibodies.	Acute asthma attacks associated with ABPA: **Corticosteroids**	Rx of ABPA: **Itraconazole**[1] 200 mg po bid times 16 wks or longer	Itra decreases number of exacerbations requiring corticosteroids with improved immunological markers improved lung function & exercise tolerance *(IDSA Guidelines updated CID 46:327, 2008).*
Allergic fungal sinusitis: relapsing chronic sinusitis; nasal polyps without bony invasion; asthma, eczema or allergic rhinitis; ↑ IgE levels and isolation of Aspergillus sp. or other dematiaceous sp. (Alternaria, Cladosporium, etc.)	**Rx controversial:** systemic corticosteroids + surgical debridement (relapse common).	For failures try **Itra**[1] 200 mg po bid times 12 mos or flucon nasal spray.	Controversial area.
Aspergilloma (fungus ball)	No therapy or surgical resection. Efficacy of antimicrobial agents not proven.		Aspergillus may complicate pulmonary sequestration.
Invasive, pulmonary (IPA) or extrapulmonary: Post-transplantation and post-chemotherapy in neutropenic pts (PMN <500 per mm^3) but may also present with neutrophil recovery. Most common pneumonia in transplant recipients. Usually a late (≥100 days) complication in allogeneic bone marrow & liver transplantation: High mortality *(CID 44:531, 2007).* **Typical x-ray/CT lung lesions** (halo sign, cavitation, or macronodules) *(CID 44:373, 2007).* An immunologic test that detects circulating **galactomannan antigen** is available for dx of invasive aspergillosis *(Lancet ID 4:349, 2005).* Serum galactomannan relatively insensitive; antifungal rx may decrease sensitivity *(CID 40:1762, 2005).* Improved sensitivity when performed on BAL fluid. *(Am J Respir Crit Care Med 177:27, 2008).* **False-pos. tests occur with serum from pts receiving PIP-TZ, Amox-Clav** & other beta lactams, infection with other fungi & some blood product conditioning fluid *(CID 55:e22, 2012).* **Better diagnostic strategy:** combination of serum galactomannan & aspergillus PCR (not routinely available) *(LnID 13:519, 2013).* **Beta D-Glucan:** in fungal cell wall. Can detect with immunoassay. Many false positives + low sensitivity *(JCM 51:3478, 2013).*	**Primary therapy** *(See CID 46:327, 2008):* **Voriconazole 6 mg/kg IV q12h on day 1; then either (4 mg/kg IV q12h) or (200 mg po q12h for body weight ≥40 kg, but 100 mg po q12h for body weight <40 kg) (use actual wt). Goal trough (day 4): 1.0–5.5 mg/L associated with improved response rates and reduced adverse effects *(Clin Infect Dis 55:1080, 2012).*** **Alternative therapies:** **Liposomal ampho B** (L-AmB) 3-5 mg/kg/day IV; OR **Ampho B lipid complex** (ABLC) 5 mg/kg/d IV; OR **Caspofungin** 70 mg/day then 50 mg/day thereafter; OR **Micafungin**[NAI] 100 mg bid *(JAC 64:840, 2009– based on PK/PD study);* OR **Posaconazole**[NAI] 200 mg qid, then 400 mg bid after stabilization of disease; OR **Itraconazole** capsules 600 mg/day for 3 days, then 400 mg/day (or 2.5 mg/kg of oral solution once daily).		**Voriconazole** more effective than ampho B. Vori, both a substrate and an inhibitor of CYP2C19, CYP2C9, and CYP3A4, has potential for deleterious drug interactions (e.g., with protease inhibitors) and careful review of concomitant medications is mandatory. Measurement of serum concentrations advisable with prolonged therapy or for patients with possible drug-drug interactions. In patients with CrCl < 50 mL/min, po may be preferred due to concerns for nephrotoxicity of IV vehicle in renal dysfunction. However, it is likely less toxic than previously thought *(Clin Infect Dis 54:913, 2012)* **Ampho B: not recommended except as a lipid formulation,** either L-AMB or ABLC. 10 mg/kg and 3 mg/kg doses of L-AMB are equally efficacious with greater toxicity of higher dose *(CID 2007; 44:1289–97).* One comparative trial found much greater toxicity with ABLC than with L-AMB: 34.6% vs 9.4% adverse events and 21.2% vs 2.8% nephrotoxicity *(Cancer 112:1282, 2008).* Vori preferred as primary therapy. **Caspo:** ~50% response rate in IPA. Licensed for salvage therapy. **Micafungin:** Favorable responses to micafungin as a single agent in 6/12 patients in primary therapy group and 9/22 in the salvage therapy group of an open-label, non-comparative trial *(J Infect 53: 337, 2006).* **Posaconazole:** 42% response rate in open-label trial of patients refractory/intolerant to conventional therapy *(Clin Infect Dis 44:2, 2007).* Concern exists for cross-resistance with azole-non-responders. Measurement of serum concentrations advisable. *(Continued on next page)*

[1] **Oral solution preferred to tablets because of ↑ absorption** *(see Table 11B, page 125).*

See page 2 for abbreviations. All dosage recommendations are for adults (unless otherwise indicated) and assume normal renal function

TABLE 11A (2)

TYPE OF INFECTION/ORGANISM/ SITE OF INFECTION	ANTIMICROBIAL AGENTS OF CHOICE		COMMENTS
	PRIMARY	ALTERNATIVE	
Aspergillosis *(continued from previous page)*			
			(Continued from previous page) **Itraconazole:** Itraconazole formulated as capsules, oral solution in hydroxypropyl-beta-cyclodextrin (HPCD), and parenteral solution with HPCD as a solubilizer; oral solution and parenteral formulation not licensed for treatment of invasive aspergillosis. 2.5 mg/kg oral solution provides dose equivalent to 400 mg capsules. Measurements of plasma concentrations recommended during oral therapy of invasive aspergillosis; target troughs concentrations > 0.25 mcg/mL. Itraconazole is a substrate of CYP3A4 and non-competitive inhibitor of CYP3A4 with potential for significant drug-drug interactions. Do not use for azole-non-responders. **Combination therapy:** A possible benefit of adding an echinocandin to Voriconazole or Amphotericin B has been suggested by animal studies and retrospective studies, primarily as salvage therapy *(Clin Infect Dis. 39:797, 2004; Cancer. 110:2740, 2007)*.
Blastomycosis *(CID 46: 1801, 2008)* (Blastomyces dermatitidis) Cutaneous, pulmonary or extrapulmonary.	**LAB,** 3-5 mg/kg per day; OR **Ampho B**, 0.7-1 mg/kg per day, for 1-2 weeks, **then itra**[2] 200 mg tid for 3 days followed by itra 200 mg bid for 6 -12 months	**Itra** 200 mg tid for 3 days then once or twice per day for 6-12 months for mild to moderate disease; OR **Flu** 400-800 mg per day for those intolerant to itra	Serum levels of **itra** should be determined after 2 weeks to ensure adequate drug exposure. Flu less effective than itra; role of vori or posa unclear but active in vitro.
Blastomycosis: CNS disease *(CID 50:797, 2010)*	**LAB** 5 mg/kg per day for 4–6 weeks, followed by **Flu** 800 mg per day	**Itra** 200 mg bid or tid; OR **Vori** 200-400 mg q12h	Flu and vori have excellent CNS penetration, perhaps counterbalance their slightly reduced activity compared to itra. Treat for at least 12 months and until CSF has normalized. Document serum itra levels to assure adequate drug concentrations. Recent study suggests more favorable outcome with Voriconazole *(CID 50:797, 2010)*.

[2] **Oral solution preferred to tablets because of ↑ absorption** *(see Table 11B, page 125)*.

See page 2 for abbreviations. All dosage recommendations are for adults (unless otherwise indicated) and assume normal renal function

TABLE 11A (3)

TYPE OF INFECTION/ORGANISM/ SITE OF INFECTION	ANTIMICROBIAL AGENTS OF CHOICE		COMMENTS
	PRIMARY	ALTERNATIVE	
Candidiasis: Candida is a common cause of nosocomial bloodstream infection. A decrease in *C. albicans* & increase in non-albicans species show ↓ susceptibility among candida species to antifungal agents (esp. fluconazole). These changes have predominantly affected immunocompromised pts in environments where antifungal prophylaxis (esp. fluconazole) is widely used. Oral, esophageal, or vaginal candidiasis is a major manifestation of advanced HIV & represents one of the most common AIDS-defining diagnoses. *See CID 48:503, 2009 for updated IDSA Guidelines.*			
Candidiasis: Bloodstream infection			
Bloodstream: non-neutropenic patient Remove all intravascular catheters if possible; replace catheters at a new site (not over a wire). Higher mortality associated with delay in therapy *(CID 43:25, 2006).*	**Capsofungin** 70 mg IV loading dose, then 50 mg IV daily; OR **Micafungin** 100 mg IV daily; OR **Anidulafungin** 200 mg IV loading dose then 100 mg IV daily.	**Fluconazole** 800 mg (12 mg/kg) loading dose, then 400 mg daily IV OR **Lipid-based ampho B** 3-5 mg/kg IV daily; OR **Ampho B** 0.7 mg/kg IV daily; OR **Voriconazole** 400 mg (6 mg/kg) twice daily for 2 doses then 200 mg q12h.	**Echinocandin** for patients with recent azole exposure or with moderately severe or severe illness, hemodynamic instability. An echinocandin should be used for treatment of *Candida glabrata* unless susceptibility to fluconazole or voriconazole has been confirmed. Echinocandin may be preferred empirical therapy in centers with high prevalence of non-albicans candida species. Echinocandin compared to polyenes or an azole was associated with better survival and is considered the first-line drug of choice by some *(Clin Infect Dis 54:1110, 2012).* A double-blind randomized trial of anidulafungin (n=127) and fluconazole (n=118) showed an 88% microbiologic response rate (119/135 candida species) with anidulafungin vs a 76% (99/130 candida species) with fluconazole (p=0.02) *(NEJM 356: 2472, 2007).* **Fluconazole** recommended for patients with mild-to-moderate illness, hemodynamically stable, with no recent azole exposure. Fluconazole not recommended for treatment of documented *C. kruseii*: use an echinocandin or voriconazole or posaconazole (note: echinocandins have better in vitro activity than either vori or posa against *C. glabrata*). Fluconazole recommended for treatment of *Candida parapsilosis* because of reduced susceptibility of this species to echinocandins. Transition from echinocandin to fluconazole for stable patients with *Candida albicans* or other azole-susceptible species. **Voriconazole** with little advantage over fluconazole (more drug-drug interactions) except for oral step-down therapy of *Candida krusei* or voriconazole-susceptible *Candida glabrata*. Recommended **duration of therapy** is 14 days after last positive blood culture. Duration of systemic therapy should be extended to 4-6 weeks for eye involvement. **Funduscopic examination** within first week of therapy to exclude ophthalmic involvement. Ocular disease present in ~15% of patients with candidemia, but endophthalmitis is uncommon (~2%) *(CID 53:262, 2011).* Intraocular injections of ampho B may be required for endophthalmitis; echinocandins have poor penetration into the eye. For **septic thrombophlebitis,** catheter removal and incision and drainage and resection of the vein, as needed, are recommended; duration of therapy at least 2 weeks after last positive blood culture.

TABLE 11A (4)

TYPE OF INFECTION/ORGANISM/ SITE OF INFECTION	ANTIMICROBIAL AGENTS OF CHOICE		COMMENTS
	PRIMARY	ALTERNATIVE	
Candidiasis: Bloodstream infection *(continued)*			
Bloodstream: neutropenic patient Remove all intravascular catheters if possible; replace catheters at a new site (not over a wire).	**Capsofungin** 70 mg IV loading dose, then 50 mg IV daily, 35 mg for moderate hepatic insufficiency; OR **Micafungin** 100 mg IV daily; OR **Anidulafungin** 200 mg IV loading dose then 100 mg IV daily; OR **Lipid-based ampho B** 3-5 mg/kg IV daily.	**Fluconazole** 800 mg (12 mg/kg) loading dose, then 400 mg daily IV or PO; OR **Voriconazole** 400 mg (6 mg/kg) twice daily for 2 doses then 200 mg (3 mg/kg) q12h.	Fluconazole may be considered for less critically ill patients without recent azole exposure. Duration of therapy in absence of metastatic complications is for 2 weeks after last positive blood culture, resolution of signs, and resolution of neutropenia. Perform funduscopic examination after recovery of white count as signs of ophthalmic involvement may not be seen during neutropenia. *See comments above for recommendations concerning choice of specific agents.*
Candidiasis: Bone and joint infections			
Osteomyelitis	**Fluconazole** 400 mg (6 mg/kg) daily IV or PO; OR **Lipid-based ampho B** 3–5 mg/kg daily for several weeks, then oral fluconazole.	An **echinocandin** (as above) or **ampho** B 0.5–1 mg/kg daily for several weeks then oral **fluconazole.**	Treat for a total of 6-12 months. **Surgical debridement** often necessary; **remove hardware** whenever possible.
Septic arthritis	**Fluconazole** 400 mg (6 mg/kg) daily IV or PO; OR **Lipid-based ampho B** 3–5 mg/kg daily for several weeks, then oral fluconazole.	An **echinocandin** or **ampho** B 0.5–1 mg/kg daily for several weeks then oral **fluconazole.**	**Surgical debridement** in all cases; removal of prosthetic joints whenever possible. Treat for at least 6 weeks and indefinitely if retained hardware.
Candidiasis: Cardiovascular infections			
Endocarditis *(See Eur J Clin Microbiol Infect Dis 27:519, 2008)*	**An echinocandin:** **Caspofungin** 50–150 mg/day; OR **Micafungin** 100–150 mg/day; OR **Anidulafungin** 100–200 mg/day; OR **Lipid-based ampho B** 3–5 mg/kg daily + **5-FC** 25 mg/kg qid.	**Ampho B** 0.6–1 mg/kg daily + **5-FC** 25 mg/kg qid	Consider use of higher doses of echinocandins for endocarditis or other endovascular infections. Can switch to **fluconazole 400-800 mg orally in stable patients** with negative blood cultures and fluconazole susceptible organism. *See Med 90:237, 2011* for review of Fluconazole for candida endocarditis. Valve replacement strongly recommended, particularly in those with prosthetic valve endocarditis. Duration of therapy not well defined, but treat for at least 6 weeks after valve replacement and longer in those with complications (e.g., perivalvular or myocardial abscess, extensive disease, delayed resolution of candidemia). Long-term (life-long?) suppression with fluconazole 400-800 mg daily for native valve endocarditis and no valve replacement; life-long suppression for prosthetic valve endocarditis if no valve replacement.
Myocarditis	**Lipid-based ampho B** 3–5 mg/kg daily; OR **Fluconazole** 400–800 mg (6–12 mg/kg) daily IV or PO; OR **An echinocandin** *(see endocarditis)*.		Can switch to **fluconazole 400-800 mg orally in stable patients** with negative blood cultures and fluconazole susceptible organism. Recommended duration of therapy is for several months.

TABLE 11A (5)

TYPE OF INFECTION/ORGANISM/ SITE OF INFECTION	ANTIMICROBIAL AGENTS OF CHOICE		COMMENTS
	PRIMARY	ALTERNATIVE	
Candidiasis: Cardiovascular infections *(continued)*			
Pericarditis	**Lipid-based ampho B** 3–5 mg/kg daily; OR **Fluconazole** 400–800 mg (6–12 mg/kg) daily IV or po; OR **An echinocandin** *(see endocarditis)*		**Pericardial window or pericardiectomy** also is recommended. Can switch to **fluconazole 400-800 mg orally in stable patients** with negative blood cultures and fluconazole susceptible organism. Recommended duration of therapy is for several months.
Candidiasis: Mucosal, esophageal, and oropharyngeal			
Candida esophagitis Primarily encountered in HIV-positive patients	**Fluconazole** 200-400 (3-6 mg/kg) mg daily; OR **echinocandin** (**caspofungin** 50 mg IV daily; OR **micafungin** 150 mg IV daily; OR **anidulafungin** 200 mg IV loading dose then 100 mg IV daily); OR **Ampho B** 0.5 mg/kg daily.	An azole (**itraconazole** solution 200 mg daily; or **posaconazole** suspension 400 mg bid for 3 days then 400 mg daily or **voriconazole** 200 mg q12h.	**Duration of therapy** 14-21 days. IV echinocandin or ampho B for patients unable to tolerate oral therapy. For fluconazole refractory disease, itra (80% will respond), posa, vori, an echinocandin, or ampho B. Echinocandins associated with higher relapse rate than fluconazole. ARV therapy recommended. Suppressive therapy with fluconazole 200 mg 3x/wk for recurrent infections. Suppressive therapy may be discontinued once CD4 > 200/mm^3.
Oropharyngeal candidiasis			
Non-AIDS patient	**Clotrimazole troches** 10 mg 5 times daily; OR **Nystatin suspension** or pastilles qid; OR **Fluconazole** 100-200 mg daily.	**Itraconazole** solution 200 mg daily; OR **posaconazole** suspension 400 mg bid for 3 days then 400 mg daily; or **voriconazole** 200 mg q12h; OR an echinocandin (**capsofungin** 70 mg loading dose then 50 mg IV daily; or **micafungin** 100 mg IV daily; or **anidulafungin** 200 mg IV loading dose then 100 mg IV daily); OR **Ampho B** 0.3 mg/kg daily.	**Duration of therapy** 7-14 days. Clotrimazole or nystatin recommended for mild disease; fluconazole preferred for moderate-to-severe disease. Alternative agents reserved for refractory disease.
AIDS patient	**Fluconazole** 100-200 mg daily for 7-14 days.	Same as for non-AIDS patient, above, for 7-14 days.	Antiretroviral therapy (ARV) recommended in HIV-positive patients to prevent recurrent disease. Suppressive therapy not necessary, especially with ARV therapy and CD4 > 200/mm^3, but if required fluconazole 100 mg thrice weekly recommended. Itra, posa, or vori for 28 days for fluconazole-refractory disease. IV echinocardin also an option. Dysphagia or odynophagia predictive of esophageal candidiasis.

TABLE 11A (6)

TYPE OF INFECTION/ORGANISM/ SITE OF INFECTION	ANTIMICROBIAL AGENTS OF CHOICE		COMMENTS
	PRIMARY	ALTERNATIVE	
Candidiasis: Mucosal, esophageal, and oropharyngeal *(continued)*			
Vulvovaginitis			
Non-AIDS Patient	**Topical azole therapy: Butoconazole 2% cream** (5 gm) q24h at bedtime x 3 days or 2% cream SR 5 gm x 1; OR **Clotrimazole 100 mg vaginal tabs** (2 at bedtime x 3 days) or 1% cream (5 gm) at bedtime times 7 days (14 days may ↑ cure rate) or 100 mg vaginal tab x 7 days or 500 mg vaginal tab x 1; OR **Miconazole 200 mg vaginal suppos** (1 at bedtime x 3 days) or 100 mg vaginal suppos. q24h x 7 days or 2% cream (5 gm) at bedtime x 7 days; OR **Terconazole 80 mg vaginal tab** (1 at bedtime x 3 days) or 0.4% cream (5 gm) at bedtime x 7 days or 0.8% cream 5 gm intravaginal q24h x 3 days; or tioconazole 6.5% vag. ointment x 1 dose. **Oral therapy:** **Fluconazole** 150 mg po x 1; OR **Itraconazole** 200 mg po bid x 1 day.		**Recurrent vulvovaginal candidiasis:** fluconazole 150 mg weekly for 6 months.
AIDS Patient	Topical **azoles** (clotrimazole, buto, mico, tico, or tercon) x3–7d; OR Topical **nystatin** 100,000 units/day as vaginal tablet x14d; OR Oral **flu** 150 mg x1 dose.		For recurrent disease 10-14 days of topical azole or oral flu 150 mg, then flu 150 mg weekly for 6 mos.
Candidiasis: Other infections			
CNS Infection	**Lipid-based ampho B** 3–5 mg/kg daily ± 5-FC 25 mg/kg qid.	**Fluconazole** 400–800 mg (6–12 mg/kg) IV or po.	Removal of **intraventricular devices** recommended. Flu 400-800 mg as step-down therapy in the stable patient and in patient intolerant of ampho B. Experience too limited to recommend echinocandins at this time. **Treatment duration** for several weeks until resolution of CSF, radiographic, and clinical abnormalities.
Cutaneous *(including paronychia, Table 1, page 28)*	Apply topical ampho B, clotrimazole, econazole, miconazole, or nystatin 3-4 x daily for 7–14 days or ketoconazole 400 mg po once daily x 14 days. Ciclopirox olamine 1% cream/lotion; apply topically bid x 7–14 days.		
Endophthalmitis • Occurs in 10% of candidemia, thus ophthalmological consult for all pts • Diagnosis: typical white exudates on retinal exam and/or isolation by vitrectomy • Chorioretinitis accounts for 85% of ocular disease while endophthalmitis occurs in only 15% *(Clin Infect Dis 53:262, 2011)*.	Chorioretinitis or Endophthalmitis: Lipid-based **Amphotericin B** 3-5 mg/kg daily + **Flucytosine** 25 mg/kg qid OR **Voriconazole** 6 mg/kg po/IV q12 x 2 doses and then 4 mg/kg po/IV q12. Consider intravitreal **Amphotericin B** 5–10 mcg in 0.1 mL or intravitreal **Voriconazole** 100 mcg in 0.1 mL for sight threatening disease.	Chorioretinitis or Endophthalmitis: **Fluconazole** 6-12 mg/kg daily (poor activity against C. glabrata or C. krusei) and consider intravitreal **Amphotericin B** 5-10 mcg in 0.1 mL for sight-threatening disease. Consider vitrectomy in advanced disease. *Clin Infect Dis. 52:648, 2011.*	**Duration of therapy:** 4-6 weeks or longer, based on resolution determined by repeated examinations. Patients with chorioretinitis only often respond to systemically administered antifungals. Intravitreal amphotericin and/or vitrectomy may be necessary for those with vitritis or endophthalmitis *(Br J Ophthalmol 92:466, 2008; Pharmacotherapy 27:1711, 2007)*.

TABLE 11A (7)

TYPE OF INFECTION/ORGANISM/ SITE OF INFECTION	ANTIMICROBIAL AGENTS OF CHOICE		COMMENTS
	PRIMARY	ALTERNATIVE	
Candidiasis: Other infections *(continued)*			
Neonatal candidiasis	**Ampho B** 1 mg/kg daily; OR **Fluconazole** 12 mg/kg daily.	**Lipid-based ampho B** 3-5 mg/kg daily.	**Lumbar puncture** to rule out CNS disease, **dilated retinal examination,** and **intravascular catheter removal** strongly recommended. Lipid-based ampho B used only if there is no renal involvement. Echinocandins considered 3rd line therapy. Duration of therapy is at least 3 weeks.
Peritonitis (Chronic Ambulatory Peritoneal Dialysis) *See Table 19, page 220.*	**Fluconazole** 400 mg po q24h x 2–3 wks; or **caspofungin** 70 mg IV on day 1 followed by 50 mg IV q24h for 14 days; or **micafungin** 100 mg q24h for 14 days.	**Ampho B,** continuous intraperitoneal dosing at 1.5 mg/L of dialysis fluid times 4–6 wks.	Remove cath immediately or if no clinical improvement in 4–7 days.
Candidiasis: Urinary tract infections			
Cystitis **Asymptomatic** *See CID 52:s427, 2011; CID 52:s452, 2011.*	**If possible, remove catheter or stent. No therapy indicated except in patients at high risk for dissemination or undergoing a urologic procedure.**		**High risk patients** include neonates and neutropenic patients; these patients should be managed as outlined for treatment of bloodstream infection. For patients undergoing urologic procedures, flu 200 mg (3 mg/kg) daily or ampho B 0.5 mg/kg daily (for flu-resistant organisms) for several days pre- and post-procedure.
Symptomatic	**Fluconazole** 200 mg (3 mg/kg) daily for 14 days.	**Ampho B** 0.5 mg/kg daily (for fluconazole resistant organisms) for 7-10 days.	Concentration of echinocandins in urine is low; case reports of efficacy versus azole resistant organisms *(Can J Infect Dis Med Microbiol 18:149, 2007; CID 44:e46, 2007).* Persistent candiduria in immunocompromised pt warrants ultrasound or CT of kidneys to rule out fungus ball.
Pyelonephritis	**Fluconazole** 200–400 mg (3–6 mg/kg) once daily orally.	**Ampho B** 0.5 mg/kg daily IV ± 5-FC 25 mg/kg orally qid.	**Treat for 2 weeks.** For suspected disseminated disease treat as if bloodstream infection is present.
Chromoblastomycosis *(Clin Exp Dermatol, 34:849, 2009).* (Cladophialophora, Phialophora, or Fonsecaea); Cutaneous (usually feet, legs): raised scaly lesions, most common in tropical areas	If lesions small & few, **surgical excision or cryosurgery with liquid nitrogen.** If lesions chronic, extensive, burrowing: **itraconazole.**	**Itraconazole:** 200-400 mg po q24h or 400 mg pulse therapy once daily for 1 week monthly for 6-12 months (or until response)[NAI].	**Terbinafine**[NAI] 500-1000 mg once daily alone or in combination with itraconazole 200-400 mg; or **posaconazole** (800 mg/d) also may be effective.

TABLE 11A (8)

TYPE OF INFECTION/ORGANISM/ SITE OF INFECTION	ANTIMICROBIAL AGENTS OF CHOICE		COMMENTS
	PRIMARY	ALTERNATIVE	
Coccidioidomycosis (Coccidioides immitis) *(IDSA Guidelines 2005: CID 41:1217, 2005; see also Mayo Clin Proc 83:343, 2008)*			
Primary pulmonary (San Joaquin or Valley Fever): **Pts low risk persistence/complication**	**Antifungal rx not generally recommended.** Treat if fever, wt loss and/or fatigue do not resolve within several wks to 2 mos *(see below)*		Uncomplicated pulmonary in normal host common in endemic areas *(Emerg Infect Dis 12:958, 2006)* Influenza -like illness of 1–2 wks duration.
Primary pulmonary in pts with ↑ risk for complications or dissemination. Rx indicated: • Immunosuppressive disease, post-transplantation, hematological malignancies or therapies (steroids, TNF-α antagonists) • Pregnancy in 3rd trimester • Diabetes • CF antibody >1:16 • Pulmonary Infiltrates • Dissemination (identification of spherules or culture of organism from ulcer, joint effusion, pus from subcutaneous abscess or bone biopsy, etc.)	**Mild to moderate severity:** **Itraconazole** solution 200 mg po or IV bid; OR **Fluconazole** 400 mg po q24h for 3–12 mos **Locally severe or disseminated disease** **Ampho B** 0.6–1 mg/kg per day x 7 days then 0.8 mg/kg every other day or **liposomal ampho B** 3-5 mg/kg/d IV or **ABLC** 5 mg/kg/d IV, until clinical improvement (usually several wks or longer in disseminated disease), followed by **itra** or **flu** for at least 1 year. Some use combination of Ampho B & Flu for progressive severe disease; controlled series lacking. **Consultation with specialist recommended:** surgery may be required. Lifetime suppression in HIV+ patients or until CD4 >250 & infection controlled: flu 200 mg po q24h or itra 200 mg po bid *(Mycosis 46:42, 2003)*.		**Ampho B cure rate 50–70%. Responses to azoles are similar. Itra** may have slight advantage esp. in soft tissue infection. Relapse rates after rx 40%: Relapse rate ↑ if ↑ CF titer ≥1:256. Following CF titers after completion of rx important; rising titers warrant retreatment. **Posaconazole** reported successful in 73% of pts with refractory non-meningeal cocci *(Chest 132:952, 2007)*. Not frontline therapy. Treatment of pediatric cocci to include salvage therapy with Vori & Caspo *(CID 56:1573, 1579 & 1587, 2013)*.
Meningitis: occurs in 1/3 to 1/2 of pts with disseminated coccidioidomycosis			
Adult *(CID 42:103, 2006)*	**Fluconazole** 400–1,000 mg po q24h indefinitely	**Ampho B** IV as for pulmonary *(above)* + 0.1–0.3 mg daily intra-thecal (intraventricular) via reservoir device. **OR itra** 400–800 mg q24h **OR voriconazole** *(see Comment)*	**80% relapse rate, continue flucon indefinitely. Voriconazole** successful in high doses (6 mg/kg IV q12h) followed by oral suppression (200 mg po q12h)
Child	**Fluconazole** (po) (Pediatric dose not established, 6 mg per kg q24h used)		
Cryptococcosis *(IDSA Guideline: CID 30:710, 2000)*. New Guidelines CID 50:291, 2010. Excellent review: *Brit Med Bull 72:99, 2005*			
Non-meningeal (non-AIDS) Risk 57% in organ transplant & those receiving other forms of immunosuppressive agents *(EID 13:953, 2007)*.	**Fluconazole** 400 mg/day IV or po for 8 wks to 6 mos **For more severe disease:** **Ampho B** 0.5–0.8 mg/kg per day IV till response then change to **fluconazole** 400 mg po q24h for 8–10 wks course	**Itraconazole** 200-400 mg solution q24h for 6-12 mos OR **Ampho B** 0.3 mg/kg per day IV + **flucytosine** 37.5 mg/kg[3] po qid times 6 wks (use ideal body wt)	**Flucon alone 90% effective for meningeal and non-meningeal forms.** Fluconazole as effective as ampho B. Addition of **interferon-γ** (IFN-γ-lb 50 mcg per M² subcut. 3x per wk x 9 wks) to liposomal ampho B assoc. with response in pt failing antifungal rx *(CID 38: 910, 2004)*. Posaconazole 400-800 mg also effective in a small series of patients *(CID 45:562, 2007; Chest 132:952, 2007)*
Meningitis (non-AIDS)	**Ampho B** 0.5–0.8 mg/kg per day IV + **flucytosine** 37.5 mg/kg[3] po q6h until pt afebrile & cultures neg (~6 wks) *(NEJM 301:126, 1979)*, then stop ampho B/flucyt, start **fluconazole** 200 mg po q24h *(AnIM 113:183, 1990)*; OR **Fluconazole** 400 mg po q24h x 8–10 wks (less severely ill pt). Some recommend flu for 2 yrs to reduce relapse rate *(CID 28:297, 1999)*. Some recommend Ampho B plus fluconazole as induction Rx. Studies underway.		If CSF opening pressure >25 cm H_2O, repeat LP to drain fluid to control pressure. Outbreaks of C. gattii meningitis have been reported in the Pacific Northwest *(EID 13:42, 2007)*; severity of disease and prognosis appear to be worse than with C. neoformans; initial therapy with ampho B + flucytosine recommended. C. gattii less susceptible to flucon than C. neoformans *(Clin Microbiol Inf 14:727, 2008)*. Outcomes in both AIDS and non-AIDS cryptococcal meningitis improved with Ampho B + 5-FC induction therapy for 14 days in those with neurological abnormalities or high organism burden *(PLoS ONE 3:e2870, 2008)*.

[3] Some experts would reduce to 25 mg per kg q6h

See page 2 for abbreviations. *All dosage recommendations are for adults (unless otherwise indicated) and assume normal renal function*

TABLE 11A (9)

TYPE OF INFECTION/ORGANISM/ SITE OF INFECTION	ANTIMICROBIAL AGENTS OF CHOICE		COMMENTS
	PRIMARY	ALTERNATIVE	
Cryptococcosis *(continued)*			
HIV+/AIDS: Cryptococcemia and/or Meningitis			
Treatment *See Clin Infect Dis 50:291, 2010 (IDSA Guidelines).* ↓ with ARV but still common presenting OI in newly diagnosed AIDS pts. Cryptococcal infection may be manifested by positive blood culture or positive serum cryptococcal antigen (CRAG: >95% sens). CRAG no help in monitoring response to therapy. With ARV, symptoms of acute meningitis may return: immune reconstitution inflammatory syndrome (IRIS). ↑ CSF pressure **(> 250 mm H_2O)** associated with high mortality: lower with CSF removal. If frequent LPs not possible, ventriculoperitoneal shunts an option *(Surg Neurol 63:529 & 531, 2005).*	**Ampho B** 0.7 mg/kg IV q24H + **flucytosine**[4] 25 mg/kg po q6h for at least two weeks or longer until CSF is sterilized. *See Comment.* **Then** **Consolidation therapy: Fluconazole** 400-800 mg po q24h to complete a 10-wks course then suppression *(see below).* Start Antiretroviral Therapy (ART) if possible.	**Amphotericin B** or **liposomal ampho B** + **fluconazole** 400 mg po or IV daily; **OR** **Amphotericin B** 0.7 mg/kg **or liposomal ampho B** 4 mg/kg IV q24h alone; **OR Fluconazole** ≥ 800 mg/day (1200 mg preferred) (po or IV) **plus flucytosine** 25 mg/kg po q6h for 4–6 weeks.	Outcome of treatment: treatment failure associated with dissemination of infection & high serum antigen titer, indicative of high burden of organisms and lack of 5FC use during inductive Rx, abnormal neurological evaluation & underlying hematological malignancy. Mortality rates still high, particularly in those with concomitant pneumonia *(Postgrad Med 121:107, 2009).* Early Dx essential for improved outcome *(PLOS Medicine 4:e47, 2007).* Ampho B + 5FC treatment ↓ crypto CFUs more rapidly than ampho + flu or ampho + 5FC + flu. Ampho B 1 mg/kg/d alone much more rapidly fungicidal in vivo than flu 400 mg/d *(CID 45:76&81, 2007).* Use of lipid-based ampho B associated with lower mortality compared to ampho B deoxycholate in solid organ transplant recipients *(CID 48:1566, 2009).* Monitor 5-FC levels: peak 70-80 mg/L, trough 30-40 mg/L. Higher levels assoc. with bone marrow toxicity. No difference in outcome if given IV or po *(AAC 51:1038, 2007).* Failure of flu may rarely be due to resistant organism, especially if burden of organism high at initiation of Rx. Although 200 mg qd = 400 mg qd of flu: median survival 76 & 82 days respectively, authors prefer 400 mg po qd *(BMC Infect Dis 6:118, 2006).* Trend toward improved outcomes with fluconazole 400-800 mg combined with ampho B versus ampho B alone in AIDS patients *(CID 48:1775, 2009).* Role of other azoles uncertain: successful outcomes were observed in 14/29 (48%) subjects with cryptococcal meningitis treated with posaconazole *(JAC 56:745, 2005).* Voriconazole also may be effective. Survival probably improved with ART but IRIS may complicate its use. There is considerable controversy as to the timing of initiation of ART *(see CID 50:1532, 2010 and CID 51: 984, 985, 986, 987, 2010).* One study suggests higher mortality with initiation of ART within 72 hrs of diagnosis *(CID 50:1532, 2010),* but the generalization of this study is an issue. Among others, most authorities continue to recommend ART within 2-6 wks of diagnosis.
Suppression (chronic maintenance therapy) Discontinuation of antifungal rx can be considered among pts who remain asymptomatic, with CD4 >100–200/mm^3 for ≥6 months. Some perform a lumbar puncture before discontinuation of maintenance rx. Reappearance of pos. serum CRAG may predict relapse	**Fluconazole** 200 mg/day po [If CD4 count rises to >100/mm^3 with effective antiretroviral rx, some authorities recommend dc suppressive rx. *See www.hivatis.org.* Authors would only dc if CSF culture negative.]	**Itraconazole** 200 mg po q12h if flu intolerant or failure. No data on Vori for maintenance.	Itraconazole less effective than fluconazole & not recommended because of higher relapse rate (23% vs 4%). Recurrence rate of 0.4 to 3.9 per 100 patient-years with discontinuation of suppressive therapy in 100 patients on ARV with CD4 >100 cells/mm^3.

[4] Flucytosine = 5-FC

TABLE 11A (10)

TYPE OF INFECTION/ORGANISM/ SITE OF INFECTION	ANTIMICROBIAL AGENTS OF CHOICE		COMMENTS
	PRIMARY	ALTERNATIVE	
Dermatophytosis *(See Mycopathologia 166:353, 2008)*			
Onychomycosis (Tinea unguium) (primarily cosmetic) Ciclopirox olamine 8% lacquer daily for 48 weeks; best suited for superficial and distal infections (overall cure rates of approx 30%).	**Fingernail Rx Options:** **Terbinafine**[5] 250 mg po q24h [children <20 kg: 67.5 mg/day, 20–40 kg: 125 mg/day, >40 kg: 250 mg/day] x 6 wks (79% effective) OR **Itraconazole**[6] 200 mg po q24h x 3 mos.[NAI] OR **Itraconazole** 200 mg po bid x 1 wk/mo x 2 mos OR **Fluconazole** 150–300 mg po q wk x 3–6 mos.[NAI]		**Toenail Rx Options:** **Terbinafine**[5] 250 mg po q24h [children <20 kg: 67.5 mg/day, 20–40 kg: 125 mg/day, >40 kg: 250 mg/day] x 12 wks (76% effective) OR **Itraconazole** 200 mg po q24h x 3 mos (59% effective) OR **Itraconazole** 200 mg bid x 1 wk/mo. x 3–4 mos (63% effective)[NAI] OR **Fluconazole** 150–300 mg po q wk x 6–12 mos (48% effective)[NAI] **Laser rx FDA approved:** modestly effective, expensive *(Med Lett 55:15, 2013)*.
Tinea capitis ("ringworm") (Trichophyton tonsurans, Microsporum canis, N. America; other sp. elsewhere) *(PIDJ 18:191, 1999)*	**Terbinafine**[5] 250 mg po q 24h x 2-4 wks (adults); 5 mg/kg/day x 4 wks (children).	**Itraconazole**[6] 5 mg/kg per day x 4 wks[NFDA]. **Fluconazole** 6 mg/kg q wk x 8-12 wks.[NAI] Cap at 150 mg po q wk for adults **Griseofulvin:** adults 500 mg po q24h x 6-8 wks, children 10–20 mg/kg per day until hair regrows.	Durations of therapy are for T. tonsurans; treat for approx. twice as long for M. canis. All agents with similar cure rates (60-100%) in clinical studies. Addition of topical ketoconazole or selenium sulfate shampoo reduces transmissibility *(Int J Dermatol 39:261, 2000)*
Tinea corporis, cruris, or pedis (Trichophyton rubrum, T. mentagrophytes, Epidermophyton floccosum) "Athlete's foot, jock itch," and ringworm	**Topical rx:** Generally applied 2x/day. Available as creams, ointments, sprays, by prescription & "over the counter." Apply 2x/day for 2–3 wks. Recommend: Lotrimin Ultra or Lamisil AT; contain butenafine & terbinafine—both are fungicidal	**Terbinafine** 250 mg po q24h x 2 wks[NAI] OR **ketoconazole** 200 mg po q24h x 4 wks OR **fluconazole** 150 mg po 1x/wk for 2–4 wks[NAI] **Griseofulvin:** adults 500 mg po q24h times 4–6 wks, children 10–20 mg/kg per day. Duration: 2-4 wks for corporis, 4-8 wks for pedis.	**Keto** po often effective in severe recalcitrant infection. Follow for hepatotoxicity; many drug-drug interactions.
Tinea versicolor (Malassezia furfur or Pityrosporum orbiculare) Rule out erythrasma—*see Table 1, page 54*	**Ketoconazole** (400 mg po single dose)[NAI] or (200 mg q24h x 7 days) or (2% cream 1x q24h x 2 wks)	**Fluconazole** 400 mg po single dose or **Itraconazole** 400 mg po q24h x 3–7 days	**Keto** (po) times 1 dose was 97% effective in 1 study. Another alternative: **Selenium sulfide** (Selsun), 2.5% lotion, apply as lather, leave on 10 min then wash off, 1/day x 7 day or 3–5/wk times 2–4 wks
Fusariosis Third most common cause of invasive mould infections, after *Aspergillus* and *Mucorales* and related molds, in patients with hematologic malignancies *(Mycoses 52:197, 2009)*. Pneumonia, skin infections, bone and joint infections, and disseminated disease occur in severely immunocompromised patients. In contrast to other moulds, blood cultures are frequently positive. *Fusarium solani*, *F. oxysporum*, *F. verticillioides* and *F. moniliforme* account for approx. 90% of isolates *(Clin Micro Rev 20: 695, 2007)* Frequently fatal, outcome depends on decreasing the level of immunosuppression.			
Laser rx FDA approved: modestly effective, expensive *(Med Lett 55:15, 2013)*. *(NEJM 360:2108, 2009)*	**Lipid-based ampho B** 5-10 mg/kg/d; OR **Ampho B** 1-1.5 mg/kg/d.	**Posaconazole** 400 mg po bid with meals (if not taking meals, 200 mg qid); OR **Voriconazole** IV: 6 mg per kg q12h times 1 day, then 4 mg per kg q12h; PO: 400 mg q12h, then 200 mg q12h. *See comments.*	**Surgical debridement** for localized disease. *Fusarium* spp. resistance to most antifungal agents, including echinocandins. *F. solani* and *F. verticillioides* typically are resistant to azoles. *F. oxysporum* and *F. moniliforme* may be susceptible to voriconazole and posaconazole. Role of combination therapy not well defined but case reports of response *(Mycoses 50: 227, 2007)*. Given variability in susceptibilities can consider combination therapy with vori and ampho B awaiting speciation. Outcome dependent on reduction or discontinuation of immunosuppression. Duration of therapy depends on response; long-term suppressive therapy for patients remaining on immunosuppressive therapy.

[5] **Serious but rare cases of hepatic failure** have been reported in pts receiving terbinafine & should not be used in those with chronic or active liver disease *(see Table 11B, page 127)*.
[6] Use of itraconazole has been associated with myocardial dysfunction and with onset of congestive heart failure.

See page 2 for abbreviations. All dosage recommendations are for adults (unless otherwise indicated) and assume normal renal function

TABLE 11A (11)

TYPE OF INFECTION/ORGANISM/ SITE OF INFECTION	ANTIMICROBIAL AGENTS OF CHOICE		COMMENTS
	PRIMARY	ALTERNATIVE	
Histoplasmosis (Histoplasma capsulatum): *See IDSA Guideline: CID 45:807, 2007.* Best diagnostic test is urinary, serum, or CSF histoplasma antigen: MiraVista Diagnostics (1-866-647-2847)			
Acute pulmonary histoplasmosis	**Mild to moderate disease, symptoms <4 wks:** No rx; If symptoms last over one month: **Itraconazole** 200 mg po tid for 3 days then once or twice daily for 6-12 wks. **Moderately severe or severe: Liposomal ampho B,** 3-5 mg/kg/d or **ABLC** 5 mg/kg/d IV or ampho B 0.7-1.0 mg/kg/d for 1-2 wks, then itra 200 mg tid for 3 days, then bid for 12 wks. + **methylprednisolone** 0.5-1 mg/kg/d for 1-2 wks.		Ampho B for patients at low risk of nephrotoxicity.
Chronic cavitary pulmonary histoplasmosis	**Itra** 200 mg po tid for 3 days then once or twice daily for at least 12 mos (some prefer 18-24 mos).		Document therapeutic itraconazole blood levels at 2 wks. Relapses occur in 9-15% of patients.
Mediastinal lymphadenitis, mediastinal granuloma, pericarditis; and rheumatologic syndromes	**Mild cases:** Antifungal therapy not indicated. Nonsteroidal anti-inflammatory drug for pericarditis or rheumatologic syndromes. If no response to non-steroidals, **Prednisone** 0.5-1.0 mg/kg/d tapered over 1-2 weeks for 1) pericarditis with hemodynamic compromise, 2) lymphadenitis with obstruction or compression syndromes, or 3) severe rheumatologic syndromes. **Itra** 200 mg po once or twice daily for 6-12 wks for moderately severe to severe cases, or if prednisone is administered.		Check itra blood levels to document therapeutic concentrations.
Progressive disseminated histoplasmosis	**Mild to moderate disease: itra** 200 mg po tid for 3 days then bid for at least 12 mos **Moderately severe to severe disease: Liposomal ampho B,** 3 mg/kg/d or **ABLC** 5 mg/kg/d for 1-2 weeks then **itra** 200 mg tid for 3 days, then bid for at least 12 mos.		**Ampho B** 0.7-1.0 mg/kg/d may be used for patients at low risk of nephrotoxicity. Confirm therapeutic itra blood levels. Azoles are teratogenic; itra should be avoided in pregnancy; use a lipid ampho formulation. Urinary antigen levels useful for monitoring response to therapy and relapse
CNS histoplasmosis	**Liposomal ampho B,** 5 mg/kg/d, for a total of 175 mg/kg over 4-6 wks, then **itra** 200 mg 2-3x a day for at least 12 mos. Vori likely effective for CNS disease or Itra failures. *(Arch Neurology 65: 666, 2008; J Antimicro Chemo 57:1235, 2006).*		Monitor CNS histo antigen, monitor itra blood levels. PCR may be better for Dx than histo antigen. Absorption of Itra (check levels) and CNS penetration may be an issue; case reports of success with Fluconazole *(Braz J Infect Dis 12:555, 2008)* and Posaconazole *(Drugs 65:1553, 2005)* following Ampho B therapy.
Prophylaxis (immunocompromised patients)	**Itra** 200 mg po daily		Consider primary **prophylaxis in HIV-infected** patients with < 150 CD4 cells/mm^3 in high prevalence areas. Secondary prophylaxis (i.e., suppressive therapy) indicated in HIV-infected patients with < 150 CD4 cells/mm^3 and other immunocompromised patients in who immunosuppression cannot be reversed

TABLE 11A (12)

TYPE OF INFECTION/ORGANISM/ SITE OF INFECTION	ANTIMICROBIAL AGENTS OF CHOICE		COMMENTS
	PRIMARY	ALTERNATIVE	
Madura foot *(See Nocardia & Scedosporium)*			
Mucormycosis & other related species—Rhizopus, Rhizomucor, Lichtheimia *(CID 54:1629, 2012)*. Rhinocerebral, pulmonary due to angioinvasion with tissue necrosis. Key to successful rx: early dx with symptoms suggestive of sinusitis (or lateral facial pain or numbness): think mucor with palatal ulcers, &/or black eschars, onset unilateral blindness in immunocompromised or diabetic pt. Rapidly fatal without rx. Dx by culture of tissue or stain: wide ribbon-like, non-septated with variation in diameter & right angle branching. Diabetics are predisposed to mucormycosis due to microangiopathy & ketoacidosis. Iron overload also predisposes: iron stimulates fungal growth.	**Liposomal ampho B** 5-10 mg/kg/day; OR **Ampho B** 1-1.5 mg/kg/day.	**Posaconazole** 400 mg po bid with meals (if not taking meals, 200 mg po qid)[NAI].	**Ampho B** (ABLC) monotherapy relatively ineffective with 20% success rate vs 69% for other polyenes *(CID 47:364, 2008)*. Complete or partial response rates of 60-80% in **posaconazole** salvage protocols *(JAC 61, Suppl 1, i35, 2008)*. Resistant to **voriconazole:** prolonged use of voriconazole prophylaxis predisposes to mucormycosis infections. Total duration of therapy based on response: continue therapy until 1) resolution of clinical signs and symptoms of infection, 2) resolution or stabilization of radiographic abnormalities; and 3) resolution of underlying immunosuppression. Posaconazole for secondary prophylaxis for those on immunosuppressive therapy *(CID 48:1743, 2009)*.
Paracoccidioidomycosis (South American blastomycosis) P. brasiliensis *(Dermatol Clin 26:257, 2008; Expert Rev Anti Infect Ther 6:251, 2008)*. Important cause of death from fungal infection in HIV-infected patients in Brazil *(Mem Inst Oswaldo Cruz 104:513, 2009)*.	**TMP/SMX** 800/160 mg bid-tid for 30 days, then 400/80 mg/day indefinitely (up to 3-5 years); OR **Itraconazole** (100 or 200 mg orally daily)	**Ketoconazole** 200-400 mg daily for 6-18 months; OR **Ampho B** total dose > 30 mg/kg	Improvement in >90% pts on itra or keto.[NAI] **Ampho B** reserved for severe cases and for those intolerant to other agents. TMP-SMX suppression life-long in HIV+.
Lobomycosis (keloidal blastomycosis)/ P. loboi	**Surgical excision**, **clofazimine** or **itraconazole**.		
Penicilliosis (Penicillium marneffei): Common disseminated fungal infection in AIDS pts in SE Asia (esp. Thailand & Vietnam).	**Ampho B** 0.5–1 mg/kg per day times 2 wks followed by **itraconazole** 400 mg/day for 10 wks followed by 200 mg/day po **indefinitely for HIV-infected pts.**	For less sick patients **Itra** 200 mg po tid x 3 days, then 200 mg po bid x 12 wks, then 200 mg po q24h.[7] (IV if unable to take po)	3rd most common OI in AIDS pts in SE Asia following TBc and cryptococcal meningitis. Prolonged fever, lymphadenopathy, hepatomegaly. Skin nodules are umbilicated (mimic cryptococcal infection or molluscum contagiosum). Preliminary data suggests vori effective: *CID 43:1060, 2006.*
Phaeohyphomycosis, Black molds, Dematiaceous fungi *(See CID 48:1033, 2009)* Sinuses, skin, bone & joint, brain abscess, endocarditis, emerging especially in HSCT pts with disseminated disease. **Scedosporium prolificans,** Bipolaris, Wangiella, Curvularia, Exophiala, Phialemonium, Scytalidium, Alternaria.	**Surgery** + **itraconazole** 400 mg/day po, duration not defined, probably 6 mo[NAI]	Case report of success with **voriconazole** + **terbinafine** *(Scand J Infect Dis 39:87, 2007)*; OR **Itraconazole** + **terbinafine** synergistic against S. prolificans. No clinical data & combination could show ↑ toxicity *(see Table 11B, page 125)*.	**Posaconazole** successful in case of brain abscess *(CID 34:1648, 2002)* and refractory infection *(Mycosis: 519, 2006)*. **Notoriously resistant to antifungal rx including amphotericin & azoles.** 44% of patients in compassionate use/salvage therapy study responded to voriconazole *(AAC 52:1743, 2008)*. >80% mortality in immunocompromised hosts.
Pneumocystis pneumonia (PCP) caused by **Pneumocystis jiroveci**. *Ref: JAMA 301:2578, 2009.*			
Not acutely ill, able to take po meds. PaO_2 >70 mmHg Diagnosis: sputum PCR. Serum Beta-D Glucan may help; reasonable sensitivity & specificity, but also many false positives *(JCM 51:3478, 2013)*.	(**TMP-SMX-DS**, 2 tabs po q8h x21 days) OR (**Dapsone** 100 mg po q24h + **trimethoprim** 5 mg/kg po tid x21 days)	[**Clindamycin** 300–450 mg po q6h + **primaquine** 15 mg base po q24h] x21 days OR **Atovaquone** suspension 750 mg po bid with food x21 days	Mutations in gene of the enzyme target (dihydropteroate synthetase) of sulfamethoxazole identified. Unclear whether mutations result in resist to TMP-SMX or dapsone + TMP *(EID 10:1721, 2004)*. Dapsone ref.: *CID 27:191, 1998.* **After 21 days, chronic suppression in AIDS pts *(see below—post-treatment suppression)*.**
	NOTE: Concomitant use of corticosteroids usually reserved for sicker pts with PaO_2 <70 *(see below)*		

[7] **Oral solution preferred to tablets because of ↑ absorption** *(see Table 11B, page 125)*.

See page 2 for abbreviations. All dosage recommendations are for adults (unless otherwise indicated) and assume normal renal function

TABLE 11A (13)

TYPE OF INFECTION/ORGANISM/ SITE OF INFECTION	ANTIMICROBIAL AGENTS OF CHOICE		COMMENTS
	PRIMARY	ALTERNATIVE	
Pneumocystis pneumonia (PCP) *(continued)*			
Primary prophylaxis and post-treatment suppression	(**TMP-SMX-DS or -SS**, 1 tab po q24h or 1 DS 3x/wk) OR (**dapsone** 100mg po q24h). DC when CD4 >200 x/3 mos *(NEJM 344:159, 2001)*.	(**Pentamidine** 300mg in 6mL sterile water by aerosol q4wks) OR (**dapsone** 200mg po + **pyrimethamine** 75mg po + **folinic acid** 25mg po—**all once a week**) or **atovaquone** 1500mg po q24h with food.	TMP-SMX-DS regimen provides cross-protection vs toxo and other bacterial infections. Dapsone + pyrimethamine protects vs toxo. Atovaquone suspension 1500mg once daily as effective as daily dapsone *(NEJM 339:1889, 1998)* or inhaled pentamidine *(JID 180:369, 1999)*.
Scedosporium apiospermum (Pseudallescheria boydii) (not considered a true dematiaceous mold) *(Medicine 81:333, 2002)* Skin, subcut **(Madura foot)**, brain abscess, recurrent meningitis. May appear after near-drowning incidents. Also emerging especially in hematopoietic stem cell transplant (HSCT) pts with disseminated disease	**Voriconazole** 6 mg/kg IV q12h on day 1, then either (4 mg/kg IV q12h) or (200 mg po q12h for body weight ≥40 kg, but 100 mg po q12h for body weight <40 kg) *(AAC 52:1743, 2008)*. 300 mg bid if serum concentrations are subtherapeutic, i.e., < 1 mcg/mL *(CID 46:201, 2008)*.	Surgery + **itraconazole** 200 mg po bid until clinically well.[NAI] (Many species now resistant or refractory to itra); OR **Posa** 400 mg po bid with meals (if not taking meals, 200 mg po qid).	**Resistant to many antifungal drugs including amphotericin**. In vitro voriconazole more active than itra and posaconazole in vitro *(Clin Microbiol Rev 21:157, 2008)*. Case reports of successful rx of disseminated and CNS disease with voriconazole *(AAC 52:1743, 2008)*. Posaconazole active *in vitro* and successful in several case reports
Sporotrichosis *IDSA Guideline: CID 45:1255, 2007.*			
Cutaneous/Lymphocutaneous	**Itraconazole** po 200 mg/day for 2-4 wks after all lesions resolved, usually 3-6 mos.	If no response, **itra** 200 mg po bid or **terbinafine** 500 mg po bid or **SSKI** 5 drops (eye drops) tid & increase to 40-50 drops tid	Fluconazole 400-800 mg daily only if no response to primary or alternative suggestions. Pregnancy or nursing: local hyperthermia *(see below)*.
Osteoarticular	**Itra** 200 mg po bid x 12 mos.	**Liposomal ampho B** 3-5 mg/kg/d IV or **ABLC** 5 mg/kg/d IV or **ampho B deoxycholate** 0.7-1 mg/kg IV daily; if response, change to **itra** 200 mg po bid x total 12 mos.	After 2 wks of therapy, document adequate serum levels of itraconazole.
Pulmonary	If severe, **lipid ampho B** 3-5 mg/kg IV or **standard ampho B** 0.7-1 mg/kg IV once daily until response, then **itra** 200 mg po bid. Total of 12 mos.	Less severe: **itraconazole** 200 mg po bid x 12 mos.	After 2 weeks of therapy document adequate serum levels of itra. Surgical resection plus ampho B for localized pulmonary disease.
Meningeal or Disseminated	**Lipid ampho B** 5 mg/kg IV once daily x 4-6 wks, then—if better—**itra** 200 mg po bid for total of 12 mos.	AIDS/Other immunosuppressed pts: chronic therapy with **itra** 200 mg po once daily.	After 2 weeks, document adequate serum levels of itra.
Pregnancy and children	**Pregnancy:** Cutaneous—local hyperthermia. Severe: **lipid ampho B** 3-5 mg/kg IV once daily. **Avoid itraconazole.**	**Children:** Cutaneous: **Itra** 6-10 mg/kg (max of 400 mg) daily. Alternative is **SSKI** 1 drop tid increasing to max of 1 drop/kg or 40-50 drops tid/day, whichever is lowest.	For children with disseminated sporotrichosis: Standard ampho B 0.7 mg/kg IV once daily & after response, itra 6-10 mg/kg (max 400 mg) once daily.

TABLE 11B – ANTIFUNGAL DRUGS: DOSAGE, ADVERSE EFFECTS, COMMENTS

DRUG NAME, GENERIC (TRADE)/USUAL DOSAGE	ADVERSE EFFECTS/COMMENTS
Non-lipid amphotericin B deoxycholate (Fungizone): 0.5-0.7 mg/kg per day as single infusion **Ampho B predictably not active vs. Scedosporium, Candida lusitaniae & Aspergillus terreus** *(TABLE 11C, page 128)*	**Admin:** Ampho B is a colloidal suspension that must be prepared in electrolyte-free D5W at 0.1 mg/mL to avoid precipitation. No need to protect suspensions from light. Infusions cause chills/fever, myalgia, anorexia, nausea, rarely hemodynamic collapse/hypotension. Postulated due to proinflammatory cytokines, doesn't appear to be histamine release *(Pharmacol 23:966, 2003)*. Infusion duration usu. 4+ hrs. No difference found in 1 vs 4 hr infus. except chills/fever occurred sooner with 1 hr infus. Febrile reactions ↓ with repeat doses. Rare pulmonary reactions (severe dyspnea & focal infiltrates suggest pulmonary edema) assoc with rapid infus. **Severe rigors respond to meperidine (25–50 mg IV).** Premedication with acetaminophen, diphenhydramine, hydrocortisone (25–50 mg) and heparin (1000 units) had no influence on rigors/fever. If cytokine postulate correct, NSAIDs or high-dose steroids may prove efficacious but their use may risk worsening infection under rx or increased risk of **nephrotoxicity** (i.e., NSAIDs). Clinical side effects ↓ with ↑ age. **Toxicity:** Major concern is nephrotoxicity. Manifest initially by kaliuresis and **hypokalemia**, then fall in serum bicarbonate (may proceed to renal tubular acidosis), ↓ in renal erythropoietin and anemia, and rising BUN/serum creatinine. Hypomagnesemia may occur. Can reduce risk of renal injury by **(a) pre- & post-infusion hydration with 500 mL saline (if clinical status allows salt load), (b)** avoidance of other nephrotoxins, eg, radiocontrast, aminoglycosides, cis-platinum, **(c)** use of lipid prep of ampho B.
Lipid-based ampho B products[1]: **Amphotericin B lipid complex (ABLC)** (Abelcet): 5 mg/kg per day as single infusion	**Admin:** Consists of ampho B complexed with 2 lipid bilayer ribbons. Compared to standard ampho B, larger volume of distribution, rapid blood clearance and high tissue concentrations (liver, spleen, lung). Dosage: **5 mg/kg once daily;** infuse at 2.5 mg/kg per hr; adult and ped. dose the same. Do NOT use an in-line filter. Do not dilute with saline or mix with other drugs or electrolytes.[2] **Toxicity:** Fever and chills 14–18%; nausea 9%, vomiting 8%; serum creatinine ↑ in 11%; renal failure 5%; anemia 4%; ↓ K 5%; rash 4%. A fatal fat embolism following ABLC infusion *(Exp Mol Path 177:246, 2004)*. Majority of pts intolerant of liposomal ampho B can tolerate lipid ampho B *(CID 56:701, 2013)*.
Liposomal amphotericin B (**LAB**, AmBisome)**:** 3–5 mg/kg per day as single infusion. If intolerant, majority OK with lipid form *(CID 56:701, 2013)*.	**Admin:** Consists of vesicular bilayer liposome with ampho B intercalated within the membrane. Dosage: **3–5 mg/kg per day** IV as single dose infused over a period of approx. 120 min. If tolerated, infusion time reduced to 60 min. *(see footnote*[2]*)*. Tolerated well in elderly pts *(J Inf 50:277, 2005)*. **Major toxicity:** Gen less than ampho B. Nephrotoxicity 18.7% vs 33.7% for ampho B, chills 47% vs 75%, nausea 39.7% vs 38.7%, vomiting 31.8% vs 43.9%, rash 24% for both, ↓ Ca 18.4% vs 20.9%, ↓ K 20.4% vs 25.6%, ↓ mg 20.4% vs 25.6%. Acute reactions common with liposomal ampho B, 20– 40%. 86% occur within 5 min of infusion, incl chest pain, dyspnea, hypoxia or severe abdom, flank or leg pain; 14% dev flushing & urticaria near end of 4 hr infusion. All responded to diphenhydramine (1 mg/kg) & interruption of infusion. Reactions may be due to complement activation by liposome *(CID 36:1213, 2003)*.
Caspofungin (Cancidas) 70 mg IV on day 1 followed by 50 mg IV q24h (reduce to 35 mg IV q24h with moderate hepatic insufficiency)	An echinocandin which inhibits synthesis of β-(1,3)-D-glucan. Fungicidal against candida (MIC <2 mcg/mL) including those resistant to other antifungals & active against aspergillus (MIC 0.4–2.7 mcg/mL). Approved indications for caspo incl: empirical rx for febrile, neutropenic pts; rx of candidemia, candida intraabdominal abscesses, peritonitis, & pleural space infections; esophageal candidiasis; & invasive aspergillosis in pts refractory to or intolerant of other therapies. Serum levels on rec. dosages = peak 12, trough 1.3 (24 hrs) mcg/mL. **Toxicity:** remarkably non-toxic. Most common adverse effect: pruritus at infusion site & headache, fever, chills, vomiting, & diarrhea assoc with infusion. ↑ serum creatinine in 8% on caspo vs 21% short-course ampho B in 422 pts with candidemia *(Ln, Oct. 12, 2005, online)*. Drug metab in liver & dosage ↓ to 35 mg in moderate to severe hepatic failure. Class C for preg (embryotoxic in rats & rabbits). *See Table 22, page 224 for drug-drug interactions, esp. cyclosporine (hepatic toxicity) & tacrolimus (drug level monitoring recommended)*. Reversible thrombocytopenia reported *(Pharmacother 24:1408, 2004)*. **No drug in CSF or urine.**
Micafungin (Mycamine) 50 mg/day for prophylaxis post-bone marrow stem cell trans; 100 mg candidemia, 150 mg candida esophagitis.	The 2nd echinocandin approved by FDA for rx of esophageal candidiasis & prophylaxis against candida infections in HSCT[3] recipients. Active against most strains of candida sp. & aspergillus sp. incl those resist to fluconazole such as C. glabrata & C. krusei. No antagonism seen when combo with other antifungal drugs. No dosage adjust for severe renal failure or moderate hepatic impairment. Watch for drug-drug interactions with sirolimus or nifedipine. Micafungin well tolerated & common adverse events incl nausea 2.8%, vomiting 2.4%, & headache 2.4%. Transient ↑ LFTs, BUN, creatinine reported; rare cases of significant hepatitis & renal insufficiency. *See CID 42:1171, 2006.* **No drug in CSF or urine.**

1 Published data from patients intolerant of or refractory to conventional ampho B deoxycholate (Amp B d). **None of the lipid ampho B preps has shown superior efficacy compared to ampho B in prospective trials (except liposomal ampho B was more effective vs ampho B in rx of disseminated histoplasmosis at 2 wks). Dosage equivalency has not been established** *(CID 36:1500, 2003)*. Nephrotoxicity ↓ with all lipid ampho B preps.
2 Comparisons between Abelcet & AmBisome suggest higher infusion-assoc. toxicity (rigors) & febrile episodes with Abelcet (70% vs 36%) but higher frequency of mild hepatic toxicity with AmBisome (59% vs 38%, p=0.05). Mild elevations in serum creatinine were observed in 1/3 of both *(BJ Hemat 103:198, 1998; Focus on Fungal Inf #9, 1999; Bone Marrow Tx 20:39, 1997; CID 26:1383, 1998)*.
3 HSCT = hematopoietic stem cell transplant.

See page 2 for abbreviations. *All dosage recommendations are for adults (unless otherwise indicated) and assume normal renal function*

TABLE 11B (2)

DRUG NAME, GENERIC (TRADE)/USUAL DOSAGE	ADVERSE EFFECTS/COMMENTS
Anidulafungin (Eraxis) For Candidemia; 200 mg IV on day 1 followed by 100 mg/day IV). Rx for EC; 100 mg IV x 1, then 50 mg IV once/d.	An echinocandin with antifungal activity (cidal) against candida sp. & aspergillus sp. including ampho B- & triazole-resistant strains. FDA approved for treatment of esophageal candidiasis (EC), candidemia, and other complicated Candida infections. Effective in clinical trials of esophageal candidiasis & in 1 trial was superior to fluconazole in rx of invasive candidiasis/candidemia in 245 pts (75.6% vs 60.2%). Like other echinocandins, remarkably non-toxic; most common side-effects: nausea, vomiting, ↓ mg, ↓ K & headache in 11–13% of pts. No dose adjustments for renal or hepatic insufficiency. *See CID 43:215, 2006*. **No drug in CSF or urine.**
Fluconazole (Diflucan) 100 mg tabs 150 mg tabs 200 mg tabs 400 mg IV Oral suspension: 50 mg per 5 mL.	IV=oral dose because of excellent bioavailability. **Pharmacology:** absorbed po, water solubility enables IV. For peak serum levels *(see Table 9A, page 86)*. T½ 30hr (range 20–50 hr). 12% protein bound. **CSF levels 50–90% of serum in normals,** ↑ in meningitis. No effect on mammalian steroid metabolism. **Drug-drug interactions common,** *see Table 22*. Side-effects overall 16% [more common in HIV+ pts (21%)]. Nausea 3.7%, headache 1.9%, skin rash 1.8%, abdominal pain 1.7%, vomiting 1.7%, diarrhea 1.5%, ↑ SGOT 20%. Alopecia (scalp, pubic crest) in 12–20% pts on ≥400 mg po q24h after median of 3 mos (reversible in approx. 6mo). Rare: severe hepatotoxicity *(CID 41:301, 2005)*, exfoliative dermatitis. **Note: Candida krusei and Candida glabrata resistant to Flu.**
Flucytosine (Ancobon) 500 mg cap	AEs: Overall 30%. GI 6% (diarrhea, anorexia, nausea, vomiting); hematologic 22% [leukopenia, thrombocytopenia, when serum level >100 mcg/mL (esp. in azotemic pts)]; hepatotoxicity (asymptomatic ↑ SGOT, reversible); skin rash 7%; aplastic anemia (rare—2 or 3 cases). False ↑ in serum creatinine on EKTACHEM analyzer.
Griseofulvin (Fulvicin, Grifulvin, Grisactin) 500 mg, susp 125 mg/mL.	Photosensitivity, urticaria, GI upset, fatigue, leukopenia (rare). Interferes with warfarin drugs. Increases blood and urine porphyrins, should not be used in patients with porphyria. Minor disulfiram-like reactions. Exacerbation of systemic lupus erythematosus.
Imidazoles, topical For vaginal and/or skin use	Not recommended in 1st trimester of pregnancy. Local reactions: 0.5-1.5%: dyspareunia, mild vaginal or vulvar erythema, burning, pruritus, urticaria, rash. Rarely similar symptoms in sexual partner.
Itraconazole (Sporanox) 100 mg cap 10 mg/mL oral solution IV usual dose 200 mg bid x 4 doses followed by 200 mg q24h for a max of 14 days	**Itraconazole tablet & solution forms not interchangeable, solution preferred.** Many authorities recommend measuring drug serum concentration after 2 wks to ensure satisfactory absorption. To obtain highest plasma concentration, tablet is given with food & acidic drinks (e.g., cola) while solution is taken in fasted state; under these conditions, the peak conc. of capsule is approx. 3 mcg/mL & of solution 5.4 mcg/mL. Peak levels reached faster (2.2 vs 5 hrs) with solution. **Peak plasma concentrations after IV injection (200 mg) compared to oral capsule (200 mg): 2.8 mcg/mL (on day 7 of rx) vs 2 mcg/mL (on day 36 of rx).** Protein-binding for both preparations is over 99%, which explains virtual absence of penetration into CSF **(do not use to treat meningitis).** Adverse effects: dose-related nausea 10%, diarrhea 8%, vomiting 6%, & abdominal discomfort 5.7%. Allergic rash 8.6%, ↑ bilirubin 6%, edema 3.5%, & hepatitis 2.7% reported. ↑ doses may produce hypokalemia 8% & ↑ blood pressure 3.2%. Delirium, peripheral neuropathy & tremor reported *(J Neur Neurosurg Psych 81:327, 2010)*. **Reported to produce impairment in cardiac function.** Severe liver failure req transplant in pts receiving pulse rx for onychomycosis: FDA reports 24 cases with 11 deaths out of 50 mill people who received the drug prior to 2001. Other concern, as with fluconazole and ketoconazole, is **drug-drug interactions;** *see Table 22*. Some can be life-threatening.
Ketoconazole (Nizoral) 200 mg tab	Gastric acid required for absorption—cimetidine, omeprazole, antacids block absorption. In achlorhydria, dissolve tablet in 4 mL 0.2N HCl, drink with a straw. Coca-Cola ↑ absorption by 65%. CSF levels "none." **Drug-drug interactions important,** *see Table 22*. **Some interactions can be life-threatening.** **Dose- dependent nausea and vomiting.** Liver toxicity of hepatocellular type reported in about 1:10,000 exposed pts—usually after several days to weeks of exposure. At doses of ≥800 mg per day serum testosterone and plasma cortisol levels fall. With high doses, adrenal (Addisonian) crisis reported.
Miconazole (Monistat IV) 200 mg—*not available in U.S.*	IV miconazole indicated in patient critically ill with Scedosporium (Pseudallescheria boydii) infection. Very toxic due to vehicle needed to get drug into solution.
Nystatin (Mycostatin) 30 gm cream 500,000 units oral tab	Topical: virtually no adverse effects. Less effective than imidazoles and triazoles. PO: large doses give occasional GI distress and diarrhea.

TABLE 11B (3)

DRUG NAME, GENERIC (TRADE)/USUAL DOSAGE	ADVERSE EFFECTS/COMMENTS
Posaconazole *(Noxafil)* 400 mg po bid with meals (if not taking meals, 200 mg qid). 200 mg po tid (with food) for prophylaxis. 40 mg/mL suspension. 100 mg delayed-release tabs **Takes 7-10 days to achieve steady state. No IV formulation.**	An oral triazole with activity against a wide range of fungi refractory to other antifungal rx including: aspergillosis, mucormycosis (variability by species), fusariosis, Scedosporium (Pseudallescheria), phaeohyphomycosis, histoplasmosis, refractory candidiasis, refractory coccidioidomycosis, refractory cryptococcosis, & refractory chromoblastomycosis. **Should be taken with high fat meal for maximum absorption.** Approved for prophylaxis of invasive aspergillus and candidiasis. Clinical response in 75% of 176 AIDS pts with azole-refractory oral/esophageal candidiasis. Posaconazole has similar toxicities as other triazoles: nausea 9%, vomiting 6%, abd. pain 5%, headache 5%, diarrhea, ↑ ALT, AST, & rash (3% each). In pts rx for >6 mos., serious side-effects have included adrenal insufficiency, nephrotoxicity, & QTc interval prolongation. Significant drug-drug interactions; inhibits CYP3A4 *(see Table 22)*. Consider monitoring serum concentrations *(AAC 53:24, 2009)*. **100 mg delayed-release tablets:** loading dose of 300 mg (three 100 mg delayed-release tablets) twice daily on the first day, followed by a once-daily maintenance dose of 300 mg (three 100 mg delayed-release tablets) starting on the second day of therapy. Approved for prophylaxis only and not treatment. The tablet and solution are not interchangeable.
Terbinafine (Lamisil) 250 mg tab	In pts given terbinafine for onychomycosis, rare cases (8) of idiosyncratic & symptomatic hepatic injury & more rarely liver failure leading to death or liver transplant. The drug is **not recommended** for pts with **chronic or active liver disease;** hepatotoxicity may occur in pts with or without pre-existing disease. Pretreatment serum transaminases (ALT & AST) advised & alternate rx used for those with abnormal levels. Pts started on terbinafine should be warned about symptoms suggesting liver dysfunction (persistent nausea, anorexia, fatigue, vomiting, RUQ pain, jaundice, dark urine or pale stools). If symptoms develop, drug should be discontinued & liver function immediately evaluated. In controlled trials, changes in ocular lens and retina reported—clinical significance unknown. Major drug-drug interaction is 100% ↑ in rate of clearance by rifampin. AEs: usually mild, transient and rarely caused discontinuation of rx. % with AE, terbinafine vs placebo: nausea/diarrhea 2.6–5.6 vs 2.9; rash 5.6 vs 2.2; taste abnormality 2.8 vs 0.7. Inhibits CYP2D6 enzymes *(see Table 22)*. An acute generalized exanthematous pustulosis and subacute cutaneous lupus erythematosus reported.
Voriconazole (Vfend) **IV: Loading dose 6 mg per kg q12h times 1 day, then 4 mg per kg q12h IV** for invasive aspergillus & serious mold infections; **3 mg per kg IV q12h** for serious candida infections. **Oral: >40 kg body weight:** 400 mg po q12h, then 200 mg po q12h. **<40 kg body weight:** 200 mg po q12h, then 100 mg po q12h **Take oral dose 1 hour before or 1 hour after eating.** Oral suspension (40 mg per mL). Oral suspension dosing: Same as for oral tabs. Reduce to ½ maintenance dose for moderate hepatic insufficiency	A triazole with activity against Aspergillus sp., **including Ampho resistant strains of A. terreus.** Active vs Candida sp. (including krusei), Fusarium sp., & various molds. Steady state serum levels reach 2.5–4 mcg per mL. Up to 20% of patients with subtherapeutic levels with oral administration: check levels for suspected treatment failure, life threatening infections. 300 mg bid oral dose or 8 mg/kg/d IV dose may be required to achieve target steady-state drug concentrations of 1-6 mcg/mL. **Toxicity** similar to other azoles/triazoles including uncommon serious hepatic toxicity (hepatitis, cholestasis & fulminant hepatic failure. Liver function tests should be monitored during rx & drug dc'd if abnormalities develop. Rash reported in up to 20%, occ. photosensitivity & rare Stevens-Johnson, hallucinations & anaphylactoid infusion reactions with fever and hypertension. 1 case of QT prolongation with ventricular tachycardia in a 15 y/o pt with ALL reported. **Approx. 21% experience a transient visual disturbance** following IV or po ("altered/enhanced visual perception", blurred or colored visual change or photophobia) within 30–60 minutes. Visual changes resolve within 30–60 min. after administration & are attenuated with repeated doses **(do not drive at night for outpatient rx)**. Persistent visual changes occur rarely. Cause unknown. In patients with ClCr <50 mL per min., the intravenous vehicle (SBECD-sulfobutylether-B cyclodextrin) may accumulate but not obviously toxic *(CID 54:913, 2012)*. Hallucinations, hypoglycemia, electrolyte disturbance & pneumonitis attributed to ↑ drug concentrations. Potential for drug-drug interactions high—*see Table 22*. **With prolonged use, fluoride in drug can cause a painful periostitis.** **NOTE: Not in urine in active form. No activity vs. mucormycosis.**

See page 2 for abbreviations. All dosage recommendations are for adults (unless otherwise indicated) and assume normal renal function

TABLE 11C – AT A GLANCE SUMMARY OF SUGGESTED ANTIFUNGAL DRUGS AGAINST TREATABLE PATHOGENIC FUNGI

Microorganism	Antifungal[1, 2, 3, 4]					
	Fluconazole[5]	Itraconazole	Voriconazole	Posaconazole	Echinocandin[6]	Amphotericin
Candida albicans	+++	+++	+++	+++	+++	+++
Candida dubliniensis	+++	+++	+++	+++	+++	+++
Candida glabrata	±	±	+	+	+++	++
Candida tropicalis	+++	+++	+++	+++	+++	+++
Candida parapsilosis[7]	+++	+++	+++	+++	++ (higher MIC)	+++
Candida krusei	-	+	++	++	+++	++
Candida guilliermondii	+++	+++	+++	+++	++ (higher MIC)	++
Candida lusitaniae	+	+	++	++	++	-[8]
Cryptococcus neoformans	+++	+	+++	+++	-	+++
Aspergillus fumigatus[9]	-	++	+++	++	++	+++
Aspergillus flavus[9]	-	++	+++	+++	++	++ (higher MIC)
Aspergillus terreus	-	++	+++	+++	++	-
Fusarium sp.	-	±	++	++	-	++ (lipid formulations)
Scedosporium apiospermum (*Pseudoallescheria boydii*)	-	-	+++	++	-	-
Scedosporium prolificans[10]	-	-	±	±	-	-
Trichosporon spp.	±	+	++	++	-	+
Mucormycosis (e.g., Mucor, Rhizopus, Lichtheimia)	-	-	-	++	-	+++ (lipid formulations)
Dematiaceous molds[11] (e.g., *Alternaria, Bipolaris, Curvularia, Exophiala*)	-	++	+++	+++	+	+
Dimorphic Fungi						
Blastomyces dermatitidis	+	+++	++	++	-	+++
Coccidioides immitis/posadasii	+++	+++	++	++	-	+++
Histoplasma capsulatum	+	+++	++	++	-	+++
Sporothrix schenckii	-	++	-	+	-	+++

- = no activity; ± = possibly activity; + = active, 3rd line therapy (least active clinically)
++ = Active, 2nd line therapy (less active clinically); +++ = Active, 1st line therapy (usually active clinically)

1 Minimum inhibitory concentration values do not always predict clinical outcome.
2 Echinocandins, voriconazole, posaconazole and polyenes have poor urine penetration.
3 During severe immune suppression, success requires immune reconstitution.
4 **Flucytosine** has activity against *Candida* sp., *Cryptococcus* sp., and dematiaceous molds, but is primarily used in combination therapy.
5 For infections secondary to *Candida* sp., patients with prior triazole therapy have higher likelihood of triazole resistance.
6 Echinocandin pharmacodynamics, *see JAC 65:1108, 2010.*
7 Successful treatment of infections from *Candida parapsilosis* requires removal of foreign body or intravascular device.
8 Treatment failures reported, even for susceptible strains.
9 Lipid formulations of amphotericin may have greater activity against *A. fumigatus* and *A. flavus* (+++).
10 *Scedosporium prolificans* is poorly susceptible to single agents and may require combination therapy (e.g., addition of terbinafine).
11 Infections from mucormycosis, some *Aspergillus* sp., and dematiaceous molds often require surgical debridement.

TABLE 12A – TREATMENT OF MYCOBACTERIAL INFECTIONS*

Tuberculin skin test (TST). Same as PPD *[Chest 138:1456, 2010].*

Criteria for positive TST after 5 tuberculin units (intermediate PPD) read at 48–72 hours:

- ≥5 mm induration: + HIV, immunosuppressed, ≥15 mg prednisone per day, healed TBc on chest x-ray, recent close contact
- ≥10 mm induration: foreign-born, countries with high prevalence; IVD Users; low income; NH residents; chronic illness; silicosis
- ≥15 mm induration: otherwise healthy

Two-stage to detect sluggish positivity: If 1st PPD + but <10 mm, repeat intermediate PPD in 1 wk. Response to 2nd PPD can also happen if pt received BCG in childhood.

BCG vaccine as child: if ≥10 mm induration, & from country with TBc, should be attributed to MTB. Prior BCG may result in booster effect in 2-stage TST.

Routine anergy testing not recommended.

Interferon Gamma Release Assays (IGRAs): IGRAs detect sensitivities to MTB by measuring IFN-γ release in response to MTB antigens. May be used in place of TST in all situations in which TST may be used *(MMWR 59 (RR-5), 2010)*. FDA approved tests available in the U.S.:

- QuantiFERON-TB Gold (QFT-G) (approved 2005)
- QuantiFERON-TB Gold In-Tube Test (QFT-GIT) (approved 2007)
- T-Spot (approved 2008)

IGRAs are relatively specific for MTB and do not cross-react with BCG or most nontuberculous mycobacteria. CDC recommends IGRA over TST for persons unlikely to return for reading TST & for persons who have received BCG. TST is preferred in children age < 5 yrs (but IGRA is acceptable). IGRA or TST may be used without preference for recent contacts of TB with special utility for follow-up testing since IGRAs do not produce "booster effect". May also be used without preference over TBc for occupational exposures. As with TST, testing with IGRAs in low prevalence populations will result in false-positive results *(CID 53:234, 2011)*. For detailed discussion of IGRAs, *see MMWR 59 (RR-5), 2010 and JAMA 308:241, 2012.*

Rapid (24-hr or less) diagnostic tests for MTB: (1) the Amplified Mycobacterium tuberculosis Direct Test amplifies and detects MTB ribosomal RNA; (2) the AMPLICOR Mycobacterium tuberculosis Test amplifies and detects MTB DNA. Both tests have sensitivities & specificities >95% in sputum samples that are AFB-positive. In negative smears, specificity remains >95% but sensitivity is 40–77% *(MMWR 58:7, 2009; CID 49:46, 2009)* to 60-90% *(see: http://www.cdc.gov/tb/publications/guidelines/amplification_tests/default.htm).*

Xpert MTB/RIF is a rapid test (2 hrs) for MTB in sputum samples which also detects RIF resistance with specificity of 99.2% and sensitivity of 72.5% in smear negative patients *(NEJM 363:1005, 2010)*. Current antibody-based and ELISA-based rapid tests for TBc not recommended by WHO because they are less accurate than microscopy ± culture *(Lancet ID 11:736, 2011)*.

CAUSATIVE AGENT/DISEASE	MODIFYING CIRCUMSTANCES	SUGGESTED REGIMENS	
		INITIAL THERAPY	CONTINUATION PHASE OF THERAPY
I. **Mycobacterium tuberculosis exposure baseline TST/IGRA negative** (household members & other close contacts of potentially infectious cases)	Neonate- Rx essential NOTE: If fever, abnormal CXR (pleural effusion, hilar adenopathy, infiltrate) at baseline, treat for active TBc and not with INH alone.	**INH** (10 mg/kg/ day for 8-10 wks)	Repeat tuberculin skin test (TST) in 8-12 wks: if TST neg & CXR normal & infant age at exposure > 6 mos., stop INH, if TST (≥ 5 mm) or age ≤ 6 mos, treat with INH for total of 9 mos. If follow-up CXR abnormal, treat for active TBc.
	Children <5 years of age—Rx indicated	As for neonate for 1st 8-10 wks.	If repeat TST at 8-10 wks is negative, stop. If repeat TST ≥ 5 mm, continue INH for total of 9 mos. If INH not given initially, repeat TST at 3 mos, **if + rx** with INH for 9 mos. *(see Category II below)*.
	Older children & adults— Risk 2–4% 1st yr		Pts at high risk of progression (e.g., HIV+, immunosuppressed or on immunosuppressive therapy) and no evidence of active infection should be treated for LTBI (see below). For others repeat TST/IGRA at 8-10 wks: no rx if repeat TST/IGRA neg.

See page 2 for abbreviations, page 139 for footnotes

* Dosages are for adults (unless otherwise indicated) and assume normal renal function

† **DOT** = directly observed therapy

TABLE 12A (2)

CAUSATIVE AGENT/DISEASE	MODIFYING CIRCUMSTANCES	SUGGESTED REGIMENS	
		INITIAL THERAPY	**ALTERNATIVE**
II. Latent tuberculosis). infection (LTBI, positive TST or IGRA as above, active TB ruled out *See FIGURE 1 for treatment algorithm for pt with abnormal baseline CXR (e.g., upper lobe fibronodular disease) suspected active Tbc.)* *Review: NEJM 364:1414, 2011.*	Age no longer an exclusion, all persons with LTBI should be offered therapy	**INH** po once daily (adult: 5 mg/kg/day, max 300 mg/day; child: 10-15 mg/kg/day not to exceed 300 mg/day) x 9 mos. For current recommendations for monitoring hepatotoxicity on INH *see MMWR 59:227, 2010.* Supplemental pyridoxine 50 mg/day for HIV+ patients. A 12 dose once weekly DOT[†] **INH** + **Rifapentine** (RFP): **INH** po 15 mg/kg (max dose 900 mg); **RFP** po (wt-based dose): 10-14 kg: 300 mg; 14.1-25 kg: 450 mg; 25.1-32 kg: 600 mg; 32.1-49.9 kg: 750 mg; ≥50 kg: 900 mg. Not recommended for children age < 2 yrs; pts with HIV/AIDS on ART; pregnant women; or pts presumed infected with INH- or RIF-resistant MTB *(MMWR 60:1650, 2011, NEJM 365:2155, 2011).*	**INH** 300 mg once daily for 6 mo (but slightly less effective than 9 mos.; not recommended in children, HIV+ persons, or those with fibrotic lesions on chest film). **INH** 2x/wk (adult: 15 mg/kg, max 900 mg; child: 20-30 mg/kg, max dose 900 mg) x 9 mo. **RIF** once daily po (adult: 10 mg/kg/day, max dose 600 mg/day; child: 10-20 mg/kg/day, max dose 600 mg/day) for 4 mos. **INH** + **RIF** once daily x 3 mos.
	Pregnancy	Regimens as above. Once active disease is excluded may delay initiation of therapy until after delivery unless patient is recent contact to an active case, HIV+. Supplemental pyridoxine 10-25 mg/d recommended	
LTBI, suspected INH-resistant organism		**RIF** once daily po (adult: 10 mg/kg/day, max dose 600 mg/day; child: 10-20 mg/kg/day, max dose 600 mg/day) for 4 mos.	**RFB** 300 mg once daily po may be substituted for RIF (in HIV+ patient on anti-retrovirals, dose may need to be adjusted for drug interactions).
LTBI, suspected INH and RIF resistant organism		**Moxi**. 400 mg ± **EMB** 15 mg/kg once daily x 12 months	**Levo**. 500 mg once daily + (**EMB** 15 mg/kg or **PZA** 25 mg/kg) once daily x 12 months.

 * Dosages are for adults (unless otherwise indicated) and assume normal renal function [†] **DOT** = directly observed therapy

TABLE 12A (3)

CAUSATIVE AGENT/DISEASE	MODIFYING CIRCUMSTANCES	SUGGESTED REGIMENS: INITIAL THERAPY[8] Regimen: in order of preference	Drugs	Interval/Doses[1] (min. duration)	CONTINUATION PHASE OF THERAPY[7] (in vitro susceptibility known): Regimen	Drugs	Interval/Doses[1,2] (min. duration)	Range of Total Doses (min. duration)
		SEE COMMENTS FOR DOSAGE AND DIRECTLY OBSERVED THERAPY (DOT) REGIMENS						
III. Mycobacterium tuberculosis **A. Pulmonary TB** General reference on rx in adults & children: *MMWR 52 (RR-11):1, 2003*. In pts with newly diagnosed HIV and TB, Rx for both should be started as soon as possible *(NEJM 362:697, 2010)*. **Isolation essential!** Hospitalized pts with suspected or documented active TB should be isolated in single rooms using airborne precautions until deemed non-infectious. ***See footnotes, page 139*** **USE DOT REGIMENS IF POSSIBLE** *(continued on next page)*	**Rate of INH resistance known to be <4%** (drug-susceptible organisms)	1 *(See, Figure 2 page 135)*	INH RIF PZA EMB	7 days per wk times 56 doses (8 wks) or 5 days per wk times 40 doses (8 wks)[3] Fixed dose combination of INH, RIF, PZA & EMB currently being evaluated *(JAMA 305:1415, 2011)*.	1a	INH/ RIF[9]	7 days per wk times 126 doses (18 wks) or 5 days per wk times 90 doses (18 wks)[3]	182–130 (26 wks)
					1b	INH/ RIF	2 times per wk times 36 doses (18 wks)	92–76 (26 wks)[4]
					1c[5]	INH/ RFP	1 time per wk times 18 doses (18 wks)	74–58 (26 wks)
		2 *(See Figure 2 page 135)*	INH RIF PZA EMB	7 days per wk times 14 doses (2 wks), then 2 times per wk times 12 doses (6 wk) or 5 days per wk times 10 doses (2 wks)[3] then 2 times per wk times 12 doses (6 wks)	2a	INH/ RIF	2 times per wk times 36 doses (18 wks)	62–58 (26 wks)[4]
					2b[5]	INH/ RFP	1 time per wk times 18 doses (18 wks)	44–40 (26 wks)
		3 *(See Figure 2 page 135)*	INH RIF PZA EMB	3 times per wk times 24 doses (8 wks)	3a	INH/ RIF	3 times per wk times 54 doses (18 wks)	78 (26 wks)
		4 *(See Figure 2 page 135)*	INH RIF EMB	7 days per wk times 56 doses (8 wks) or 5 days per wk times 40 doses (8 wks)[3]	4a	INH/ RIF[6]	7 days per wk times 217 doses (31 wks) or 5 days per wk times 155 doses (31 wks)[3]	273–195 (39 wks)
					4b	INH/ RIF[6]	2 times per wk times 62 doses (31 wks)	118–102 (39 wks)

COMMENTS

Regimen*	INH	RIF	PZA	EMB	SM	RFB
	Dose in mg per kg (max. q24h dose)					
Q24h:						
Child	10–20 (300)	10–20 (600)	15–30 (2000)	15–25	20–40 (1000)	10–20 (300)
Adult	5 (300)	10 (600)	15–30 (2000)	15–25	15 (1000)	5 (300)
2 times per wk (DOT):						
Child	20–40 (900)	10–20 (600)	50–70 (4000)	50	25–30 (1500)	10–20 (300)
Adult	15 (900)	10 (600)	50–70 (4000)	50	25–30 (1500)	5 (300)
3 times per wk (DOT):						
Child	20–40 (900)	10–20 (600)	50–70 (3000)	25–30	25–30 (1500)	NA
Adult	15 (900)	10 (600)	50–70 (3000)	25–30	25–30 (1500)	NA

Second-line anti-TB agents can be dosed as follows to facilitate DOT: Cycloserine 500–750 mg po q24h (5 times per wk)
Ethionamide 500–750 mg po q24h (5 times per wk)
Kanamycin or capreomycin 15 mg per kg IM/IV q24h (3–5 times per wk)
Ciprofloxacin 750 mg po q24h (5 times per wk)
Ofloxacin 600–800 mg po q24h (5 times per wk)
Levofloxacin 750 mg po q24h (5 times per wk)
(CID 21:1245, 1995)

Risk factors for drug-resistant (MDR) TB: Recent immigration from Latin America or Asia or living in area of ↑ resistance (≥4%) or previous rx without RIF; exposure to known MDR TB. Incidence of MDR TB in **US steady** at 0.7%. Incidence of primary drug resistance is particularly high (>25%) in parts of China, Thailand, Russia, Estonia & Latvia; ~80% of US MDR cases in foreign born.

(continued on next page)

  * Dosages are for adults (unless otherwise indicated) and assume normal renal function † **DOT** = directly observed therapy

TABLE 12A (4)

CAUSATIVE AGENT/DISEASE	MODIFYING CIRCUM-STANCES	SUGGESTED REGIMEN[8]	DURATION OF TREATMENT (mos.)[8]	SPECIFIC COMMENTS[8]	COMMENTS
III. Mycobacterium tuberculosis **A. Pulmonary TB** *(continued from previous page)*	**INH (± SM) resistance**	**RIF**, **PZA**, **EMB** (a **FQ** may strengthen the regimen for pts with extensive disease).	6	INH should be stopped in cases of INH resistance. Outcome similar for drug susceptible and INH-mono-resistant strains *(CID 48:179, 2009)*.	*(continued from previous page)* **Moxi** and **levo** are **FQs of choice**, not CIP. FQ resistance may be seen in pts previously treated with FQ. WHO recommends using moxi (if MIC ≤ 2) if resistant to earlier generation FQs *(AAC 54:4765, 2010)*. **Linezolid** has excellent in vitro activity, including MDR strains and effective in selected cases of MDR TB and XDR TB but watch for toxicity *(NEJM 367:1508, 2012)*. **Bedaquiline** recently FDA approved for treatment of MDR TB based on efficacy in Phase 2 trials *(NEJM 360:2397, 2009; AAC 56:3271, 2012)*. Dose is 400 mg once daily for 2 weeks then 200 mg tiw for 22 weeks administered as directly observed therapy (DOT), taken with food, and always in combination with other anti-TB meds. **Consultation with an expert in MDR-TB management** strongly advised before use of this agent.
Multidrug-Resistant Tuberculosis (MDR TB): Defined as resistant to at least 2 drugs including INH & RIF. Pt clusters with high mortality *(NEJM 363:1050, 2010)*.	**Resistance to INH & RIF (± SM)**	**FQ**, **PZA**, **EMB**, **AMK or capreomycin (SM only if confirmed susceptible)**, ± alternative agent[7]	18–24	Extended rx is needed to ↓ the risk of relapse. In cases with extensive disease, the use of an additional agent (alternative agents) may be prudent to ↓ the risk of failure & additional acquired drug resistance. Resectional surgery may be appropriate.	
Extensively Drug-Resistant TB (XDR-TB): Defined as resistant to INH & RIF plus any FQ and at least 1 of the 3 second-line drugs: capreomycin, kanamycin or amikacin *(MMWR 56:250, 2007; CID 51:379, 2010)*.	**Resistance to INH, RIF (± SM), & EMB or PZA**	**FQ** (**EMB** or **PZA** if active), **AMK or capreomycin (SM only if confirmed susceptible)**, & 2 alternative agents[7]	24	Use the first-line agents to which there is susceptibility. Add 2 or more alternative agents in case of extensive disease. Surgery should be considered. Survival ↑ in pts receiving active FQ & surgical intervention *(AJRCCM 169:1103, 2004)*.	
See footnotes, page 139 Reviews of therapy for MDR TB: *JAC 54:593, 2004; Med Lett 7:75, 2009. For XDR-TB see MMWR 56:250, 2007 ; NEJM 359:563, 2008*	**Resistance to RIF**	**INH**, **EMB**, **FQ**, supplemented with **PZA** for the first 2 mos (an IA may be included for the first 2–3 mos. for pts with extensive disease)	12–18	Extended use of an IA may not be feasible. An all-oral regimen times 12–18 mos. should be effective but for more extensive disease &/or to shorten duration (e.g., to 12 mos.), an IA may be added in the initial 2 mos. of rx.	
	XDR-TB	Expert consultation strongly advised. Wee Specific Comments	18-24	Therapy requires administration of 4-6 drugs to which infecting organism is susceptible, including multiple second-line drugs *(MMWR 56:250, 2007)*. Increased mortality seen primarily in HIV+ patients. Cure with outpatient therapy likely in non-HIV+ patients when regimens of 4 or 5 or more drugs to which organism is susceptible are employed *(NEJM 359:563, 2008; CID 47:496, 2008)*. Successful sputum culture conversion correlates to initial susceptibility to FQs and kanamycin *(CID 46:42, 2008)*. Bedaquiline and Linezolid are options.	

     * Dosages are for adults (unless otherwise indicated) and assume normal renal function   † **DOT** = directly observed therapy

TABLE 12A (5)

CAUSATIVE AGENT/DISEASE; MODIFYING CIRCUMSTANCES	SUGGESTED REGIMENS: INITIAL THERAPY	SUGGESTED REGIMENS: CONTINUATION PHASE OF THERAPY (in vitro susceptibility known)	COMMENTS
III. Mycobacterium tuberculosis *(continued)*			
B. Extrapulmonary TB	**INH** + **RIF** (or **RFB**) + **PZA** + **EMB** q24h times 2 months	**INH** + **RIF** (or **RFB**)	6 mos regimens probably effective in most cases. IDSA recommends 6 mos for lymph node, pleural, pericarditis, disseminated disease, genitourinary & peritoneal TBc; 6–9 mos for bone & joint; 9-12 mos for CNS (including meningeal) TBc. Corticosteroids "strongly rec" only for pericarditis & meningeal TBc *[MMWR 52(RR-11):1, 2003]*.
	Authors add **pyridoxine** 25–50 mg po q24h to regimens that include INH.		
C. Tuberculous meningitis Excellent summary of clinical aspects and therapy (including steroids): *CMR 21:243, 2008*. Also *J Infect 59:167, 2009*.	(**INH** + **RIF** + **EMB** + **PZA**) + prednisone 60 mg/day x 4 wks, then 30 mg/day x 4 wks, then 15 mg/day x 2 wks, then 5 mg/day x 1 wk	May omit **EMB** when susceptibility to **INH** and **RIF** established. *See Table 9, page 86*, for CSF drug penetration. Initial reg of **INH + RIF + SM + PZA** also effective, even in patients with INH resistant organisms.	**3 drugs often rec for initial rx; we prefer 4** *(J Infect 59:167, 2009)*. Infection with MDR TB ↑ mortality & morbidity. **Dexamethasone** (for 1st mo) shown to ↓ complications & ↑ survival *(NEJM 351:1741, 2004)*. FQs (Levo, Gati, CIP) may be useful if started early *(AAC 55:3244, 2011)*.
D. Tuberculosis during pregnancy	**INH** + **RIF** + **EMB** for 9 mos	SM should not be substituted for EMB due to toxicity. AMK, capreomycin, kanamycin, FQs also contraindicated. PZA is recommended for routine use in pregnant women by the WHO but has not been recommended for general use in U.S. due to lack of safety data, although PZA has been used in some US health jurisdictions without reported adverse events. Breast-feeding should not be discouraged. If PZA is not included in the initial treatment regimen, the minimum duration of therapy is 9 months. Pyridoxine, 25 mg/ day, should be administered.	
E. Treatment failure or relapse: Usually due to poor compliance or resistant organisms, or subtherapeutic drug levels *(CID 55:169, 2012)*.	Directly observed therapy (DOT). Check susceptibilities. *(See section III. A, page 131 & above)*	Pts whose sputum is culture-positive after 5–6 mos. = treatment failures. Failures may be due to non-compliance or resistant organisms. Confirm susceptibilities of original isolates and obtain susceptibility to first and second line agents on current isolates. Non-compliance common, therefore institute DOT. If isolates show resistance, modify regimen to include at least 2 (preferably 3) new active agents, ones that the patient has not previously received if at all possible. Patients with MDR-TB usually convert sputum within 12 weeks of successful therapy.	
F. HIV infection or AIDS—pulmonary or extrapulmonary	**INH** + **RIF** (or **RFB**) + **PZA** q24h x 2 mos.	**INH** + **RIF** (or **RFB**) q24h times 4 months (total 6 mos.). Treat up to 9 mos. in pts with delayed response, cavitary disease.	1. Co-administration of RIF not recommended for these anti-retroviral drugs: nevirapine, etravirine, rilpivirine; maraviroc, elvitegravir (integrase inhibitor in four drug combination Stribild®), all HIV protease inhibitors. Use RFB instead). 2. RIF may be coadministered with efavirenz; nucleoside reverse transcriptase inhibitors. Coadministration of RIF with raltegravir best avoided (use RFB instead) but if necessary increase raltegravir dose to 800 mg q12h: RIF + dolutegravir OK at 50 mg bid of latter. 3. Because of possibility of developing resistance to RIF or RFB in pts with low CD4 cell counts who receive wkly or biwkly (2x/wk) therapy, daily dosing (preferred), or at a min 3x/wk dosing (failure rate likely higher) recommended for initial or continuation phase of rx. 4. Clinical & microbiologic response similar to that of HIV-neg patient 5. Post-treatment suppression not necessary for drug-susceptible strains.
	Add pyridoxine 50 mg po q24h to regimens that include INH		
Concomitant protease inhibitor (PI) therapy	**INH** 300 mg q24h + **RFB** (150 mg q24h or 300 mg tiw) + **EMB** 15 mg/kg q24h + **PZA** 25 mg/kg q24h x 2 mos.; then INH + RFB times 4 mos. (up to 7 mos.)	**INH** + **RFB** x 4 mos. (7 mos. in slow responders, cavitary disease)	Rifamycins induce cytochrome CYP450 enzymes (RIF > RFP > RFB) & reduce serum levels of concomitantly administered PIs. Conversely, PIs inhibit CYP450 & cause ↑ serum levels of RFP & RFB. If dose of RFB is not reduced, toxicity ↑.
	Alternative: **INH** + **FQ** + **PZA** + **EMB** x2 mos.	**INH** + **FQ** + **PZA** for additional 10 mos (up to 16 months if delayed response).	FQ either **levo** 500 mg q24h or **moxi** 400 mg q24h. May be used with any PI regimen.

See page 2 for abbreviations, page 139 for footnotes * Dosages are for adults (unless otherwise indicated) and assume normal renal function † **DOT** = directly observed therapy

TABLE 12A (6)

FIGURE 1 ALGORITHM FOR MANAGEMENT OF AT-RISK PATIENT WITH LOW OR HIGH SUSPICION OF ACTIVE TUBERCULOSIS WHILE CULTURES ARE PENDING *(modified from MMWR 52(RR-11):1, 2003).*

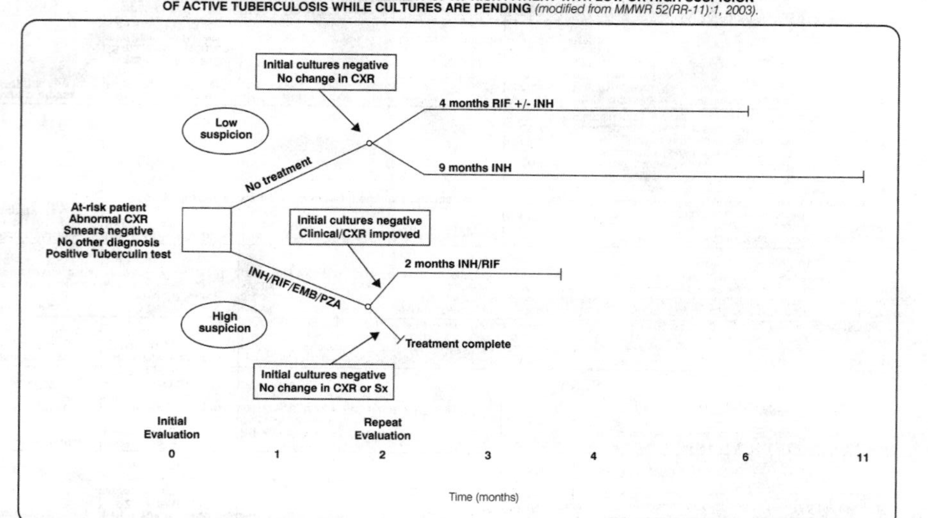

Patients at high clinical suspicion of active TB should be started on 4-drug therapy, pending results of cultures. If cultures are negative and there is no change in symptoms or CXR, the 4-drug regimen can be stopped and no further therapy is required. If cultures are negative and there is clinical or CXR improvement, continue INH/RIF for 2 additional months. For patients at low suspicion for active TB, treat for LTBI once cultures are negative.

See page 2 for abbreviations, page 139 for footnotes

* Dosages are for adults (unless otherwise indicated) and assume normal renal function

[†] **DOT** = directly observed therapy

TABLE 12A (7)

FIGURE 2 *[Modified from MMWR 52(RR-11):1, 2003]*

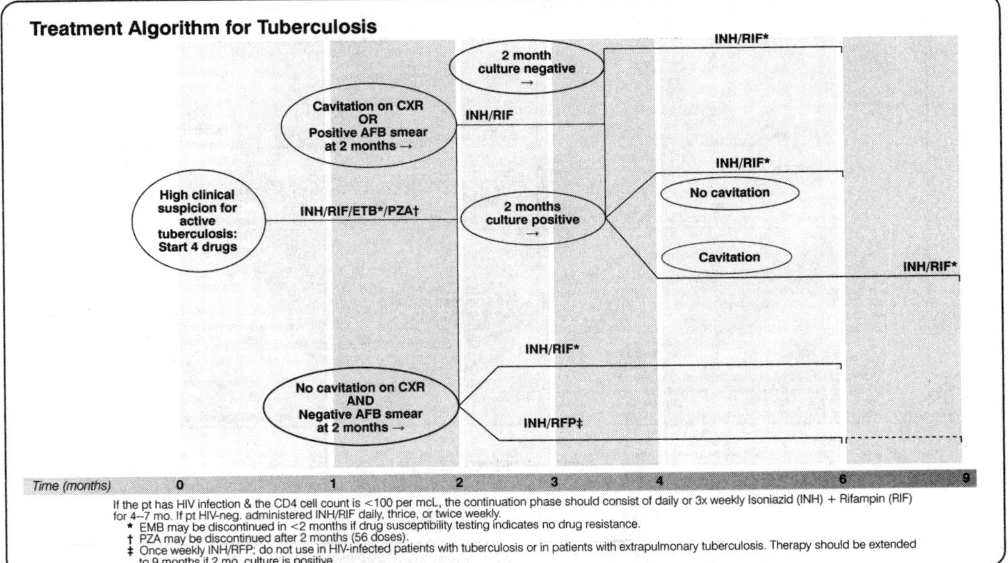

If the pt has HIV infection & the CD4 cell count is <100 per mcL, the continuation phase should consist of daily or 3x weekly Isoniazid (INH) + Rifampin (RIF) for 4--7 mo. If pt HIV-neg. administered INH/RIF daily, thrice, or twice weekly.

* EMB may be discontinued in <2 months if drug susceptibility testing indicates no drug resistance.

† PZA may be discontinued after 2 months (56 doses).

‡ Once weekly INH/RFP; do not use in HIV-infected patients with tuberculosis or in patients with extrapulmonary tuberculosis. Therapy should be extended to 9 months if 2 mo. culture is positive.

See page 2 for abbreviations.

TABLE 12A (8)

CAUSATIVE AGENT/DISEASE	MODIFYING CIRCUMSTANCES	SUGGESTED REGIMENS PRIMARY/ALTERNATIVE		COMMENTS
IV. Other Mycobacterial Disease ("Atypical") *(See ATS Consensus: AJRCCM 175:367, 2007; EID 17:506, 2011)*				
A. M. bovis		**INH + RIF + EMB**		The M. tuberculosis complex includes M. bovis. **All isolates resistant to PZA**. 9–12 months of rx used by some authorities. Isolation not required. Increased prevalence of extrapulmonary disease in U.S. born Hispanic populations and elsewhere *(CID 47:168, 2008; EID 14:909, 2008; EID 17:457, 2011)*.
B. Bacillus Calmette-Guerin (BCG) (derived from M. bovis)	Only fever (>38.5°C) for 12–24 hrs	**INH** 300 mg q24h times 3 months		Intravesical BCG effective in superficial bladder tumors and carcinoma in situ. With sepsis, consider initial adjunctive prednisolone. Also susceptible to RFB, CIP, oflox, levo, moxi, streptomycin, amikacin, capreomycin *(AAC 53:316, 2009)*. BCG may cause regional adenitis or pulmonary disease in HIV-infected children *(CID 37:1226, 2003)*. **Resistant to PZA.**
	Systemic illness or sepsis	**INH** 300 mg + **RIF** 600 mg + **EMB** 1200 mg po q24h times 6 mos.		
C. M. avium-intracellulare complex (MAC, MAI, or Battey bacillus) *ATS/IDSA Consensus Statement: AJRCCM 175:367, 2007; alternative ref: CID 42:1756, 2006.* Anti-tumor necrosis factor-α increases risk of infection with MAI and other non-tuberculous mycobacteria *(EID 15:1556, 2009)*.	**Immunocompetent patients**			See AJRCCM 175:367, 2007 for details of dosing and duration of therapy. Intermittent (tiw) therapy not recommended for patients with cavitary disease, patients who have been previously treated or patients with moderate of severe disease. The primary microbiologic goal of therapy is 12 months of negative sputum cultures on therapy. **"Classic" pulmonary MAC:** Men 50–75, smokers, COPD. May be associated with hot tub use *(Clin Chest Med 23:675, 2002)*. **"New" pulmonary MAC:** Women 30–70, scoliosis, mitral valve prolapse, (bronchiectasis), pectus excavatum ("Lady Windermere syndrome") and fibronodular disease in elderly women *(EID 16:1576, 2010)*. May also be associated with interferon gamma deficiency *(AJM 113:756, 2002)*. For cervicofacial lymphadenitis (localized) in immunocompetent children, surgical excision is as effective as chemotherapy *(CID 44:1057, 2007)*. Moxifloxacin and gatifloxacin, active in vitro & in vivo *(AAC 51:4071, 2007)*.
	Nodular/Bronchiectatic disease	[**Clarithro** 1000 mg or **azithro** 500 mg] tiw + **EMB** 25 mg/kg tiw + [**RIF** 600 mg or **RFB** 300 mg] tiw		
	Cavitary disease or severe nodular/bronchiectatic disease	[**Clarithro** 500-1000 mg/day (lower dose for wt <50 kg) or **azithro** 250 mg/day] + **EMB** 15 mg/kg/day + [**RIF** 600 mg/day or **RFB** 150-300 mg/day] ± [**strep** or **AMK**]		
	Immunocompromised pts: Primary prophylaxis—Pt's CD4 count <50–100 per mm³ Discontinue when CD4 count >100 per mm³ in response to ART	**Azithro** 1200 mg po weekly OR **Clarithro** 500 mg po bid	**RFB** 300 mg po q24h OR **Azithro** 1200 mg po weekly + **RIF** 300 mg po q24h	**Many drug-drug interactions,** *see Table 22, pages 226, 229*. Drug-resistant MAI disease seen in 29–58% of pts in whom disease develops while taking clarithro prophylaxis & in 11% of those on azithro but has not been observed with RFB prophylaxis. Clarithro resistance more likely in pts with extremely low CD4 counts at initiation. Need to be sure no active MTB; RFB used for prophylaxis may promote selection of rifamycin-resistant MTB.
	Treatment Either presumptive dx or after + culture of blood, bone marrow, or usually, sterile body fluids, eg liver	(**Clarithro** 500 mg* po bid + **EMB** 15 mg/kg/day ± **RFB** 300 mg po q24h (adjust dose) *** Higher doses of clari (1000 mg bid) may be associated with ↑ mortality**	**Azithro** 500 mg po/day + **EMB** 15 mg/kg/day +/- **RFB** 300-450 mg po/day	Adjust RFB dose as needed for drug-drug interactions. *(continued on next page)*

    * Dosages are for adults (unless otherwise indicated) and assume normal renal function   † **DOT** = directly observed therapy

TABLE 12A (9)

CAUSATIVE AGENT/DISEASE	MODIFYING CIRCUMSTANCES	SUGGESTED REGIMENS PRIMARY/ALTERNATIVE		COMMENTS
IV. Other Mycobacterial Disease ("Atypical") *(continued)*				
C. M. avium-intracellulare complex *(continued)*				*(continued from previous page)* Addition of a third or fourth drug should be considered for patients with advanced immunosuppression (CD4+ count <50 cells/μL), high mycobacterial loads (>2 log CFU/mL of blood), or in the absence of effective ART: AMK 10–15 mg/kg IV daily; Strep 1 gm IV or IM daily; CIP 500–750 mg PO bid; Levo 500 mg PO daily; Moxi 400 mg PO daily. Testing of susceptibility to clarithromycin and azithromycin is recommended. In ART-naïve patients, may consider withholding initiation of ART until after 2 weeks of MAC treatment to lessen drug interactions, reduce pill burden, and potentially lower occurrence of immune reconstitution inflammatory syndrome (IRIS). Short term (4–8 weeks) of systemic corticosteroid (equivalent to 20–40 mg of prednisone) can be used for IRIS.
	Chronic post-treatment suppression—secondary prophylaxis	**Always necessary.** [**Clarithro** or azithro] + **EMB** 15 mg/ kg/day *(dosage above)*	**Clarithro** or **azithro** or **RFB** *(dosage above)*	Recurrences almost universal without chronic suppression. However, in patients on ART with robust CD4 cell response, it is possible to discontinue chronic suppression *(MMWR 58/No. RR-4)*
D. Mycobacterium celatum	Treatment; optimal regimen not defined	May be susceptible to **clarithro**, **FQ** *(Clin Micro Inf 3:582, 1997)*. Suggest rx "like MAI" but often resistant to RIF *(J Inf 38:157, 1999)*. Most reported cases received 3 or 4 drugs, usually clarithro + EMB + CIP ± RFB *(EID 9:399, 2003)*.		Isolated from pulmonary lesions and blood in AIDS patients *(CID 24:144, 1997)*. Easily confused with M. xenopi (and MAC). Susceptibilities similar to MAC, but highly resistant to RIF *(CID 24:140, 1997)*.
E. Mycobacterium abscessus **Mycobacterium chelonae**	Treatment; Surgical excision may facilitate clarithro rx in subcutaneous abscess and is important adjunct to rx. For role of surgery in M. abscessus pulmonary disease, *see CID 52:565, 2011.*	Cutaneous: **Clarithro** 500 mg po bid x 6 months. Pulmonary/disseminated: 2 or 3 IV drugs (check susceptibility) (Amikacin, IMP, Cefoxitin, Tigecycline). Watch out for inducible resistance to Clarithro		M. abscessus susceptible to AMK (70%), clarithro (95%), cefoxitin (70%), CLO, cefmetazole, RFB, FQ, IMP, azithro, CIP, doxy, mino, tigecycline *(CID 42:1756, 2006; JIC 15:46, 2009)*. Single isolates of M. abscessus often not associated with disease. Clarithro-resistant strains now described. M. chelonae susceptible to AMK (80%), clarithro, azithro, tobramycin (100%), IMP (60%), moxifloxacin *(AAC 46:3283, 2002)*, CIP, mino, doxy, linezolid (94%) *(CID 42:1756, 2006)*. Resistant to cefoxitin, FQ. Tigecycline highly active in vitro *(AAC 52:4184, 2008; CID 49:1358, 2009)*.
F. Mycobacterium fortuitum	Treatment; optimal regimen not defined. Surgical excision of infected areas.	**AMK** + **cefoxitin** + **probenecid** 2–6 wks, then po **TMP- SMX**, or **doxy** 2–6 mos. Usually responds to 6–12 mos of oral rx with 2 drugs to which it is susceptible.		**Resistant to all standard anti-TBc drugs.** Sensitive in vitro to doxycycline, minocycline, cefoxitin, IMP, AMK, TMP-SMX, CIP, oflox, azithro, clarithro, linezolid, tigecycline *(Clin Micro Rev 15:716, 2002)*, but some strains resistant to azithromycin, rifabutin. For M. fortuitum pulmonary disease treat with at least 2 agents active in vitro until sputum cultures negative for 12 months *(AJRCCM 175:367, 2007)*.
G. Mycobacterium haemophilum	Regimen(s) not defined. In animal model, **clarithro** + **rifabutin** effective *(AAC 39:2316, 1995)*. Combination of **CIP** + **RFB** + **clarithro** reported effective but clinical experience limited *(Clin Micro Rev 9:435, 1996; CID 52:488, 2011)*. Surgical debridement may be necessary *(CID 26:505, 1998)*.			Clinical: Ulcerating skin lesions, synovitis, osteomyelitis, cervicofacial lymphadenitis in children. Associated with permanent eyebrow makeup *(CID 52:488, 2011)*. Lab: Requires supplemented media to isolate. Sensitive in vitro to: CIP, cycloserine, rifabutin, moxifloxacin. Over ½ resistant to: INH, RIF, EMB, PZA. For localized cervicofacial lymphadenitis in immunocompetent children, surgical excision as effective as chemotherapy *(CID 44:1057, 2007)* or "watchful waiting" *(CID 52:180, 2011)*.

See page 2 for abbreviations, page 139 for footnotes   * Dosages are for adults (unless otherwise indicated) and assume normal renal function   † **DOT** = directly observed therapy

TABLE 12A (10)

CAUSATIVE AGENT/DISEASE	MODIFYING CIRCUMSTANCES	SUGGESTED REGIMENS PRIMARY/ALTERNATIVE	COMMENTS
IV. Other Mycobacterial Disease ("Atypical") *(continued)*			
H. Mycobacterium genavense	Regimens used include ≥2 drugs: **EMB**, **RIF**, **RFB**, **CLO**, **clarithro**. In animal model, **clarithro** & **RFB** (& to lesser extent amikacin & **EMB**) shown effective in reducing bacterial counts; CIP not effective *(JAC 42:483, 1998)*.		Clinical: CD4 <50. Symptoms of fever, weight loss, diarrhea. Lab: Growth in BACTEC vials slow (mean 42 days). Subcultures grow only on Middlebrook 7H11 agar containing 2 mcg per mL mycobactin J—growth still insufficient for in vitro sensitivity testing.
I. Mycobacterium gordonae	Regimen(s) not defined, but consider **RIF** + **EMB** + **KM** or **CIP** (or **linezolid** *(AJRCCM 175:367, 2007)*		Frequent colonizer, not associated with disease. In vitro: sensitive to EMB, RIF, AMK, CIP, clarithro, linezolid *(AAC 47:1736, 2003)*. Resistant to INH. Surgical excision.
J. Mycobacterium kansasii	Q24h po: **INH** (300 mg) + **RIF** (600 mg) + **EMB** (25 mg per kg times 2 mos., then 15 mg per kg). Rx for 18 mos. (until culture-neg. sputum times 12 mos; 15 mos. if HIV+ pt.) *(See Comment)*	For **RIF** resistant organism: (**INH** 900 mg + **pyridoxine** 50 mg + **EMB** 25 mg/kg) po q24h + **Sulfamethoxazole** 1000 mg tid (if sulfamethoxazole is unavailable options include **TMP-SMX** two double strength tablets (320 mg **TMP** and 1600 mg SMX) bid OR **Clarithromycin** 500 mg po bid OR **Moxifloxacin** 400 mg po once daily. Treat for 12-15 mos or until 12-15 mos of culture-negative sputum.	**All isolates are resistant to PZA.** Highly susceptible to linezolid in vitro *(AAC 47:1736, 2003)* and to clarithro and moxifloxacin *(JAC 55:950, 2005)*. If HIV+ pt taking protease inhibitor, substitute either clarithro (500 mg bid) or RFB (150 mg per day) for RIF. Because of variable susceptibility to INH, some substitute clarithro 500–750 mg q24h for INH. Resistance to clarithro reported, but most strains susceptible to clarithro as well as moxifloxacin *(JAC 55:950, 2005)* & levofloxacin *(AAC 48:4562, 2004)*.
K. Mycobacterium marinum	(**Clarithro** 500 mg bid) or (**minocycline** 100–200 mg q24h) or (**doxycycline** 100–200 mg q24h), or (**TMP-SMX** 160/800 mg po bid), or (**RIF** + **EMB**) for 3 mos. *(AJRCCM 156:S1, 1997; Eur J Clin Microbiol ID 25:609, 2006)*. Surgical excision.		Resistant to INH & PZA. Also susceptible in vitro to linezolid *(AAC 47: 1736, 2003)*. CIP, moxifloxacin also show moderate in vitro activity *(AAC 46:1114, 2002)*.
L. Mycobacterium scrofulaceum	Surgical excision. Chemotherapy seldom indicated. Although regimens not defined, **clarithro** + **CLO** with or **without EMB**. **INH**, **RIF**, **strep** + **cycloserine** have also been used.		In vitro resistant to INH, RIF, EMB, PZA, AMK, CIP. Susceptible to clarithro, strep, erythromycin.
M. Mycobacterium simiae	Regimen(s) not defined. Start 4 drugs as for disseminated MAI.		Most isolates resistant to all 1st-line anti-tbc drugs. Isolates often not clinically significant.
N. Mycobacterium ulcerans (Buruli ulcer)	WHO recommends **RIF** + **SM** for 8 weeks. **RIF**+ **CIP** recommended as alternatives by WHO *(CMN 31:119, 2009)*. Recent small studies document similar effectiveness of 4 wks of **RIF** + **SM** followed by 4 weeks of **RIF** + **Clarithro** *(Lancet 375:664, 2010)* and a regimen of 8 wks of **RIF** + **Clarithro** (No relapse in 30 pts) *(CID 52:94, 2011)*.		Susceptible in vitro to RIF, strep, CLO, clarithro, CIP, oflox, amikacin, moxi, linezolid. Monotherapy with RIF selects resistant mutants in mice *(AAC 47:1228, 2003)*. RIF + moxi; RIF + clarithro; moxi + clarithro similar to RIF + SM in mice *(AAC 51:3737, 2007)*.
O. Mycobacterium xenopi	Regimen(s) not defined *(CID 24:226 & 233, 1997)*. Some recommend a **macrolide** + (**RIF** or **rifabutin**) + **EMB** ± **SM** *(AJRCCM 156:S1, 1997)* or **RIF** + **INH** ± **EMB** *(Resp Med 97:439, 2003)* but recent study suggests no need to treat in most pts with HIV *(CID 37:1250, 2003)*.		In vitro: sensitive to clarithro *(AAC 36:2841, 1992)* and rifabutin *(JAC 39:567, 1997)* and many standard antimycobacterial drugs. Clarithro-containing regimens more effective than RIF/INH/EMB regimens in mice *(AAC 45:3229, 2001)*. FQs, linezolid also active in vitro.
Mycobacterium leprae (leprosy) Classification: *CID 44:1096, 2007*. Clinical mgmt of leprosy reactions: *IDCP 18:235, 2010*. Overview: *Lancet ID 11:464, 2011*.	There are 2 sets of therapeutic recommendations here: one from USA (National Hansen's Disease Programs [NHDP], Baton Rouge, LA) and one from WHO. Both are based on expert recommendations and neither has been subjected to controlled clinical trial.		

See page 2 for abbreviations, page 139 for footnotes

* Dosages are for adults (unless otherwise indicated) and assume normal renal function

† **DOT** = directly observed therapy

TABLE 12A (11)

Type of Disease	NHDP Regimen	WHO Regimen	COMMENTS
Paucibacillary Forms: (Intermediate, Tuberculoid, Borderline tuberculoid)	(**Dapsone** 100 mg/day + **RIF** 600 mg po/day) for 12 months	(**Dapsone** 100 mg/day (unsupervised) + **RIF** 600 mg 1x/mo (supervised)) for 6 mos	Side effects overall 0.4%
Single lesion paucibacillary	Treat as paucibacillary leprosy for 12 months.	Single dose ROM therapy: (RIF 600 mg + Oflox 400 mg + Mino 100 mg) *(Ln 353:655, 1999)*.	
Multibacillary forms: Borderline Borderline-lepromatous Lepromatous *See Comment for erythema nodosum leprosum* Rev.: *Lancet 363:1209, 2004*	(**Dapsone** 100 mg/day + **CLO** 50 mg/day + **RIF** 600 mg/day) for 24 mos **Alternative regimen:** (**Dapsone** 100 mg/day + **RIF** 600 mg/day + **Minocycline** 100 mg/day) for 24 mos if CLO is refused or unavailable.	(**Dapsone** 100 mg/day + **CLO** 50 mg/day (both unsupervised) + **RIF** 600 mg + **CLO** 300 mg once monthly (supervised)). Continue regimen for 12 months.	Side-effects overall 5.1%. For **erythema nodosum leprosum:** prednisone 60–80 mg/day or thalidomide 100-400 mg/day. Thalidomide available in US at 1-800-4-CELGENE. Altho thalidomide effective, WHO no longer rec because of potential toxicity however the majority of leprosy experts feel thalidomide remains drug of choice for ENL under strict supervision. **CLO (Clofazimine)** available from NHDP under IND protocol; contact at 1-800-642-2477. **Ethionamide** (250 mg q24h) or prothionamide (375 mg q24h) may be subbed for CLO. Etanercept effective in one case refractory to above standard therapy *(CID 52:e133, 2011)*. Regimens incorporating clarithro, minocycline, dapsone monotherapy have been abandoned due to emergence of resistance *(CID 52:e127, 2011)*, but older patients previously treated with dapsone monotherapy may remain on lifelong maintenance therapy. Moxi highly active in vitro and produces rapid clinical response *(AAC 52:3113, 2008)*.

FOOTNOTES:

1. When DOT is used, drugs may be given 5 days/wk & necessary number of doses adjusted accordingly. Although no studies compare 5 with 7 q24h doses, extensive experience indicates this would be an effective practice.
2. Patients with cavitation on initial chest x-ray & positive cultures at completion of 2 mos of rx should receive a 7 mos (31 wks; either 217 doses [q24h] or 62 doses [2x/wk]) continuation phase.
3. 5 day/wk admin is always given by DOT.
4. Not recommended for HIV-infected pts with CD4 cell counts <100 cells/mcL.
5. Options 1c & 2b should be used only in HIV-neg. pts who have neg. sputum smears at the time of completion of 2 mos rx & do not have cavitation on initial chest x-ray. For pts started on this regimen & found to have a + culture from 2 mos specimen, rx should be extended extra 3 mos.
6. Options 4a & 4b should be considered only when options 1–3 cannot be given.
7. Alternative agents = ethionamide, cycloserine, p-aminosalicylic acid, clarithromycin, AM-CL, linezolid.
8. Modified from *MMWR 52(RR-11):1, 2003. See also IDCP 11:329, 2002.*
9. Continuation regimen with INH/EMB less effective than INH/RIF *(Lancet 364:1244, 2004)*.

TABLE 12B – DOSAGE AND ADVERSE EFFECTS OF ANTIMYCOBACTERIAL DRUGS

AGENT (TRADE NAME)[1]	USUAL DOSAGE*	ROUTE/1° DRUG RESISTANCE (RES) US[2,§]	SIDE-EFFECTS, TOXICITY AND PRECAUTIONS	SURVEILLANCE
FIRST LINE DRUGS				
Ethambutol (Myambutol) (100, 400 mg tab)	25 mg/kg/day for 2 mos then 15 mg/ kg/day q24h as 1 dose (<10% protein binding) [Bacteriostatic to both extra-cellular & intracellular organisms]	RES: 0.3% (0–0.7%) po 400 mg tab	**Optic neuritis** with decreased visual acuity, central scotomata, and loss of green and red perception; peripheral neuropathy and headache (~1%), rashes (rare), arthralgia (rare), hyperuricemia (rare). Anaphylactoid reaction (rare). *Comment:* Primarily used to inhibit resistance. Disrupts outer cell membrane in M. avium with ↑ activity to other drugs.	Monthly visual acuity & red/ green with dose >15 mg/kg/ day. ≥10% loss considered significant. Usually reversible if drug discontinued.
Isoniazid (INH) (Nydrazid, Laniazid, Teebaconin) (50, 100, 300 mg tab)	Q24h dose: 5–10 mg/kg/day up to 300 mg/day as 1 dose. 2x/wk dose: 15 mg/kg (900 mg max dose) (< 10% protein binding) [Bactericidal to both extracellular and intracellular organisms] Add pyridoxine in alcoholic, pregnant, or malnourished pts.	RES: 4.1% (2.6–8.5%) po 300 mg tab IM 100 mg/mL in 10 mL (IV route not FDA-approved but has been used, esp. in AIDS)	Overall ~1%. Liver: **Hep** (children 10% mild ↑ SGOT, normalizes with continued rx, age <20 yrs rare, 20–34 yrs 1.2%, ≥50 yrs 2.3%) [also ↑ with q24h alcohol & previous exposure to Hep C (usually asymptomatic—*CID 36:293, 2003*)]. May be fatal. With prodromal sx, dark urine do LFTs; discontinue if SGOT >3–5xnormal. **Peripheral neuropathy** (17% on 6 mg/kg per day, less on 300 mg, incidence ↑ in slow acetylators); **pyridoxine 10 mg q24h will decrease incidence;** other neurologic sequelae, convulsions, optic neuritis, toxic encephalopathy, psychosis, muscle twitching, dizziness, coma (all rare); allergic skin rashes, fever, minor disulfiram-like reaction, flushing after Swiss cheese; blood dyscrasias (rare); + antinuclear (20%). **Drug-drug interactions** common, *see Table 22*.	Pre-rx liver functions. Repeat if symptoms (fatigue, weakness, malaise, anorexia, nausea or vomiting) >3 days *(AJRCCM 152: 1705, 1995)*. Some recommend SGOT at 2, 4, 6 mos esp. if age >50 yrs. Clinical evaluation every mo.
Pyrazinamide (500 mg tab)	25 mg per kg per day (maximum 2.5 gm per day) q24h as 1 dose [Bactericidal for intracellular organisms]	po 500 mg tab	**Arthralgia; hyperuricemia** (with or without symptoms); hepatitis (not over 2% if recommended dose not exceeded); gastric irritation; photosensitivity (rare).	Pre-rx liver functions. Monthly SGOT, uric acid. Measure serum uric acid if symptomatic gouty attack occurs.
Rifamate®— combination tablet	2 tablets single dose q24h	po (1 hr before meal)	1 tablet contains 150 mg INH, 300 mg RIF	As with individual drugs
Rifampin (Rifadin, Rimactane, Rifocin) (100, 300, 450, 600 mg cap)	10.0 mg per kg per day up to 600 mg per day q24h as 1 dose (60–90% protein binding) [Bactericidal to all populations of organisms]	RES: 0.2% (0–0.3%) po 300 mg cap (IV available, Merrell-Dow)	INH/RIF dc'd in ~3% for toxicity; gastrointestinal irritation, antibiotic-associated colitis, drug fever (1%), pruritus with or without skin rash (1%), anaphylactoid reactions in HIV+ pts, mental confusion, thrombocytopenia (1%), leukopenia (1%), hemolytic anemia, transient **abnormalities in liver function. "Flu syndrome"** (fever, chills, headache, bone pain, shortness of breath) seen if RIF taken irregularly or if q24h dose restarted after an interval of no rx. **Discolors urine, tears, sweat, contact lens an orange-brownish color.** May cause drug-induced lupus erythematosus *(Ln 349: 1521, 1977)*.	Pre-rx liver function. Repeat if symptoms. **Multiple significant drug-drug interactions,** *see Table 22*.
Rifater®— combination tablet *(See Side-Effects)*	Wt ≥55 kg, 6 tablets single dose q24h	po (1 hr before meal)	1 tablet contains 50 mg INH, 120 mg RIF, 300 mg PZA. Used in 1st 2 months of rx (PZA 25 mg per kg). Purpose is convenience in dosing, ↑ compliance *(AnIM 122: 951, 1995)* but cost 1.58 more. Side-effects = individual drugs.	As with individual drugs, PZA 25 mg per kg
Streptomycin (IV/IM soln)	15 mg per kg IM q24h, 0.75–1.0 gm per day initially for 60–90 days, then 1.0 gm 2–3 times per week (15 mg per kg per day) q24h as 1 dose	RES: 3.9% (2.7–7.6%) IM (or IV)	Overall 8%. **Ototoxicity:** vestibular dysfunction (vertigo); paresthesias; dizziness & nausea (all less in pts receiving 2–3 doses per week); tinnitus and high frequency loss (1%); nephrotoxicity (rare); peripheral neuropathy (rare); allergic skin rashes (4–5%); drug fever. Available from X-Gen Pharmaceuticals, 607-732-4411. Ref. re: IV—*CID 19:1150, 1994*. Toxicity similar with qd vs tid dosing *(CID 38:1538, 2004)*.	Monthly audiogram. In older pts, serum creatinine or BUN at start of rx and weekly if pt stable

[1] Note: Malabsorption of antimycobacterial drugs may occur in patients with AIDS enteropathy. For review of adverse effects, *see AJRCCM 167:1472, 2003.*

[2] **RES** = % resistance of M. tuberculosis

See page 2 for abbreviations.

* Dosages are for adults (unless otherwise indicated) and assume normal renal function

§ Mean (range) (higher in Hispanics, Asians, and patients <10 years old)

† **DOT** = directly observed therapy

TABLE 12B (2)

AGENT (TRADE NAME)[1]	USUAL DOSAGE*	ROUTE/1° DRUG RESISTANCE (RES) US[2,§]	SIDE-EFFECTS, TOXICITY AND PRECAUTIONS	SURVEILLANCE
SECOND LINE DRUGS (more difficult to use and/or less effective than first line drugs)				
Amikacin (Amikin) (IV sol'n)	7.5–10.0 mg per kg q24h [Bactericidal for extracellular organisms]	RES: (est. 0.1%) IM/IV 500 mg vial	*See Table 10B, pages 103 & 109* Toxicity similar with qd vs tid dosing *(CID 38:1538, 2004)*.	Monthly audiogram. Serum creatinine or BUN weekly if pt stable
Bedaquiline (Sirturo) (100 mg tab)	Directly observed therapy (DOT): 400 mg once daily for 2 weeks, then 200 mg 3 times weekly for 22 weeks, taken with food and always used in combination with other anti-TB medications.	Does not exhibit cross-resistance to other TB drugs; always use in combination with other TB drugs to prevent selection of resistant mutants	Most common: nausea, vomiting, arthralgia, headache, hyperuricemia. Elevated transaminases. Bedaquiline in clinical trials was administered as one component of a multiple drug regimen, so side-effects were common, yet difficult to assign to a particular drug.	Moderate QTc increases (average of 10-16 ms over the 24 weeks of therapy. Potential risks of pancreatitis, myopathy, myocardial injury, severe hepatotoxicity.
Capreomycin sulfate (Capastat sulfate)	1 gm per day (15 mg per kg per day) q24h as 1 dose	RES: 0.1% (0–0.9%) IM/IV	Nephrotoxicity (36%), ototoxicity (auditory 11%), eosinophilia, leukopenia, skin rash, fever, hypokalemia, neuromuscular blockade.	Monthly audiogram, biweekly serum creatinine or BUN
Ciprofloxacin (Cipro) (250, 500, 750 mg tab)	750 mg bid	po 500 mg or 750 mg ER IV 200-400 mg vial	TB not a FDA-approved indication for CIP. Desired CIP serum levels 4–6 mcg per mL, requires median dose 800 mg *(AJRCCM 151:2006, 1995)*. Discontinuation rates 6–7%. CIP well tolerated *(AJRCCM 151:2006, 1995)*. FQ-resistant M. Tb identified in New York *(Ln 345:1148, 1995). See Table 10A, page 99 & Table 10B, page 106 for adverse effects.*	None
Clofazimine (Lamprene) (50, 100 mg cap)	50 mg per day (unsupervised) + 300 mg 1 time per month supervised or 100 mg per day	po 50 mg (with meals)	Skin: **pigmentation (pink-brownish black)** 75–100%, dryness 20%, pruritus 5%. GI: abdominal pain 50% (rarely severe leading to exploratory laparoscopy), splenic infarction (VR), bowel obstruction (VR), GI bleeding (VR). Eye: conjunctival irritation, retinal crystal deposits.	None
Cycloserine (Seromycin) (250 mg tab)	750–1000 mg per day (15 mg per kg per day) 2–4 doses per day [Bacteriostatic for both extra-cellular & intracellular organisms]	RES: 0.1% (0–0.3%) po 250 mg cap	Convulsions, **psychoses** (5–10% of those receiving 1.0 gm per day); headache; somnolence; hyperreflexia; increased CSF protein and pressure, **peripheral neuropathy.** 100 mg pyridoxine (or more) q24h should be given concomitantly. Contraindicated in epileptics.	None
Dapsone (25, 100 mg tab)	100 mg per day	po 100 mg tab	Blood: ↓ hemoglobin (1–2 gm) & ↑ retics (2–12%), in most pts. Hemolysis in G6PD deficiency. ↑ hemolysis due to concomitant atazanavir *(AAC 56:1081, 2012)*. **Methemoglobinemia.** CNS: peripheral neuropathy (rare). GI: nausea, vomiting. Renal: albuminuria, nephrotic syndrome. Erythema nodosum leprosum in pts rx for leprosy (½ pts 1st year). Hypersensitivity syndrome in 0.5-3.6% *(See Surveillance)*.	Hypersensitivity syndrome: fever, rash, eosinophilia, lymphadenopathy, hepatitis, pneumonitis. Genetic marker identified *(NEJM 369:1620, 2013)*.
Ethionamide (Trecator-SC) (120, 250 mg tab)	500–1000 mg per day (15–20 mg per kg per day) 1–3 doses per day [Bacteriostatic for extracellular organisms only]	RES: 0.8% (0–1.5%) po 250 mg tab	**Gastrointestinal irritation** (up to 50% on large dose); goiter; peripheral neuropathy (rare); convulsions (rare); changes in affect (rare); difficulty in diabetes control; rashes; hepatitis; purpura; stomatitis; gynecomastia; menstrual irregularity. Give drug with meals or antacids; 50–100 mg pyridoxine per day concomitantly; SGOT monthly. Possibly teratogenic.	

See page 2 for abbreviations.

* Dosages are for adults (unless otherwise indicated) and assume normal renal function
§ Mean (range) (higher in Hispanics, Asians, and patients <10 years old)

† **DOT** = directly observed therapy

TABLE 12B (3)

AGENT (TRADE NAME)[1]	USUAL DOSAGE*	ROUTE/1° DRUG RESISTANCE (RES) US[2,§]	SIDE-EFFECTS, TOXICITY AND PRECAUTIONS	SURVEILLANCE
SECOND LINE DRUGS *(continued)*				
Linezolid (Zyvox) (600 mg tab, oral suspension 100 mg/mL)	600 mg qd	PO or IV	Not FDA-approved indication. High rate of adverse events (>80% with 4 months or longer of therapy: myelosuppression, peripheral neuropathy, optic neuropathy. Avoid tyramine-containing foods, soy products, adrenergic agents (e.g., pseudoephedrine, phenylpropanolamine) MOA inhibitors, SSRIs. 600 mg > 300 mg dose for toxicity; consider reducing dose to 300 mg for toxicity or after 4 mos of therapy or culture-conversion to reduce toxicity.	Baseline and monthly complete blood count, visual acuity checks, screen for symptoms of peripheral neuropathy, neurologic examination.
Moxifloxacin (Avelox) (400 mg tab)	400 mg qd	po 400 mg cap IV	Not FDA-approved indication. Concomitant administration of rifampin reduces serum levels of moxi *(CID 45:1001, 2007)*.	None
Ofloxacin (Floxin) (200, 300, 400 mg tab)	400 mg bid	po 400 mg cap IV	Not FDA-approved indication. Overall adverse effects 11%, 4% discontinued due to side-effects. GI: nausea 3%, diarrhea 1%. **CNS:** insomnia 3%, headache 1%, dizziness 1%.	
Para-aminosalicylic acid (PAS, Paser) (Na^+ or K^+ salt) (4 gm cap)	4–6 gm bid (200 mg per kg per day) [Bacteriostatic for extracellular organisms only]	RES: 0.8% (0–1.5%) po 450 mg tab *(see Comment)*	**Gastrointestinal irritation** (10–15%); goitrogenic action (rare); depressed prothrombin activity (rare); G6PD-mediated hemolytic anemia (rare), drug fever, rashes, hepatitis, myalgia, arthralgia. Retards hepatic enzyme induction, may ↓ INH hepatotoxicity. Available from CDC, (404) 639-3670, Jacobus Pharm. Co. (609) 921-7447.	None
Rifabutin (Mycobutin) (150 mg cap)	300 mg per day (prophylaxis or treatment)	po 150 mg tab	Polymyalgia, polyarthralgia, leukopenia, granulocytopenia. Anterior uveitis when given with concomitant clarithromycin; avoid 600 mg dose *(NEJM 330:438, 1994)*. Uveitis reported with 300 mg per day *(AnIM 12:510, 1994)*. Reddish urine, orange skin (pseudojaundice).	None
Rifapentine (Priftin) (150 mg tab)	600 mg twice weekly for 1st 2 mos., then 600 mg q week	po 150 mg tab	Similar to other rifabutins. *(See RIF, RFB)*. Hyperuricemia seen in 21%. Causes red-orange discoloration of body fluids. Note ↑ prevalence of RIF resistance in pts on weekly rx *(Ln 353:1843, 1999)*.	None
Thalidomide (Thalomid) (50, 100, 200 mg cap)	100–300 mg po q24h (may use up to 400 mg po q24h for severe erythema nodosum leprosum)	po 50 mg tab	**Contraindicated in pregnancy. Causes severe life-threatening birth defects. Both male and female patients must use barrier contraceptive methods (Pregnancy Category X). Frequently causes drowsiness or somnolence. May cause peripheral neuropathy.** *(AJM 108:487, 2000)* For review, *see Ln 363:1803, 2004*.	Available only through pharmacists participating in System for Thalidomide Education and Prescribing Safety (S.T.E.P.S.)

See page 2 for abbreviations.

* Dosages are for adults (unless otherwise indicated) and assume normal renal function
§ Mean (range) (higher in Hispanics, Asians, and patients <10 years old)

† **DOT** = directly observed therapy

TABLE 13A– TREATMENT OF PARASITIC INFECTIONS

- ***See Table 13D* for sources for antiparasitic drugs not otherwise commercially available.**
- The following resources are available through the Centers for Disease Control and Prevention (CDC) in Atlanta. Website is www.cdc.gov. General advice for parasitic diseases other than malaria: (+1) (404) 718-4745 (day), (+1) (770) 488-7100 (after hours). For CDC Drug Service 8:00 a.m. – 4:30 p.m. EST: (+1) (404) 639-3670; fax: (+1) (404) 639-3717. *See www.cdc.gov/laboratory/drugservice/index.html* For malaria: Prophylaxis advice (+1) (770) 488-7788; treatment (+1) (770) 488-7788; or after hours (+1) (770) 488-7100; toll-free (US) 1-855-856-4713; website: www.cdc.gov/malaria
- **NOTE: All dosage regimens are for adults with normal renal function unless otherwise stated.** Many of the suggested regimens are not FDA approved.
- For licensed drugs, suggest checking package inserts to verify dosage and side-effects. Occasionally, post-licensure data may alter dosage as compared to package inserts.

INFECTING ORGANISM	SUGGESTED REGIMENS		COMMENTS
	PRIMARY	ALTERNATIVE	
PROTOZOA—INTESTINAL (non-pathogenic: E. hartmanni, E. dispar, E. coli, Iodamoeba bütschlii, Endolimax nana, Chilomastix mesnili)			
Balantidium coli	**Tetracycline** 500 mg po qid x 10 days	**Metronidazole** 750 mg po tid times 5 days	Another alternative: Iodoquinol 650 mg po tid x 20 days.
Blastocystis hominis Ref: *J Clin Gastro 44:85, 2010.*	**Metronidazole** 1.5 gm po 1x/day x 10 days or 750 mg po tid x 10 days (need to treat is dubious).	**Alternatives: iodoquinol*** 650 mg po tid x 20 days or **TMP-SMX-DS,** one bid x 7 days or **Nitazoxanide** 500 mg po bid x 3 days	Role as pathogen unclear; may serve as marker of exposure to contaminated food/water.
Cryptosporidium parvum & hominis Treatment is unsatisfactory Ref.: *Curr Opin Infect Dis 23:494, 2010*	**Immunocompetent—No HIV: Nitazoxanide** 500 mg po bid x 3 days (expensive)	**HIV with immunodeficiency:** Effective antiretroviral therapy best therapy. **Nitazoxanide** no clinical or parasite response compared to placebo.	**Nitazoxanide:** Approved in liquid formulation for rx of children & 500 mg tabs for adults who are immunocompetent. Ref.: *CID 40:1173, 2005.* **C. hominis** assoc. with ↑ in post-infection eye & joint pain, recurrent headache, & dizzy spells (*CID 39:504, 2004*).
Cyclospora cayetanensis; cyclosporiasis (*Clin Micro Rev 23:218, 2010*)	**Immunocompetent pts: TMP-SMX-DS** tab 1 po bid x 7–10 days. Other options: *see Comments.*	**AIDS pts: TMP-SMX-DS** tab 1 po qid for up to 3-4 wks. Immunocompromised pts: may require suppressive rx with **TMP-SMX** DS 1 tab 3x/wk	If sulfa-allergic: **CIP** 500 mg po bid x 7 days but results inconsistent. Anecdotal success with nitazoxanide. Biliary disease described in HIV pts.
Dientamoeba fragilis See *AJTMH 82:614, 2010; Clin Micro Infect 14:601, 2008.*	**Iodoquinol*** 650 mg po tid x 20 days or **Paromomycin*** 25-35 mg/kg/day po in 3 div doses x 7 days or **Metronidazole** 750 mg tid x 10 days.	For treatment failures: **Tetracycline** 500 mg po qid x 10 days + **Iodoquinol*** 650 mg po tid x 10 days OR (**Iodoquinol*** + **Paromomycin***)	**Metronidazole** associated with high failure rates in some studies.
Entamoeba histolytica; amebiasis. Reviews: *Ln 361:1025, 2003; NEJM 348:1563, 2003.*			
Asymptomatic cyst passer	**Paromomycin*** 25-35 mg/kg/day po in 3 divided doses x 7 days OR **iodoquinol*** 650 mg po tid x 20 days	**Diloxanide furoate*** (Furamide) 500 mg po tid x 10 days.	Note: E. hartmanni and E. dispar are non-pathogenic.
Patient with diarrhea/dysentery; mild/moderate disease. Oral therapy possible	**Metronidazole** 500–750 mg po tid x 7-10 days or **tinidazole** 2 gm po daily x 3 days, followed by: Either [**paromomycin*** 25-35 mg/kg/day po divided in 3 doses x 7 days] or [**iodoquinol*** 650 mg po tid x 20 days] to clear intestinal cysts. *See comment.*		Colitis can mimic ulcerative colitis; ameboma can mimic adenocarcinoma of colon. **Nitazoxanide** 500 mg po bid x 3 days may be effective (*JID 184:381, 2001 & Tran R Soc Trop Med & Hyg 101:1025, 2007*)
Severe or extraintestinal infection, e.g., hepatic abscess	(**Metronidazole** 750 mg **IV to PO** tid x 10 days or **tinidazole** 2 gm 1x/day x 5 days) followed by **paromomycin*** 25-35 mg/kg/day po divided in 3 doses x 7 days or **Iodoquinol*** 650 mg po tid x 20 days.		**Serology positive (antibody present) with extraintestinal disease.**
Giardia intestinalis, Giardia lamblia, Giardia duodenalis: giardiasis	(**Tinidazole** 2 gm po x 1) OR (**nitazoxanide** 500 mg po bid x 3 days). **Metro** & **Paromomycin** are alternatives	**Metronidazole** 250 mg po tid x 5 days (high frequency of GI side-effects). *See Comment.* **Pregnancy: Paromomycin*** 25-35 mg/kg/day po in 3 divided doses x 5-10 days or **Albendazole** 400 mg po once daily with food x 5 days.	**Refractory pts: (metro 750 mg po + quinacrine 100 mg po)** or (**Paromomycin** 10 mg/kg po) 3x/day x 3 wks (*CID 33:22, 2001*) or furazolidone 100 mg po qid x 7 days. **Nitazoxanide** ref.: *CID 40:1173, 2005.*

* For source of drug, see *Table 13D, page 157.*

TABLE 13A (2)

INFECTING ORGANISM	SUGGESTED REGIMENS		COMMENTS
	PRIMARY	ALTERNATIVE	
PROTOZOA—INTESTINAL *(continued)*			
Cystoisospora belli (formerly Isospora belli) (AIDS ref: MMWR 58 (RR-4):1, 2009)	**Immunocompetent: TMP-SMX-DS** tab 1 po bid x 7-10 days; **Immunocompromised: TMP-SMX-DS** qid for up to 4 wks. If CD4<200 may not respond; need ART.	**CIP** 500 mg po bid x 7 days is second-line alternative *(AnIM 132:885, 2000)* OR **Pyrimethamine** 50-75 mg/day + **Folinic acid** 10-25 mg/day (po).	**Chronic suppression in AIDS pts:** either **TMP-SMX-DS** 1 tab po 3x/wk OR tab 1 po daily OR (**pyrimethamine** 25 mg/day po + **folinic acid** 10 mg/day po) OR as 2nd-line alternative: **CIP** 500 mg po 3x/wk.
Microsporidiosis	For HIV pts: antiretroviral therapy key		
Ocular: Encephalitozoon hellum or cuniculi, Vittaforma (Nosema) corneae, Nosema ocularum	**Albendazole** 400 mg po bid x 3 wks plus fumagillin eye drops *(see Comment)*.	In HIV+ pts, reports of response of E. hellum to **fumagillin*** eyedrops *(see Comment)*. For V. corneae, may need keratoplasty	To obtain fumagillin: 800-292-6773 or www.leiterrx.com. Neutropenia & thrombocytopenia serious adverse events. Dx: Most labs use modified trichrome stain. Need electron micrographs for species identification. FA and PCR methods in development. Peds dose ref.: *PIDJ 23:915, 2004*
Intestinal (diarrhea): Enterocytozoon bieneusi, Encephalitozoon (Septata) intestinalis	**Albendazole** 400 mg po bid x 3 wks; peds dose: 15 mg/kg per day div. into 2 daily doses x 7 days for **E. intestinalis.** Fumagillin equally effective.	Oral **fumagillin* 20 mg po tid** reported effective for **E. bieneusi** *(NEJM 346:1963, 2002) — see Comment*	
Disseminated: E. hellum, cuniculi or intestinalis; Pleistophora sp., *others in Comment*	**Albendazole** 400 mg po bid x 3 wks. Fumagillin 20 mg po tid (not available in US)	No established rx for Pleistophora sp.	For Trachipleistophora sp., try itraconazole + albendazole *(NEJM 351:42, 2004)*. Other pathogens: Brachiola vesicularum & algerae *(NEJM 351:42, 2004)*.
PROTOZOA—EXTRAINTESTINAL			
Amebic meningoencephalitis *(Clin Infect Dis 51:e7, 2010 (Balamuthia))*			
Acanthamoeba sp.— no proven rx Rev.: *FEMS Immunol Med Micro 50:1, 2007*	Success with IV **pentamidine** + **sulfadiazine** + **flucytosine** + (either **fluconazole** or **itraconazole**) *(FEMS Immunol Med Micro 50:1, 2007)*. 2 children responded to po rx: **TMP-SMX** + **rifampin**+ **keto** *(PIDJ 20:623, 2001)*.		For Acanthamoeba keratitis: miltefosine or voriconazole.
Balamuthia mandrillaris	[**Pentamidine** + **Albendazole** + (**Fluconazole** or **Itraconazole**)] or [**Liposomal Ampho B** + **Sulfadiazine** + (**Azithro** or **Clarithro**)]. *See CID 51:e7, 2010.*		Anecdotal response to miltefosine.
Naegleria fowleri. >95% mortality. Ref. *MMWR 57:573, 2008.*	**Ampho B** 1.5 mg/kg per day in 2 div. doses x 3 days; then 1 mg/kg/day x 6 days plus 1.5 mg/day intrathecal x 2 days; then 1 mg/day intrathecal qod x 8 days.		For Naegleria: Ampho B + azithro synergistic in vitro & in mouse model *(AAC 51:23, 2007)*. Ampho B + fluconazole + rifampin may work *(Arch Med Res 36:83, 2005)*.
Sappinia diploidea	**Azithro** + **pentamidine** + **itra** + **flucytosine** *(JAMA 285:2450, 2001)*		
Babesia microti (US) and **Babesia divergens** (EU) *(NEJM 366:366:2397, 2012)*	**For mild/moderate disease: Atovaquone** 750 mg po bid + **Azithro** 500 mg po on day 1, then 250-1000 mg po daily for total of 7-10 days. If relapse, treat x 6 wks & until blood smear neg x 2 wks.	**For severe babesiosis:** (**Clindamycin** 600 mg po tid) + (**quinine** 650 mg po tid) x 7–10 days For adults, can give **clinda** IV as 1.2 gm bid.	Overwhelming infection in asplenic patients. In immunocompromised patients, treat for 6 or more weeks *(CID 46:370, 2008)*. Transfusion related cases occur.
Leishmaniasis *(Suggest consultation – CDC (+1) 404-718-4745; see LnID 7:581, 2007; CID 43:1089, 2006)*			
Cutaneous: Mild Disease (< 4 lesions, none > 5 cm diameter, no lesions in cosmetically sensitive area, none over joints). Otherwise, consider Moderate Disease	**Mild Disease** (< 4 lesions, none > 5 cm): **Paromomycin*** ointment bid x 20 days (investigational); cryotherapy (freeze up to 3x with liquid nitrogen); intralesional Antimony 20 mg/kg into lesions weekly x 8-10 wks. Heat therapy ref, *see www.thermosurgery.com.*	**Moderate Disease: Sodium stibogluconate*** (Pentostam) or **Meglumine antimoniate** (Glucantime) 20 mg/kg/day IV/IM x 20 days. Dilute in 120 mL of D5W and infuse over 2 hrs. Alternative: **Fluconazole** 200 mg po daily x 6 weeks (for L. mexicanus, L. panamensis, L. major) or **Ketoconazole** 600 mg po daily x 30 days (L. mexicanus)	Oral therapy, Topical paromomycin* & other topical treatment only when low potential for mucosal spread; never use for L. brasiliensis or L. guyanensis cutaneous lesions. Generic pentavalent antimony varies in quality and safety. Leishmania in travelers frequently responds to observation and local therapy *(CID 57:370, 2013)*.

* For source of drug, *see Table 13D, page 157*.

TABLE 13A (3)

INFECTING ORGANISM	SUGGESTED REGIMENS		COMMENTS
	PRIMARY	ALTERNATIVE	
PROTOZOA—EXTRAINTESTINAL *(continued)*			
Leishmaniasis, Mucosal (Espundia). All cutaneous lesions due to L. brasiliensis.	**Pentavalent antimony (Sb)*** 20 mg/kg/day IV or IM x 28 days or **liposomal amphotericin B** (regimens vary) with total cumulative dose of 20-60 mg/kg or **amphotericin B** 0.5-1 mg/kg IV daily or qod to total dose of 20-40 mg/kg. *See J Am Acad Dermatol 68:284, 2013.*	No good alternative; variable efficacy of oral Miltefosine: **Miltefosine*** 2.5 mg/kg/day (to maximum of 150 mg/day) po divided tid x 28 days *(AJTMH 81:387, 2009)*.	Antimony available from CDC drug service; miltefosine available from Paladin Labs. *See Table 13D for contact information.*
Visceral leishmaniasis – Kala-Azar – New World & Old World *L. donovani*: India, Africa *L. infantum*: Mediterranean *L. chagasi*: New World	**Liposomal ampho B** FDA-approved in immunocompetent hosts: 3 mg/kg once daily days 1-5 & days 14, 21. Alternative regimens: 3 mg/kg IV daily on days 1-5 and day 10 or 10 mg/kg on days 1 and 2.	**Standard Ampho B** 1 mg/kg IV daily x 15-20 days or qod x 8 wks (to total of 15-20 mg/kg) OR **Miltefosine*** 2.5 mg/kg/day (max 150 mg/day) po x 28 days OR **pentavalent antimony*** 20 mg/kg/day IV/IM x 28 days.	In HIV patients, may need lifelong suppression with Amphotericin B q 2-4 wks
Malaria (Plasmodia species) —NOTE: CDC Malaria info— prophylaxis/treatment (770) 488-7788. After hours: 770-488-7100. US toll-free 1-855-856-4713. CDC offers species confirmation and drug resistance testing. Refs: *JAMA 297:2251, 2264 & 2285, 2007.* Websites: *www.cdc.gov/malaria; www.who.int/health-topics/malaria.htm.* Review of rapid diagnostic tests: *CID 54:1637, 2012.*			
Prophylaxis—Drugs plus personal protection: screens, nets, 30–35% DEET skin repellent (avoid > 50% DEET) *(Med Lett 54:75, 2012)*, permethrin spray on clothing and mosquito nets. Country risk in CDC Yellow Book.			
For areas free of chloroquine (CQ)-resistant P. falciparum: Central America (west of Panama Canal), Caribbean, Korea, Middle East (most)	**CQ** phosphate 500 mg (300 mg base) po per wk starting 1–2 wks before travel, during travel, & 4 wks post-travel **or atovaquone-proguanil (AP)** 1 adult tab per day (1 day prior to, during, & 7 days post-travel). Another option for P. vivax only countries: **primaquine (PQ)** 30 mg base po daily in non-pregnant. G6PD-normal travelers; >92% effective vs P. vivax *(CID 33:1990, 2001)*. Note: **CQ** may exacerbate psoriasis.	**CQ Peds dose:** 8.3 mg/kg (5 mg/kg of base) po 1x/wk up to 300 mg (base) max. dose **or AP** by weight (peds tabs): 11–20 kg, 1 tab; 21–30 kg, 2 tabs; 31–40 kg, 3 tabs; >40 kg, 1 adult tab per day. **Adults: Doxy** or **MQ** as below.	CQ safe during pregnancy. **The areas free of CQ-resistant falciparum malaria continue to shrink:** *See CDC or WHO maps for most current information on CQ resistance.* **Doxy AEs:** photosensitivity, candida vaginitis, gastritis.
For areas with CQ-resistant P. falciparum	**Atovaquone** 250 mg—**proguanil** 100 mg **(Malarone)** comb. tablet, 1 per day with food 1–2 days prior to, during, & 7 days post-travel. Peds dose in footnote[1]. **Not in pregnancy.** Malarone preferred for trips of a week or less; expense may preclude use for longer trips. Native population: intermittent pregnancy prophylaxis/treatment programs in a few countries. Fansidar 1 tab po 3 times during pregnancy *(Expert Rev Anti Infect Ther 8:589, 2010)*.	**Doxycycline** 100 mg po daily for adults & children > 8 yrs of age[1]. Take 1-2 days before, during & for 4 wks after travel. **OR** **Mefloquine (MQ)**[1] 250 mg (228 mg base) po once per wk, 1-2 wks before, during, & for 4 wks after travel *(see Comment)*. *Peds dose in footnote[1]* **Doxy AEs:** photosensitivity, candida vaginitis, gastritis.	**Pregnancy: MQ current best option.** Insufficient data with **Malarone. Avoid doxycycline and primaquine. Primaquine: Can cause hemolytic anemia if G6PD deficiency present. MQ not recommended** if cardiac conduction abnormalities, seizures, or psychiatric disorders, e.g., depression, psychosis. MQ outside U.S.: 275 mg tab, contains 250 mg of base. If used, can start 3 wks before travel to assure tolerability.

[1] **Peds prophylaxis dosages** (Ref.: *CID 34:493, 2002*): **Mefloquine** weekly dose by **weight** in kg: <15 = 5 mg/kg; 15–19 = ¼ adult dose; 20–30 = ½ adult dose; 31–45 = ¾ adult dose; >45 = adult dose. **Atovaquone/proguanil** by **weight** in kg, single daily dose using peds tab (62.5 mg atovaquone & 25 mg proguanil): 5-8 kg, 1/2 tab; 8-10 kg, 3/4 tab; 11–20 kg, 1 tab; 21–30 kg, 2 tabs; 31-40 kg, 3 tabs; ≥41 kg, one adult tab. **Doxycycline,** ages >8–12 yrs: 2 mg per kg per day up to 100 mg/day. Continue daily x 4 wks after leaving risk area. Side effects: photosensitivity, nausea, yeast vaginitis

* For source of drug, *see Table 13D, page 157*.

TABLE 13A (4)

INFECTING ORGANISM	SUGGESTED REGIMENS		COMMENTS
	PRIMARY	ALTERNATIVE	

PROTOZOA—EXTRAINTESTINAL/Malaria (Plasmodia species) *(continued)*

Treatment of Malaria. Diagnosis is by microscopy. Alternative: rapid antigen detection test (Binax NOW): detects 96-100% of P. falciparum and 50% of other plasmodia *(CID 49:908, 2009; CID 54:1637, 2012)*. Need microscopy to speciate. Can stay positive for over a month after successful treatment.

Clinical Severity/ Plasmodia sp.	Region Acquired	Suggested Treatment Regimens (Drug) – Adults	Suggested Treatment Regimens (Drug) – Peds	Comments
Uncomplicated/ P. falciparum (or species not identified)	Cen. Amer., west of Panama Canal; Haiti, Dom. Repub., & most of Mid-East **CQ-sensitive**	**CQ phosphate** 1 gm salt (600 mg base) po, then 0.5 gm in 6 hrs, then 0.5 gm daily x 2 days. Total: 2500 mg salt	**Peds: CQ** 10 mg/kg of base po; then 5 mg/kg of base at 6, 24, & 48 hrs. Total: 25 mg/kg base	**Peds dose should never exceed adult dose. CQ + MQ prolong QTc. Doses > 2x recommended may be fatal.**
Malaria rapid diagnostic test (Binax NOW) *CID 54:1637, 2012.*	CQ-resistant or unknown resistance. Note: If >5% parasitemia or Hb <7, treat as severe malaria.	**Adults: Atovaquone-proguanil** 1 gm–400 mg (4 adult tabs) po 1x/day x 3 days w/ food R **[QS** 650 mg po tid x 3 days (7 days if SE Asia)**]** + **[(Doxy** 100 mg po bid) or (**tetra** 250 mg po qid) or **clinda** 20 mg/kg/d divided tid) x 7 days**] OR** **Artemether-lumefantrine*** tabs 20/120 mg: 4 tabs po (at 0, 8 hrs) then bid x 2 days (total 6 doses); take with food **OR** a less desirable adult alternative, **mefloquine** 750 mg po x 1 dose, then 500 mg po x 1 dose 6-12 hr later. **MQ** is 2nd line alternative due to neuropsychiatric reaction. Also, resistance in SE Asia.	**Peds:** (**QS** 10 mg/kg po tid x 3 days) + (**clinda** 20 mg/kg per day div. tid) —both x 7 days. **MQ Salt:** 15 mg/kg x 1, then 6-12 hrs later, 10 mg/kg ALL po. **Artemether-lumefantrine*** • 5 kg to < 15 kg: 1 tablet (20 mg/ 120 mg) as a single dose, then 1 tablet again after 8 hours, then 1 tablet every 12 hours for 2 days • 15 kg to < 25 kg: 2 tablets (40 mg/ 240 mg) as a single dose, then 2 tablets again after 8 hours, then 2 tablets every 12 hours for 2 days • 25 kg to < 35 kg: 3 tablets (60 mg/ 360 mg) as a single dose, then 3 tablets again after 8 hours, then 3 tablets every 12 hours for 2 days • > 35 kg: as per adult dose	**Pregnancy & children:** Can substitute clinda for doxy/tetra: 20 mg/kg per day po div. tid x 7 days. In U.S., QS is only available as quinacrine 324 mg capsule, thus hard to use to treat children. **Peds atovaquone-proguanil dose** (all once daily x 3 d) by weight: 5-8 kg: 2 peds tabs; 9-10 kg: 3 peds tabs; 11-20 kg: 1 adult tab; 21-30 kg: 2 adult tabs; 31-40 kg: 3 adult tabs; >40 kg: 4 adult tabs. **Pregnancy:** Quinine + Clindamycin **Note: Oral Artemether-lumefantrine tabs FDA-approved but not widely stocked. Call 1-800-COARTEM to obtain.** IV Artesunate available from CDC Drug Service, *see Table 13D, page 157.*
Uncomplicated / P. malariae or P. knowlesi *(JID 199: 1107 & 1143, 2009).*	All regions **– CQ-sensitive**	**CQ** as above: adults & peds. In South Pacific, beware of P. knowlesi: looks like P. malariae, but behaves like P. falciparum *(CID 46:165, 2007)*.	**Artemether-lumefantrine*** (20/120 mg tab) 4 tabs po x 1 dose, repeat in 8 hrs, then repeat q12h x 2 days (take with food) OR **Atovaquone-proguanil** (1000/400 mg) 4 adult tabs po daily x 3 days	
Uncomplicated/ P. vivax or P. ovale	**CQ-sensitive** (except Papua, New Guinea, Indonesia which are CQ-resistant-*see below*)	**CQ** as above + **PQ** base: 30 mg po once daily x 14 days Each primaquine phosphate tab is 26.3 mg of salt and 15 mg of base. 30 mg of base = 2 26.3 mg tabs prim. phos.	**Peds: CQ** as above + **PQ** base 0.5 mg po once daily x 14 days	PQ added to eradicate latent parasites in liver. **Screen for G6PD def. before starting PQ;** if G6PD deficient dose PQ as 45 mg po once weekly x 8 wks. **Note: rare severe reactions.** Avoid PQ in pregnancy.
Uncomplicated/ P. vivax	**CQ-resistant:** Papua, New Guinea & Indonesia	[**QS** + (**doxy** or **tetra**) + **PQ**] as above or **Artemether-Lumefantrine** (same dose as for P. falciparum)	**MQ** + **PQ** as above. **Peds** (<8 yrs old): **QS** alone x 7 days or **MQ** alone. If latter fail, add **doxy** or **tetra**	Rarely acute. Lung injury and other serious complications: *LnID 8:449, 2008.*

* For source of drug, *see Table 13D, page 157*.

TABLE 13A (5)

INFECTING ORGANISM	SUGGESTED REGIMENS			COMMENTS
	PRIMARY		ALTERNATIVE	
PROTOZOA—EXTRAINTESTINAL/Malaria (Plasmodia species) /Treatment of Malaria *(continued)*				
Clinical Severity/ Plasmodia sp.	**Region Acquired**	**Suggested Treatment Regimens (Drug)**		**Comments**
		Primary—Adults	**Alternative & Peds**	
Uncomplicated Malaria/Alternatives for Pregnancy Ref: *LnID 7:118 & 136, 2007*	CQ-sensitive areas	**CQ** as above		Doxy or tetra used if benefits outweigh risks. No controlled studies of AP in pregnancy. If P. vivax or P. ovale, after pregnancy check for G6PD deficiency & give PQ 30 mg po daily times 14 days.
	CQ-resistant P. falciparum	**QS** + **clinda** as above	If failing or intolerant, **QS** + **doxy**	
	CQ-resistant P. vivax	**QS** 650 mg po tid x 7 days		
	Intermittent pregnancy treatment (empiric)	Give treatment dose of [Sulfadoxine 500 mg + Pyrimethamine 25 mg (Fansidar) po] at 3 times during pregnancy to decrease maternal & fetal morbidity & mortality		
Severe malaria, i.e., impaired consciousness, severe anemia, renal failure, pulmonary edema, ARDS, DIC, jaundice, acidosis, seizures, parasitemia >5%. One or more of latter. **Almost always P. falciparum.** *Ref: NEJM 358:1829, 2008; Science 320:30, 2008.*	All regions Note: •Artesunate is effective but not FDA-approved. Available from CDC Drug Service under specific conditions. •IV quinidine rarely available. Possible emergency availability from Eli Lilly.	**Quinidine gluconate** in normal saline: 10 mg/kg (salt) IV over 1 hr then 0.02 mg/ kg/min by constant infusion OR 24 mg/kg IV over 4 hrs & then 12 mg/kg over 4 hrs q8h. Continue until parasite density <1% & can take po QS. **QS** 650 mg po tid x 3 days (7 days if SE Asia) + [(**Doxy** 100 mg IV q12h x 7 days) **OR** (**clinda** 10 mg/kg IV load & then 5 mg/kg IV q8h x 7 days)]	**Peds: Quinidine gluconate IV**—same mg/kg dose as for adults **PLUS** (**Doxy:** if <45 kg, 4 mg per kg IV q12h; if ≥45 kg, dose as for adults) OR **Clinda,** same mg/kg dose as for adults **Artesunate*** 2.4 mg/kg IV at 0, 12, 24, 48 hrs, then **Doxy** 100 mg IV q12h x 7 days *(see Comment)*	During quinidine IV: monitor BP, EKG (prolongation of QTc), & blood glucose (hypoglycemia). Consider exchange transfusion if parasitemia >10%. Switch to QS po + (Doxy or Clinda) when patient able to take oral drugs. **Steroids not recommended for cerebral malaria.** If quinidine not available, or patient intolerant or high level parasitemia, **IV artesunate*** available from CDC Malaria Branch (8 hr transport time post-approval), *see Table 13D (Ref: CID 44:1067 & 1075, 2007).* Substitute Clinda for Doxy in pregnancy.
Malaria—self-initiated treatment: Only for people at high risk. Carry a reliable supply of recommended treatment (to avoid counterfeit meds). Use only if malaria is lab-diagnosed and no available reliable meds.	**Artemether-lumefantrine** (20/120 mg tab) 4 tabs po x 1 dose, repeat in 8 hrs, then repeat q12h x 2 days (take with food) OR **Atovaquone-proguanil (AP)** 4 adult tabs (1 gm/400 mg) po daily x 3 days		**Peds:** Using adult **AP** tabs for 3 consecutive days: 11–20 kg, 1 tab; 21–30 kg, 2 tabs; 31–40 kg, 3 tabs; >41 kg, 4 tabs. For Peds dosing of Artemether-lumefantrine, *see Uncomplicated/ P. falciparum, page 146.*	Do not use for renal insufficiency pts. Do not use if weight <11 kg, pregnant, or breast-feeding. **Artemether-lumefantrine:** sold as Riamet (EU) and Coartem (US & elsewhere).
Toxoplasma gondii (Reference: *Ln 363:1965, 2004*)				
Immunologically normal patients *(For pediatric doses, see reference)*				
Acute illness w/ lymphadenopathy	No specific rx unless severe/persistent symptoms or evidence of vital organ damage			
Acq. via transfusion (lab accident)	Treat as for active chorioretinitis.			
Active chorioretinitis; meningitis; lowered resistance due to steroids or cytotoxic drugs	[**Pyrimethamine** (pyri) 200 mg po once on 1st day, then 50–75 mg q24h] + [**sulfadiazine** *(see footnote[2])* S 1–1.5 gm po qid] + [**leucovorin (folinic acid)** 5–20 mg 3x/wk]—*see Comment.* Treat 1–2 wks beyond resolution of signs/symptoms; continue leucovorin 1 wk after stopping pyri.			For congenital toxo, toxo meningitis in adults, & chorioretinitis, **add prednisone 1 mg/kg/day in 2 div. doses** until CSF protein conc. falls or vision-threatening inflammation subsides. Adjust folinic acid dose by following CBC results.

[2] Sulfonamides for toxo. Sulfadiazine now commercially available. Sulfisoxazole much less effective.

* For source of drug, *see Table 13D, page 157.*

TABLE 13A (6)

INFECTING ORGANISM	SUGGESTED REGIMENS		COMMENTS
	PRIMARY	ALTERNATIVE	
PROTOZOA—EXTRAINTESTINAL/Toxoplasma gondii/ Immunologically normal patients *(continued)*			
Acute in pregnant women. Ref: *CID 47:554, 2008.*	**If <18 wks gestation at diagnosis: Spiramycin*** 1 gm po q8h until 16-18 wks; dc if amniotic fluid PCR is negative. Positive PCR: treat as below. **If >18 wks gestation & documented fetal infection by positive amniotic fluid PCR: (Pyrimethamine** 50 mg po q12h x 2 days, then 50 mg/day + **sulfadiazine** 75 mg/kg po x 1 dose, then 50 mg/kg q12h (max 4 gm/day) + **folinic acid** 10-20 mg po daily) for minimum of 4 wks or for duration of pregnancy.		Screen patients with IgG/IgM serology at commercial lab. IgG+ /IgM neg = remote past infection; IgG+/IgM+ = seroconversion. For Spiramycin, consult with Palo Alto Medical Foundation Toxoplasma Serology Lab: 650-853-4828 or toxlab@pamf.org
Fetal/congenital	Mgmt complex. Combo rx with pyrimethamine + sulfadiazine + leucovorin—*see Comment*		Details in *Ln 363:1965, 2004.* **Consultation advisable.**
AIDS			
Cerebral toxoplasmosis *Ref: MMWR 58(RR-4) 1, 2009.*	[**Pyrimethamine** (pyri) 200 mg x 1 po, then 75 mg/day po] + (**sulfadiazine** [Wt based dose: 1 gm if <60 kg, 1.5 gm if ≥60 kg] po q6h) + (**folinic acid** 10–25 mg/day po) for minimum of 6 wks after resolution of signs/ symptoms, and then suppressive rx *(see below)* OR **TMP-SMX** 10/50 mg/kg per day po or IV div. q12h x 30 days *(AAC 42:1346, 1998)*	[**Pyri** + **folinic acid** (as in primary regimen)] + 1 of the following: (1) **Clinda** 600 mg po/IV q6h or (2) **TMP=SMX** 5/25 mg/kg/day po or IV bid or (3) **atovaquone** 750 mg po q6h. Treat 4–6 wks after resolution of signs/symptoms, then suppression.	Use alternative regimen for pts with severe sulfa allergy. If multiple ring-enhancing brain lesions (CT or MRI), >85% of pts respond to 7–10 days of empiric rx; if no response, suggest brain biopsy. Pyri penetrates brain even if no inflammation; folinic acid prevents pyrimethamine hematologic toxicity.
Primary prophylaxis, AIDS pts—IgG toxo antibody + CD4 count <100 per mcL	(**TMP-SMX-DS**, 1 tab po q24h or 3x/wk) or (**TMP-SMX-SS**, 1 tab po q24h)	[(**Dapsone** 50 mg po q24h) + (**pyri** 50 mg po q wk) + (**folinic acid** 25 mg po q wk)] OR **atovaquone** 1500 mg po q24h	Prophylaxis for pneumocystis also effective vs toxo. *Ref: MMWR 58(RR-4):1, 2009.* **Another alternative:** (Dapsone 200 mg po + pyrimethamine 75 mg po + folinic acid 25 mg po) once weekly.
Suppression after rx of cerebral toxo	(**Sulfadiazine** 2-4 gm po divided in 2-4 doses/day) + (**pyri** 25–50 mg po q24h) + (**folinic acid** 10–25 mg po q24h). DC if CD4 count >200 x 3 mos	[(**Clinda** 600 mg po q8h) + (**pyri** 25–50 mg po q24h) + (**folinic acid** 10–25 mg po q24h)] OR **atovaquone** 750 mg po q6–12h	(Pyri + sulfa) prevents PCP and toxo; (clinda + pyri) prevents toxo only. Additional drug needed to prevent PCP.
Trichomonas vaginalis	*See Vaginitis, Table 1, page 26.*		
Trypanosomiasis. Ref.: *Ln 362:1469, 2003.* **Note: Drugs for African trypanosomiasis may be obtained free from WHO or CDC.** ***See Table 13D, page 157,*** **for source information.**			
West African sleeping sickness (T. brucei gambiense)			
Early: Blood/lymphatic—CNS OK	**Pentamidine** 4 mg/kg IV/IM daily x 7-10 days	In US, free from CDC drug service: **Suramin*** 100 mg IV (test dose), then 1 gm IV on days 1, 3, 7, 14, & 21. Peds dose is 10-15 mg/kg.	
Late: Encephalitis Combination of IV eflornithine, 400 mg/kg/day divided q12h x 7 days, plus nifurtimox, 15 mg/kg/day po, divided q8h x 10 days more efficacious than standard dose eflornithine *(CID 45:1435 & 1443, 2007; Ln 374:56, 2009).*	**Eflornithine*** 100 mg/kg q6h IV x 14 days *(CID 41:748, 2005).*	**Melarsoprol*** 2.2 mg/kg per day IV x 10 days (**Nifurtimox/Eflornithine** combination superior to melarsoprol alone *(JID 195:311 & 322, 2007).*	

* For source of drug, *see Table 13D, page 157.*

TABLE 13A (7)

INFECTING ORGANISM	SUGGESTED REGIMENS		COMMENTS
	PRIMARY	ALTERNATIVE	
PROTOZOA—EXTRAINTESTINAL/Toxoplasma gondii/AIDS *(continued)*			
East African sleeping sickness (T. brucei rhodesiense)			
Early: Blood/lymphatic	**Suramin*** 100 mg IV (test dose), then 1 gm IV on days 1 3, 7, 14, & 21	Peds: Suramin* 2 mg/kg test dose, then IV on days 1, 3, 7, 14 & 21	Suramin & Melarsoprol: CDC Drug Service or WHO (at no charge) *(see Table 13D)*
Late: Encephalitis (prednisolone may prevent encephalitis) Pre-treatment with Suramin advised by some.	**Melarsoprol*** From 2–3.6 mg/kg per day IV over 3 days; repeat 3.6 mg/kg after 7 days & for 3rd time at 3.6 mg/kg 7 days after 2nd course	**Melarsoprol** 2.2 mg/kg/day IV x 10 days *(PLoS NTD 6:e1695, 2012) (preferable to standard regimen)*	Early illness: patient waiting for Suramin, use pentamidine 4 mg/kg/day IV/IM x 1-2 doses. Does not enter CSF.
T. cruzi—**Chagas disease** or acute American trypanosomiasis Ref.: *Ln 375:1388, 2010; LnID 10:556, 2010.* For chronic disease: *see Comment.*	**Benznidazole*** 5–7 mg/kg per day po div. 2x/day x 60 days. NOTE: Take with meals to alleviate G-I side effects. **Contraindicated in pregnancy.**	**Nifurtimox*** 8–10 mg/kg per day po div. 4x/day after meals x 120 days Ages 11–16 yrs: 12.5–15 mg/kg per day div. qid po x 90 days Children <11yrs: 15–20 mg/kg per day div. qid po x 90 days.	Immunosuppression for heart transplant can reactivate chronic Chagas disease *(J Card Failure 15:249, 2009)*. Can transmit by organ/transfusions *(CID 48:1534, 2009)*.
NEMATODES—INTESTINAL (Roundworms). Eosinophilia? Think Strongyloides, toxocaria and filariasis: *CID 34:407, 2005; 42:1781 & 1655, 2006-- See Table 13C.*			
Anisakis simplex (**anisakiasis**) Anisakiasis differentiated from Anisakidosis *(CID 51:806, 2010)*. Other: A. physiatry, Pseudoterranova decipiens.	Physical removal: endoscope or surgery IgE antibody test vs *A. simplex* may help diagnosis. No antimicrobial therapy.	Anecdotal reports of possible treatment benefit from albendazole *(Ln 360:54, 2002; CID 41:1825, 2005)*	Anisakiasis acquired by eating raw fish: herring, salmon, mackerel, cod, squid. Similar illness due to Pseudoterranova species acquired from cod, halibut, red snapper.
Ascaris lumbricoides (**ascariasis**) *Ln 367:1521, 2006*	**Albendazole** 400 mg po daily x 3 days or **mebendazole** 100 mg po bid x 3 days	**Ivermectin** 150–200 mcg/kg po x 1 dose	Review of efficacy of single dose: *JAMA 299:1937, 2008.*
Capillaria philippinensis (**capillariasis**)	**Albendazole** 400 mg po bid x 10 days	**Mebendazole** 200 mg po bid x 20 days	Albendazole preferred.
Enterobius vermicularis (**pinworm**)	**Mebendazole** 100 mg po x 1, repeat in 2 wks	**Pyrantel pamoate** 11 mg/kg base (to max. dose of 1 gm) po x 1 dose; repeat in 2 wks **OR Albendazole** 400 mg po x 1 dose, repeat in 2 wks.	*Side-effects in Table 13B, page 156.* Treat whole household.
Gongylonemiasis (adult worms in oral mucosa)	Surgical removal	**Albendazole** 400 mg/day po x 3 days	Ref: *CID 32:1378, 2001; J Helminth 80:425, 2006.*
Hookworm (Necator americanus and Ancylostoma duodenale)	**Albendazole** 400 mg po daily x 3 days	**Mebendazole** 100 mg po bid x 3 days OR **Pyrantel pamoate** 11 mg/kg (to max. dose of 1 gm) po daily x 3 days	NOTE: Ivermectin not effective. Eosinophilia may be absent but eggs in stool *(NEJM 351:799, 2004)*.
Strongyloides stercoralis (**strongyloidiasis**) *(Hyperinfection, See Comment)*	**Ivermectin** 200 mcg/kg per day po x 2 days	**Albendazole** 400 mg po bid x 7 days ; less effective	**For hyperinfections,** repeat at 15 days. For hyperinfection: veterinary ivermectin given subcutaneously or rectally *(CID 49:1411, 2009)*.

* For source of drug, *see Table 13D, page 157.*

TABLE 13A (8)

INFECTING ORGANISM	SUGGESTED REGIMENS		COMMENTS
	PRIMARY	ALTERNATIVE	
NEMATODES—INTESTINAL (Roundworms) *(continued)*			
Trichostrongylus orientalis, T. colubriformis	**Pyrantel pamoate** 11 mg/kg (max. 1 gm) po x 1	**Albendazole** 400 mg po x 1 dose	**Mebendazole** 100 mg po bid x 3 days
Trichuris trichiura (**whipworm**) *NEJM 370:610, 2014; PLoS One 6:e25003, 2011*	**Mebendazole** 100 mg po bid x 3 days	**Albendazole** 400 mg po qd x 3 days or **Ivermectin** 200 mcg/kg po qd x 3 days	Cure rate of 55% with one 500 mg dose of **Mebendazole** + one dose of **Ivermectin** 200 mcg/kg *(CID 51:1420, 2010)*.
NEMATODES—EXTRAINTESTINAL (Roundworms)			
Ancylostoma braziliense & caninum: causes **cutaneous larva migrans** (Dog & cat hookworm)	**Albendazole** 400 mg po bid x 3-7 days *(Ln ID 8:302, 2008)*.	**Ivermectin** 200 mcg/kg po x 1 dose/day x 1–2 days (not in children wt < 15 kg)	Also called "creeping eruption," dog and cat hookworm. Ivermectin cure rate 81-100% (1 dose) to 97% (2–3 doses) *(CID 31:493, 2000)*.
Angiostrongylus cantonensis (Angiostrongyliasis); causes eosinophilic meningitis	Mild/moderate disease: Analgesics, serial LPs (if necessary). Prednisone 60 mg/day x 14 days reduces headache & need for LPs.	Adding **Albendazole** 15 mg/kg/day to prednisone 60 mg/day both for 14 days may reduce duration of headaches and need for repeat LPs.	**Do not use Albendazole without prednisone,** see *TRSMH 102:990, 2008*. Gnathostoma and Baylisascaris also cause eosinophilic meningitis.
Baylisascariasis (Raccoon roundworm); eosinophilic meningitis	No drug proven efficacious. Try po **albendazole,** Peds: 25–50 mg/kg/day po; Adults: 400 mg po bid with corticosteroids. Treat for one month.		Steroids ref: *CID 39:1484, 2004*. Other causes of eosinophilic meningitis: Gnathostoma & Angiostrongylus.
Dracunculus medinensis: **Guinea worm** *(CMAJ 170:495, 2004)*	Slow extraction of pre-emergent worm over several days	No drugs effective. Oral analgesics, anti-inflammatory drugs, topical antiseptics/antibiotic ointments to alleviate symptoms and facilitate worm removal by gentle manual traction over several days.	
Filariasis. Wolbachia bacteria needed for filarial development. **Rx with doxy 100–200 mg/day x 6-8 wks** ↓ number of wolbachia & number of microfilaria but no effect on adult worms			
Lymphatic filariasis (**Elephantiasis**): Wuchereria bancrofti or Brugia malayi or B. timori. Ref: *Curr Opin Inf Dis 21:673, 2008 (role of Wolbachia)*.	**Diethylcarbamazine***[3](DEC): [6 mg/kg/day po in 3 divided doses x 14 days OR 6 mg/kg/day as single po dose daily x 14 days OR gradual dose increase: day 1-50 mg po, day 2-50 mg po tid, day 3-100 mg po tid, day 4 through 12-6 mg/kg po divided tid + **Doxy** 200 mg/day x 6 wks.	Interest in combining albendazole with **DEC;** no trials comparing combination vs. DEC alone. **Doxycycline** 200 mg/day x 6 wks PLUS **DEC** + **albendazole** reduced microfilaremia *(CID 46:1385, 2008)*.	**NOTE: DEC can cause irreversible eye damage if concomitant onchocerciasis.** Goal is reducing burden of adult worms. (Albendazole 400 mg po + Ivermectin 200 μg/kg po) or DEC 6 mg/kg po suppresses microfilaria but no effective on adult worms.
Cutaneous			
Loiasis: **Loa loa**, eye worm disease	**Diethylcarbamazine** (DEC)*[3]: Day 1, 50 mg; Day 2, 50 mg tid; Day 3, 100 mg tid; Days 4-21, 8-10 mg/kg/day in 3 divided doses x 21 days. **If concomitant onchocerca, treat onchocerca first.**	**Albendazole** 200 mg po bid x 21 days if still symptomatic after 2 courses of DEC.	If over 5,000 microfilaria/mL of blood, DEC can cause encephalopathy. Might start with albendazole x few days ± steroids, then DEC.
Onchocerca volvulus (**onchocerciasis**) — river blindness *(AJTMH 81:702, 2009)*	First give **doxy** 200 mg/day x 6 wks and then **Ivermectin:** Single dose of 150 mcg/kg po; repeat every 3-6 months until asymptomatic.	DEC is contraindicated	Oncho & Loa loa may both be present. Check peripheral smear; if Loa loa microfilaria present, treat oncho first with ivermectin before DEC for Loa loa.
Body cavity			
Mansonella perstans (dipetalonemiasis)	In randomized trial, doxy 200 mg po once daily x 6 weeks cleared microfilaria from blood in 67 of 69 patients *(NEJM 361:1448, 2009)*.	**Albendazole** in high dose x 3 weeks.	Efficacy of doxy believed to be due to inhibition of endosymbiont wolbachia; Ivermectin has no activity. Ref: *Trans R Soc Trop Med Hyg 100:458, 2006*.
Mansonella streptocerca	**Ivermectin** 150 μg/kg x 1 dose.	May need antihistamine or corticosteroid for allergic reaction from disintegrating organisms. Chronic pruritic hypopigmented lesions that may be confused with leprosy. Can be asymptomatic.	

[3] May need antihistamine or corticosteroid for allergic reaction from disintegrating organisms

* For source of drug, see *Table 13D, page 157*.

TABLE 13A (9)

INFECTING ORGANISM	SUGGESTED REGIMENS		COMMENTS
	PRIMARY	ALTERNATIVE	
NEMATODES—EXTRAINTESTINAL (Roundworms)/Filariasis *(continued)*			
Mansonella ozzardi	**Ivermectin** 200 μ/kg x 1 dose may be effective. Limited data but no other option.	Usually asymptomatic. Articular pain, pruritus, lymphadenopathy reported. May have allergic reaction from dying organisms.	
Dirofilariasis: **Heartworms**			
D. immitis, dog heartworm	No effective drugs; surgical removal only option		Can lodge in pulmonary artery → coin lesion. Eosinophilia rare.
D. tenuis (raccoon), D. ursi (bear), D. repens (dogs, cats)	No effective drugs	Worms migrate to conjunctivae, subcutaneous tissue, scrotum, breasts, extremities	
Gnathostoma spinigerum			
Cutaneous larva migrans	**Albendazole** 400 mg po q24h or bid times 21 days	**Ivermectin** 200 μg/kg/day po x 2 days.	Other etiology of larva migrans: Ancyclostoma sp., *see page 150*
Eosinophilic meningitis	Supportive care; monitor for cerebral hemorrhage	Case reports of steroid use: both benefit and harm from Albendazole or ivermectin *(EIN 17:1174, 2011)*.	Other causes of eosinophilic meningitis: **Angiostrongylus** *(see page 150)* & **Baylisascaris** *(see page 150)*
Toxocariasis *(Ann Trop Med Parasit 103:3, 2010)*	**Rx directed at relief of symptoms as infection self-limited, e.g., steroids & antihistamines; use of anthelmintics controversial.**		
Visceral larval migrans	**Albendazole** 400 mg po bid x 5 days ± **Prednisone** 60 mg/day	**Mebendazole** 100–200 mg po bid times 5 days	Severe lung, heart or CNS disease may warrant steroids *(Clin Micro Rev 16:265, 2003)*. Differential dx of larval migrans syndromes: Toxocara canis & catis, Ancylostoma spp., Gnathostoma spp., Spirometra spp.
Ocular larval migrans	First 4 wks of illness: (Oral **prednisone** 30–60 mg po q24h + subtenon **triamcinolone** 40 mg/wk) x 2 wks (Surgery is sometimes necessary)		No added benefit of anthelmintic drugs. Rx of little effect after 4 wks. Some use steroids *(Clin Micro Rev 16:265, 2003)*.
Trichinella spiralis (**Trichinellosis**) — muscle infection *(Review: Clin Micro Rev 22:127, 2009)*.	**Albendazole** 400 mg po bid x 8–14 days	**Mebendazole** 200–400 mg po tid x 3 days, then 400–500 mg po tid x 10 days	Use albendazole/mebendazole with caution during pregnancy. ↑ IgE, ↑ CPK, ESR 0, massive eosinophilia: >5000/μL.
	Concomitant **prednisone** 40–60 mg po q24h		
TREMATODES (Flukes) – Liver, Lung, Intestinal. All flukes have snail intermediate hosts; transmitted by injection of metacercariae on plants, fish or crustaceans.			
Clonorchis sinensis (liver fluke)	**Praziquantel** 25 mg/kg po tid x 2 days or **albendazole** 10 mg/kg per day po x 7 days		Same dose in children
Dicrocoelium dendriticum	**Praziquantel** 25 mg/kg po tid x 1 day		Ingestion of raw or undercooked sheep liver *(CID 44:145, 2007)*.
Fasciola buski (intestinal fluke)	**Praziquantel** 25 mg/kg po tid x 1 day		Same dose in children
Fasciola hepatica (sheep liver fluke), Fasciola gigantica	**Triclabendazole*** once, may repeat after 12-24 hrs. 10 mg/kg po x 1 dose. Single 10 mg/kg po dose effective in controlling endemic disease *(PLoS Negl Trop Dis 6(8):e1720)*.		Alternative: **Bithionol*** Adults and children: 30–50 mg/kg (max. dose 2 gm/day) every other day times 10–15 doses. In CDC formulary, efficacy unclear.
Heterophyes heterophyes (intestinal fluke); Metagonimus yokogawai (intestinal fluke); Metorchis conjunctus (No Amer liver fluke); Nanophyetus salmincola	**Praziquantel** 25 mg/kg po tid x 1 days		
Opisthorchis viverrini (liver fluke)	**Praziquantel** 25 mg/kg po tid x 2 days		
Paragonimus sp. (lung fluke)	**Praziquantel** 25 mg/kg po tid x 2 days or **Triclabendazole*** 10 mg/kg po x 2 doses over 12-24 hrs.		Same dose in children

* For source of drug, *see Table 13D, page 157*.

TABLE 13A (10)

INFECTING ORGANISM	SUGGESTED REGIMENS		COMMENTS
	PRIMARY	ALTERNATIVE	
TREMATODES (Flukes) – Liver, Lung, Intestinal *(continued)*			
Schistosoma haematobium; GU bilharziasis. *(NEJM 346:1212, 2002)*	**Praziquantel** 40 mg/kg po on the same day (one dose of 40 mg/kg or two doses of 20 mg/kg)		Same dose in children.
Schistosoma intercalatum	**Praziquantel** 20 mg/kg po on the same day in 1 or 2 doses		Same dose in children
Schistosoma japonicum; Oriental schisto. *(NEJM 346:1212, 2002)*	**Praziquantel** 60 mg/kg po on the same day (3 doses of 20 mg/kg)		Same dose in children. Cures 60–90% pts.
Schistosoma mansoni (intestinal bilharziasis) **Possible praziquantel resistance** *(JID 176:304, 1997) (NEJM 346:1212, 2002)*	**Praziquantel** 40 mg/kg po on the same day in (one dose of 40 mg/kg or two doses of 20 mg/kg)		Praziquantel: Same dose for children and adults. Cures 60–90% pts. Report of success treating myeloradiculopathy with single po dose of praziquantel, 50 mg/kg, + prednisone for 6 mos *(CID 39:1618, 2004)*.
Schistosoma mekongi	**Praziquantel** 60 mg per kg po on the same day (3 doses of 20 mg/kg)		Same dose for children
Toxemic schisto; Katayama fever	**Praziquantel** 20 mg per kg po bid with short course of high dose prednisone. Repeat Praziquantel in 4-6 wks *(Clin Micro Rev 16:225, 2010)*.		Reaction to onset of egg laying 4-6 wks after infection exposure in fresh water.
CESTODES (Tapeworms)			
Echinococcus granulosus (hydatid disease) *(LnID 12:871, 2012; Inf Dis Clin No Amer 26:421, 2012)*	**Liver cysts:** Meta-analysis supports percutaneous aspiration-injection-reaspiration (**PAIR**) + albendazole for uncomplicated single liver cysts. Before & after drainage: **albendazole** ≥60 kg, 400 mg po bid or <60 kg, 15 mg/kg per day div. bid, with meals. After 1-2 days puncture (P) & needle aspirate (A) cyst content. Instill (I) hypertonic saline (15–30%) or absolute alcohol, wait 20–30 min, then re-aspirate (R) with final irrigation. **Continue albendazole for at least 30 days.** Cure in 96% as comp to 90% pts with surgical resection. Albendazole ref: *Acta Tropica 114:1, 2010*.		
Echinococcus multilocularis (alveolar cyst disease) *(COID 16:437, 2003)*	**Albendazole** efficacy not clearly demonstrated, can try in dosages used for hydatid disease. Wide surgical resection only reliable rx; technique evolving. Post-surgical resection or if inoperable: Albendazole for several years *(Acta Tropic 114:1, 2010)*.		
Intestinal tapeworms Diphyllobothrium latum (fish), Dipylidium caninum (dog), Taenia saginata (beef), & Taenia solium (pork)	**Praziquantel** 5–10 mg/kg po x 1 dose for children and adults.	**Niclosamide*** 2 gm po x 1 dose	Niclosamide from Expert Compounding Pharm, *see Table 13D*.
Hymenolepis diminuta (rats) and H. nana (humans)	**Praziquantel** 25 mg/kg po x 1 dose for children and adults.	**Niclosamide*** 2 gm po daily x 7 days	
Neurocysticercosis (NCC): Larval form of T. solium Ref.: *AJTMH 72:3, 2005*	**NOTE: Treat T. solium intestinal tapeworms,** if present, with **praziquantel** 5-10 mg/kg po x 1 dose for children & adults.		
Parenchymal NCC "Viable" cysts by CT/MRI Meta-analysis: Treatment assoc with cyst resolution, ↓ seizures, and ↓ seizure recurrence. Ref: *AnIM 145:43, 2006.*	[**Albendazole** ≥60 kg: 400 mg bid with meals or 60 kg: 15 mg/kg per day in 2 div. doses (max. 800 mg/day) + **Dexamethasone** 0.1 mg/kg per day ± Anti-seizure medication] — all x 10-30 days. May need anti-seizure therapy for a year.	(**Praziquantel** 100 mg/kg per day in 3 div. doses po x 1 day, then 50 mg/kg/d in 3 doses plus **Dexamethasone** 0.1 mg/kg per day ± Anti-seizure medication) — all x 29 days. *See Comment*	Albendazole assoc. with 46% ↓ in seizures *(NEJM 350:249, 2004)*. Praziquantel less cysticidal activity. Steroids decrease serum levels of praziquantel. NIH reports methotrexate at ≤20 mg/wk allows a reduction in steroid use *(CID 44:449, 2007)*.
"Degenerating" cysts	**Albendazole + dexamethasone as above**		**Treatment improves prognosis of associated seizures.**
Dead calcified cysts	**No treatment indicated**		
Subarachnoid NCC	(**Albendazole** + **steroids** as above) + shunting for hydrocephalus prior to drug therapy. Ref: *Expert Rev Anti Infect Ther 9:123, 2011*.		
Intraventricular NCC	Neuroendoscopic removal is treatment of choice with or without obstruction. If surgery not possible, **albendazole + dexamethasone; observe closely for evidence of obstruction of flow of CSF.**		

* For source of drug, *see Table 13D, page 157*.

TABLE 13A (11)

INFECTING ORGANISM		SUGGESTED REGIMENS		COMMENTS
		PRIMARY	ALTERNATIVE	
CESTODES (Tapeworms)/Neurocysticercosis (NCC) *(continued)*				
Sparganosis (Spirometra mansonoides) Larval cysts; source—frogs/snakes		Surgical resection. No antiparasitic therapy. Can inject alcohol into subcutaneous masses.		
ECTOPARASITES. Ref.: *CID 36:1355, 2003; Ln 363:889, 2004.* **NOTE: Due to potential neurotoxicity and risk of aplastic anemia, lindane not recommended.**				
DISEASE	**INFECTING ORGANISM**			
Head lice *NEJM 367:1687 & 1750, 2012; Med Lett 54:61, 2012.*	Pediculus humanus, var. capitis	**Permethrin** 1% lotion: Apply to shampooed dried hair for 10 min.; repeat in 9-10 days. **OR** **Malathion** 0.5% lotion (Ovide): Apply to dry hair for 8–12 hrs, then shampoo. 2 doses 7-9 days apart. **OR** **Spinosad** 0.9% suspension; wash off after 10 min (85% effective). Repeat in 7 days, if needed. Use nit comb initially & repeat in 7-10 days	**Ivermectin** 200-400 µg/kg po once; 3 doses at 7 day intervals effective in 95% *(JID 193:474, 2006)*. Topical ivermectin 0.5% lotion, 75% effective. **Malathion:** Report that 1–2 20-min. applications 98% effective *(Ped Derm 21:670, 2004)*. In alcohol—potentially flammable. **Benzyl alcohol:** 76% effective	**Permethrin:** success in 78%. Resistance increasing. No advantage to 5% permethrin. **Spinosad** is effective, but expensive. Wash hats, scarves, coats & bedding in hot water, then dry in hot dryer for 20+ minutes.
Pubic lice (crabs)	Phthirus pubis	**Pubic hair: Permethrin** OR **malathion** as for head lice	**Eyelids: Petroleum jelly** applied qid x 10 days OR **yellow oxide of mercury** 1% qid x 14 days	
Body lice	Pediculus humanus, var. corporis	No drugs for the patient. Organism lives in & deposits eggs in seams of clothing. Discard clothing; if not possible, treat clothing with 1% malathion powder or 0.5% permethrin powder. Success with ivermectin in homeless shelter: 12 mg po on days 0, 7, & 14 *(JID 193:474, 2006)*		
Myiasis Due to larvae of flies		Usually cutaneous/subcutaneous nodule with central punctum. Treatment: Occlude punctum to prevent gas exchange with petrolatum, fingernail polish, makeup cream or bacon. When larva migrates, manually remove. Ref: *CID 35:336, 2002.*		
Scabies	Sarcoptes scabiei			
Immunocompetent patients Refs: *MMWR 59(RR-12):89, 2010; NEJM 362:717, 2010.*		**Permethrin** 5% cream (ELIMITE) under nails (finger and toe). Apply entire skin from chin down to and including under fingernails and toenails. Leave on 8–14 hrs. Repeat in 1-2 wks. Safe for children age >2 mos.	**Ivermectin** 250 µg/kg po x 1. As above, second dose if persistent symptoms. **Less effective: Crotamiton** 10% cream, apply x 24 hr, rinse off, then reapply x 24 hr.	Trim fingernails. Reapply cream to hands after handwashing. Treat close contacts; wash and heat dry linens. Pruritus may persist times 2 wks after mites gone.
AIDS and HTLV-infected patients (CD4 <150 per mm^3), debilitated or developmentally disabled patients (**Norwegian scabies**—*see Comments*)		For Norwegian scabies: **Permethrin** 5% cream daily x 7 days, then twice weekly until cured. Add **ivermectin** po (dose in Alternative)	**Ivermectin** 200 mcg/kg po on days 1, 2, 8, 9, 15 (and maybe 22, 29) + **Permethrin** cream.	Norwegian scabies in AIDS pts: Extensive, crusted. Can mimic psoriasis. Not pruritic. Highly contagious—isolate!

* For source of drug, *see Table 13D, page 157*.

TABLE 13B – DOSAGE AND SELECTED ADVERSE EFFECTS OF ANTIPARASITIC DRUGS

Doses vary with indication. For convenience, drugs divided by type of parasite; some drugs used for multiple types of parasites, e.g., albendazole.

CLASS, AGENT, GENERIC NAME (TRADE NAME)	USUAL ADULT DOSAGE	ADVERSE REACTIONS/COMMENTS
Antiprotozoan Drugs		
Intestinal Parasites		
Diloxanide furoate[NUS] (Furamide)	500 mg po tid x 10 days	Source: *See Table 13D, page 157*. Flatulence, N/V, diarrhea.
Iodoquinol (Yodoxin)	Adults: 650 mg po tid (or 30-40 mg/kg/day div. tid); children: 40 mg/kg per day div. tid.	Rarely causes nausea, abdominal cramps, rash, acne. Contraindicated if iodine intolerance (contains 64% bound iodine). Can cause iododerma (papular or pustular rash) and/or thyroid enlargement.
Metronidazole	Side-effects similar for all. *See metronidazole in Table 10B, page 106, & Table 10A, page 101*	
Nitazoxanide (Alinia)	Adults: 500 mg po q12h. Children 4–11: 200 mg susp. po q12h. Take with food. Expensive.	Abdominal pain 7.8%, diarrhea 2.1%. Rev.: *CID 40:1173, 2005; Expert Opin Pharmacother 7:953, 2006.* Headaches; rarely yellow sclera (resolves after treatment).
Paromomycin (Humatin) Aminosidine IV in U.K.	Up to 750 mg qid (250 mg tabs). Source: *See Table 13D.*	Aminoglycoside similar to neomycin; if absorbed due to concomitant inflammatory bowel disease can result in oto/nephrotoxicity. Doses >3 gm daily are associated with nausea, abdominal cramps, diarrhea.
Quinacrine[NUS] (Atabrine, Mepacrine)	100 mg po tid. No longer available in U.S.; 2 pharmacies will prepare as a service: (1) Connecticut (+1) 203-785-6818; (2) California 800-247-9767	Contraindicated for pts with history of psychosis or psoriasis. Yellow staining of skin. Dizziness, headache, vomiting, toxic psychosis (1.5%), hemolytic anemia, leukopenia, thrombocytopenia, urticaria, rash, fever, minor disulfiram-like reactions.
Tinidazole (Tindamax)	250-500 mg tabs, with food. Regimen varies with indication.	Chemical structure similar to metronidazole but better tolerated. Seizures/peripheral neuropathy reported. **Adverse effects:** Metallic taste 4–6%, nausea 3–5%, anorexia 2–3%.
Antiprotozoan Drugs: Non-Intestinal Protozoa		
Extraintestinal Parasites		
Antimony compounds[NUS] Stibogluconate sodium (Pentostam) from CDC or Meglumine antimonate (Glucantime—French trade names	For IV use: vials with 100 mg antimony/mL. Dilute selected dose in 50 mL of D5W shortly before use. Infuse over at least 10 minutes.	**AEs in 1st 10 days:** headache, fatigue, elevated lipase/amylase, clinical pancreatitis. After 10 days: elevated AST/ALT/ALK/PHOS. **NOTE: Reversible T wave changes in 30-60%. Risk of QTc prolongation. Renal excretion; modify dose if renal insufficiency. Metabolized in liver; lower dose if hepatic insufficiency. Generic drug may have increased toxicity due to antimony complex formation.**
Artemether-Lumefantrine, po (Coartem, FDA-approved)	Tablets contain 20 mg Artemether and 120 mg Lumefantrine. Take with food. Can be crushed and mixed with a few teaspoons of water	Can prolong QT_C: avoid in patients with congenital long QT_C, family history of sudden death or long QT_C, or need for drugs known to prolong QT_C *(see list under fluoroquinolones, Table 10A, page 99)*. Artemether induces CYP3A4 and both Artemether & Lumefantrine are metabolized by CYP3A4 *(see drug-drug interactions, Table 22A, page 224)*. Adverse effects experienced by >30% of adults: headache, anorexia, dizziness, arthralgia and myalgia.
Artesunate, IV Ref: *NEJM 358:1829, 2008*	Available from CDC Malaria Branch. 2.4 mg/kg IV at 0, 12, 24, & 48 hrs	More effective than quinine & safer than quinidine. Contact CDC at 770-488-7758 or 770-488-7100 after hours. No dosage adjustment for hepatic or renal insufficiency. No known drug interactions.
Atovaquone (Mepron) Ref.: *AAC 46:1163, 2002*	Suspension: 1 tsp (750 mg) po bid 750 mg/5 mL.	No. pts stopping rx due to side-effects was 9%; rash 22%, GI 20%, headache 16%, insomnia 10%, fever 14%
Atovaquone and proguanil (Malarone) For prophylaxis of P. falciparum; little data on P. vivax. Generic available in US.	**Prophylaxis:** 1 tab po (250 mg + 100 mg) q24h with food **Treatment:** 4 tabs po (1000 mg + 400 mg) once daily with food x 3 days Adult tab: 250/100 mg; Peds tab 62.5/25 mg. Peds dosage: *prophylaxis footnote 1 page 145; treatment see comment, page 146.*	Adverse effects in rx trials: Adults—abd. pain 17%, N/V 12%, headache 10%, dizziness 5%. Rx stopped in 1%. Asymptomatic mild ↑ in ALT/AST. Children—cough, headache, anorexia, vomiting, abd. pain. *See drug interactions, Table 22*. Safe in G6PD-deficient pts. Can crush tabs for children and give with milk or other liquid nutrients. Renal insufficiency: contraindicated if CrCl <30 mL per min.

NOTE: Drugs available from CDC Drug Service indicated by "CDC." Call (+1) (404) 639-3670 (or -2888 (Fax)). ***See Table 13D, page 157 for sources and contact information for hard-to-find antiparasitic drugs.***

TABLE 13B (2)

CLASS, AGENT, GENERIC NAME (TRADE NAME)	USUAL ADULT DOSAGE	ADVERSE REACTIONS/COMMENTS
Antiprotozoan Drugs: Non-Intestinal Protozoa/Extraintestinal Parasites *(continued)*		
Benznidazole (CDC Drug Service)	7.5 mg/kg per day po. 100 mg tabs	Photosensitivity in 50% of pts. GI: abdominal pain, nausea/vomiting/anorexia. CNS: disorientation, insomnia, twitching/seizures, paresthesias, polyneuritis. **Contraindicated in pregnancy**
Chloroquine phosphate (Aralen)	Dose varies—*see Malaria Prophylaxis and rx, pages 145-146.*	Minor: anorexia/nausea/vomiting, headache, dizziness, blurred vision, pruritus in dark-skinned pts. Major: protracted rx in rheumatoid arthritis can lead to retinopathy. Can exacerbate psoriasis. Can block response to rabies vaccine. Contraindicated in pts with epilepsy.
Dapsone *See Comment re methemoglobinemia*	100 mg po q24h	Usually tolerated by pts with rash after TMP-SMX. Dapsone is common etiology of acquired methemoglobinemia *(NEJM 364:957, 2011)*. Metabolite of dapsone converts heme iron to +3 charge (no O2 transport) from normal +2. Normal blood level 1%; cyanosis at 10%; headache, fatigue, tachycardia, dizziness at 30-40%, acidosis & coma at 60%, death at 70-80%. Low G6PD is a risk factor. Treatment: methylene blue 1-2 mg/kg IV over 5 min x 1 dose.
Eflornithine (Ornidyl) (WHO or CDC drug service)	200 mg/kg IV (slowly) q12h x 7 days for African trypanosomiasis	Diarrhea in ½ pts, vomiting, abdominal pain, anemia/leukopenia in ½ pts, seizures, alopecia, jaundice, ↓ hearing. Contraindicated in pregnancy.
Fumagillin	Eyedrops + po. 20 mg po tid. Leiter's: 800-292-6772.	Adverse events: Neutropenia & thrombocytopenia
Mefloquine	One 250 mg tab/wk for malaria prophylaxis; for rx, 1250 mg x 1 or 750 mg & then 500 mg in 6–8 hrs. In U.S.: 250 mg tab = 228 mg base; outside U.S., 275 mg tab = 250 mg base	Side-effects in roughly 3%. Minor: headache, irritability, insomnia, weakness, diarrhea. Toxic psychosis, seizures can occur. Do not use with quinine, quinidine, or halofantrine. Rare: Prolonged QT interval and toxic epidermal necrolysis *(Ln 349:101, 1997)*. Not used for self-rx due to neuropsychiatric side-effects.
Melarsoprol (Mel B, Arsobal) (CDC)	See Trypanosomiasis for adult dose. Peds dose: 0.36 mg/kg IV, then gradual ↑ to 3.6 mg/kg q1–5 days for total of 9–10 doses.	Post-rx encephalopathy (2-10%) with 50% mortality overall, risk of death 2° to rx 8-14%. Prednisolone 1 mg per kg per day po may ↓ encephalopathy. Other: Heart damage, albuminuria, abdominal pain, vomiting, peripheral neuropathy, Herxheimer-like reaction, pruritus.
Miltefosine (Impavido) *(Expert Rev Anti Infect Ther 4:177, 2006)*	100–150 mg (approx. 2.25 mg/kg per day) po divided tid x 28 days Cutaneous leishmaniasis 2.25 mg/kg po q24h x 6 wks	Source: *See Table 13D, page 157.* **Pregnancy—No;** teratogenic. Side-effects vary: kala-azar pts, vomiting in up to 40%, diarrhea in 17%; "motion sickness", headache & increased creatinine. Daily dose >150 mg can cause severe GI side effects *(Ln 352:1821, 1998)*.
Nifurtimox (Lampit) *(CDC)* (Manufactured in Germany by Bayer)	8–10 mg/kg per day po div. 4 x per day for 90-120 days	Side-effects in 40–70% of pts. GI: abdominal pain, nausea/vomiting. CNS: polyneuritis (1/3), disorientation, insomnia, twitching, seizures. Skin rash. Hemolysis with G6PD deficiency.
Pentamidine (NebuPent)	300 mg via aerosol q month. Also used IM.	Hypotension, hypocalcemia, hypoglycemia followed by hyperglycemia, pancreatitis. Neutropenia (15%), thrombocytopenia. Nephrotoxicity. Others: nausea/vomiting, ↑ liver tests, rash.
Primaquine phosphate	26.3 mg (=15 mg base). Adult dose is 30 mg of base po daily.	In G6PD def. pts, can cause hemolytic anemia with hemoglobinuria, esp. African, Asian peoples. Methemoglobinemia. Nausea/abdominal pain if pt. fasting. *(CID 39:1336, 2004)*. **Pregnancy: No.**
Pyrimethamine (Daraprim, Malocide) Also combined with sulfadoxine as **Fansidar** (25–500 mg)	100 mg po, then 25 mg/day. Cost of folinic acid (leucovorin)	Major problem is hematologic: megaloblastic anemia, ↓ WBC, ↓ platelets. Can give 5 mg folinic acid per day to ↓ bone marrow depression and not interfere with antitoxoplasmosis effect. If high-dose pyrimethamine, ↑ folinic acid to 10–50 mg/day. Pyrimethamine + sulfadiazine can cause mental changes due to carnitine deficiency *(AJM 95:112, 1993)*. Other: Rash, vomiting, diarrhea, xerostomia.
Quinidine gluconate Cardiotoxicity ref: *LnID 7:549, 2007*	Loading dose of 10 mg (equiv to 6.2 mg of quinidine base) / kg IV over 1–2 hr, then constant infusion of 0.02 mg of quinidine gluconate / kg per minute. May be available for compassionate use from Lilly.	Adverse reactions of quinidine/quinine similar: (1) IV bolus injection can cause fatal hypotension, (2) hyperinsulinemic hypoglycemia, esp. in pregnancy, (3) ↓ rate of infusion of IV quinidine if QT interval ↑ >25% of baseline, (4) reduce dose 30–50% after day 3 due to ↓ renal clearance and ↓ vol. of distribution.

NOTE: Drugs available from CDC Drug Service indicated by "CDC." Call (+1) (404) 639-3670 (or -2888 (Fax)). ***See Table 13D, page 157 for sources and contact information for hard-to-find antiparasitic drugs.***

TABLE 13B (3)

CLASS, AGENT, GENERIC NAME (TRADE NAME)	USUAL ADULT DOSAGE	ADVERSE REACTIONS/COMMENTS
Antiprotozoan Drugs: Non-Intestinal Protozoa/Extraintestinal Parasites *(continued)*		
Quinine sulfate (Qualaquin) (300 mg salt = 250 mg base).	324 mg tabs. No IV prep. in US. Oral rx of chloroquine-resistant falciparum malaria: 624 mg po tid x 3 days, then (tetracycline 250 mg po qid or doxy 100 mg bid) x 7 days	Cinchonism; tinnitus, headache, nausea, abdominal pain, blurred vision. Rarely: blood dyscrasias, drug fever, asthma, hypoglycemia. Transient blindness in <1% of 500 pts *(AnIM 136:339, 2002)*. **Contraindicated if prolonged QTc, myasthenia gravis, optic neuritis or G6PD deficiency.**
Spiramycin (Rovamycin)	1 gm po q8h *(see Comment)*.	GI and allergic reactions have occurred. Available at no cost after consultation with Palo Alto Medical Foundation Toxoplasma Serology Lab: 650-853-4828 or from U.S. FDA 301-796-1600.
Sulfadiazine	1–1.5 gm po q6h.	*See Table 10A, page 101, for sulfonamide side-effects*
Sulfadoxine & pyrimethamine combination (Fansidar)	Contains 500 mg sulfadoxine & 25 mg pyrimethamine	Long half-life of both drugs: Sulfadoxine 169 hrs, pyrimethamine 111 hrs allows weekly dosage. In African, used empirically in pregnancy for intermittent preventative treatment (ITPp) against malaria: dosing at 3 set times during pregnancy. Reduces material and fetal mortality if HIV+. See *Expert Rev Anti Infect Ther 8:589, 2010.* Fatalities reported due to Stevens-Johnson syndrome and toxic epidermal necrolysis. Renal excretion—caution if renal impairment.
DRUGS USED TO TREAT NEMATODES, TREMATODES, AND CESTODES		
Albendazole (Albenza)	Doses vary with indication. Take with food; fatty meal increases absorption.	**Pregnancy Cat. C;** give after negative pregnancy test. Abdominal pain, nausea/vomiting, alopecia, ↑ serum transaminase. Rare leukopenia.
Diethylcarbamazine *(CDC)*	Used to treat filariasis.	Headache, dizziness, nausea, fever. Host may experience inflammatory reaction to death of adult worms: fever, urticaria, asthma, GI upset (Mazzotti reaction). **Pregnancy—No.**
Ivermectin (Stromectol, Mectizan) (3 mg tab & topical 0.5% lotion for head lice)	Strongyloidiasis dose: 200 μg/kg/day po x 2 days Onchocerciasis: 150 μg/kg x 1 po Scabies: 200 μg/kg po x 1; if AIDS, wait 14 days & repeat	Mild side-effects: fever, pruritus, rash. In rx of onchocerciasis, can see tender lymphadenopathy, headache, bone/joint pain. Host may experience inflammatory reaction to death of adult worms: fever, urticaria, asthma, GI upset (Mazzotti reaction).
Mebendazole (Vermox)	Doses vary with indication.	Rarely causes abdominal pain, nausea, diarrhea. Contraindicated in pregnancy & children <2 yrs old.
Praziquantel (Biltricide)	Doses vary with parasite; *see Table 13A*.	Mild: dizziness/drowsiness, N/V, rash, fever. Only contraindication is ocular cysticercosis. Potential exacerbation of neurocysticercosis. Metab.-induced by anticonvulsants and steroids; can negate effect with cimetidine 400 mg po tid. Reduce dose if advanced liver disease.
Pyrantel pamoate (over-the-counter)	Oral suspension. Dose for all ages: 11 mg/kg (to max. of 1 gm) x 1 dose	Rare GI upset, headache, dizziness, rash
Suramin (Germanin) *(CDC)*	Drug powder mixed to 10% solution with 5 mL water and used within 30 min. First give test dose of 0.1 gm IV. Try to avoid during pregnancy.	Does not cross blood-brain barrier; no effect on CNS infection. Side-effects: vomiting, pruritus, urticaria, fever, paresthesias, albuminuria (discontinue drug if casts appear). Do not use if renal/liver disease present. Deaths from vascular collapse reported.
Triclabendazole (Egaten) (CDC)	Used for fasciola hepatica liver fluke infection: 10 mg/kg po x 1 dose. May repeat in 12-24 hrs. 250 mg tabs	AEs ≥10%: sweating and abdominal pain. AEs 1-10%: weakness, chest pain, fever, anorexia, nausea, vomiting. Note: use with caution if G6PD def. or impaired liver function.

NOTE: Drugs available from CDC Drug Service indicated by "CDC." Call (+1) (404) 639-3670 (or -2888 (Fax)). ***See Table 13D, page 157 for sources and contact information for hard-to-find antiparasitic drugs.***

TABLE 13C – PARASITES THAT CAUSE EOSINOPHILIA (EOSINOPHILIA IN TRAVELERS)

Frequent and Intense (>5000 eos/mcL)	Moderate to Marked Early Infections	During Larval Migration; Absent or Mild During Chronic Infections	Other
Strongyloides (absent in compromised hosts); Lymphatic Filariasis; Toxocaria (cutaneous larva migrans)	Ascaris; Hookworm; Clonorchis; Paragonimis	Opisthorchis	Schistosomiasis; Cysticercosis; Trichuris; Angiostrongylus; Non-lymphatic filariasis; Gnathostoma; Capillaria; Trichostrongylus

TABLE 13D – SOURCES FOR HARD-TO-FIND ANTIPARASITIC DRUGS

Source	Drugs Available	Contact Information
CDC Drug Service	Artesunate, Benznidazole, Diethylcarbamazine (DEC), Eflornithine, Melarsoprol, Nifurtimox, Sodium stibogluconate, Suramin, Triclabendazole	www.cdc.gov/laboratory/drugservice/index.html (+1) 404-639-3670
WHO	Drugs for treatment of African trypanosomiasis	simarrop@who.int; (+41) 794-682-726; (+41) 227-911-345 francoj@who.int; (+41) 796-198-535; (+41) 227-913-313
Compounding Pharmacies, Specialty Labs, Others		
Expert Compounding Pharmacy	Quinacrine, Iodoquinol, niclosamide	www.expertpharmacy.org 1-800-247-9767; (+1) 818-988-7979
Fagron Compounding Pharmacy (formerly Gallipot)	Quinacrine, Iodoquinol, Paromomycin, Diloxanide	www.fagron.com 1-800-423-6967; (+1) 651-681-9517
Leiter's Pharmacy	Fumagillin	www.leiterrx.com 1-800-292-6772, +1-408-292-6772
Paladin Labs	Miltefosine	www.paladin-labs.com
Victoria Apotheke Zurich	Paromomycin (oral and topical), Triclabendazole	www.pharmaworld.com (+41) 43-344-6060
Fast Track Research	Miltefosine (may be free under treatment IND for cutaneous, mucocutaneous leishmaniasis)	jberman@fasttrackresearch.com
Palo Alto Medical Foundation, Toxoplasma Serology Lab	Spiramycin (consultation required for release)	(+1) 650-853-4828; toxlab@pamf.org

TABLE 14A – ANTIVIRAL THERAPY*

For HIV, see *Table 14D*; for Hepatitis, *see Table 14F* and *Table 14G*

VIRUS/DISEASE	DRUG/DOSAGE	SIDE EFFECTS/COMMENTS
Adenovirus: Cause of RTIs including fatal pneumonia in children & young adults and 60% mortality in transplant pts *(CID 43:331, 2006)*. Frequent cause of cystitis in transplant patients. Adenovirus 14 associated with severe pneumonia in otherwise healthy young adults *(MMWR 56(45):1181, 2007)*. **Findings include:** fever, ↑ liver enzymes, leukopenia, thrombocytopenia, diarrhea, pneumonia, or hemorrhagic cystitis.	In severe cases of pneumonia or post HSCT[1]: **Cidofovir** • 5 mg/kg/wk x 2 wks, then q 2 wks + **probenecid** 1.25 gm/M^2 given 3 hrs before cidofovir and 3 & 9 hrs after each infusion • Or 1 mg/kg IV 3x/wk. For adenovirus hemorrhagic cystitis *(CID 40:199, 2005; Transplantation. 2006; 81:1398)*: Intravesical **cidofovir** (5 mg/kg in 100 mL saline instilled into bladder).	Successful in 3/8 immunosuppressed children *(CID 38:45, 2004 & 8 of 10 children with HSCT (CID 41; 1812, 2005)*. ↓ in virus load predicted response to cidofovir. Ribavirin has had mixed activity; appears restricted to group C serotypes. Vidarabine and Ganciclovir have in vitro activity against adenovirus; little to no clinical data. New adenovirus, "titi monkey adenovirus" (TMAdV) transmitted from a monkey to researcher and subsequently to members of his family. *PLoS Pathog 2011 Jul 14; 7:e1002155.* Brincidofovir (CMX001-Chimerix) oral cidofovir prodrug in Phase III.
Coronavirus—SARS-CoV (Severe Acute Respiratory Distress Syn.) A new coronavirus, isolated Spring 2003 *(NEJM 348:1953 & 1967, 2003)* emerged from southern China & spread to Hong Kong and 32 countries. Bats appear to be a primary reservoir for SARS virus *(PNAS 102: 14040, 2005)*.	**Therapy remains predominantly supportive care.** Therapy tried or under evaluation *(see Comments)*: • Ribavirin—ineffective. • Interferon alfa ± steroids—small case series. • Pegylated IFN-α effective in monkeys. • Low dose steroids alone successful in one Beijing hospital. High dose steroids ↑ serious fungal infections. • Inhaled nitric oxide improved oxygenation & improved chest x-ray *(CID 39:1531, 2004)*.	**Transmission by close contact:** effective infection control practices (**mask [changed frequently]**, eye protection, gown, gloves) key to stopping transmission. Other coronaviruses (HCOV-229E, OC43, NL63, etc.) implicated as cause of croup, pneumonia asthma exacerbations, & other RTIs in children *(CID 40:1721, 2005; JID 191:492, 2005)*.
Enterovirus—Meningitis: most common cause of aseptic meningitis. Rapid CSF PCR test is accurate; reduces costs and hospital stay for infants *(Peds 120:489, 2007)*	**No rx currently recommended;** however, **pleconaril** (VP 63843) still under investigation.	No clinical benefit demonstrated in double-blind placebo-controlled study in 21 infants with enteroviral aseptic meningitis *(PIDJ 22:335, 2003)*. Failed to ameliorate symptoms but did have some improvement among those with severe headache *(AAC 2006 50:2409-14)*.
Hemorrhagic Fever Virus Infections: *Review: LnID 6:203, 2006.*		
Congo-Crimean Hemorrhagic Fever (HF) Tick-borne; symptoms include N/V, fever, headache, myalgias, & stupor (1/3). Signs: *conjunctival* injection, hepatomegaly, petechiae (1/3). Lab: ↓ platelets, ↓ WBC, ↑ ALT, AST, LDH & CPK (100%).	Oral **ribavirin, 30 mg/kg** as initial loading dose & 15 mg/kg q6h x 4 days & then 7.5 mg/kg/day x 6 days (WHO recommendation) *(see Comment)*. Reviewed *Antiviral Res 78:125, 2008.*	3/3 healthcare workers in Pakistan had complete recovery *(Ln 346:472, 1995)* & 61/69 (89%) with confirmed CCHF rx with ribavirin survived in Iran *(CID 36:1613, 2003)*. Shorter time of hospitalization among ribavirin treated pts (7.7 vs. 10.3 days), but no difference in mortality or transfusion needs in study done in Turkey *(J Infection 52: 207-215, 2006)*. Suggested benefit from ribavirin & dexamethasone *(281 pts) (CID 57:1270, 2013)*.
Ebola/Marburg HF (Central Africa) Severe *outbreak* of Ebola in Angola 308 cases with 277 deaths by 5/3/05 *(NEJM 352:2155, 2005; LnID 5:331, 2005)*. Major epidemic of Marburg 1998-2000 in Congo & 2004–5 in Angola *(NEJM 355:866, 2006)*	**No effective antiviral rx** *(J Virol 77: 9733, 2003)*.	Can infect gorillas & chimps that come in contact with other dead animal carcasses *(Science 303:387, 2004)*. Marburg reported in African Fruit Bat, *Rousettus aegyptiacus (PLoS ONE 2: e764, 2007)*. Study in Gabon revealed 15% seroprevalence among 4349 healthy volunteers from 220 randomly selected villages. None recalled any illness similar to Ebola. Seroprevalence among children rises until age 15, then plateaus. Seropositive status correlates to location of fruit bats. *PLoS ONE (Feb 9); 5:e9126, 2010*
With pulmonary syndrome: Hantavirus pulmonary syndrome, "sin nombre virus"	**No benefit from ribavirin has been demonstrated** *(CID 39:1307, 2004)*. Early recognition of disease and supportive (usually ICU) care is key to successful outcome.	Acute onset of fever, headache, myalgias, non-productive cough, thrombocytopenia, increased PT and non-cardiogenic pulmonary edema with respiratory insufficiency following exposure to rodents.
With renal syndrome: Lassa, Venezuelan, Korean, HF, Sabia, Argentinian HF, Bolivian HF, Junin, Machupo	Oral **ribavirin, 30 mg/kg** as initial loading dose & 15 mg/kg q6h x 4 days & then 7.5 mg/kg x 6 days (WHO recommendation) *(see Comment)*.	Toxicity low, hemolysis reported but recovery when treatment stopped. No significant changes in WBC, platelets, hepatic or renal function. *See CID 36:1254, 2003,* for management of contacts.

[1] HSCT = Hematopoietic stem cell transplant

* *See page 2 for abbreviations. NOTE: All dosage recommendations are for adults (unless otherwise indicated) and assume normal renal function.*

TABLE 14A (2)

VIRUS/DISEASE	DRUG/DOSAGE	SIDE EFFECTS/COMMENTS
Hemorrhagic Fever Virus Infections *(continued)*		
Dengue and dengue hemorrhagic fever (DHF) *www.cdc.gov/ncidod/dvbid/dengue/dengue-hcp.htm* Think dengue in traveler to tropics or subtropics (incubation period usually 4-7 days) with fever, bleeding, thrombocytopenia, or hemoconcentration with shock. Dx by viral isolation or serology; serum to CDC (telephone 787-706-2399).	**No data on antiviral rx.** Fluid replacement with careful hemodynamic monitoring critical. Rx of **DHF** with colloids effective: 6% hydroxyethyl starch preferred in 1 study *(NEJM 353:9, 2005)*. Review in *Semin Ped Infect Dis 16: 60-65, 2005.*	Of 77 cases dx at CDC (2001–2004), recent (2-wks) travel to Caribbean island 30%, Asia 17%, Central America 15%, S. America 15% *(MMWR 54:556, June 10, 2005)*. 5 pts with severe **DHF** rx with dengue antibody-neg. gamma globulin 500 mg per kg q24h IV for 3–5 days; rapid ↑ in platelet counts *(CID 36:1623, 2003)*. New test approved by FDA in 2011: DENV Detect IgM Capture ELISA test. Has some cross-reactivity with West Nile Virus infection. Should only be used in pts with symptoms c/w Dengue Fever.
West Nile virus *(JAMA 310:308, 2013)* A flavivirus transmitted by mosquitoes, blood transfusions, transplanted organs & breast-feeding. Birds (>200 species) are main host with humans & horses incidental hosts. The US epidemic continues.	**No proven rx to date.** 2 clinical trials in progress: (1) Interferon alfa-N3 *(CID 40:764, 2005)* (this option falling out of favor). (2) IVIG from Israel with high titer antibody West Nile *(JID 188:5, 2003; Transpl Inf Dis 4:160, 2003)*. Contact NIH, 301-496-7453; *see www.clinicaltrials.gov/show/NCT00068055.* Reviewed in *Lancet Neurology 6: 171-181, 2007.*	Usually nonspecific febrile disease but 1/150 cases develops meningoencephalitis, aseptic meningitis or polio-like paralysis *(AnIM 104:545, 2004; JCI 113: 1102, 2004)*. Long-term sequelae (neuromuscular weakness & psychiatric) common *(CID 43:723, 2006)*. Dx by ↑ IgM in serum & CSF or CSF PCR (contact State Health Dept./CDC). Blood supply now tested in U.S. ↑ serum lipase in 11/17 cases *(NEJM 352:420, 2005)*.
Yellow fever	**No data on antiviral rx** **Guidelines for use of preventative vaccine:** *(MMWR 51: RR17, 2002)*	Reemergence in Africa & S. Amer. due to urbanization of susceptible population *(Lancet Inf 5:604, 2005)*. Vaccination effective. *(JAMA 276:1157, 1996)*. Vaccine safe and effective in HIV patients, especially in those with suppressed VL and higher CD4 counts *(CID 48:659, 2009)*. A purified whole-virus, inactivated, cell-culture–derived vaccine (XRX-001) produced using the 17D strain has proven safe and resulted in neutralizing antibodies after 2 doses in a de-escalation, phase I study. *(N Engl J Med 2011 Apr 7; 364:1326)*
Chikungunya fever A self-limited arbovirus illness spread by Aedes mosquito. High epidemic potential (Caribbean).	**No antiviral therapy.** Fluids, analgesics, anti-pyretics	Clinical presentation: high fever, severe myalgias & headache, macular papular rash with occ. thrombocytopenia. Rarely hemorrhagic complications. Dx by increase in IgM antibody or serum NAAT (CDC, Focus Diagnostics).
SFTSV (Severe fever with thrombocytopenia syndrome virus)	**No known therapy.**	New virus in the Bunyaviridae family described in China. Initially thought to be anaplasma infection; serology showed new virus. Possibly transmitted by Haemaphysalis longicornis ticks. *(N Engl J Med 2011; 364:1523-32)*.
Hepatitis Viral Infections	*See Tables Table 14F (Hepatitis A & B), Table 14G (Hepatitis C)*	

* *See page 2 for abbreviations.* NOTE: All dosage recommendations are for adults (unless otherwise indicated) and assume normal renal function.

TABLE 14A (3)

VIRUS/DISEASE	DRUG/DOSAGE	SIDE EFFECTS/COMMENTS
Herpesvirus Infections **Cytomegalovirus (CMV)** At risk pts: HIV/AIDS, cancer chemotherapy, post-transplant	**Primary prophylaxis** not generally recommended except in certain transplant populations *(see Table 15E)*. Preemptive therapy in pts with ↑ CMV DNA titers in plasma & CD4 <100/mm³. Recommended by some: **valganciclovir** 900 mg po q12h *(CID 32: 783, 2001)*. Authors rec. primary prophylaxis be dc if response to ART with ↑ CD4 >100 for 6 mos. *(MMWR 53:98, 2004)*.	Risk for developing CMV disease correlates with quantity of CMV DNA in plasma: each $\log_{10}$ ↑ associated with 3.1-fold ↑ in disease *(CID 28:758, 1999)*. Resistance demonstrated in 5% of transplant recipients receiving primary prophylaxis *(J Antimicrob Chemother 65:2628, 2010)*. Consensus guidelines: *Transplantation 96:333, 2013.*
Colitis, Esophagitis, Gastritis Dx by biopsy of ulcer base/edge *(Clin Gastro Hepatol 2:564, 2004)* with demonstration of CMV inclusions & other pathogen(s).	**Ganciclovir** as with retinitis except induction period extended for 3–6 wks. No agreement on use of maintenance; may not be necessary except after relapse. Responses less predictable than for retinitis. **Valganciclovir also likely effective.** Switch to oral valganciclovir when po tolerated & when symptoms not severe enough to interfere with absorption. Antiretroviral therapy is essential in long term suppression. Alternative: **Cidofovir** 5 mg/kg IV, qwk x 2 wks followed by administration q2 wks; MUST be administered with **probenecid** 2 gm po 3 hrs before each dose and further 1 gm doses 2 hrs and 8 hrs after completion of the cidofovir infusion. IV saline hydration is essential.	
Encephalitis, Ventriculitis: Treatment not defined, but should be considered the same as retinitis. Disease may develop while taking ganciclovir as suppressive therapy. *See Herpes 11 (Suppl. 12):95A, 2004.*		
Lumbosacral polyradiculopathy: diagnosis by CMV DNA in CSF	**Ganciclovir,** as with retinitis. **Foscarnet** 40 mg/kg IV q12h another option. Switch to **valganciclovir** when possible. Suppression continued until CD4 remains >100/mm³ for 6 mos. **Alternative: Cidofovir 5** mg/kg IV, qwk x 2 wks followed by administration q2 wks; MUST be administered with probenicid 2 gm po 3 hrs before each dose and further 1 gm doses 2 hrs and 8 hrs after completion of the cidofovir infusion. IV saline hydration is essential.	About 50% will respond; survival ↑ (5.4 wks to 14.6 wks) *(CID 27:345, 1998)*. Resistance can be demonstrated genotypically.
Mononeuritis multiplex	Not defined	Due to vasculitis & may not be responsive to antiviral therapy
Pneumonia (CMV)— Seen predominantly in transplants (esp. bone marrow), **rare in HIV.** Treat only when histological evidence present in AIDS & other pathogens not identified. High rate of CMV reactivation in immunocompetent ICU patients; prolonged hospitalizations and increased mortality *(JAMA 300:413, 2008)*.	**Ganciclovir/valganciclovir**, as with CMV retinitis. In bone marrow transplant pts, combination therapy with CMV or IV immune globulin. *See Comments re ganciclovir resistance.*	In bone marrow transplant pts, serial measure of pp65 antigen was useful in establishing early diagnosis of CMV interstitial pneumonia with good results if ganciclovir was initiated within 6 days of antigen positivity *(Bone Marrow Transplant 26:413, 2000)*. For preventive therapy, *see Table 15E pp65 test now replaced by quantitative CMV PCR.* Suspect ganciclovir resistance when: 1) ↑ or persistent VL, 2) ↓ VL of < 0.5 log/wk, 3) progressive disease after 21 days. Test by combination of PCR & gene sequencing. Depending on specific mutation, switch to Foscarnet and/or IVIG and/or continue ganciclovir *(CID 56:1018, 2013)*.

TABLE 14A (4)

VIRUS/DISEASE	DRUG/DOSAGE		SIDE EFFECTS/COMMENTS
Herpesvirus Infections *(continued)*			
CMV Retinitis Most common cause of blindness in AIDS patients with <50/mm³ CD4 counts. 19/30 pts (63%) with inactive CMV retinitis who responded to HAART (↑ of ≥60 CD4 cells/mL) developed immune recovery vitreitis (vision ↓ & floaters with posterior segment inflammation —vitreitis, papillitis & macular changes) an average of 43 wks after rx started *(JID 179: 697, 1999)*. Corticosteroid rx ↓ inflammatory reaction of immune recovery vitreitis without reactivation of CMV retinitis, either periocular corticosteroids or short course of systemic steroid.	**For immediate sight-threatening lesions: Ganciclovir** intraocular implant + **valganciclovir** 900 mg po q12h. **For peripheral lesions: Valganciclovir** 900 mg po q12h x 14–21d, then 900 mg po q24h for maintenance therapy	**Ganciclovir** 5 mg/kg IV q12h x 14–21d, then **valganciclovir** 900 mg po q12h **OR** **Foscarnet** 60 mg/kg IV q8h or 90 mg/kg IV q12h x 14–21d, then 90–120 mg/kg IV q24h **OR** **Cidofovir** 5 mg/kg IV x 2 wks, then 5 mg/kg every other wk; each dose should be administered with IV saline hydration & oral probenecid **OR** Repeated intravitreal injections with **fomivirsen** (for relapses only, not as initial therapy)	Differential diagnosis: HIV retinopathy, herpes simplex retinitis, varicella-zoster retinitis (rare, hard to diagnose). Valganciclovir po equal to GCV IV in induction of remission: *(NEJM 346:1119, 2002)*. Cannot use ganciclovir ocular implant alone as approx. 50% risk of CMV retinitis other eye at 6 mos. & 31% risk visceral disease. Risk ↓ with systemic rx but when contralateral retinitis does occur, ganciclovir-resistant mutation often present *(JID 189:611, 2004)*. **Concurrent systemic rx recommended!** Because of unique mode of action, **fomivirsen** may have a role if isolates become resistant to other therapies. Retinal detachments 50–60% within 1 yr of dx of retinitis. *(Ophthal 111:2232, 2004)*. Equal efficacy of IV GCV & FOS. GCV avoids nephrotoxicity of FOS; FOS avoids bone marrow suppression of GCV. Although bone marrow toxicity may be similar to ganciclovir. **Oral valganciclovir should replace both.**
Pts who discontinue suppression therapy should undergo regular eye examination for early detection of relapses!	**Post treatment suppression** (Prophylactic) if CD4 count <100/mm³: **Valganciclovir** 900 mg po q24h.		Discontinue if CD4 >100/mm³ x 6 mos on ART.
CMV in Transplant patients: *See Table 15E for discussion of prophylaxis.* CMV disease can manifest as CMV syndrome with or without end-organ disease. **Ganciclovir** 5 mg/kg IV q12h OR **Valganciclovir** 900 mg po q12h *(Am J Transplant 7:2106, 2007)* are effective treatment options. Treatment duration should be individualized. Continue treatment until (1) CMV PCR or antigenemia has become undetectable, (2) clinical evidence of disease has resolved, and (3) at least 2-3 weeks of treatment *(Am J Transplant 13(Suppl 4):93, 2013; Blood 113:5711, 2009)*. Secondary prophylaxis (**Valganciclovir** 900 mg daily) should be considered for 1-3 month course in patients recently treated with high-dose immunosuppression such as lymphocyte depleting antibodies, those with severe CMV disease, or those with >1 episode of CMV disease. In HST recipients, secondary prophylaxis should be considered in similar cases balancing the risk of recurrent infection with drug toxicity			
CMV in pregnancy: Hyperimmune globulin 200 IU/kg maternal weight as single dose during pregnancy (early), administered IV reduced complications of CMV in infant at one year of life. *(CID 55: 497, 2012)*.			
Epstein Barr Virus (EBV) — Mononucleosis *(Ln ID 3:131, 2003)*	**No treatment.** Corticosteroids for tonsillar obstruction, CNS complications, or threat of splenic rupture.		**Etiology of atypical lymphocytes:** EBV, CMV, Hep A, Hep B, toxo, measles, mumps, drugs *(Int Pediatr 18:20, 2003)*.
HHV-6—Implicated as cause of roseola (exanthem subitum) & other febrile diseases of childhood *(NEJM 352:768, 2005)*. Fever & rash documented in transplant pts *(JID 179:311, 1999)*. Reactivation in 47% of 110 U.S. hematopoietic stem cell transplant pts assoc. with delayed monocytes & platelet engraftment *(CID 40:932, 2005)*. Recognized in assoc. with meningoencephalitis in immunocompetent adults. Diagnosis made by pos. PCR in CSF. ↓ viral copies in response to **ganciclovir** rx *(CID 40:890 & 894, 2005)*. Foscarnet therapy improved thrombotic microangiopathy *(Am J Hematol 76:156, 2004)*.			
HHV-7—ubiquitous virus (>90% of the population is infected by age 3 yrs). No relationship to human disease. Infects CD4 lymphocytes via CD4 receptor; transmitted via saliva.			
HHV-8—The agent of Kaposi's sarcoma, Castleman's disease, & body cavity lymphoma. Associated with diabetes in sub-Saharan Africa *(JAMA 299:2770, 2008)*.	**No antiviral treatment.** Effective anti-HIV therapy may help.		Localized lesions: radiotherapy, laser surgery or intralesional chemotherapy. Systemic: chemotherapy. Castleman's disease responded to ganciclovir *(Blood 103:1632, 2004)* & valganciclovir *(JID 2006)*.

* *See page 2 for abbreviations.* NOTE: All dosage recommendations are for adults (unless otherwise indicated) and assume normal renal function.

TABLE 14A (5)

VIRUS/DISEASE	DRUG/DOSAGE	SIDE EFFECTS/COMMENTS
Herpes simplex virus (HSV Types 1 & 2)		
Bell's palsy H. simplex most implicated etiology. Other etiologic considerations: VZV, HHV-6, Lyme disease.	As soon as possible after onset of palsy: **Prednisone** 1 mg/kg po divided bid x 5 days then taper to 5 mg bid over the next 5 days (total of 10 days prednisone) Alternate: **Prednisone** (dose as above) + **Valacyclovir** 500 mg bid x 5 days	Prospective randomized double blind placebo controlled trial compared prednisolone vs acyclovir vs. (prednisolone + acyclovir) vs placebo. Best result with prednisolone: 85% recovery with placebo, 96% recovery with prednisolone, 93% with combination of acyclovir & prednisolone *(NEJM 357:1598 & 1653, 2007)*. **Large meta-analysis confirms: Steroids alone, effective; antiviral drugs alone, not effective; steroids + antiviral drugs, no more effective than steroids alone** *(JAMA: 302: 985, 2009)*.
Encephalitis (Excellent reviews: *CID 35: 254, 2002*). UK experience *(EID 9:234, 2003; Eur J Neurol 12:331, 2005 ; Antiviral Res: 71:141-148, 2006)*	**Acyclovir** IV 10 mg/kg IV (infuse over 1 hr) q8h x 14–21 days. 20 mg/kg q8h in children <12 yrs. Dose calculation in obese patients uncertain. To lessen risk of nephrotoxicity with larger doses seems reasonable to infuse each dose over more than 1 hour. In morbid obesity, use actual body weight.	HSV-1 is most common cause of sporadic encephalitis. Survival & recovery from neurological sequelae are related to mental status at time of initiation of rx. **Early dx and rx imperative.** Mortality rate reduced from >70% to 19% with acyclovir rx. PCR analysis of CSF for HSV-1 DNA is 100% specific & 75–98% sensitive. 8/33 (25%) CSF samples drawn before day 3 were neg. by PCR; neg. PCR assoc. with ↓ protein & <10 WBC per mm^3 in CSF *(CID 36:1335, 2003)*. All were + after 3 days. Relapse after successful rx reported in 7/27 (27%) children. Relapse was associated with a lower total dose of initial acyclovir rx (285 ± 82 mg per kg in relapse group vs. 462 ± 149 mg per kg, p <0.03) *(CID 30:185, 2000; Neuropediatrics 35:371, 2004)*.
Genital Herpes: *Sexually Transmitted Treatment Guidelines 2010: MMWR 59 (RR-12), 2010.*		
Primary (initial episode)	**Acyclovir** (Zovirax or generic) 400 mg po tid x 7–10 days OR	↓ by 2 days time to resolution of signs & symptoms, ↓ by 4 days time to healing of lesions, ↓ by 7 days duration of viral shedding. Does not prevent recurrences. For severe cases only: 5 mg per kg IV q8h times 5–7 days.
	Valacyclovir (Valtrex) 1000 mg po bid x 7-10 days OR	An ester of acyclovir, which is well absorbed, bioavailability 3–5 times greater than acyclovir.
	Famciclovir (Famvir) 250 mg po tid x 7–10 days	Metabolized to penciclovir, which is active component. Side effects and activity similar to acyclovir. **Famciclovir** 250 mg po tid **equal to acyclovir** 200 mg 5 times per day.
Episodic recurrences	**Acyclovir** 800 mg po tid **x 2 days** or 400 mg po tid **x 5 days** or **Famciclovir** 1000 mg bid **x 1 day** or 125 mg po bid x 5 days or **Valacyclovir** 500 mg po bid **x 3 days** or 1 gm po once daily **x 5 days** For HIV patients, *see Comment*	For episodic recurrences in HIV patients: **acyclovir** 400 mg po tid x 5-10 days or **famciclovir** 500 mg po bid x 5-10 days or **valacyclovir** 1 gm po bid x 5-10 days
Chronic daily suppression	**Suppressive therapy reduces the frequency of genital herpes recurrences by 70–80% among pts who have frequent recurrences (i.e., >6 recurrences per yr) & many report no symptomatic outbreaks.** **Acyclovir** 400 mg po bid , **or famciclovir** 250 mg po bid, **or valacyclovir** 1 gm po q24h; pts with <9 recurrences per yr could use 500 mg po q24h and then use valaciclovir 1 gm po q24h if breakthrough at 500 mg. For HIV patients, *see Comment*	For chronic suppression in HIV patients: **acyclovir** 400-800 mg po bid or tid or **famciclovir** 500 mg po bid or **valacyclovir** 500 mg po bid
Genital, immunocompetent		
Gingivostomatitis, primary (children)	**Acyclovir** 15 mg/kg po 5x/day x 7 days	Efficacy in randomized double-blind placebo-controlled trial *(BMJ 314:1800, 1997)*.
Keratoconjunctivitis and recurrent epithelial keratitis	**Trifluridine** (Viroptic), 1 drop 1% solution q2h (max. 9 drops per day) for max. of 21 days *(see Table 1, page 13)*	In controlled trials, response % > idoxuridine. Suppressive rx with acyclovir (400 mg bid) reduced recurrences of ocular HSV from 32% to 19% *(NEJM 339:300, 1998)*.
Mollaret's recurrent "aseptic" meningitis (usually HSV-2) *(Ln 363:1772, 2004)*	No controlled trials of antiviral rx & resolves spontaneously. If therapy is to be given, **acyclovir** (15–30 mg/kg/day IV) or **valacyclovir** 1-2 gm po qid should be used.	Pos. PCR for HSV in CSF confirms dx *(EJCMID 23:560, 2004)*. Daily suppression rx might ↓ frequency of recurrence but no clinical trials. Oral Valacyclovir ref: *JAC 47:855, 2001*.

* *See page 2 for abbreviations.* NOTE: All dosage recommendations are for adults (unless otherwise indicated) and assume normal renal function.

TABLE 14A (6)

VIRUS/DISEASE	DRUG/DOSAGE	SIDE EFFECTS/COMMENTS
Herpes simplex virus (HSV Types 1 & 2) *(continued)*		
Mucocutaneous *(for genital see previous page)*		
Oral labial, "fever blisters":		
Normal host *See Ann Pharmacotherapy 38:705, 2004; JAC 53:703, 2004*	Start rx with prodrome symptoms (tingling/burning) before lesions show. **Drug** / **Dose** / **Sx Decrease** **Oral: Valacyclovir** 2 gm po q12h x 1 day ↓ 1 day **Famciclovir**[2] 500 mg po bid x 7 days ↓ 2 days **Acyclovir**[NFDA] 400 mg po 5 x per day (q4h while awake) x 5 days) ↓ ½ day **Topical:** **Penciclovir** 1% cream q2h during day x 4 days ↓ 1 day **Acyclovir** 5% cream[3] 6x/day (q3h) x 7 days ↓ ½ day	Penciclovir *(J Derm Treat 13:67, 2002; JAMA 277:1374, 1997; AAC 46: 2848, 2002)*. Docosanol *(J Am Acad Derm 45:222, 2001)*. Oral acyclovir 5% cream *(AAC 46:2238, 2002)*. Oral famciclovir *(JID 179:303, 1999)*. Topical fluocinonide (0.05% Lidex gel) q8h times 5 days in combination with famciclovir ↓ lesion size and pain when compared to famciclovir alone *(JID 181:1906, 2000)*.
Herpes Whitlow	*See Table 1, page 28*	
Oral labial or genital: Immunocompromised (includes pts with AIDS) and critically ill pts in ICU setting/large necrotic ulcers in perineum or face. *(See Comment)*	**Acyclovir** 5 mg per kg IV (infused over 1 hr) q8h times 7 days (250 mg per M²) or 400 mg po 5 times per day times 14–21 days *(see Comment if suspect acyclovir-resistant)* **OR** **Famciclovir:** In HIV infected, 500 mg po bid for 7 days for recurrent episodes of genital herpes **OR** **Valacyclovir**[NAI]**:** In HIV-infected, 500 mg po bid for 5–10 days for recurrent episodes of genital herpes or 500 mg po bid for chronic suppressive rx.	**Acyclovir-resistant HSV: IV foscarnet** 90 mg/kg IV q12h x 7 days. Suppressive therapy with famciclovir (500 mg po bid), valacyclovir (500 mg po bid) or acyclovir (400-800 mg po bid) reduces viral shedding and clinical recurrences.
Pregnancy and genital H. simplex	Acyclovir safe even in first trimester. No proof that acyclovir at delivery reduces risk/severity of neonatal Herpes. In contrast, C-section in women with active lesions reduces risk of transmission. Ref. *Obstet Gyn 106:845, 2006.*	
Herpes simiae (Herpes B virus): **Monkey bite** *CID 35:1191, 2002*	**Postexposure prophylaxis: Valacyclovir** 1 gm po q8h times 14 days or acyclovir 800 mg po 5 times per day times 14 days. **Treatment of disease:** (1) CNS symptoms absent: **Acyclovir** 12.5–15 mg per kg IV q8h or ganciclovir 5 mg per kg IV q12h. (2) CNS symptoms present: **Ganciclovir** 5 mg per kg IV q12h	Fatal human cases of myelitis and hemorrhagic encephalitis have been reported following bites, scratches, or eye inoculation of saliva from monkeys. Initial sx include fever, headache, myalgias and diffuse adenopathy, incubation period of 2–14 days *(EID 9:246, 2003)*. In vitro ACV and ganciclovir less active than other nucleosides (penciclovir or 5-ethyldeoxyuridine may be more active; clinical data needed) *(AAC 51:2028, 2007)*.

[2] FDA approved only for HIV pts

[3] Approved for immunocompromised pts

* *See page 2 for abbreviations.* NOTE: All dosage recommendations are for adults (unless otherwise indicated) and assume normal renal function.

TABLE 14A (7)

VIRUS/DISEASE	DRUG/DOSAGE	SIDE EFFECTS/COMMENTS
Herpesvirus Infections *(continued)*		
Varicella-Zoster Virus (VZV)		
Varicella: Vaccination has markedly ↓ incidence of varicella & morbidity *(NEJM 352:450, 2005; NEJM 353:2377, 2005 & NEJM 356:1338, 2007)*. Guidelines for VZV vaccine *(MMWR 56(RR-4) 2007)*.		
Normal host (chickenpox) Child (2–12 years)	**In general, treatment not recommended.** Might use oral **acyclovir** for healthy persons at ↑ risk for moderate to severe varicella, i.e., >12 yrs of age; chronic cutaneous or pulmonary diseases; chronic salicylate rx (↑ risk of Reye syndrome), **acyclovir** dose: 20 mg/kg po qid x 5 days (start within 24 hrs of rash) or **valacyclovir** 20 mg/kg tid x 5 days.	Acyclovir slowed development and ↓ number of new lesions and ↓ duration of disease in children: 9 to 7.6 days *(PIDJ 21:739, 2002)*. Oral dose of acyclovir in children should not exceed 80 mg per kg per day or 3200 mg per day.
Adolescents, young adults	Start within 24 hrs of rash: **Valacyclovir** 1000 mg po tid x 5-7 days or **Famciclovir** 500 mg po tid (probably effective, but data lacking)	↓ duration of fever, time to healing, and symptoms *(AnIM 130:922, 1999)*.
Pneumonia or chickenpox in 3rd trimester of pregnancy	**Acyclovir** 800 mg po 5 times per day or 10 mg per kg IV q8h times 5 days. Risks and benefits to fetus and mother still unknown. Many experts recommend rx, especially in 3rd trimester. Some would add VZIG (varicella-zoster immune globulin).	Varicella pneumonia associated with 41% mortality in pregnancy Acyclovir ↓ incidence and severity *(JID 185:422, 2002)*. If varicella-susceptible mother exposed and respiratory symptoms develop within 10 days after exposure, start acyclovir
Immunocompromised host	**Acyclovir** 10–12 mg per kg (500 mg per M^2) IV (infused over 1 hr) q8h times 7 days	Disseminated 1° varicella infection reported during infliximab rx of rheumatoid arthritis *(J Rheum 31:2517, 2004)*. Continuous infusion of high-dose acyclovir (2 mg per kg per hr) successful in 1 pt with severe hemorrhagic varicella *(NEJM 336:732, 1997)*. Mortality high (43%) in AIDS pts *(Int J Inf Dis 6:6, 2002)*.
Prevention—Postexposure prophylaxis Varicella deaths still occur in unvaccinated persons *(MMWR 56 (RR-4) 1-40, 2007)*	**CDC Recommendations for Prevention:** Since <5% of cases of varicella but >50% of varicella-related deaths occur in adults >20 yrs of age, the CDC recommends a more aggressive approach in this age group: **1st, varicella-zoster immune globulin** (VZIG) (125 units/10 kg (22 lbs) body weight IM up to a max. of 625 units; minimum dose is 125 units) is recommended for postexposure prophylaxis in susceptible persons at greater risk for complications (immunocompromised such as HIV, malignancies, pregnancy, and steroid therapy) as soon as possible after exposure (<96 hrs). If varicella develops, initiate treatment quickly (<24 hrs of rash) with **acyclovir** as below. Some would rx presumptively with acyclovir in high-risk pts. **2nd,** susceptible adults should be vaccinated. Check antibody in adults with negative or uncertain history of varicella (10–30% will be Ab-neg.) and vaccinate those who are Ab-neg. **3rd,** susceptible children should receive vaccination. Recommended routinely before age 12–18 mos. but OK at any age.	

* *See page 2 for abbreviations.* NOTE: All dosage recommendations are for adults (unless otherwise indicated) and assume normal renal function.

TABLE 14A (8)

VIRUS/DISEASE	DRUG/DOSAGE	SIDE EFFECTS/COMMENTS
Herpesvirus Infections *(continued)*		
Herpes zoster (shingles) *(See NEJM 369:255, 2013)*		
Normal host ▪ Effective therapy most evident in pts >50 yrs. ▪ *(For treatment of post-herpetic neuralgia, see CID 36: 877, 2003; Ln 374:1252, 2009)* ▪ New vaccine ↓ herpes zoster & post-herpetic neuralgia *(NEJM 352: 2271, 2005; JAMA 292:157, 2006)*. Reviewed *in J Am Acad Derm 58:361, 2008.* ▪ Analgesics for acute pain associated with Herpes zoster *(NEJM 369:255, 2013)*	**[NOTE: Trials showing benefit of therapy: only in pts treated within 3 days of onset of rash]** **Valacyclovir** 1000 mg po tid times 7 days (adjust dose for renal failure) *(See Table 17A)* **OR**	
	Famciclovir 500 mg tid x 7 days. Adjust for renal failure *(see Table 17A)* **OR**	Time to healing more rapid. Reduced incidence of post-herpetic neuralgia (PHN) vs placebo in pts >50 yrs of age. Famciclovir similar to acyclovir in reduction of acute pain and incidence of PHN *(J Micro Immunol Inf 37:75, 2004)*.
	Acyclovir 800 mg po 5 times per day times 7–10 days Add **Prednisone** in pts over 50 yrs old to decrease discomfort during acute phase of zoster. Does not decrease incidence of post-herpetic neuralgia. Dose: 30 mg po bid days 1–7, 15 mg bid days 8–14 and 7.5 mg bid days 15–21.	A meta-analysis of 4 placebo-controlled trials (691 pts) demonstrated that acyclovir accelerated by approx. 2-fold pain resolution by all measures employed and reduced incidence of post-herpetic neuralgia at 3 & 6 mos *(CID 22:341, 1996)*; med. time to resolution of pain 41 days vs 101 days in those >50 yrs. Prednisone added to acyclovir improved quality of life measurements (↓ acute pain, sleep, and return to normal activity) *(AnIM 125:376, 1996)*. In post-herpetic neuralgia, controlled trials demonstrated effectiveness of gabapentin, the lidocaine patch (5%) & opioid analgesic in controlling pain *(Drugs 64:937, 2004; J Clin Virol 29:248, 2004)*. Nortriptyline & amitriptyline are equally effective but nortriptyline is better tolerated *(CID 36:877, 2003)*. Role of antiviral drugs in rx of PHN unproven *(Neurol 64:21, 2005)* but 8 of 15 pt improved with IV acyclovir 10 mg/kg q 8 hrs x 14 days followed by oral valacyclovir 1 gm 3x a day for 1 month *(Arch Neur 63:940, 2006)*
Immunocompromised host Not severe	**Acyclovir** 800 mg po 5 times per day times 7 days. (**Options: Famciclovir** 750 mg po q24h or 500 mg bid or 250 mg 3 times per day times 7 days **OR valacyclovir** 1000 mg po tid times 7 days, though both are not FDA-approved for this indication)	If progression, switch to IV. RA pts on TNF-alpha inhibitors at high risk for VZV. Zoster more severe, but less post-herpetic neuralgia *(JAMA 301:737, 2009)*.
Severe: >1 dermatome, trigeminal nerve or disseminated	**Acyclovir** 10–12 mg per kg IV (infusion over 1 hr) q8h times 7–10 days. In older pts, ↓ to 7.5 mg per kg. If nephrotoxicity and pt improving, ↓ to 5 mg per kg q8h.	A common manifestation of immune reconstitution following HAART in HIV-infected children *(J All Clin Immun 113:742, 2004)*. Rx must be begun within 72 hrs. For Acyclovir-resistant VZV in HIV+ pts previously treated with acyclovir: **Foscarnet** (40 mg per kg IV q8h for 14–26 days).

* *See page 2 for abbreviations.* NOTE: All dosage recommendations are for adults (unless otherwise indicated) and assume normal renal function.

TABLE 14A (9)

Influenza A & B and novel influenza viruses

- Refs: *http://www.cdc.gov/flu/professionals/antivirals/index.htm* *http://www.cdc.gov/flu/weekly/*
- Guidelines: ACIP: *(MMWR 60 (RR01);1-24 2011) IDSA (CID 48:1003-1032, 2009)*
- Novel H1N1 (referred to as pandemic H1N1, pH1N1, H1N1pdm and formerly swine flu) emerged in 2009 and now is the dominant H1N1 strain worldwide. Old distinction from seasonal H1N1 is still sometimes used but not relevant
- Rapid influenza tests are can be falsely negative in 20-50%
- Initiate therapy as close to the onset of symptoms as possible, and certainly within 48 hrs of onset of symptoms. Starting therapy after 48 hours of onset of symptoms is associated with reduced therapeutic benefit. However, starting therapy up to 5 days after onset in patients who are hospitalized is associated with improved survival *(Clin Infect Dis 55:1198, 2012)*.
- Oseltamivir and zanamivir are recommended drugs. Amantadine and rimantidine should not be used because of widespread resistance.
- Empiric therapy should be started for all patients who are hospitalized, have severe or progressive influenza or are at higher risk of complications due to age or underlying medical conditions.
- Rapid test/PCR confirmation of influenza infection recommended unless diagnosis is clear (e.g. typical symptoms when flu is circulating widely). Can start therapy while waiting on results.
- Vaccine info *(http://www.cdc.gov/flu/professionals/acip/index.htm)*
- Other important influenza viruses causing human disease
  - **H3N2v influenza:** 159 cases of influenza A/H3N2v reported over the summer of 2012. Most of the cases of influenza A/H3N2v occurred in children under the age of 10 with direct contact with pigs. This variant is susceptible to the neuraminidase inhibitors, oseltamivir and zanamivir. *See MMWR 61:619, 2012.*
  - **Avian influenza H5N1:** Re-emerged in Asia in 2003 and human cases detected in 15 countries mostly in Asia as well as Egypt, Nigeria and Djibouti. Circulation associated with massive poultry die off. Imported cases rare – one in Canada. As of January 2014, 648 confirmed cases and 384 deaths (59%). Human infection associated with close contact with poultry; very limited human to human transmission. Mortality associated with high viral load, disseminated virus and high cytokine activity *(Nature Medicine 12:1203-1207 2006)*. Sensitive to oseltamivir but oseltamivir resistance has emerged on therapy *(NEJM 353:267-272 2005)*. Use oseltamivir and consider IV zanamivir
  - **Avian influenza H7N9:** Emerged in Eastern China in March 2013 and 132 cases documented during Spring 2013 with 44 deaths (33%). Cases appeared again in early winter 2013-2014 and continue to increase. Infection associated with close contact with live bird markets; extremely limited human to human transmission to date. Mortality highest among older persons and those with medical conditions. Oseltamivir active against most but not all strains. No zanamivir resistance documented to date.

Virus/Disease	Susceptible to (Recommended Drug/Dosage):	Resistant to:	Side Effects/Comments
A/H1N1 (current seasonal resembles pandemic H1N1)	**Oseltamivir** Adult: Oseltamivir 75 mg po bid x 5 days Pediatric (child age 1-12 years): Infant 2 wks-11 months: 3 mg/kg bid x 5 days ≤15 kg: 30 mg bid x 5 days >15 kg to 23 kg: 45 mg bid x 5 days >23 kg to 40 kg: 60 mg bid x 5 days >40 kg: 75 mg bid x 5 days or **Zanamivir** 2 inhalations (5 mg each) bid x 5 days	Amantadine and rimantidine (100%)	• **A/H1N1:** Higher dose (150 mg bid) not more effective for H1N1 • **Zanamivir** not recommended for children < 7 years or those with reactive airway disease • **IV zanamivir** is available under compassionate use IND and clinical trials for hospitalized influenza patients with suspected or known gastric stasis, gastric malabsorption, gastrointestinal bleeding, or for patients suspected or confirmed with oseltamivir-resistant influenza virus infection. For compassionate use, contact GlaxoSmithKline at (+1) 919-315-5215 or email: gskclinicalsupportHD@GSK.com. • Another investigational drug for severe, life-threatening disease is **IV Peramivir** (Biocryst/Shionogi) 600 mg IV daily for a minimum of 5 days. For access to compassionate use call 205-989-3262 or website: *http://www.biocryst.com/e_ind* *(Continued on next page)*

* *See page 2 for abbreviations.* NOTE: All dosage recommendations are for adults (unless otherwise indicated) and assume normal renal function.

TABLE 14A (10)

Virus/Disease	Susceptible to (Recommended Drug/Dosage):	Resistant to:	Side Effects/Comments
Influenza (A & B) *(continued)*			
A/H3N2 **A/H3N2v**	**Oseltamivir** Adult: Oseltamivir 75 mg po bid x 5 days Pediatric (child age 1-12 years): Infant 2 wks-11 months: 3 mg/kg bid x 5 days ≤15 kg: 30 mg bid x 5 days >15 kg to 23 kg: 45 mg bid x 5 days >23 kg to 40 kg: 60 mg bid x 5 days >40 kg: 75 mg bid x 5 days or **Zanamivir** 2 inhalations (5 mg each) bid x 5 days	Amantadine and rimantidine (100%)	*(Continued from previous page)* • **Influenza B:** One study suggested virologic benefit to higher dose oseltamivir for critically ill patients with influenza B. • **A/H5N1:** Given high mortality, consider obtaining investigational drug. Zanamivir retains activity against most oseltamivir resistant H5N1
B	**Oseltamivir** Adult: Oseltamivir 75 mg po bid x 5 days Pediatric (child age 1-12 years): Infant 2 wks-11 months: 3 mg/kg bid x 5 days ≤15 kg: 30 mg bid x 5 days >15 kg to 23 kg: 45 mg bid x 5 days >23 kg to 40 kg: 60 mg bid x 5 days >40 kg: 75 mg bid x 5 days or **Zanamivir** 2 inhalations (5 mg each) bid x 5 days	Amantadine and rimantidine (intrinsically resistant)	
H5N1	**Oseltamivir** Adult: Oseltamivir 75 mg po bid x 5 days Pediatric (child age 1-12 years): Infant 2 wks-11 months: 3 mg/kg bid x 5 days ≤15 kg: 30 mg bid x 5 days >15 kg to 23 kg: 45 mg bid x 5 days >23 kg to 40 kg: 60 mg bid x 5 days >40 kg: 75 mg bid x 5 days or **Zanamivir** 2 inhalations (5 mg each) bid x 5 days	Amantadine and rimantidine	
H7N9	**Oseltamivir** Adult: Oseltamivir 75 mg po bid x 5 days Pediatric (child age 1-12 years): Infant 2 wks-11 months: 3 mg/kg bid x 5 days ≤15 kg: 30 mg bid x 5 days >15 kg to 23 kg: 45 mg bid x 5 days >23 kg to 40 kg: 60 mg bid x 5 days >40 kg: 75 mg bid x 5 days or **Zanamivir** 2 inhalations (5 mg each) bid x 5 days	Amantadine and rimantidine, rarely oseltamivir	

* *See page 2 for abbreviations.* NOTE: All dosage recommendations are for adults (unless otherwise indicated) and assume normal renal function.

TABLE 14A (11)

VIRUS/DISEASE	DRUG/DOSAGE	SIDE EFFECTS/COMMENTS
Measles While measles in the US is at the lowest rates ever (55/100,000) much higher rates reported in developing countries *(CID 42:322, 2006)*. Imported measles in US on the rise *(MMWR 57: 169, 2008)*. High attack rates in the unvaccinated *(CID 47:1143, 2008)*. Concern about lack of vaccine effectiveness in developing countries *(Lancet 373:1543, 2009)*.		
Children	No therapy or **vitamin A** 200,000 units po daily times 2 days	Vitamin A may ↓ severity of measles.
Adults	No rx or **ribavirin** IV: 20–35 mg per kg per day times 7 days	↓ severity of illness in adults *(CID 20:454, 1994)*.
Metapneumovirus (HMPV) A paramyxovirus isolated from pts of all ages, with mild bronchiolitis/bronchospasm to pneumonia. Can cause lethal pneumonia in HSCT pts *(Ann Intern Med 144:344, 2006)*	**No proven antiviral therapy** (intravenous ribavirin used anecdotally with variable results)	Human metapneumovirus isolated from 6-21% of children with RTIs *(NEJM 350:443, 2004)*. Dual infection with RSV assoc. with severe bronchiolitis *(JID 191:382, 2005)*. Nucleic acid test now approved to detect 12 respiratory viruses *(xTAG Respiratory Viral Panel, Luminex Molecular Diagnostics)*.
Monkey pox (orthopox virus) *(see LnID 4:17, 2004)* Outbreak from contact with ill prairie dogs. Source likely imported Gambian giant rats *(MMWR 42:642, 2003)*.	**No proven antiviral therapy.** Cidofovir is active in vitro & in mouse model *(AAC 46:1329, 2002; Antiviral Res 57:13, 2003)* *(Potential new drugs Virol J 4:8, 2007)*	Incubation period of 12 days, then fever, headache, cough, adenopathy, & a vesicular papular rash that pustulates, umbilicates, & crusts on the head, trunk, & extremities. Transmission in healthcare setting rare *(CID 40:789, 2005; CID 41:1742, 2005, CID 41;1765, 2005)*.
Norovirus (Norwalk-like virus, or NLV) Vast majority of outbreaks of non-bacterial gastroenteritis *(NEJM 368:1121, 2013)*.	**No antiviral therapy.** Replete volume. Transmission by contaminated food, fecal-oral contact with contaminated surfaces, or fomites.	Sudden onset of nausea, vomiting, and/or watery diarrhea lasting 12–60 hours. Ethanol-based hand rubs effective *(J Hosp Inf 60:144, 2005)*.
Papillomaviruses: Warts **External Genital Warts**	**Patient applied:** **Podofilox** (0.5% solution or gel): apply 2x/day x 3 days, 4th day no therapy, repeat cycle 4x; OR **Imiquimod** 5% cream: apply once daily hs 3x/wk for up to 16 wks. **Provider administered:** Cryotherapy with liquid nitrogen; repeat q1-2 wks; OR **Podophyllin resin** 10-25% in tincture of benzoin. Repeat weekly as needed; OR **Trichloroacetic acid** (TCA): repeat weekly as needed; OR surgical removal.	**Podofilox:** Inexpensive and safe (pregnancy safety not established). Mild irritation after treatment. **Imiquimod:** Mild to moderate redness & irritation. Topical imiquimod effective for treatment of vulvar intraepithelial neoplasms *(NEJM 358:1465, 2008)*. Safety in pregnancy not established. **Cryotherapy:** Blistering and skin necrosis common. **Podophyllin resin:** Must air dry before treated area contacts clothing. Can irritate adjacent skin. **TCA:** Caustic. Can cause severe pain on adjacent normal skin. Neutralize with soap or sodium bicarbonate.
Warts on cervix	Need evaluation for evolving neoplasia	Gynecological consult advised.
Vaginal warts	Cryotherapy with liquid nitrogen or **TCA**	
Urethral warts	Cryotherapy with liquid nitrogen or **Podophyllin resin** 10-25% in tincture of benzoin	
Anal warts	Cryotherapy with liquid nitrogen or **TCA** or surgical removal	Advise anoscopy to look for rectal warts.
Skin papillomas	**Topical α-lactalbumin. Oleic acid** (from human milk) applied 1x/day for 3 wks	↓ lesion size & recurrence vs placebo ($p < 0.001$) *(NEJM 350:2663, 2004)*. Further studies warranted.

* *See page 2 for abbreviations.* NOTE: All dosage recommendations are for adults (unless otherwise indicated) and assume normal renal function.

TABLE 14A (12)

VIRUS/DISEASE	DRUG/DOSAGE	SIDE EFFECTS/COMMENTS
Parvo B19 Virus (Erythrovirus B19). *Review: NEJM 350:586, 2004. Wide range of manifestation.* **Treatment options for common symptomatic infections:**		
Erythema infectiosum	Symptomatic treatment only	Diagnostic tools: IgM and Igb antibody titers. Perhaps better: blood parvovirus PCR. Dose of IVIG not standardized; suggest 400 mg/kg IV of commercial IVIG for 5 or 10 days or 1000 mg/kg IV for 3 days. Most dramatic anemias in pts with pre-existing hemolytic anemia. Bone marrow shown erythrocyte maturation arrest with giant pronormoblasts.
Arthritis/arthralgia	Nonsteroidal anti-inflammatory drugs (NSAID)	
Transient aplastic crisis	Transfusions and oxygen	
Fetal hydrops	Intrauterine blood transfusion	
Chronic infection with anemia	**IVIG** and transfusion *(CID 56:968, 2013)*	
Chronic infection without anemia	Perhaps **IVIG**	
Papovavirus/Polyomavirus		
Progressive multifocal leukoencephalopathy (PML) Serious demyelinating disease due to JC virus in immunocompromised pts.	No specific therapy for JC virus. Two general approaches: 1. In HIV pts: HAART. Cidofovir may be effective. 2. Stop or decrease immunosuppressive therapy.	Failure of treatment with interferon alfa-2b, cytarabine and topotecan. Immunosuppressive natalizumab temporarily removed from market due to reported associations with PML. Mixed reports on cidofovir. Most likely effective in ART-experienced pts.
BK virus induced nephropathy in immunocompromised pts and hemorrhagic cystitis	Decrease immunosuppression if possible. Suggested antiviral therapy based on anecdotal data. If progressive renal dysfunction: 1. **Fluoroquinolone** first; 2. **IVIG** 500 mg/kg IV; 3. **Leflunomide** 100 mg po daily x 3 days, then 10-20 mg po daily; 4. **Cidofovir** only if refractory to all of the above *(see Table 14B for dose).*	Use PCR to monitor viral "load" in urine and/or plasma. Report of cidofovir as potentially effective for BK hemorrhagic cystitis *(CID 49:233, 2009).*
Rabies *(see Table 20B, page 222; see MMWR 54: RR-3:1, 2005, CDC Guidelines for Prevention and Control 2006, MMWR/55/RR-5, 2006)*		
Rabid dogs account for 50,000 cases per yr worldwide. Most cases in the U.S. are cryptic, i.e., no documented evidence of bite or contact with a rabid animal *(CID 35:738, 2003)*. 70% assoc. with 2 rare bat species *(EID 9:151, 2003)*. An organ donor with early rabies infected 4 recipients (2 kidneys, liver & artery) who all died of rabies avg. 13 days after transplant *(NEJM 352:1103, 2005)*.	**Mortality 100% with only survivors those who receive rabies vaccine before the onset of illness/symptoms** *(CID 36:61, 2003)*. A 15-year-old female who developed rabies 1 month post-bat bite survived after drug induction of coma (+ other rx) for 7 days; did not receive immunoprophylaxis *(NEJM 352:2508, 2005)*.	Corticosteroids ↑ mortality rate and ↓ incubation time in mice. Therapies that have failed after symptoms develop include rabies vaccine, rabies immunoglobulin, rabies virus neutralizing antibody, ribavirin, alfa interferon, & ketamine.
Respiratory Syncytial Virus (RSV) Major cause of morbidity in neonates/infants. Nucleic acid test now approved to detect 12 respiratory viruses *(xTAG Respiratory Viral Panel, Luminex Molecular Diagnostics). Ref: CID 56:258, 2013 (immunocompromised host)*	Hydration, supplemental oxygen. Ribavirin: routine use not recommended in normal host due to high cost, toxicity, absence of controlled data. In bone marrow stem cell transplants given by aerosol, IV or po (with or without IVIG), RSV antibody or palivizumab *(Blood 117:2755, 2011; CID 56:258, 2013)*. In retrospective risk stratified study of bone marrow stem cell patients with RSV, aerosolized RBV reduced mortality *(CID 57:1731, 2013)*.	In adults, RSV accounted for 10.6% of hospitalizations for pneumonia, 11.4% for COPD, 7.2% for asthma & 5.4% for CHF in pts >65 yrs of age *(NEJM 352:1749, 2005)*. RSV caused 11% of clinically important respiratory illnesses in military recruits *(CID 41:311, 2005)*. Palivizumab (Synagis) 15 mg/kg IM once per month November-April. Timing of coverage may need to be adjusted in some regions based on reported cases in the region, as opposed to using fixed dosing schedules *(Pediatrics 126:e116, 2010)*.
Prevention of RSV in: (1) Children <24 mos. old with chronic lung disease of prematurity (formerly bronchopulmonary dysplasia) requiring supplemental O_2 or (2) Premature infants (<32 wks gestation) and <6 mos. old at start of RSV season or (3) Children with selected congenital heart diseases	**Palivizumab** (Synagis) 15 mg per kg IM q month Nov-Apr. *See Pediatrics 126:e16, 2010.*	Expense argues against its use, but in 2004 approx. 100,000 infants received drug annually in U.S. *(PIDJ 23:1051, 2004)*. Significant reduction in RSV hospitalization among children with congenital heart disease *(Expert Opin Biol Ther. 7:1471-80, 2007)*

* *See page 2 for abbreviations.* NOTE: All dosage recommendations are for adults (unless otherwise indicated) and assume normal renal function.

TABLE 14A (13)

VIRUS/DISEASE	DRUG/DOSAGE	SIDE EFFECTS/COMMENTS
Rhinovirus (Colds) *See Ln 361:51, 2003* Found in 1/2 of children with community-acquired pneumonia; role in pathogenesis unclear *(CID 39:681, 2004)*. High rate of rhinovirus identified in children with significant lower resp tract infections *(Ped Inf Dis 28:337, 2009)*	No antiviral rx indicated *(Ped Ann 34:53, 2005)*. Symptomatic rx: • Ipratropium bromide nasal (2 sprays per nostril tid) • Clemastine 1.34 mg 1–2 tab po bid–tid (OTC). Avoid zinc products *(see Comment)*.	Sx relief: ipratropium nasal spray ↓ rhinorrhea and sneezing vs placebo *(AnIM 125:89, 1996)*. Clemastine (an antihistamine) ↓ sneezing, rhinorrhea but associated with dry nose, mouth & throat in 6–19% *(CID 22:656, 1996)*. Oral **pleconaril** given within 24 hrs of onset reduced duration (1 day) & severity of "cold symptoms" in DBPCT ($p < .001$) *(CID 36:1523, 2003)*. Echinacea didn't work *(CID 38:1367, 2004 & 40:807, 2005)* —put it to rest! Public health advisory advising that three over-the-counter cold remedy products containing zinc (e.g., Zicam) should not be used because of multiple reports of permanent anosmia *(www.fda.gov/Safety/MedWatch/SafetyInformation/SafetyAlertsforHumanMedicalProducts/ucm166996.htm)*.
Rotavirus: Leading recognized cause of diarrhea-related illness among infants and children world-wide and kills ½ million children annually.	No antiviral rx available; oral hydration life-saving. In one study, **Nitazoxanide** 7.5 mg/kg 2x/d x 3 days reduced duration of illness from 75 to 31 hrs in Egyptian children. Impact on rotavirus or other parameters not measured. *(Lancet 368:100 & 124, 2006)*. Too early to recommend routine use *(Lancet 368:100, 2006)*	Two live-attenuated vaccines highly effective (85 and 98%) and safe in preventing rotavirus diarrhea and hospitalization *(NEJM 354; 1 & 23, 2006)*. ACIP recommends either of the two vaccines, RV1 or RV5, for infants *(MMWR 58(RR02): 1, 2009)*.
SARS-CoV: *See page 158*		
Smallpox *(NEJM 346:1300, 2002)*	Smallpox vaccine (if within 4 days of exposure) + cidofovir (dosage uncertain but likely similar to CMV (5 mg/kg IV once weekly for 2 weeks followed by once weekly dosing. Must be used with hydration and Probenecid; *contact CDC: 770-488-7100)*	
Contact vaccinia *(JAMA 288:1901, 2002)*	From vaccination: Progressive vaccinia—vaccinia immune globulin may be of benefit. To obtain immune globulin, contact CDC: 770-488-7100. *(CID 39:759, 776 & 819, 2004)*	
West Nile virus: *See page 159*		

* *See page 2 for abbreviations.* NOTE: All dosage recommendations are for adults (unless otherwise indicated) and assume normal renal function.

TABLE 14B – ANTIVIRAL DRUGS (NON-HIV)

DRUG NAME(S) GENERIC (TRADE)	DOSAGE/ROUTE IN ADULTS*	COMMENTS/ADVERSE EFFECTS
CMV *(See Sanford Guide to HIV/AIDS Therapy)*		
Cidofovir (Vistide)	5 mg per kg IV once weekly for 2 weeks, then once every other week. **Properly timed IV prehydration with normal saline & Probenecid must be used with each cidofovir infusion:** 2 gm po 3 hrs before each dose and further 1 gm doses 2 & 8 hrs after completion of the cidofovir infusion. Renal function (serum creatinine and urine protein) must be monitored prior to each dose *(see pkg insert for details)*. Contraindicated if creatinine >1.5 mg/dL, CrCl ≤55 mL/min or urine protein ≥100 mg/dL.	**Adverse effects: Nephrotoxicity;** dose-dependent proximal tubular injury (Fanconi-like syndrome): proteinuria, glycosuria, bicarbonaturia, phosphaturia, polyuria (nephrogenic diabetic insipidus, *Ln 350:413, 1997*), acidosis, ↑ creatinine. Concomitant saline prehydration, probenecid, extended dosing intervals allow use but still highly nephrotoxic. Other toxicities: nausea 69%, fever 58%, alopecia 27%, myalgia 16%, probenecid hypersensitivity 16%, neutropenia 29%. Iritis and uveitis reported; also ↓ intraocular pressure. **Black Box warning.** Renal impairment can occur after ≤2 doses. Contraindicated in pts receiving concomitant nephrotoxic agents. Monitor for ↓ WBC. In animals, carcinogenic, teratogenic, causes ↓ sperm and ↓ fertility. FDA indication only CMV retinitis in HIV pts. **Comment:** Recommended dosage, frequency or infusion rate must not be exceeded. Dose must be reduced or discontinued if changes in renal function occur during rx. For ↑ of 0.3–0.4 mg per dL in serum creatinine, cidofovir dose must be ↓ from 5 to 3 mg per kg; discontinue cidofovir if ↑ of 0.5 mg per dL above baseline or 3+ proteinuria develops (for 2+ proteinuria, observe pts carefully and consider discontinuation).
Foscarnet (Foscavir)	<u>Induction</u>: 90 mg per kg IV, over 1.5-2 hours, q12h **OR** 60 mg per kg, over 1 hour, q8h <u>Maintenance</u>: 90 –120 mg per kg IV, over 2 hours, q24h Dosage adjustment with renal dysfunction *(see Table 17A)*.	Use infusion pump to control rate of administration. **Adverse effects: Major toxicity is renal impairment (1/3 of patients)** --↑ creatinine, proteinuria, nephrogenic diabetes insipidus, ↓K+, ↓Ca++, ↓ Mg++. Toxicity ↑ with other nephrotoxic drugs [ampho B, aminoglycosides or pentamidine (especially severe ↓ Ca++)]. Adequate hydration may ↓ toxicity. Other: headache, mild (100%); fatigue (100%), nausea (80%), fever (25%). CNS: seizures. Hematol: ↓ WBC, ↓ Hgb. Hepatic: liver function tests ↑. Neuropathy. Penile and oral ulcers.
Ganciclovir (Cytovene)	IV: 5 mg per kg q12h times 14 days (induction) 5 mg per kg IV q24h or 6 mg per kg 5 times per wk (maintenance) Dosage adjust. with renal dysfunction *(see Table 17A)*	**Adverse effects: Black Box warnings:** cytopenias, carcinogenicity/teratogenicity & aspermia in animals. Absolute neutrophil count dropped below 500 per mm³ in 15%, thrombocytopenia 21%, anemia 6%. Fever 48%. GI 50%: nausea, vomiting, diarrhea, abdominal pain 19%, rash 10%. Retinal detachment 11% (likely due to underlying diseases). Confusion, headache, psychiatric disturbances and seizures. Neutropenia may respond to granulocyte colony stimulating factor (G-CSF or GM-CSF). Severe myelosuppression may be ↑ with coadministration of zidovudine or azathioprine. 32% dc/interrupted rx, principally for neutropenia. Avoid extravasation.
	Oral: 1.0 gm tid with food (fatty meal) (250 mg & 500 mg cap)	Hematologic less frequent than with IV. Granulocytopenia 18%, anemia 12%, thrombocytopenia 6%. GI, skin same as with IV. Retinal detachment 8%.
Ganciclovir (Vitrasert)	Intraocular implant, 4.5 mg	**Adverse effects:** Late retinal detachment (7/30 eyes). Does not prevent CMV retinitis in good eye or visceral dissemination. **Comment:** Replacement every 6 months recommended.
Valganciclovir (Valcyte)	Treatment (induction): 900 mg po q12h; Prophylaxis (maintenance): 900 mg po q24h. Dosage adjustment for renal dysfunction *(See Table 17A)*.	A prodrug of ganciclovir with better bioavailability than oral ganciclovir: 60% with food. **Adverse effects:** Similar to ganciclovir. **CMV retinitis** (sight-threatening lesions): 900 mg po q12h + Ganciclovir intraocular implant; (peripheral lesions): 900 mg po q12h x 14-21 days, then 900 mg po q24h for maintenance

* *See page 2 for abbreviations. NOTE: All dosage recommendations are for adults (unless otherwise indicated) and assume normal renal function.*

TABLE 14B (2)

DRUG NAME(S) GENERIC (TRADE)	DOSAGE/ROUTE IN ADULTS*	COMMENTS/ADVERSE EFFECTS
Herpesvirus (non-CMV)		
Acyclovir (Zovirax or generic)	Doses: *see Table 14A for various indications* 400 mg or 800 mg tab 200 mg cap Suspension 200 mg per 5 mL Ointment or cream 5% IV injection Dosage adjustment for renal dysfunction *(See Table 17A)*.	**po:** Generally well-tolerated with occ. diarrhea, vertigo, arthralgia. Less frequent rash, fatigue, insomnia, fever, menstrual abnormalities, acne, sore throat, muscle cramps, lymphadenopathy. **IV:** Phlebitis, caustic with vesicular lesions with IV infiltration, CNS (1%): lethargy, tremors, confusion, hallucinations, delirium, seizures, coma—all reversible. Renal (5%): ↑ creatinine, hematuria. With high doses may crystallize in renal tubules → obstructive uropathy (rapid infusion, dehydration, renal insufficiency and ↑ dose ↑ risk). Adequate pre-hydration may prevent such nephrotoxicity. Hepatic: ↑ ALT, AST. Uncommon: neutropenia, rash, diaphoresis, hypotension, headache, nausea.
Famciclovir (Famvir)	125 mg, 250 mg, 500 mg tabs Dosage depends on indication: *(see label and Table 14A)*.	Metabolized to penciclovir. **Adverse effects:** similar to acyclovir, included headache, nausea, diarrhea, and dizziness but incidence does not differ from placebo. May be taken without regard to meals. Dose should be reduced if CrCl <60 mL per min *(see package insert & Table 14A, page 162 & Table 17A, page 217)*. May be taken with or without food.
Penciclovir (Denavir)	Topical 1% cream	Apply to area of recurrence of herpes labialis with start of sx, then q2h while awake times 4 days. Well tolerated.
Trifluridine (Viroptic)	Topical 1% solution: 1 drop q2h (max. 9 drops/day) until corneal re-epithelialization, then dose is ↓ for 7 more days (one drop q4h for at least 5 drops/day), not to exceed 21 days total rx.	Mild burning (5%), palpebral edema (3%), punctate keratopathy, stromal edema. For HSV keratoconjunctivitis or recurrent epithelial keratitis.
Valacyclovir (Valtrex)	500 mg, 1 gm tabs Dosage depends on indication and renal function *(see label, Table 14A & Table 17A)*	An ester pro-drug of acyclovir that is well-absorbed, bioavailability 3–5 times greater than acyclovir. **Adverse effects** similar to acyclovir *(see JID 186:540, 2002)*. Thrombotic thrombocytopenic purpura/hemolytic uremic syndrome reported in pts with advanced HIV disease and transplant recipients participating in clinical trials at doses of 8 gm per day.
Hepatitis		
Adefovir dipivoxil (Hepsera)	10 mg po q24h (with normal CrCl); *see Table 17A if renal impairment*. 10 mg tab	Adefovir dipivoxil is a prodrug of adefovir. It is an acyclic nucleotide analog with activity against hepatitis B (HBV) at 0.2–2.5 mM (IC_{50}). *See Table 9* for Cmax & T½. Active against YMDD mutant lamivudine-resistant strains and in vitro vs. entecavir- resistant strains. To minimize resistance, package insert recommends using in combination with lamivudine for lamivudine-resistant virus; consider alternative therapy if viral load remains > 1,000 copies/mL with treatment. Primarily renal excretion—adjust dose. No food interactions. Generally few side effects, but **Black Box warning** regarding lactic acidosis/hepatic steatosis with nucleoside analogs and severe exacerbation of hepB on discontinuing therapy; monitoring required after discontinuation. At 10 mg per day potential for delayed nephrotoxicity. Monitor renal function, esp. with pts with pre-existing or other risks for renal impairment. Pregnancy Category C. Hepatitis may exacerbate when treatment discontinued; Up to 25% of pts developed ALT ↑ 10 times normal within 12 wks; usually responds to re-treatment or self-limited, but hepatic decompensation has occurred.
Boceprevir (Victrelis)	For HCV genotype 1 800 mg po TID (with food) in combination with pegIFN + RBV*	* Initiate boceprevir 4 weeks after starting pegIFN +RBV. Use response guided therapy *(see table 14A for details)* Most Common AEs: Fatigue, anemia, nausea, headache, and dysgeusia. Difficult to distinguish between AEs caused by pegIFN or RBV
Entecavir (Baraclude)	0.5 mg q24h. If refractory or resistant to lamivudine or telbivudine: 1 mg per day Tabs: 0.5 mg & 1 mg. Oral solution: 0.05 mg/mL. Administer on an empty stomach.	A nucleoside analog active against HBV including lamivudine-resistant mutants. Minimal adverse effects reported: headache, fatigue, dizziness, & nausea reported in 22% of pts. Alopecia, anaphylactoid reactions reported. Potential for lactic acidosis and exacerbation of hepB at discontinuation (**Black Box warning**) as above. Do not use as single anti-retroviral agent in HIV co-infected pts; M134 mutation can emerge *(NEJM 356:2614, 2007)*. Adjust dosage in renal impairment *(see Table 17A, page 217)*.

* *See page 2 for abbreviations. NOTE: All dosage recommendations are for adults (unless otherwise indicated) and assume normal renal function.*

TABLE 14B (3)

DRUG NAME(S) GENERIC (TRADE)	DOSAGE/ROUTE IN ADULTS*	COMMENTS/ADVERSE EFFECTS
Hepatitis *(continued)*		
Interferon alfa is available as alfa-2a (Roferon-A), **alfa-2b** (Intron-A)	For hepC, usual Roferon-A and Intron-A doses are 3 million international units 3x weekly subQ.	Depending on agent, available in pre-filled syringes, vials of solution, or powder. **Black Box warnings:** include possibility of causing or aggravating serious neuropsychiatric effects, autoimmune disorders, ischemic events, infection. Withdraw therapy if any of these suspected. **Adverse effects:** Flu-like syndrome is common, esp. during 1st wk of rx: fever 98%, fatigue 89%, myalgia 73%, headache 71%. **GI:** anorexia 46%, diarrhea 29%. CNS: dizziness 21%. Hemorrhagic or ischemic stroke. Rash 18%, may progress to Stevens Johnson or exfoliative dermatitis. Profound fatigue & psychiatric symptoms in up to ½ of pts *(J Clin Psych 64:708, 2003)* (depression, anxiety, emotional lability & agitation); consider prophylactic antidepressant in pts with history. Alopecia. ↑ TSH, autoimmune thyroid disorders with ↓- or ↑- thyroidism. Hematol: ↓ WBC 49%, ↓ Hgb 27%, ↓ platelets 35%. Post-marketing reports of antibody-mediated pure red cell aplasia in patients receiving interferon/ribavirin with erythropoiesis-stimulating agents. Acute reversible hearing loss &/or tinnitus in up to 1/3 *(Ln 343:1134, 1994)*. Optic neuropathy (retinal hemorrhage, cotton wool spots, ↓ in color vision) reported *(AIDS 18:1805, 2004)*. Doses may require adjustment (or dc) based on individual response or adverse events, and can vary by product, indication (eg, HCV or HBV) and mode of use (mono- or combination-rx). (Refer to labels of individual products and to ribavirin if used in combination for details of use.)
PEG interferon alfa-2b (PEG-Intron)	0.5–1.5 mcg/kg subQ q wk	
Pegylated-40k interferon alfa-2a (Pegasys)	180 mcg subQ q wk	
Lamivudine (3TC) (Epivir-HBV)	Hepatitis B dose: 100 mg po q24h Dosage adjustment with renal dysfunction *(see label)*. Tabs 100 mg and oral solution 5 mg/mL.	**Black Box warnings:** caution, dose is lower than HIV dose, so must exclude co-infection with HIV before using this formulation; lactic acidosis/hepatic steatosis; severe exacerbation of liver disease can occur on dc. YMDD-mutants resistant to lamivudine may emerge on treatment. **Adverse effects:** *See Table 14D.*
Ribavirin (Rebetol, Copegus)	For use with an interferon for hepatitis C. Available as 200 mg caps and 40 mg/mL oral solution (Rebetol) or 200 mg and 400 mg tabs (Copegus) *(See Comments regarding dosage)*.	**Black Box warnings:** ribavirin monotherapy of HCV is ineffective; hemolytic anemia may precipitate cardiac events; teratogenic/ embryocidal (**Preg Category X**). Drug may persist for 6 mos, avoid pregnancy for at least 6 mos after end of rx of women *or their partners*. Only approved for pts with Ccr > 50 mL/min. Also should not be used in pts with severe heart disease or some hemoglobinopathies. ARDS reported *(Chest 124:406, 2003)*. **Adverse effects:** hemolytic anemia (may require dose reduction or dc), dental/periodontal disorders, and all adverse effects of concomitant interferon used *(see above)*. Postmarketing: retinal detachment, ↓ hearing, hypersensitivity reactions. See *Table 14A* for specific regimens, but dosing depends on: interferon used, weight, HCV genotype, and is modified (or dc) based on side effects (especially degree of hemolysis, with different criteria in those with/without cardiac disease). For example, initial Rebetrol dose with Intron A (interferon alfa-2b) is wt-based: 400 mg am & 600 mg pm for ≤ 75 kg, and 600 mg am & 600 mg pm for wt > 75 kg, but with Pegintron approved dose is 400 mg am & 400 mg pm with meals. Doses and duration of Copegus with peg-interferon alfa-2a are less in pts with genotype 2 or 3 (800 mg per day divided into 2 doses, for 24 wks) than with genotypes 1 or 4 (1000 mg per day divided into 2 doses for wt < 75 kg and 1200 mg per day divided into 2 doses for ≥ 75 kg for 48 wks); in HIV/HCV co-infected pts, dose is 800 mg per day regardless of genotype. *(See individual labels for details, including initial dosing and criteria for dose modification in those with/without cardiac disease.)*
Telaprevir (Incivek)	For HCV genotype 1 750 mg q8h (with food) in combination with INF+RBV	Must be given in combination with PegIFN/RBV. D/c telaprevir after 12 weeks of Rx. Use response guided therapy *(see table 14A for details)* Most common AEs: **Black Box Warning:** Rash (inc rare Steven's Johnson reaction, DRESS, and TEN, each of which may be fatal), pruritis, nausea, anorexia, headache, fatigue, anemia, insomnia, and depression. Difficult to dissect telaprevir AEs from IFN/ribavirin.
Telbivudine (Tyzeka)	600 mg orally q24h, without regard to food. Dosage adjustment with renal dysfunction, Ccr < 50 mL/min *(see label)*. 600 mg tabs; 100 mg per 5 mL solution.	An oral nucleoside analog approved for Rx of Hep B. It has ↑ rates of response and superior viral suppression than lamivudine *(NEJM 357:2576, 2007)*. **Black Box warnings** regarding lactic acidosis/hepatic steatosis with nucleosides and potential for severe exacerbation of HepB on dc. Generally well-tolerated with ↓ mitochondrial toxicity vs other nucleosides and no dose limiting toxicity observed *(Ann Pharmacother 40:472, 2006; Medical Letter 49:11, 2007)*. Myalgias, myopathy and rhabdomyolysis reported. Peripheral neuropathy. Genotypic resistance rate was 4.4% by one yr, ↑ to 21.5% by 2 yrs of rx of eAg+ pts. Selects for YMDD mutation like lamivudine. Combination with lamivudine was inferior to monotherapy *(Hepatology 45:507, 2007)*.

* *See page 2 for abbreviations. NOTE: All dosage recommendations are for adults (unless otherwise indicated) and assume normal renal function.*

TABLE 14B (4)

DRUG NAME(S) GENERIC (TRADE)	DOSAGE/ROUTE IN ADULTS*	COMMENTS/ADVERSE EFFECTS
Influenza A. Treatment and prophylaxis of influenza has become more complicated. Many circulating strains are resistant to adamantanes (amantadine & rimantidine), while others are resistant to the neuraminidase inhibitor, oseltamivir, but susceptible to adamantane. Resistance to the neuraminidase inhibitor, zanamivir, is very rare, but there are limitations to the use of this inhalation agent. In this rapidly evolving area, close attention to guidance from public health authorities is warranted. In patients severely ill with influenza, combination therapy, higher than usual doses of oseltamivir and/or longer than usual treatment courses may be considered in appropriate circumstances *(MMWR 58: 749-752, 2009; NEJM 358:261-273, 2008)*.		
Amantadine (Symmetrel) **or Rimantadine** (Flumadine)	**Amantadine** 100 mg caps, tabs; 50 mg/mL oral solution & syrup. Treatment or prophylaxis: 100 mg bid; or 100 mg daily if age ≥65 y; dose reductions with CrCl starting at ≤50 mL/min. **Rimantadine** 100 mg tabs, 50 mg/5 mL syrup. Treatment or prophylaxis: 100 mg bid, or 100 mg daily in elderly nursing home pts, or severe hepatic disease, or CrCl ≤10 mL/min. For children, rimantadine only approved for prophylaxis.	**Side-effects/toxicity:** CNS (nervousness, anxiety, difficulty concentrating, and lightheadedness). Symptoms occurred in 6% on rimantadine vs 14% on amantadine. They usually ↓ after 1st week and disappear when drug dc. GI (nausea, anorexia). Some serious side-effects—delirium, hallucinations, and seizures—are associated with high plasma drug levels resulting from renal insufficiency, esp. in older pts, those with prior seizure disorders, or psychiatric disorders. Activity restricted to influenza A viruses.
Influenza A and B—For both drugs, initiate within 48 hrs of symptom onset		
Zanamivir (Relenza) For pts ≥ 7 yrs of age (treatment) or ≥ 5 yrs (prophylaxis)	Powder is inhaled by specially designed inhalation device. Each blister contains 5 mg zanamivir. **Treatment:** oral inhalation of 2 blisters (10 mg) bid for 5 days. **Prophylaxis:** oral inhalation of 2 blisters (10 mg) once daily for 10 days (household outbreak) to 28 days (community outbreak).	Active by inhalation against neuraminidase of both influenza A and B and inhibits release of virus from epithelial cells of respiratory tract. Approx. 4–17% of inhaled dose absorbed into plasma. Excreted by kidney but with low absorption, dose reduction not necessary in renal impairment. Minimal side-effects: <3% cough, sinusitis, diarrhea, nausea and vomiting. **Reports of respiratory adverse events in pts with or without h/o airways disease, should be avoided in pts with underlying respiratory disease.** Allergic reactions and neuropsychiatric events have been reported. **Caution: do not reconstitute zanamivir powder for use in nebulizers or mechanical ventilators** (MedWatch report of death). Zanamivir for IV administration is available for compassionate use through an emergency IND application. Contact GSK *(919-315-5215)* for forms, then contact FDA *(301-796-1500 or 301-796-9900)*.
Oseltamivir (Tamiflu) For pts ≥ 1 yr (treatment or prophylaxis)	For adults: **Treatment,** 75 mg po bid for 5 days; 150 mg po bid has been used for critically ill or morbidly obese patients but this dose is not FDA-approved. **Prophylaxis,** 75 mg po once daily for 10 days to 6 wks. *(See label for pediatric weight-based dosing.)* Adjust doses for CrCl ≤30 mL/min. 30 mg, 45 mg, 75 mg caps; powder for oral suspension.	Well absorbed (80% bioavailable) from GI tract as ethyl ester of active compound GS 4071. T½ 6–10 hrs; excreted unchanged by kidney. Adverse effects include diarrhea, nausea, vomiting, headache. Nausea ↓ with food. Rarely, severe skin reactions (toxic epidermal necrolysis, Stevens-Johnson syndrome, erythema multiforme). **Delirium** & abnormal behavior reported *(CID 48:1003, 2009)*. No benefit from higher dose; not recommended *(CID 57:1511, 2013)*.
Respiratory Syncytial Virus (RSV)		
Palivizumab (Synagis) Used for prevention of RSV infection in high-risk children	15 mg per kg IM q month throughout RSV season Single dose 100 mg vial	A monoclonal antibody directed against the F glycoprotein on surface of virus; side-effects are uncommon, occ. ↑ ALT. Anaphylaxis <1/10^5 pts; acute hypersensitivity reaction <1/1000. Postmarketing reports: URI, otitis media, fever, ↓ plts, injection site reactions. Preferred over polyclonal immune globulin in high risk infants & children.
Warts *(See CID 28:S37, 1999)*	Regimens are from drug labels specific for external genital and/or perianal condylomata acuminata only *(see specific labels for indications, regimens, age limits)*.	
Interferon alfa-2b (IntronA)	Injection of 1 million international units into base of lesion, thrice weekly on alternate days for up to 3 wks. Maximum 5 lesions per course.	Interferons may cause "flu-like" illness and other systemic effects. 88% had at least one adverse effect. **Black box warning:** alpha interferons may cause or aggravate neuropsychiatric, autoimmune, ischemic or infectious disorders.
Interferon alfa-N3 (Alferon N)	Injection of 0.05 mL into base of each wart, up to 0.5 mL total per session, twice weekly for up to 8 weeks.	Flu-like syndrome and hypersensitivity reactions. Contraindicated with allergy to mouse IgG, egg proteins, or neomycin.
Imiquimod (Aldara)	5% cream. Thin layer applied at bedtime, washing off after 6-10 hr, thrice weekly to maximum of 16 wks.	Erythema, itching & burning, erosions. Flu-like syndrome, increased susceptibility to sunburn (avoid UV).
Podofilox (Condylox)	0.5% gel or solution twice daily for 3 days, no therapy for 4 days; can use up to 4 such cycles.	Local reactions—pain, burning, inflammation in 50%. Can ulcerate. Limit surface area treated as per label.
Sinecatechins (Veregen)	15% ointment. Apply 0.5 cm strand to each wart three times per day until healing but not more than 16 weeks.	Application site reactions, which may result in ulcerations, phimosis, meatal stenosis, superinfection.

* *See page 2 for abbreviations. NOTE: All dosage recommendations are for adults (unless otherwise indicated) and assume normal renal function.*

TABLE 14C – AT A GLANCE SUMMARY OF SUGGESTED ANTIVIRAL AGENTS AGAINST TREATABLE PATHOGENIC VIRUSES

Virus	ANTIVIRAL AGENT														
	Acyclovir	**Amantadine**	**Adefovir Entecavir Lamivudine Tenofovir**	**Sofosbuvir Simeprevir**	**Cidofovir**	**Famciclovir**	**Foscarnet**	**Ganciclovir**	**αInterferon Or PEG INF**	**Oseltamivir**	**Ribavirin**	**Rimantadine**	**Valacyclovir**	**Valganciclovir**	**Zanamivir**
Adenovirus	-	-	-	-	+	-	-	±	-	-	-	-	-	±	-
BK virus	-	-	-	-	+	-	-	-	-	-	-	-	-	-	-
Cytomegalo-virus	±	-	-	-	+++	±	+++	+++	-	-	-	-	±	+++	-
Hepatitis B	-	-	+++	-	-	-	-	-	+++	-	±	-	-	-	-
Hepatitis C	-	-	-	+++	-	-	-	-	+++*	-	+++*	-	-	-	-
Herpes simplex virus	+++	-	-	-	++	+++	++	++	-	-	-	-	+++	++	-
Influenza A Influenza B	-	±**	-	-	-	-	-	-	- -	+++*** ++	-	±**	-	-	+++ ++
JC Virus	-	-	-	-	+	-	-	-	-	-	-	-	-	-	-
Respiratory Syncytial Virus	-	-	-	-	-	-	-	-	-	-	+	-	-	-	-
Varicella-zoster virus	+	-	-	-	+	++	++	+	-	-	-	-	+++	+	-

* 1st line rx = *see Table 14G* ** not CDC recommended due to high prevalence of resistance *** High level resistance H1N1 (non-swine) in 2008; Swine H1N1 susceptible.

- = no activity; ± = possible activity; + = active, 3rd line therapy (least active clinically)
++ = Active, 2nd line therapy (less active clinically); +++ = Active, 1st line therapy (usually active clinically)

TABLE 14D – ANTIRETROVIRAL THERAPY (ART) IN TREATMENT-NAÏVE ADULTS (HIV/AIDS)

The U.S. Dept of Health & Human Svcs (DHHS) provides updated guidelines on a regular basis. Current guidelines, as well as recommendations for anti-retroviral therapy (ART) in pregnant women and in children, are available at *www.aidsinfo.nih.gov*. These documents provide detailed recommendations and explanations, drug characteristics, and additional alternatives concerning the use of ART. The new Guidelines include: (1) recommendations to start therapy at any CD4 count for asymptomatic patients unless there is a reason to defer treatment; the strength of the recommendation increases with lower CD4 count values; (2) A simplified recommendation scheme for choice of initial therapy for naive patients (incorporated into 6A (2) below (3) Revised definitions for regimen failure (4) TB recommendations remain unchanged. For patients with CD4 counts <50 cells/mm^3, ART should be initiated within 2 weeks of starting TB treatment **(AI)**.

- For patients with CD4 counts ≥50 cells/mm^3 with clinical disease of major severity as indicated by clinical evaluation (including low Karnofsky score, low body mass index [BMI], low hemoglobin, low albumin, organ system dysfunction, or extent of disease), the Panel recommends initiation of ART within 2 to 4 weeks of starting TB treatment (**BI** for CD4 count 50–200 cells/mm^3 and **BIII** for CD4 count >200 cells/mm^3).
- For other patients with CD4 counts ≥50 cells/mm^3, ART can be delayed beyond 2 to 4 weeks but should be initiated by 8 to 12 weeks of TB therapy (**AI** for CD4 count 50–500 cells/mm^3; **BIII** for CD4 count >500 cells/mm^3). Note that immune reconstitution syndromes (IRS or IRIS) may result from initiation of any ART, and may require medical intervention.

The following principles and concepts guide therapy:

- **The goal of rx is to inhibit maximally viral replication, allowing re-establishment & persistence of an effective immune response that will prevent or delay HIV-related morbidity.**
- **Fully undetectable levels of virus are the target of therapy for ALL patients, regardless of stage of disease or number/type of prior regimens.**
- **The lower the viral RNA can be driven, the lower the rate of accumulation of drug resistance mutations & the longer the therapeutic effect will last.**
- **To achieve maximal & durable suppression of viral RNA, combinations of potent antiretroviral agents are required, as is a high degree of adherence to the chosen regimens.**
- **Virologic failure is defined as confirmed virus > 200 c/mL.**
- **Treatment regimens must be tailored to the individual as well as to the virus. Resistance testing (genotype) should be performed prior to the initiation of ARV therapy. Antiretroviral drug toxicities can compromise adherence in the short term & can cause significant negative health effects over time. Carefully check for specific risks to the individual, for interactions between the antiretrovirals selected & between those & concurrent drugs, & adjust doses as necessary for body weight, for renal or hepatic dysfunction, & for possible pharmacokinetic interactions.**

A. **When to start therapy?** *(www.aidsinfo.nih.gov)*

Guidelines	Any symptoms or CD4 <200/μL	CD4 200-350/μL	CD4 350-500/μL	CD4 > 500/μL
IAS-USA: *JAMA 308: 387, 2012*	Treat	Treat	Treat	Consider Treatment* * No Apparent Harm in treating earlier
DHHS: *www.aidsinfo.nih.gov*	Treat	Treat	Treat	Treat* * Strength of rating increases as CD4 count decreases

Life Cycle of HIV with Sites of Action of Antiretrovirals

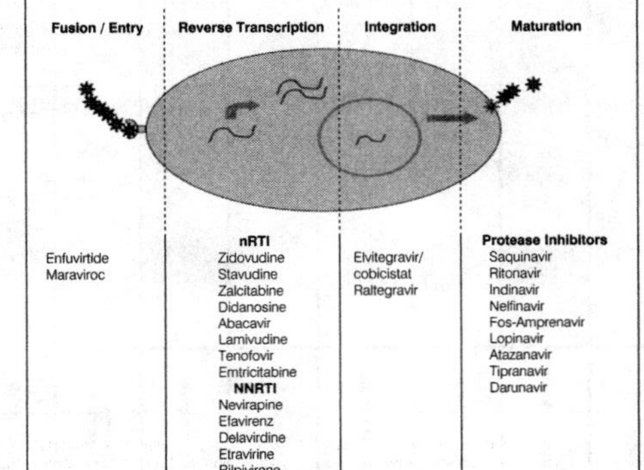

TABLE 14D (2)

B. **Recommended Antiretroviral Regimen Options for Antiretroviral Therapy-Naive Patients** *(modified from DHHS Guidelines, www.AIDSinfo.gov)*

Combination antiretroviral therapy (ART) regimens typically consist of two NRTIs plus one active 'anchor' drug. Anchor drugs are either a NNRTI, a PI (usually boosted with RTV), an INSTI, or a CCR5 antagonist. Refer to *section E (Table 14D)* below for characteristics of each drug and their usual doses, and *Table 14E* for common adverse events and safety discussion. The regimens in each category are listed in **alphabetical order.**

Recommended Initial ART Regimens for All Patients, regardless of Pre-ART Viral Load

NNRTI-Based Regimen
- EFV/TDF/ FTC

PI-Based Regimens
- ATV/r + TDF/FTC[a] **(AI)**
- DRV/r + TDF/FTC[a] **(AI)**

INSTI-Based Regimen
- DTG + ABC/3TC – **only** for patients who are HLA-B*5701 negative
- DTG + TDF/FTC
- EVG/COBI/TDF/FTC – **only** for patients with pre-treatment estimated CrCl > 70 mL/min
- RAL + ABC/3TC – **only** for patients who are HLA-B*5701 negative
- RAL + TDF/FTC[a]

Recommended Initial ART Regimens patients with pre-ART plasma HIV RNA < 100,000 copies/mL
(in addition to the regimens listed above for all patients regardless of Pre-ART VL)

NNRTI-Based Regimen
- EFV + ABC/3TC[a] – **only** for patients with HIV RNA < 100,000 copies/mL **and** who are HLA-B*5701 negative
- RPV/TDF/FTC[a] – **only** for patients with pre-treatment HIV RNA < 100,000 copies/mL **and** CD4 cell count > 200 cells/mm^3

PI-Based Regimens)
- ATV/r + ABC/3TC[a] – **only** for patients with HIV RNA < 100,000 copies/mL **and** who are HLA-B*5701 negative

Alternative Initial ART Regimen Options
Regimens that are effective and tolerable, but have potential disadvantages when compared with the recommended regimens listed above or for which there is limited data from randomized clinical trials. An alternative regimen may be the preferred regimen for some patients.

NNRTI-Based Regimens
- RPV + ABC/3TC[a] – **only** for patients who are HLA-B*5701 negative, **and** with pre-ART HIV RNA < 100,000 copies/mL, **and** CD4 count > 200 cells/mm^3

PI-Based Regimens
- DRV/r + ABC/3TC[a] – **only** for patients who are HLA-B*5701 negative
- LPV/r (once or twice daily) + ABC/3TC[a] – **only** for patients who are HLA-B*5701 negative
- LPV/r (once or twice daily) + TDF/FTC[a]

TABLE 14D (3)

Regimens that may be selected for some patients but are less satisfactory than recommended or alternative regimens
NNRTI-Based Regimen • EFV + ZDV/3TC[a] • NVP + (TDF/FTC[a] or ZDV/3TC) – **only** for ART-naive women with pre-ART CD4 count < 250 cells/mm^3 or males with pre-ART CD4 count < 400 cells/mm^3 • NVP + ABC/3TC[a] – **only** for ART-naive women with pre-ART CD4 count < 250 cells/mm^3 or males with pre-ART CD4 count < 400 cells/mm^3, who are HLA-B*5701 negative, and with pre-ART HIV RNA < 100,000 copies/mL • RPV + ZDV/3TC[a] – **only** for patients with pre-ART HIV RNA < 100,000 copies/mL and CD4 count > 200 cells/mm^3
PI-Based Regimens • (ATV or ATV/r or DRV/r or FPV/r or LPV/r or SQV/r) + ZDV/3TC[a] • ATV + ABC/3TC[a] – **only** for patients who are HLA-B*5701 negative and with pre-ART HIV RNA < 100,000 copies/mL • FPV/r + ABC/3TC[a] – **only** for patients who are HLA-B*5701 negative and with pre-ART HIV RNA < 100,000 copies/mL • FPV + TDF/FTC[a] • SQV/r + ABC/3TC[a] – **only** for patients who are HLA-B*5701 negative, with pre-ART HIV RNA < 100,000 copies/mL, and pretreatment QT interval < 450 msec • SQV/r + TDF/FTC[a] – **only** for patients with pretreatment QT interval < 450 msec
INSTI-Based Regimen • RAL + ZDV/3TC[a] • DTG + ZDV/3TC[a]
CCR5 Antagonist-Based Regimens • MVC + (TDF/FTC or ZDV/3TC[a]) – **only** for patients with CCR5 tropic HIV • MVC + ABC/3TC[a] – **only** for patients with CCR5 tropic HIV, who are HLA-B*5701 negative, and with pre-ART HIV RNA < 100,000 copies/mL

[a] 3TC may substitute for FTC or vice versa. The following combinations in the recommended list above are available as co-formulated fixed-dose combinations: ABC/3TC, EFV/TDF/FTC, EVG/COBI/TDF/FTC, LPV/r, RPV/TDF/FTC, TDF/FTC, and ZDV/3TC.

Key to Abbreviations: 3TC = lamivudine, ABC = abacavir, ART = antiretroviral therapy, ARV = antiretroviral, ATV/r = atazanavir/ritonavir, COBI = cobicistat, CrCl = creatinine clearance, DTG = dolutegravir, DRV/r = darunavir/ritonavir, EFV = efavirenz, EVG = elvitegravir, FDA = Food and Drug Administration, FPV/r = fosamprenavir/ritonavir, FTC = emtricitabine, INSTI = integrase strand transfer inhibitor, LPV/r = lopinavir/ritonavir, NNRTI = non-nucleoside reverse transcriptase inhibitor, NRTI = nucleoside reverse transcriptase inhibitor, PI = protease inhibitor, PPI = proton pump inhibitor, RAL = raltegravir, RPV = rilpivirine, RTV = ritonavir, TDF = tenofovir disoproxil fumarate.

TABLE 14D (4)

C. **During pregnancy.** Expert consultation mandatory. Timing of rx initiation & drug choice must be individualized. Viral resistance testing should be strongly considered. Long-term effects of agents unknown. Certain drugs hazardous or contraindicated. For additional information & alternative options, *see www.aidsinfo.nih.gov*. For regimens to prevent perinatal transmission, see *Table 8*. For additional information & alternative options, *see www.aidsinfo.nih.gov.*

D. **Antiretroviral Therapies That Should NOT Be Offered** *(Modified from www.aidsinfo.nih.gov)*

1. **Regimens not recommended**

	Regimen	Logic	Exception
a.	Monotherapy with NRTI	Rapid development of resistance & inferior antiviral activity	Perhaps ZDV to reduce peripartum mother-to-child transmission. *See Perinatal Guidelines at www.aidsinfo.nih.gov and Table 8B*, SANFORD GUIDE TO HIV/AIDS THERAPY
b.	Dual NRTI combinations	Resistance and Inferior antiretroviral activity compared with standard drug combinations	Perhaps ZDV to reduce peripartum mother-to-child transmission. *See Perinatal Guidelines at www.aidsinfo.nih.gov and Table 8B*, SANFORD GUIDE TO HIV/AIDS THERAPY
c.	Triple NRTI combinations	Triple-NRTI regimens have shown inferior virologic efficacy in clinical trials: (tenofovir + lamivudine + abacavir) & (didanosine + lamivudine + tenofovir) & others	(Zidovudine + lamivudine + abacavir) or (zidovudine + lamivudine + tenofovir) might be used if no alternative exists.
d.	Double Boosted PIs	Using 2 or more PI agents boosted with ritonavir adds nothing in terms of anti-HIV activity but can add extra toxicity	No exceptions
e.	2 NNRTI agents	Increased rate of side effects. Drug-drug interaction between etravirine and nevirapine and etravirine and efavirenz	No exceptions

2. **Drug, or drugs, not recommended as part of antiretroviral regimen**

	Regimen	Logic	Exception
a.	Saquinavir hard gel cap or tab (Invirase), darunavir, or tipranavir as single (unboosted) PI	Bioavailability only 4%; inferior antiretroviral activity	No exceptions
b.	Stavudine + didanosine	High frequency of toxicity: peripheral neuropathy, pancreatitis & mitochondrial toxicity (lactic acidosis). In pregnancy: lactic acid acidosis, hepatic steatosis, ± pancreatitis	Toxicity partially offset by potent antiretroviral activity of the combination. Use only when potential benefits outweigh the sizeable risks.
c.	Stavudine + zidovudine	Antagonistic	No exceptions
d.	Atazanavir + indinavir	Additive risk of hyperbilirubinemia	No exceptions
e.	Emtricitabine + lamivudine	Same target and resistance profile	No exceptions
f.	Abacavir + tenofovir	Rapid development of K65R mutation; loss of effect	Can avoid if zidovudine also used in the regimen; might be an option for salvage therapy but not earlier lines of therapy.
g.	Tenofovir + didanosine	Reduced CD4 cell count increase; concern of K 65R development	Use with caution. Likely increases ddI concentrations and serious ddI toxicities.
h.	Abacavir + didanosine	Insufficient data in naïve patients	Use with caution

TABLE 14D (5)

E. **Selected Characteristics of Antiretroviral Drugs** (CPE = CSF penetration effectiveness)

1. **Selected Characteristics of Nucleoside or Nucleotide Reverse Transcriptase Inhibitors (NRTIs)**

All agents have Black Box warning: Risk of lactic acidosis/hepatic steatosis. Also, labels note risk of fat redistribution/accumulation with ARV therapy. For combinations, *see warnings for component agents.*

*** CPE (CNS Penetration Effectiveness) value:** 1= Low Penetration; 2 - 3 = Intermediate Penetration; 4 = Highest Penetration into CNS *(Letendre, et al, CROI 2010, abs #430)*

Generic/ Trade Name	Pharmaceutical Prep.	Usual Adult Dosage & Food Effect	% Absorbed, po	Serum T½, hrs	Intracellular T½, hrs	CPE*	Elimination	Major Adverse Events/Comments *(See Table 14E)*
Abacavir (ABC; Ziagen)	300 mg tabs or 20 mg/mL oral solution	300 mg po bid or 600 mg po q24h. Food OK	83	1.5	20	1	Liver metab., renal excretion of metabolites, 82%	**Hypersensitivity reaction:** fever, rash, N/V, malaise, diarrhea, abdominal pain, respiratory symptoms. (Severe reactions may be ↑ with 600 mg dose.) **Do not rechallenge!** Report to 800-270-0425. **Test HLA-B*5701 before use.** ***See Comment Table 14E.*** Studies raise concerns re ABC/3TC regimens in pts with VL ≥ 100,000 *(www.niaid.nih.gov/news/newsreleases/2008/actg5202bulletin.htm).* Controversy re increased CV events with use of ABC. Large meta-analysis shows no increased risk *(JAIDS 61, 441, 2012)*
Abacavir (ABC)/lamivudine (Epzicom or Kivexa)	Film coated tabs ABC 600 mg + 3TC 300 mg	1 tab once daily (not recommended)	*(See individual components)*					*(See Comments for individual components)* Note: **Black Box warnings** for ABC hypersensitivity reaction & others. Should only be used for regimens intended to include these 3 agents. Black Box warning— limited data for VL >100,000 copies/mL. Not recommended as initial therapy because of inferior virologic efficacy.
Abacavir (ABC)/ lamivudine (3TC)/ zidovudine (AZT) (Trizivir)	Film-coated tabs: ABC 300 mg + 3TC 150 mg + ZDV 300 mg	1 tab po bid (not recommended for wt <40 kg or CrCl <50 mL/min or impaired hepatic function)						
Didanosine (ddI; Videx or Videx EC)	125, 200, 250, 400 enteric-coated caps; 100, 167, 250 mg powder for oral solution;	≥60 kg Usually 400 mg enteric-coated po q24h 0.5 hr before or 2 hrs after meal. Do not crush. <60 kg: 250 mg EC po q24h. Food ↓ levels. *See Comment*	30–40	1.6	25–40	2	Renal excretion, 50%	**Pancreatitis,** peripheral neuropathy, lactic acidosis & hepatic steatosis (rare but life-threatening, esp. combined with stavudine in pregnancy). Retinal, optic nerve changes. **The combination ddI + TDF is generally avoided, but if used,** reduce dose of ddI-EC from 400 mg to 250 mg EC q24h (or from 250 mg EC to 200 mg EC for adults <60 kg). **Monitor for ↑ toxicity & possible ↓ in efficacy of this combination; may result in ↓ CD4.** Possibly associated with noncirrhotic portal hypertension.

TABLE 14D (6)

Generic/ Trade Name	Pharmaceutical Prep.	Usual Adult Dosage & Food Effect	% Absorbed, po	Serum T½, hrs	Intracellular T½, hrs	CPE*	Elimination	Major Adverse Events/Comments *(See Table 14E)*
E. Selected Characteristics of Antiretroviral Drugs (CPE = CSF penetration effectiveness)								
1. Selected Characteristics of Nucleoside or Nucleotide Reverse Transcriptase Inhibitors (NRTIs) *(continued)*								
Emtricitabine (FTC, Emtriva)	200 mg caps; 10 mg per mL oral solution.	200 mg po q24h. Food OK	93 (caps), 75 (oral sol'n)	Approx. 10	39	3	Renal excretion 86%, minor bio-transformation, 14% excretion in feces	Well tolerated; headache, nausea, vomiting & diarrhea occasionally, skin rash rarely. Skin hyperpigmentation. Differs only slightly in structure from lamivudine (5-fluoro substitution). **Exacerbation of Hep B reported in pts after stopping FTC.** Monitor at least several months after stopping FTC in Hep B pts; some may need anti-HBV therapy.
Emtricitabine/ tenofovir disoproxil fumarate (Truvada)	Film-coated tabs: FTC 200 mg + TDF 300 mg	1 tab po q24h for CrCl ≥50 mL/min. Food OK	92/25	10/17	—	*(See individual components)*	Primarily renal/renal	*See Comments for individual agents* **Black Box warning—Exacerbation of HepB after stopping FTC;** but preferred therapy for those with Hep B.
Emtricitabine/ tenofovir/efavirenz (Atripla)	Film-coated tabs: FTC 200 mg + TDF 300 mg + efavirenz 600 mg	1 tab po q24h on an empty stomach, preferably at bedtime. Do not use if CrCl <50 mL/min	*(See individual components)*					Not recommended for pts <18 yrs. *(See warnings for individual components).* **Exacerbation of Hep B** reported in pts discontinuing component drugs; some may need anti-HBV therapy (preferred anti-Hep B therapy). **Pregnancy category D-** may cause fetal harm. Avoid in pregnancy or in women who may become pregnant.
Emtricitabine/ tenofovir/rilpivirine (Complera/ Eviplera)	Film-coated tabs: FTC 200 mg + TDF 300 mg + RPL 25 mg	1 tab po q24h with food	*(See individual components)*					*See individual components.* Preferred use in pts with HIV RNA level <100,000 c/mL. Should not be used with PPI agents.
Lamivudine (3TC; Epivir)	150, 300 mg tabs; 10 mg/mL oral solution	150 mg po bid or 300 mg po q24h. Food OK	86	5–7	18	2	Renal excretion, minimal metabolism	**Use HIV dose, not Hep B dose.** Usually well-tolerated. **Risk of exacerbation of Hep B after stopping 3TC.** Monitor at least several months after stopping 3TC in Hep B pts; some may need anti-HBV therapy.
Lamivudine/ abacavir (Epzicom)	Film-coated tabs: 3TC 300 mg + abacavir 600 mg	1 tab po q24h. Food OK Not recommended for CrCl <50 mL/min or impaired hepatic function	86/86	5–7/1.5	16/20	*(See individual components)*	Primarily renal/ metabolism	*See Comments for individual agents.* **Note abacavir hypersensitivity Black Box warnings** (severe reactions may be somewhat more frequent with 600 mg dose) and 3TC Hep B warnings. Test HLA-B*5701 before use.
Lamivudine/ zidovudine (Combivir)	Film-coated tabs: 3TC 150 mg + ZDV 300 mg	1 tab po bid. Not recommended for CrCl <50 mL/min or impaired hepatic function Food OK	86/64	5-7/ 0.5-3	—	*(See individual components)*	Primarily renal/ metabolism with renal excretion of glucuronide	*See Comments for individual agents* **Black Box warning**—exacerbation of Hep B in pts stopping 3TC

TABLE 14D (7)

Generic/ Trade Name	Pharmaceutical Prep.	Usual Adult Dosage & Food Effect	% Absorbed, po	Serum T½, hrs	Intracellular T½, hrs	CPE*	Elimination	Major Adverse Events/Comments *(See Table 14E)*
E. **Selected Characteristics of Antiretroviral Drugs** (CPE = CSF penetration effectiveness)								
1. **Selected Characteristics of Nucleoside or Nucleotide Reverse Transcriptase Inhibitors (NRTIs)** *(continued)*								
Stavudine (d4T; Zerit)	15, 20, 30, 40 mg capsules; 1 mg per mL oral solution	≥60 kg: 40 mg po bid <60 kg: 30 mg po bid Food OK	86	1.2–1.6	3.5	2	Renal excretion, 40%	Not recommended by DHHS as initial therapy because of adverse reactions. **Highest incidence of lipoatrophy, hyperlipidemia, & lactic acidosis of all NRTIs.** Pancreatitis. Peripheral neuropathy. *(See didanosine comments.)*
Tenofovir disoproxil fumarate (TDF; Viread)—a nucleotide	300 mg tabs	CrCl ≥50 mL/min: 300 mg po q24h. Food OK; high-fat meal ↑ absorption	39 (with food) 25 (fasted)	17	>60	1	Renal excretion	Headache, N/V. **Cases of renal dysfunction reported:** check renal function before using (dose reductions necessary if CrCl <50 cc/min); avoid concomitant nephrotoxic agents. One study found ↑ renal function at 48-wk in pts receiving TDF with a PI (mostly lopinavir/ritonavir) than with a NNRTI *(JID 197:102, 2008)*. Must adjust dose of ddI (↓) if used concomitantly but best to avoid this combination *(see ddI Comments)*. Atazanavir & lopinavir/ritonavir ↑ tenofovir concentrations: monitor for adverse effects. **Black Box warning—exacerbations of Hep B reported after stopping tenofovir.** Monitor several months after stopping TDF in Hep B pts; some may need anti-HBV Rx.
Zidovudine (ZDV, AZT; Retrovir)	100 mg caps, 300 mg tabs; 10 mg per mL IV solution; 10 mg/mL oral syrup	300 mg po q12h. Food OK	64	1.1	11	4	Metabolized to glucuronide & excreted in urine	Bone marrow suppression, GI intolerance, headache, insomnia, malaise, myopathy.
2. **Selected Characteristics of Non-Nucleoside Reverse Transcriptase Inhibitors (NNRTIs)**								
Delavirdine (Rescriptor)	100, 200 mg tabs	400 mg po three times daily. Food OK	85	5.8	3		Cytochrome P450 (3A inhibitor). 51% excreted in urine (<5% unchanged), 44% in feces	Rash severe enough to stop drug in 4.3%. ↑ AST/ALT; headaches. **Use of this agent is not recommended.**

TABLE 14D (8)

Generic/ Trade Name	Pharmaceutical Prep.	Usual Adult Dosage & Food Effect	% Absorbed, po	Serum T½, hrs	Intracellular T½, hrs	CPE*	Elimination	Major Adverse Events/Comments (*See Table 14E*)
E. Selected Characteristics of Antiretroviral Drugs (CPE = CSF penetration effectiveness)								
2. Selected Characteristics of Non-Nucleoside Reverse Transcriptase Inhibitors (NNRTIs) *(continued)*								
Efavirenz (Sustiva)	50, 100, 200 mg capsules; 600 mg tablet	600 mg po q24h at bedtime, without food. Food may ↑ serum conc., which can lead to ↑ in risk of adverse events.	42	40–55 *See Comment*	3		Cytochrome P450 2B6 (3A mixed inducer/ inhibitor). 14–34% of dose excreted in urine as glucuronidated metabolites, 16–61% in feces	Rash severe enough to dc use of drug in 1.7%. High frequency of diverse CNS AEs: somnolence, dreams, confusion, agitation. Serious psychiatric symptoms. Certain CYP2B6 polymorphisms may predict exceptionally high plasma levels with standard doses *(CID 45:1230, 2007)*. False-pos. cannabinoid screen. **New Guidelines indicate is OK to use in pregnant women (WHO Guidelines) or continue EFV in women identified as pregnant (HHS Guidelines).** Very long tissue T½. **If rx to be discontinued, stop efavirenz 1–2 wks before stopping companion drugs.** Otherwise, risk of developing efavirenz resistance, as after 1–2 days only efavirenz in blood &/or tissue. Some authorities bridge this gap by adding a PI to the NRTI backbone if feasible after efavirenz is discontinued. *(CID 42:401, 2006)*
Etravirine (Intelence)	100 mg tabs 200 mg tabs	200 mg twice daily after a meal. May also be given as 400 mg once daily	Unknown (↓ systemic exposure if taken fasting)	41	2		Metabolized by CYP 3A4 (inducer) & 2C9, 2C19 (inhibitor). Excreted into feces (>90%), mostly unchanged drug.	For pts with HIV-1 resistant to NNRTIs & others. Active in vitro against most such isolates. Rash common, but rarely can be severe. Potential for multiple drug interactions. Generally, multiple mutations are required for high-level resistance. *See Table 14E, page 190 for specific mutations and effects.* Because of interactions, do not use with boosted atazanavir, boosted tipranavir, unboosted PIs, or other NNRTIs.
Nevirapine (Viramune) Viramune XR	200 mg tabs; 50 mg per 5 mL oral suspension; XR 400 mg tabs	200 mg po q24h x 14 days & then 200 mg po bid *(see comments & **Black Box warning**)* Food OK. **If using Viramune XR, Still need the lead in dosing of 200 mg q24h prior to using 400 mg/d**	>90	25–30	4		Cytochrome P450 (3A4, 2B6) inducer; 80% of dose excreted in urine as glucuronidated metabolites, 10% in feces	**Black Box warning—fatal hepatotoxicity.** Women with CD4 >250 esp. vulnerable, inc. pregnant women. Avoid in this group unless benefits clearly > risks *(www.fda.gov/cderdrug/advisory/nevirapine.htm)*. If used, intensive monitoring required. Men with CD4 >400 also at ↑ risk. Rash severe enough to stop drug in 7%, **severe or life-threatening skin reactions** in 2%. Do not restart if any suspicion of such reactions. 2 wk dose escalation period may ↓ skin reactions. As with efavirenz, because of long T½, consider continuing companion agents for several days if nevirapine is discontinued.

TABLE 14D (9)

Generic/ Trade Name	Pharmaceutical Prep.	Usual Adult Dosage & Food Effect	% Absorbed, po	Serum T½, hrs	Intracellular T½, hrs	CPE*	Elimination	Major Adverse Events/Comments *(See Table 14E)*
E. **Selected Characteristics of Antiretroviral Drugs** (CPE = CSF penetration effectiveness)								
2. **Selected Characteristics of Non-Nucleoside Reverse Transcriptase Inhibitors (NNRTIs)** *(continued)*								
Rilpivirine (Edurant)	25 mg tabs	25 mg daily with food	absolute bio-availability unknown; 40% lower Cmax in fasted state	50	unknown		Metabolized by Cyp3A4 majority of drug metabolized by liver; 25% of dose excreted unchanged in feces.	QTc prolongation with doses higher than 50 mg per day. Most common side effects are depression, insomnia, headache, and rash. Rilpivirine should not be co-administered with carbamazepine, phenobarbitol, phenytoin, rifabutin, rifampin, rifapentine, proton pump inhibitors, or multiple doses of dexamethasone. A fixed dose combination of rilpivirine + TDF/FTC (Complera/Eviplera) is approved. **Needs stomach acid for absorption. Do not administer with PPI.**

3. **Selected Characteristics of Protease Inhibitors (PIs).**

All PIs: Glucose metabolism: new diabetes mellitus or deterioration of glucose control; fat redistribution; possible hemophilia bleeding; hypertriglyceridemia or hypercholesterolemia. Exercise caution re: potential drug interactions & contraindications. QTc prolongation has been reported in a few pts taking PIs; some PIs can block HERG channels in vitro *(Lancet 365:682, 2005)*.

Generic/ Trade Name	Pharmaceutical Prep.	Usual Adult Dosage & Food Effect	% Absorbed, po	Serum T½, hrs	CPE*	Elimination	Major Adverse Events/Comments *(See Table 14E)*
Atazanavir (Reyataz)	100, 150, 200, 300 mg capsules	400 mg po q24h with food. Ritonavir-boosted dose (atazanavir 300 mg po q24h + ritonavir 100 mg po q24h), with food, is recommended for ART-experienced pts. The boosted dose is also used when combined with either efavirenz 600 mg po q24h or TDF 300 mg po q24h. If used with buffered ddI, take with food 2 hrs pre or 1 hr post ddI.	Good oral bioavailability; food enhances bioavailability & ↓ pharmacokinetic variability. Absorption ↓ by antacids, H_2-blockers, proton pump inhibitors. Avoid unboosted drug with PPIs/H2-blockers. Boosted drug can be used with or >10 hr after H2-blockers or >12 hr after a PPI, as long as limited doses of the acid agents are used *(see 2008 drug label changes)*.	Approx. 7	2	Cytochrome P450 (3A4, 1A2 & 2C9 inhibitor) & UGT1A1 inhibitor, 13% excreted in urine (7% unchanged), 79% excreted in feces (20% unchanged)	Lower potential for ↑ lipids. Asymptomatic unconjugated hyperbilirubinemia common; jaundice especially likely in Gilbert's syndrome *(JID 192:1381, 2005)*. Headache, rash, GI symptoms. Prolongation of PR interval (1st degree AV block) reported. Caution in pre-existing conduction system disease. Efavirenz & tenofovir ↓ atazanavir exposure; use atazanavir/ritonavir regimen; also, atazanavir ↑ tenofovir concentrations—watch for adverse events. In rx-experienced pts taking TDF and needing H2 blockers, atazanavir 400 mg with ritonavir 100 mg can be given; do not use PPIs. Rare reports of renal stones.
Darunavir (Prezista)	400 mg, 600 mg, 800 mg tablets	[600 mg darunavir + 100 mg ritonavir] po bid, with food or **[800 mg darunavir (two 400 mg tabs or one 800 mg tab) + 100 mg ritonavir] po once daily with food (Preferred regimen in ART naïve pts)**	82% absorbed (taken with ritonavir). Food ↑ absorption.	Approx 15 hr (with ritonavir)	3	Metabolized by CYP3A and is a CYP3A inhibitor	Once daily dosing regimen mostly in 1st line therapy. Contains sulfa moiety. Rash, nausea, headaches seen. Coadmin of certain drugs cleared by CYP3A is contraindicated *(see label)*. Use with caution in pts with hepatic dysfunction. (Recent FDA warning about occasional hepatic dysfunction early in the course of treatment). Monitor carefully, esp. first several months and with pre-existing liver disease. May cause hormonal contraception failure.

TABLE 14D (10)

Generic/ Trade Name	Pharmaceutical Prep.	Usual Adult Dosage & Food Effect	% Absorbed, po	Serum T½, hrs	CPE*	Elimination	Major Adverse Events/Comments *(See Table 14E)*
E. **Selected Characteristics of Antiretroviral Drugs** (CPE = CSF penetration effectiveness)							
3. **Selected Characteristics of Protease Inhibitors (PIs).** *(continued)*							
Fosamprenavir (Lexiva)	700 mg tablet, 50 mg/mL oral suspension	1400 mg (two 700 mg tabs) po bid **OR** with ritonavir: [1400 mg fosamprenavir (2 tabs) + ritonavir 200 mg] po q24h **OR** [1400 mg fosamprenavir (2 tabs) + ritonavir 100 mg] po q24h **OR** [700 mg fosamprenavir (1 tab) + ritonavir 100 mg] po bid	Bioavailability not established. Food OK	7.7 Amprenavir	3	Hydrolyzed to amprenavir, then acts as cytochrome P450 (3A4 substrate, inhibitor, inducer)	Amprenavir prodrug. Contains sulfa moiety. Potential for serious drug interactions *(see label)*. Rash, including Stevens-Johnson syndrome. Once daily regimens: (1) not recommended for PI-experienced pts, (2) additional ritonavir needed if given with efavirenz *(see label)*. Boosted twice daily regimen is recommended for PI-experienced pts. Potential for PI cross-resistance with darunavir.
Indinavir (Crixivan)	100, 200, 400 mg capsules Store in original container with desiccant	Two 400 mg caps (800 mg) po q8h, without food or with light meal. Can take with enteric-coated Videx. *[If taken with ritonavir (e.g., 800 mg indinavir + 100 mg ritonavir po q12h), no food restrictions]*	65	1.2–2	4	Cytochrome P450 (3A4 inhibitor)	**Maintain hydration. Nephrolithiasis,** nausea, inconsequential ↑ of indirect bilirubin (jaundice in Gilbert syndrome), ↑ AST/ALT, headache, asthenia, blurred vision, metallic taste, hemolysis. ↑ urine WBC (>100/hpf) has been assoc. with nephritis/ medullary calcification, cortical atrophy.
Lopinavir + ritonavir (Kaletra)	(200 mg lopinavir + 50 mg ritonavir), and (100 mg lopinavir + 25 mg ritonavir) tablets. Tabs do not need refrigeration. Oral solution: (80 mg lopinavir + 20 mg ritonavir) per mL. Refrigerate, but can be kept at room temp. (≤77 °F) x 2 mos.	(400 mg lopinavir + 100 mg ritonavir)—2 tabs po bid. Higher dose may be needed in non-rx-naïve pts when used with efavirenz, nevirapine, or unboosted fosamprenavir. [Dose adjustment in concomitant drugs may be necessary; *see Table 22B.*	No food effect with tablets.	5–6	3	Cytochrome P450 (3A4 inhibitor)	Nausea/vomiting/diarrhea (worse when administered with zidovudine), ↑ AST/ ALT, pancreatitis. Oral solution 42% alcohol. Lopinavir + ritonavir can be taken as a single daily dose of 4 tabs (total 800 mg lopinavir + 200 mg ritonavir), except in treatment-experienced pts or those taking concomitant efavirenz, nevirapine, amprenavir, or nelfinavir. Possible PR and QT prolongation. Use with caution in those with cardiac conduction abnormalities or when used with drugs with similar effects.
Nelfinavir (Viracept)	625, 250 mg tabs; 50 mg/gm oral powder	Two 625 mg tabs (1250 mg) po bid, with food	20–80 Food ↑ exposure & ↓ variability	3.5–5	1	Cytochrome P450 (3A4 inhibitor)	Diarrhea. Coadministration of drugs with life-threatening toxicities & which are cleared by CYP34A is contraindicated. Not recommended in initial regimens because of inferior efficacy; **prior concerns about EMS now resolved. Acceptable choice in pregnant women although it has inferior virologic efficacy than most other ARV anchor drugs.**

TABLE 14D (11)

Generic/ Trade Name	Pharmaceutical Prep.	Usual Adult Dosage & Food Effect	% Absorbed, po	Serum T½, hrs	CPE*	Elimination	Major Adverse Events/Comments *(See Table 14E)*
E. **Selected Characteristics of Antiretroviral Drugs** (CPE = CSF penetration effectiveness)							
3. **Selected Characteristics of Protease Inhibitors (PIs).** *(continued)*							
Ritonavir (Norvir)	100 mg capsules; 600 mg per 7.5 mL solution. Refrigerate caps but not solution. Room temperature for 1 mo. is OK.	Full dose not recommended *(see comments)*. **With rare exceptions, used exclusively to enhance pharmacokinetics of other PIs, using lower ritonavir doses.**	Food ↑ absorption	3–5	1	Cytochrome P450. Potent 3A4 & 2 d6 inhibitor	Nausea/vomiting/diarrhea, extremity & circumoral paresthesias, hepatitis, pancreatitis, taste perversion, ↑ CPK & uric acid. **Black Box warning**—potentially fatal drug interactions. Many drug interactions— *see Table 22A–Table 22B.*
Saquinavir (Invirase—hard gel caps or tabs) **+ ritonavir**	Saquinavir 200 mg caps, 500 mg film-coated tabs; ritonavir 100 mg caps	[2 tabs saquinavir (1000 mg) + 1 cap ritonavir (100 mg)] po bid with food	Erratic, 4 (saquinavir alone). Much more reliably absorbed when boosted with ritonavir.	1–2	1	Cytochrome P450 (3A4 inhibitor)	Nausea, diarrhea, headache, ↑ AST/ALT. Avoid rifampin with saquinavir + ritonavir: ↑ hepatitis risk. **Black Box warning**—Invirase to be used only with ritonavir. Possible QT prolongation. Use with caution in those with cardiac conduction abnormalities or when used with drugs with similar effects.
Tipranavir (Aptivus)	250 mg caps. Refrigerate unopened bottles. Use opened bottles within 2 mo. 100 mg/mL solution	[500 mg (two 250 mg caps) + ritonavir 200 mg] po bid with food.	Absorption low, ↑ with high fat meal, ↓ with Al^{+++} & Mg^{++} antacids.	5.5-6	1	Cytochrome 3A4 but with ritonavir, most of drug is eliminated in feces.	Contains sulfa moiety. **Black Box warning—reports of fatal/nonfatal intracranial hemorrhage, hepatitis, fatal hepatic failure.** Use cautiously in liver disease, esp. hepB, hepC; contraindicated in Child-Pugh class B-C. Monitor LFTs. Coadministration of certain drugs contraindicated *(see label)*. **For highly ART-experienced pts or for multiple-PI resistant virus.** Do not use tipranavir and etravirine together owing to 76% reduction in etravirine levels.

4. **Selected Characteristics of Fusion Inhibitors**

Generic/ Trade Name	Pharmaceutical Prep.	Usual Adult Dosage	% Absorbed	Serum T½, hrs	CPE*	Elimination	Major Adverse Events/Comments *(See Table 14E)*
Enfuvirtide (T20, Fuzeon)	Single-use vials of 90 mg/mL when reconstituted. Vials should be stored at room temperature. Reconstituted vials can be refrigerated for 24 hrs only.	90 mg (1 mL) subcut. bid. Rotate injection sites, avoiding those currently inflamed.	84	3.8	1	Catabolism to its constituent amino acids with subsequent recycling of the amino acids in the body pool. Elimination pathway(s) have not been performed in humans. Does not alter the metabolism of CYP3A4, CYP2 d6, CYP1A2, CYP2C19 or CYP2E1 substrates.	Local reaction site reactions 98%, 4% discontinue; erythema/induration ~80–90%, nodules/cysts ~80%. **Hypersensitivity reactions reported** (fever, rash, chills, N/V, ↓ BP, &/or ↑ AST/ALT)—do not restart if occur. Including background regimens, peripheral neuropathy 8.9%, insomnia 11.3%, ↓ appetite 6.3%, myalgia 5%, lymphadenopathy 2.3%, eosinophilia ~10%. ↑ incidence of bacterial pneumonias: Alone offers little benefit to a failing regimen *(NEJM 348:2249, 2003)*.

TABLE 14D (12)

Generic/ Trade Name	Pharmaceutical Prep.	Usual Adult Dosage & Food Effect	% Absorbed, po	Serum T½, hrs	CPE*	Elimination	Major Adverse Events/Comments *(See Table 14E)*
E. **Selected Characteristics of Antiretroviral Drugs** (CPE = CSF penetration effectiveness) *(continued)*							
5. **Selected Characteristics of CCR-5 Co-receptor Antagonists**							
Maraviroc (Selzentry)	150 mg, 300 mg film-coated tabs	Without regard to food: - 150 mg bid if concomitant meds include CYP3A inhibitors including PIs (except tipranavir/ritonavir) and delavirdine (with/without CYP3A inducers) - 300 mg bid without significantly interacting meds including NRTIs, tipranavir/ritonavir, neverapine - 600 mg bid if concomitant meds include CYP3A inducers, including efavirenz (without strong CYP3A inhibitors)	Est. 33% with 300 mg dosage	14-18	3	CYP3A and P-glycoprotein substrate. Metabolites (via CYP3A) excreted feces > urine	**Black Box Warning-Hepatotoxicity,** may be preceded by rash, ↑ eos or IgE. NB: no hepatoxicity was noted in MVC trials. Black box inserted owing to concern about potential CCR5 class effect. Data lacking in hepatic/renal insufficiency; ↑ concern with either could ↑ risk of ↓BP. Currently for treatment-experienced patients with multi-resistant strains. **Document CCR-5-tropic virus before use, as treatment failures assoc. with appearance of CXCR-4 or mixed-tropic virus.**
6. **Selected Characteristics of Integrase Inhibitors**							
Raltegravir (Isentress)	400 mg film-coated tabs	400 mg po bid, without regard to food	Unknown	~ 9	3	Glucuronidation via UGT1A1, with excretion into feces and urine. (Therefore does NOT require ritonavir boosting)	For naïve patients and treatment experienced pts with multiply-resistant virus. Well-tolerated. Nausea, diarrhea, headache, fever similar to placebo. CK↑ & rhabdomyolysis reported: unclear relationship. Increased depression in those with a history of depression. Low genetic barrier to resistance. Increase in CPK, myositis, rhabdomyolysis have been reported. Rare Stevens Johnson Syndrome. Better oral absorption if chewed *(CID 57:480, 2013)*.
Elvitegravir/ cobicistat (Stribild)	150 mg - 150 mg	150 mg-150 mg once daily with or without food	<10%	12.9 (Cobi), 3.5 (ELV)	Un-known	The majority of **elvitegravir** metabolism is mediated by CYP3A enzymes. Elvitegravir also undergoes glucuronidation via UGT1A1/3 enzymes. **Cobicistat** is metabolized by CYP3A and to a minor extent by CYP2D6	For both treatment naive patients and treatment experienced pts with multiply-resistant virus. Generally well-tolerated. Use of cobicistat increases serum creatinine by ~ 0.1 mg/dl via inhibition of proximal tubular enzyme; this does not result in reduction in true GFR but will result in erroneous apparent reduction in eGFR by MDRD or Cockcroft Gault calculations. Usual AEs are similar to those observed with ritonavir (cobi) and tenofovir/FTC.
Dolutegravir (Tivicay)	50 mg	50 mg po once daily 50 mg po BID (if STII resistance present or if co-admin with EFV, FOS, TIP, or Rif	Unknown	14	4	Glucuronidation via UGT1A1 (therefore does not require ritonavir or cobicistat boosting)	Hypersensitivity (rare); Most common: insomnia (3%) headache (2%), N/V (1%), rash (<1%). Watch for IRIS; Watch for elevated LFTs in those with HCV

* **CPE (CNS Penetration Effectiveness) value:** 1= Low Penetration; 2 - 3 = Intermediate Penetration; 4 = Highest Penetration into CNS *(Letendre, et al, CROI 2010, abs #430)*

TABLE 14D (13)

F. **Other Considerations in Selection of Therapy**

Caution: Initiation of ART may result in immune reconstitution syndrome with significant clinical consequences. *See Table 11B, of SANFORD GUIDE TO HIV/AIDS THERAPY (AIDS Reader 16:199, 2006).*

1. Resistance testing: Given current rates of resistance, resistance testing is recommended in all patients prior to initiation of therapy, including those with acute infection syndrome (may initiate therapy while waiting for test results and adjusting Rx once results return), at time of change of therapy owing to antiretroviral failure, when suboptimal virologic response is observed, and in pregnant women. **Resistance testing NOT recommended if pt is off ART for > 4 weeks or if HIV RNA is < 1000 c/mL.** *See Table 6F of SANFORD GUIDE TO HIV/AIDS THERAPY.*
2. Drug-induced disturbances of glucose & lipid metabolism *(see Table 14E)*
3. Drug-induced lactic acidosis & other FDA "box warnings" *(see Table 14E)*
4. Drug-drug interactions *(see Table 22B)*
5. Risk in pregnancy *(see Table 8)*
6. Use in women & children *(see Table 14D)*
7. Dosing in patients with renal or hepatic dysfunction *(see Table 17A & Table 17B)*

TABLE 14E– ANTIRETROVIRAL DRUGS & ADVERSE EFFECTS
(www.aidsinfo.nih.gov)
See also www.aidsinfo.nih.gov; for combinations, see individual components

DRUG NAME(S): GENERIC (TRADE)	MOST COMMON ADVERSE EFFECTS	MOST SIGNIFICANT ADVERSE EFFECTS
Nucleoside Reverse Transcriptase Inhibitors (NRTI) Black Box warning for all nucleoside/nucleotide RTIs: lactic acidosis/hepatic steatosis, potentially fatal. Also carry Warnings that fat redistribution and immune reconstitution syndromes (including autoimmune syndromes with delayed onset) have been observed		
Abacavir (Ziagen)	Headache 7–13%, nausea 7–19%, diarrhea 7%, malaise 7-12%	**Black Box warning-Hypersensitivity reaction (HR)** in 8% with malaise, fever, GI upset, rash, lethargy & respiratory symptoms most commonly reported; myalgia, arthralgia, edema, paresthesia less common. **Discontinue immediately if HR suspected. Rechallenge contraindicated; may be life-threatening.** Severe HR may be more common with once-daily dosing. **HLA-B*5701 allele** predicts ↑ risk of HR in Caucasian pop.; excluding pts with B*5701 markedly ↓'d HR incidence *(NEJM 358:568, 2008; CID 46:1111-1118, 2008)*. DHHS guidelines recommend testing for B*5701 and use of abacavir-containing regimens only if HLA-B*5701 negative; Vigilance essential in all groups. Possible increased risk of MI with use of abacavir had been suggested *(JID 201:318, 2010)*. Other studies found no increased risk of MI *(CID 52: 929, 2011)*. A meta-analysis of randomized trials by FDA also did not show increased risk of MI *(www.fda.gov/drugs/drugsafety/ucm245164.htm)*. Nevertheless, care is advised to optimize potentially modifiable risk factors when abacavir is used.
Didanosine (ddI) (Videx)	Diarrhea 28%, nausea 6%, rash 9%, headache 7%, fever 12%, hyperuricemia 2%	**Pancreatitis 1–9%. Black Box warning—Cases of fatal & nonfatal pancreatitis** have occurred in pts receiving ddI, especially when used in combination with d4T or d4T + hydroxyurea. Fatal lactic acidosis in pregnancy with ddI + d4T. Peripheral neuropathy in 20%, 12% required dose reduction. ↑ toxicity if used with ribavirin. Use with TDF generally avoided (but would require dose reduction of ddI) because of ↑ toxicity and possible ↓ efficacy; may result in ↓ CD4. Rarely, retinal changes or optic neuropathy. Diabetes mellitus and rhabdomyolysis reported in post-marketing surveillance. Possible increased risk of MI under study *(www.fda.gov/CDER; JID 201:318, 2010)*. Non-cirrhotic portal hypertension with ascites, varices, splenomegaly reported in post-marketing surveillance. *See also Clin Infect Dis 49:626, 2009; Amer J Gastroenterol 104:1707, 2009.*
Emtricitabine (FTC) (Emtriva)	Well tolerated. Headache, diarrhea, nausea, rash, skin hyperpigmentation	Potential for lactic acidosis (as with other NRTIs). Also **in Black Box—severe exacerbation of hepatitis B on stopping drug reported—monitor clinical/labs for several months after stopping in pts with hepB.** Anti-HBV rx may be warranted if FTC stopped.
Lamivudine (3TC) (Epivir)	Well tolerated. Headache 35%, nausea 33%, diarrhea 18%, abdominal pain 9%, insomnia 11% (all in combination with ZDV). Pancreatitis more common in pediatrics.	**Black Box warning.** Make sure to use HIV dosage, not Hep B dosage. **Exacerbation of hepatitis B on stopping drug. Patients with hepB who stop lamivudine require close clinical/lab monitoring for several months.** Anti-HBV rx may be warranted if 3TC stopped.
Stavudine (d4T) (Zerit)	Diarrhea, nausea, vomiting, headache	**Peripheral neuropathy** 15–20%. Pancreatitis 1%. Appears to produce lactic acidosis, hepatic steatosis and lipoatrophy/lipodystrophy more commonly than other NRTIs. **Black Box warning—Fatal & nonfatal pancreatitis with d4T + ddI.** Use with TDF generally avoided (but would require dose reduction of ddI) because of ↑ toxicity and possible ↓ efficacy; may result in ↓ CD4. Rarely, retinal changes or optic neuropathy. Diabetes mellitus and rhabdomyolysis reported in post-marketing surveillance. **Fatal lactic acidosis/steatosis in pregnant women receiving d4T + ddI.** Fatal and non-fatal lactic acidosis and severe hepatic steatosis can occur in others receiving d4T. Use with particular caution in patients with risk factors for liver disease, but lactic acidosis can occur even in those without known risk factors. Possible ↑ toxicity if used with ribavirin. Motor weakness in the setting of lactic acidosis mimicking the clinical presentation of Guillain-Barré syndrome (including respiratory failure) (rare).
Zidovudine (ZDV, AZT) (Retrovir)	Nausea 50%, anorexia 20%, vomiting 17%, **headache 62%.** Also reported: asthenia, insomnia, myalgias, nail pigmentation. Macrocytosis expected with all dosage regimens.	**Black Box warning—hematologic toxicity, myopathy. Anemia** (<8 gm, 1%), granulocytopenia (<750, 1.8%). Anemia may respond to epoetin alfa if endogenous serum erythropoietin levels are ≤500 milliUnits/mL. Possible ↑ toxicity if used with ribavirin. Co-administration with Ribavirin not advised. Hepatic decompensation may occur in HIV/HCV co-infected patients receiving zidovudine with interferon alfa ± ribavirin.

TABLE 14E (2)

DRUG NAME(S): GENERIC (TRADE)	MOST COMMON ADVERSE EFFECTS	MOST SIGNIFICANT ADVERSE EFFECTS
Nucleotide Reverse Transcriptase Inhibitor (NtRTI) Black Box warning for all nucleoside/nucleotide RTIs: lactic acidosis/hepatic steatosis, potentially fatal. Also carry Warnings that fat redistribution and immune reconstitution syndromes (including autoimmune syndromes with delayed onset) have been observed *(continued)*		
Tenofovir disoproxil fumarate (TDF) (Viread)	Diarrhea 11%, nausea 8%, vomiting 5%, flatulence 4% (generally well tolerated)	**Black Box Warning—Severe exacerbations of hepatitis B reported in pts who stop tenofovir.** Monitor carefully if drug is stopped; anti-HBV rx may be warranted if TDF stopped. Reports of renal injury from TDF, including Fanconi syndrome *(CID 37:e174, 2003; J AIDS 35:269,204; CID 42:283, 2006)*. Fanconi syndrome and diabetes insipidus reported with TDF + ddI *(AIDS Reader 19:114, 2009)*. Modest decline in renal function appears greater with TDF than with NRTIs (CID 51:296, 2010) and may be greater in those receiving TDF with a PI instead of an NNRTI *(JID 197:102, 2008; AIDS 26:567, 2012)*. In a VA study that followed >10,000 HIV-infected individuals, TDF exposure was significantly associated with increased risk of proteinuria, a more rapid decline in renal function and chronic kidney disease *(AIDS 26:867, 2012)*. Monitor Ccr, serum phosphate and urinalysis, especially carefully in those with pre-existing renal dysfunction or nephrotoxic medications. TDF also appears to be associated with increased risk of bone loss. In a substudy of an ACTG comparative treatment trial, those randomized to TDF-FTC experienced greater decreases in spine and hip bone mineral density (BMD) at 96 weeks compared with those treated with ABC-3TC *(JID 203:1791, 2011)*. Consider monitoring BMD in those with history of pathologic fractures, or who have risks for osteoporosis or bone loss.
Non-Nucleoside Reverse Transcriptase Inhibitors (NNRTI). Labels caution that fat redistribution and immune reconstitution can occur with ART.		
Delavirdine (Rescriptor)	Nausea, diarrhea, vomiting, headache	**Skin rash** has occurred in 18%; can continue or restart drug in most cases. Stevens-Johnson syndrome & erythema multiforme have been reported rarely. ↑ in liver enzymes in <5% of patients.
Efavirenz (Sustiva)	**CNS side effects 52%;** symptoms include dizziness, insomnia, somnolence, impaired concentration, psychiatric sx, & abnormal dreams; symptoms are worse after 1st or 2nd dose & improve over 2–4 weeks; discontinuation rate 2.6%. Rash 26% (vs. 17% in comparators); often improves with oral antihistamines; discontinuation rate 1.7%. Can cause false-positive urine test results for cannabinoid with CEDIA DAU multi-level THC assay. Metabolite can cause false-positive urine screening test for benzodiazepines *(CID 48:1787, 2009)*.	**Caution:** CNS effects may impair driving and other hazardous activities. Serious neuropsychiatric symptoms reported, including severe depression (2.4%) & suicidal ideation (0.7%). Elevation in liver enzymes. Fulminant hepatic failure has been reported *(see FDA label)*. **Teratogenicity reported in primates; pregnancy category D—may cause fetal harm, avoid in pregnant women or those who might become pregnant.** NOTE: No single method of contraception is 100% reliable. Barrier + 2nd method of contraception advised, continued 12 weeks after stopping efavirenz. Contraindicated with certain drugs metabolized by CYP3A4. Slow metabolism in those homozygous for the CYP-2B6 G516T allele can result in exaggerated toxicity and intolerance. This allele much more common in blacks and women *(CID 42:408, 2006)*. Stevens-Jonson syndrome and erythema multiforme reported in post-marketing surveillance.
Etravirine (Intelence)	Rash 9%, generally mild to moderate and spontaneously resolving; 2% dc clinical trials for rash. More common in women. Nausea 5%.	Severe rash (erythema multiforme, toxic epidermal necrolysis, Stevens-Johnson syndrome) has been reported. Hypersensitivity reactions can occur with rash, constitutional symptoms and organ dysfunction, including hepatic failure *(see FDA label)*. Potential for CYP450-mediated drug interactions. Rhabdomyolysis has been reported in post-marketing surveillance.
Nevirapine (Viramune)	**Rash 37%:** usually occurs during 1st 6 wks of therapy. Follow recommendations for 14-day lead-in period to ↓ risk of rash *(see Table 14D)*. Women experience 7-fold ↑ in risk of severe rash *(CID 32:124, 2001)*. 50% resolve within 2 wks of dc drug & 80% by 1 month. 6.7% discontinuation rate.	**Black Box warning—Severe life-threatening skin reactions reported:** Stevens-Johnson syndrome, toxic epidermal necrolysis, & hypersensitivity reaction or drug rash with eosinophilia & systemic symptoms (DRESS) *(ArIM 161:2501, 2001)*. For severe rashes, dc drug immediately & do not restart. In a clinical trial, the use of prednisone ↑ the risk of rash. **Black Box warning—Life-threatening hepatotoxicity reported,** 2/3 during the first 12 wks of rx. Overall 1% develops hepatitis. Pts with pre-existing ↑ in ALT or AST &/or history of chronic Hep B or C ↑ susceptible *(Hepatol 35:182, 2002)*. Women with CD4 >250, including pregnant women, at ↑ risk. Avoid in this group unless no other option. Men with CD4 >400 also at ↑ risk. Monitor pts intensively (clinical & LFTs), esp. during the first 12 wks of rx. If clinical hepatotoxicity, severe skin or hypersensitivity reactions occur, dc drug & never rechallenge.

TABLE 14E (3)

DRUG NAME(S): GENERIC (TRADE)	MOST COMMON ADVERSE EFFECTS	MOST SIGNIFICANT ADVERSE EFFECTS
Non-Nucleoside Reverse Transcriptase Inhibitors (NNRTI) *(continued)*		
Rilpivirine (Edurant)	Headache (3%), rash (3%; led to discontinuation in 0.1%), insomnia (3%), depressive disorders (4%). Psychiatric disorders led to discontinuation in 1%. Increased liver enzymes observed.	Drugs that induce CYP3A or increase gastric pH may decrease plasma concentration of rilpivirine and co-administration with rilpivirine should be avoided. Among these are certain anticonvulsants, rifamycins, PPIs, dexamethasone and St. John's wort. At supra-therapeutic doses, rilpivirine can increase QTc interval; use with caution with other drugs known to increase QTc. May cause depressive disorder, including suicide attempts or suicidal ideation. Overall, appears to cause fewer neuropsychiatric side effects than efavirenz *(JAIDS 60:33, 2012)*.
Protease inhibitors (PI) Diarrhea is common AE (**crofelemer** 125 mg bid may help, but expensive). Abnormalities in glucose metabolism, dyslipidemias, fat redistribution syndromes are potential problems. Pts taking PI may be at increased risk for developing osteopenia/osteoporosis. Spontaneous bleeding episodes have been reported in HIV+ pts with hemophilia being treated with PI. Rheumatoid complications have been reported *(An Rheum Dis 61:82, 2002)*. Potential for QTc prolongation *(Lancet 365:682, 2005)*. **Caution for all PIs**—Coadministration with drugs dependent on CYP3A or other enzymes for elimination & for which ↑ levels can cause serious toxicity may be contraindicated. ART may result in immune reconstitution syndromes, which may include early or late presentations of autoimmune syndromes. Increased premature births among women receiving ritonavir-boosted PIs as compared with those receiving other antiretroviral therapy, even after accounting for other potential risk factors *(CID 54: 1348, 2012)*.		
Atazanavir (Reyataz)	Asymptomatic unconjugated hyperbilirubinemia in up to 60% of pts, jaundice in 7–9% [especially with Gilbert syndrome *(JID 192: 1381, 2005)*]. Moderate to severe events: Diarrhea 1–3%, nausea 6–14%, abdominal pain 4%, headache 6%, rash 20%.	Prolongation of PR interval (1st degree AV block in 5-6%) reported; rarely 2° AV block. QTc increase and torsades reported *(CID 44:e67, 2007)*. Acute interstitial nephritis *(Am J Kid Dis 44:E81, 2004)* and urolithiasis (atazanavir stones) reported *(AIDS 20:2131, 2006; NEJM 355:2158, 2006)*. Potential ↑ transanimases in pts co-infected with HBV or HCV. Severe skin eruptions (Stevens-Johnson syndrome, erythema multiforme, and toxic eruptions, or DRESS syndrome) have been reported.
Darunavir (Prezista)	With background regimens, headache 15%, nausea 18%, diarrhea 20%, ↑ amylase 17%. Rash in 10% of treated; 0.5% discontinuation.	Hepatitis in 0.5%, some with fatal outcome. Use caution in pts with HBV or HCV co-infections or other hepatic dysfunction. Monitor for clinical symptoms and LFTs. Stevens-Johnson syndrome, toxic epidermal necrolysis, erythema multiforme. Contains sulfa moiety. Potential for major drug interactions. May cause failure of hormonal contraceptives.
Fosamprenavir (Lexiva)	Skin rash ~ 20% (moderate or worse in 3–8%), nausea, headache, diarrhea.	Rarely Stevens-Johnson syndrome, hemolytic anemia. Pro-drug of amprenavir. Contains sulfa moiety. Angioedema and nephrolithiasis reported in post-marketing experience. Potential increased risk of MI *(see FDA label)*. Angioedema, oral paresthesias, myocardial infarction and nephrolithiasis reported in post-marketing experience. Elevated LFTs seen with higher than recommended doses; increased risk in those with pre-existing liver abnormalities. Acute hemolytic anemia reported with amprenavir.
Indinavir (Crixivan)	↑ in indirect bilirubin 10–15% (≥2.5 mg/dl, with overt jaundice especially likely in those with Gilbert syndrome *(JID 192: 1381, 2005)*. Nausea 12%, vomiting 4%, diarrhea 5%. Metallic taste. Paronychia and ingrown toenails reported *(CID 32:140, 2001)*.	**Kidney stones.** Due to indinavir crystals in collecting system. Nephrolithiasis in 12% of adults, higher in pediatrics. Minimize risk with good hydration (at least 48 oz. water/day) *(AAC 42:332, 1998)*. Tubulointerstitial nephritis/renal cortical atrophy reported in association with asymptomatic ↑ urine WBC. Severe hepatitis reported in 3 cases *(Ln 349:924, 1997)*. Hemolytic anemia reported.
Lopinavir/Ritonavir (Kaletra)	GI: **diarrhea** 14–24%, nausea 2–16%. More diarrhea with q24h dosing.	Lipid abnormalities in up to 20–40%. Possible increased risk of MI with cumulative exposure *(JID 201:318, 2010)*. ↑ PR interval, 2° or 3° heart block described. Post-marketing reports of ↑ QTc and torsades: avoid use in congenital QTc prolongation or in other circumstances that prolong QTc or increase susceptibility to torsades. Hepatitis, with hepatic decompensation; caution especially in those with pre-existing liver disease. Pancreatitis. Inflammatory edema of legs *(AIDS 16:673, 2002)*. Stevens-Johnson syndrome & erythema multiforme reported. Note high drug concentration in oral solution. Toxic potential of oral solution (contains ethanol and propylene glycol) in neonates.
Nelfinavir (Viracept)	Mild to moderate **diarrhea** 20%. Oat bran tabs, calcium, or oral anti-diarrheal agents (e.g., loperamide, diphenoxylate/atropine sulfate) can be used to manage diarrhea.	Potential for drug interactions. Powder contains phenylalanine.

TABLE 14E (4)

DRUG NAME(S): GENERIC (TRADE)	MOST COMMON ADVERSE EFFECTS	MOST SIGNIFICANT ADVERSE EFFECTS
Protease Inhibitors (PI) *(continued)*		
Ritonavir (Norvir) (Currently, primary use is to enhance levels of other anti-retrovirals, because of ↑ toxicity/ interactions with full-dose ritonavir)	GI: bitter aftertaste ↓ by taking with chocolate milk, Ensure, or Advera; nausea 23%, ↓ by initial dose esc (titration) regimen; vomiting 13%; diarrhea 15%. Circumoral paresthesias 5–6%. Dose >100 mg bid assoc. with ↑ GI side effects & ↑ in lipid abnormalities.	**Black Box** warning relates to many important drug-drug interactions—inhibits P450 CYP3A & CYP2 D6 system—may be life-threatening *(see Table 22A)*. Several cases of iatrogenic Cushing's syndrome reported with concomitant use of ritonavir and corticosteroids, including dosing of the latter by inhalation, epidural injection or a single IM injection. Rarely Stevens-Johnson syndrome, toxic epidermal necrolysis anaphylaxis. Primary A-V block (and higher) and pancreatitis have been reported. Hepatic reactions, including fatalities. Monitor LFTs carefully during therapy, especially in those with pre-existing liver disease, including HBV and HCV.
Saquinavir (Invirase: hard cap, tablet)	**Diarrhea,** abdominal discomfort, nausea, headache	**Warning—Use Invirase only with ritonavir.** Avoid garlic capsules (may reduce SQV levels) and use cautiously with proton-pump inhibitors (increased SQV levels significant. Use of saquinavir/ritonavir can prolong QTc interval or may rarely cause 2° or 3° heart block; torsades reported. Contraindicated in patients with prolonged QTc or those taking drugs or who have other conditions (e.g., low K+ or Mg++) that pose a risk with prolonged QTc *(http://www.fda.gov/drugs/DrugSafety/ucm230096.htm, accessed May 25, 2011)*. Contraindicated in patients with complete AV block, or those at risk, who do not have pacemaker. Hepatic toxicity encountered in patients with pre-existing liver disease or in individuals receiving concomitant rifampin. Rarely, Stevens Johnson syndrome.
Tipranavir (Aptivus)	Nausea & vomiting, diarrhea, abdominal pain. Rash in 8-14%, more common in women, & 33% in women taking ethinyl estradiol. Major lipid effects.	**Black Box Warning—associated with hepatitis & fatal hepatic failure.** Risk of hepatotoxicity increased in hepB or hepC co-infection. Possible photosensitivity skin reactions. Contraindicated in Child-Pugh Class B or C hepatic impairment. **Associated with fatal/nonfatal intracranial hemorrhage (can inhibit platelet aggregation).** Caution in those with bleeding risks. Potential for major drug interactions. Contains sulfa moiety and vitamin E.
Fusion Inhibitor		
Enfuvirtide (T20, Fuzeon)	Local injection site reactions (98% at least 1 local ISR, 4% dc because of ISR) (pain & discomfort, induration, erythema, nodules & cysts, pruritus, & ecchymosis). Diarrhea 32%, nausea 23%, fatigue 20%.	↑ Rate of bacterial pneumonia (3.2 pneumonia events/100 pt yrs), **hypersensitivity reactions** ≤1% (rash, fever, nausea & vomiting, chills, rigors, hypotension, & ↑ serum liver transaminases); can occur with reexposure. Cutaneous amyloid deposits containing enfuvirtide peptide reported in skin plaques persisting after discontinuation of drug *(J Cutan Pathol 39:220, 2012)*.
CCR5 Co-receptor Antagonists		
Maraviroc (Selzentry)	With ARV background: Cough 13%, fever 12%, rash 10%, abdominal pain 8%. Also, dizziness, myalgia, arthralgias. ↑ Risk of URI, HSV infection.	**Black box warning-Hepatotoxicity.** May be preceded by allergic features (rash, ↑eosinophils or ↑IgE levels). Use with caution in pt with HepB or C. Cardiac ischemia/infarction in 1.3%. May cause ↓BP, orthostatic syncope, especially in patients with renal dysfunction. Significant interactions with CYP3A inducers/inhibitors. Long-term risk of malignancy unknown. Stevens-Johnson syndrome reported post-marketing. Generally favorable safety profile during trial of ART-naïve individuals *(JID 201: 803, 2010)*.
Integrase Inhibitors		
Raltegravir (Isentress)	Diarrhea, headache, insomnia, nausea. LFT ↑ may be more common in pts co-infected with HBV or HCV.	Hypersensitivity reactions can occur. Rash, Stevens-Johnson syndrome, toxic epidermal necrolysis reported. Hepatic failure reported. ↑CK, myopathy and rhabdomyolysis reported *(AIDS 22:1382, 2008)*. ↑ of preexisting depression reported in 4 pts; all could continue raltegravir after adjustment of psych. meds *(AIDS 22:1890, 2008)*. Chewable tablets contain phenylalanine.
Elvitegravir (Stribild)	Nausea and diarrhea are the two most common AEs. An increase in serum creatinine of 0.1 - 0.15 mg/dl with use of cobicistat (related to inhibition of prox. tubular enzymes, not a true reduction in GFR).	Same Black Box warnings as ritonavir and tenofovir. Rare lactic acidosis syndrome. Owing to renal toxicity, should not initiate Rx when pre-Rx eGFR is < 70 cc/min. Follow serial serum creatinine and urinary protein and glucose. Discontinue drug if serum Cr rises > 0.4 mg/dl above baseline value.

TABLE 14F– HEPATITIS A & HBV TREATMENT

Hepatitis A Virus (HAV) *(Ln 351:1643, 1998)*

1. **Drug/Dosage:** No therapy recommended. If within 2 wks of exposure, IVIG 0.02 mL per kg IM times 1 protective. Hep A vaccine equally effective as IVIG in randomized trial and is emerging as preferred Rx *(NEJM 357:1685, 2007)*.
2. **HAV Superinfection:** 40% of pts with chronic Hepatitis C virus (HCV) infection who developed superinfection with HAV developed fulminant hepatic failure *(NEJM 338:286, 1998)*. Similar data in pts with chronic Hepatitis B virus (HBV) infection that suffer acute HAV *(Ann Trop Med Parasitol 93:745, 1999)*. Hence, need to vaccinate all HBV and HCV pts with HAV vaccine.

HBV Treatment

When to Treat HBV

HBeAg status	HBV DNA: "viral load"	ALT	Fibrosis*	Treatment** IFN = interferon; NUC = nucleoside/ tide analogue	Comments
+	**> 20,000**	**< 2xULN**	**F0 –F2**	Observe	Low efficacy with current Rx; biopsy helpful in determining whether to Rx. Lean toward Rx if older age or + Family Hx HCC
+	**> 20,000**	**< 2x ULN**	**F3-F4**	**Treat: IFN or NUC**	**No IFN if decompensated cirrhosis**
+	**>20,000**	**> 2x ULN**	**Any**	**Treat: IFN or NUC**	INF has higher chance of seroconversion to HBeAg Negative and HBsAg Negative status.
-	**< 2000**	**< 1xULN**	**Any**	Observe	Might Treat if F4; **No IFN if decompensated cirrhosis.**
-	**2000-20,000**	**< 2x ULN**	**F0 – F2**	Observe	
-	**2000-20,000**	**< 2x ULN**	**F3 – F4**	**Treat: NUC or (IFN)**	NUCs favored if HBeAg negative; Treatment duration ill-defined. Certainly > 1 year, likely chronic Rx (indefinitely)
-	**> 20,000**	**> 2xULN**	**Any**	**Treat: NUC or IFN**	NUCs favored if HBeAg negative; Treatment duration chronic / indefinite

Modified from *AASLD HBV Treatment Guidelines (www.aasld.org); Lok/ McMahon, Hepatology .2009; 50. p. 1-36*

* Liver Biopsy or fibrosure assay is helpful in determining when and how to treat

** Treatment options listed below

Treatment Regimens. Single drug therapy is usually sufficient; combination therapy used with HIV co-infection.

	Drug/Dose	Comments
Preferred Regimens	**Pegylated-Interferon-alpha 2a** 180 μg sc once weekly OR **Entecavir** 0.5 mg po once daily OR **Tenofovir** 300 mg po once daily	PEG-IFN: Treat for 48 weeks Entecavir: Do not use Entecavir if Lamivudine resistance present. Entecavir/Tenofovir: Treat for at least 24-48 weeks after seroconversion from HBeAg to anti-HBe. Indefinite chronic therapy for HBeAg negative patients. Renal impairment dose adjustments necessary.
Alternative Regimens	**Lamivudine** 100 mg po once daily OR **Telbivudine** 600 mg po once daily OR **Emtricitabine** 200 mg po once daily (investigational) OR **Adefovir** 10 mg po once daily	These alternative agents are rarely used except in combination. When used, restrict to short term therapy owing to high rates of development of resistance. Not recommended as first-line therapy. Use of Adefovir has mostly been replaced by Tenofovir.
Preferred Regimen for HIV-HBV Co-Infected Patient	**Truvada** (Tenofovir 300 mg + Emtricitabine 200 mg) po once daily + another anti-HIV drug	ALL patients if possible as part of a fully suppressive anti-HIV/anti-HBV regimen. Continue therapy indefinitely.

TABLE 14G– HCV TREATMENT REGIMENS AND RESPONSE

1. **Hepatitis C (HCV) Treatment Setting.** Indications for treatment of HCV must take into account both relative and absolute contraindications. Response to therapy reflects defined terms. Duration of therapy is response guided based on Genotype. Recommended follow-up during and post-treatment.
2. **Indications for Treatment.** New Direct Acting Agents (DAAs) create opportunity for interferon-free treatment. Pegylated interferon (Peg-IFN) remains a preferred regimen with a DAA for certain genotypes (eg. 1a), but for those unable to tolerate IFN or who are ineligible for IFN therapy (see contraindications below), all DAA regimens are the preferred choice. Assuming use of Pegylated Interferon (Peg-IFN) + Ribavirin in the regimen: motivated patient, acute HCV infection,

TABLE 14G (2)

biopsy: chronic hepatitis and significant fibrosis, cryoglobulinemic vasculitis, cryoglobulinemic glomerulonephritis, stable HIV infection, compensated liver disease, acceptable hematologic parameters, creatinine < 1.5 (GFR > 50).

3. **Contraindications for Treatment.** Contraindications (both relative and absolute) also assume use of Pegylated Interferon (Peg-IFN) + Ribavirin in the regimen. In this setting use of an all DAA regimen is recommended for those in whom treatment is desired.
   a. **Relative Contraindications.** Hgb < 10, ANC < 1000, PTLs < 50K, hemodialysis and/or GFR < 50, active substance and alcohol use, anticipated poor compliance, untreated mental health disorder, e.g. depression, stable auto-immune disease, Thalassemia and sickle cell anemia, sarcoidosis, HIV co-infection (CD4 < 200, concurrent zidovudine)
   b. **Absolute Contraindications.** Uncontrolled, active, major psychiatric illness, especially depression; hepatic decompensation (encephalopathy, coagulopathy, ascitis); severe uncontrolled medical disease (DM, CHF, CAD, HTN, TB, cancer); untreated thyroid disease; pregnancy, nursing, child-bearing potential (anticipated pregnancy, no birth control); active untreated autoimmune disease; HIV co-infection (CD4 < 100, concurrent ddI)
4. **Response to Therapy.** Predictors of successful response to therapy include: recent infection with HCV, Genotype 2 or 3 infection, favorable IL-28B haplotype, less severe liver disease on biopsy, HCV viral load < 800,000.
5. **Definitions of Response to Therapy.**

Null	Failure to decrease HCV VL by >2 log at week 12.
Non-Responder	Failure to clear HCV RNA by week 24.
Partial Response	>2 log ↓ HIV RNA by week 12 but not undetectable at week 24.
Early Virologic Response (EVR)	>2 log ↓ at week 12 and undetectable at week 24; **Complete EVR** = undetectable at both week 12 and 24.
Rapid Virologic Response (RVR)	Undetectable by week 4 and sustained through course of Rx
Extended Rapid Virologic Response (eRVR)	New terminology with Direct Acting Agents (DAAs). Undetectable after 4 weeks of DAA treatment (e.g., week 4 for telaprevir or week 8 for boceprevir), with sustained undetectable HCV RNA at weeks 12 and 24.
End of Treatment Response (ETR)	Undetectable at end of treatment.
Relapse	Undetectable at end of therapy (ETR) but rebound (detectable) virus within 24 weeks after therapy stopped.
Sustained Virologic Response (SVR)	CURE! Still undetectable at end of therapy and beyond 24 weeks after therapy is stopped.

6. **HCV Treatment Regimens**
   - Biopsy is a 'gold standard' for staging HCV infection and is helpful in some settings to determine the ideal timing of HCV treatment. When bx not obtained, "non-invasive" tests are often employed to assess the relative probability of advanced fibrosis or cirrhosis. Fibroscan (elastography) is now approved in the US and most of the world as a means of assessing liver fibrosis. Elastography values of > 10 kPa (Kilopascals) correlates with significant fibrosis (F3 or F4 disease).
   - Resistance tests: Genotypic resistance assays are available that can determine polymorphisms associated with reduction in susceptibility to some DAAs (Direct Acting Agents, e.g., protease inhibitors). **However, resistance tests are not routinely recommended since response to therapy is typically still preserved even when resistance conferring mutations are identified for most DAAs.**
   - **IMPORTANT NOTE REGARDING TREATMENT DECISION-MAKING:** Newer drugs are in development. **Emerging data suggest a high probability that newer regimens that spare the use of pegylated Interferon (peg-IFN) and/or Ribavirin (RBV) are quite successful and available now, with more very effective drugs coming on the market.** Therefore, the timing of the decision to initiate HCV therapy needs to be individualized based on: the patient's current clinical status, the viral genotype, the pt's ability to tolerate peg-IFN/RBV based therapies or the availability of newly released DAAs, and the likelihood of disease progression over the next 5 years while newer treatments are developed. The Ultimate Goal for treatment of HCV: no Interferon or Ribavirin, only Direct Acting Agents (DAA). Monitor updates at *webedition.sanfordguide.com or hcvguidelines.org.*

Initial therapy for HCV mono-infection

Genotype	Recommended	Alternative	Comments
1 (1a and 1b)	*For Interferon-eligible patients*: **Peg-INF** (180 μg) SQ weekly + **sofosbuvir** (400 mg) po daily + **ribavirin** (1000 mg to 1200 mg) po daily administered for 12 weeks *For Interferon-ineligible patients*: **Sofosbuvir** (400 mg) po daily + **simeprevir** (150 mg) po daily, with or without **ribavirin** (1000 mg to 1200 mg) po daily, administered for 12 weeks (this regimen may work best for those with cirrhosis)	*For Interferon-eligible patients*: **Simeprevir** (150 mg) po daily (for 12 weeks) + **Peg-INF** (180 μg) SQ weekly + **ribavirin** (1000 mg to 1200 mg) po daily, administered for 24 weeks *For Interferon-ineligible patients*: **Sofosbuvir** (400 mg) po daily + **ribavirin** (1000 mg to 1200 mg) po daily, administered for 24 weeks	The following **regimens are not recommended** for use: - PEG + RBV alone - PEG + RBV + either telaprevir or boceprevir - Monotherapy with PEG, RBV, or any direct acting agent (DAA) - Simeprevir should not be used in treatment of genotype 2 or 3 infection - DO NOT TREAT PATIENTS WITH DE-COMPENSATED CIRRHOSIS
2	**Sofosbuvir** (400 mg) po daily + **ribavirin** (1000 mg to 1200 mg) po daily, administered for 12 weeks	None	

TABLE 14G (3)

Genotype	Recommended	Alternative	Comments
Initial therapy for HCV mono-infection			
3	**Sofosbuvir** (400 mg) po daily + **ribavirin** (1000 mg to 1200 mg) po daily, administered for 24 weeks	**Peg-INF** (180 μg) SQ weekly + **sofosbuvir** (400 mg) po daily + **ribavirin** (1000 mg to 1200 mg) po daily administered for 12 weeks	
4	**Peg-INF** (180 μg) SQ weekly + **sofosbuvir** (400 mg) po daily + **ribavirin** (1000 mg to 1200 mg) po daily administered for 12 weeks *For Interferon-ineligible patients*: **Sofosbuvir** (400 mg) po daily + **ribavirin** (1000 mg to 1200 mg) po daily, administered for 24 weeks	**Simeprevir** (150 mg) po daily for 12 weeks PLUS **Peg-INF** (180 μg) SQ weekly + **ribavirin** (1000 mg to 1200 mg) po daily, both administered for 24 weeks	
5, 6	**Peg-INF** (180 μg) SQ weekly + **sofosbuvir** (400 mg) po daily + **ribavirin** (1000 mg to 1200 mg) po daily administered for 12 weeks	None	
Initial therapy for HCV-HIV co-infection			
1 (1a and 1b)	*For Interferon-eligible patients*: **Peg-INF** (180 μg) SQ weekly + **sofosbuvir** (400 mg) po daily + **ribavirin** (1000 mg to 1200 mg) po daily administered for 12 weeks *For Interferon-ineligible patients*: **Sofosbuvir** (400 mg) po daily + **ribavirin** (1000 mg to 1200 mg) po daily, administered for 24 weeks OR **Sofosbuvir** (400 mg) po daily + simeprevir (150 mg) po daily, with or without **ribavirin** (1000 mg to 1200 mg) po daily, administered for 12 weeks *(See Comment)*	*For Interferon-eligible patients*: **Peg-INF** (180 μg) SQ weekly + **Simeprevir** (150 mg) po daily + **ribavirin** (1000 mg to 1200 mg) po daily, administered for 24 weeks (See Comment)	**Simeprevir:** can only be used with select antiretrovirals: raltegravir, rilpivirine, maraviroc, tenofovir, emtricitabine, lamivudine, and abacavir The following **regimens are not recommended** for use: - PEG + RBV alone - PEG + RBV + either telaprevir or boceprevir - Monotherapy with PEG, RBV, or any direct acting agent (DAA) - Simeprevir should not be used in treatment of genotype 2 or 3 infection - DO NOT TREAT PATIENTS WITH DE-COMPENSATED CIRRHOSIS
2	**Sofosbuvir** (400 mg) po daily + **ribavirin** (1000 mg to 1200 mg) po daily, administered for 12 weeks (patients with cirrhosis may benefit from extension of Rx to 16 weeks)	None	
3	**Sofosbuvir** (400 mg) po daily + **ribavirin** (1000 mg to 1200 mg) po daily, administered for 24 weeks	None	
4,5,6	Not enough experience. If treatment is required, treat the same as for mono-infected patients	None	
Patients with Decompensated Cirrhosis (Initial Therapy)			
Any	**Sofosbuvir** (400 mg) po daily + **ribavirin** (weight based dosing adjusted for creatinine clearance and hemoglobin level) po daily, administered for up to 48 weeks	None	Regimens not recommended: - Any Interferon-based regimen - Monotherapy with PEG, RBV or any DAA
Post Liver Transplant Patients (Initial Therapy)			
1	**Sofosbuvir** (400 mg) po daily + **simeprevir** (150 mg) po daily, with or without **ribavirin** (initial dose 600 mg/day, increased monthly by 200 mg/day as tolerated to weight based dose of 1000 mg [<75 kg] to 1200 mg [≥75 kg] 1200 mg) po daily, administered for 12–24 weeks	None	

TABLE 14G (4)

Initial therapy for HCV mono-infection			
Genotype	**Recommended**	**Alternative**	**Comments**
2, 3	**Sofosbuvir** (400 mg) po daily + **ribavirin** (initial dose 600 mg/day, increased monthly by 200 mg/day as tolerated to weight based dose of 1000 mg [<75 kg] to 1200 mg [≥75 kg] 1200 mg) po daily, administered for 24 weeks	None	
4, 5, 6	Not enough experience to make recommendations; seek expert consultation	None	

TABLE 15A – ANTIMICROBIAL PROPHYLAXIS FOR SELECTED BACTERIAL INFECTIONS*

CLASS OF ETIOLOGIC AGENT/DISEASE/CONDITION	PROPHYLAXIS AGENT/DOSE/ROUTE/DURATION	COMMENTS
Group B streptococcal disease (GBS), neonatal: Approaches to management [CDC Guidelines, *MMWR 59 (RR-10):1, 2010***]:**		
Pregnant women—intrapartum antimicrobial prophylaxis procedures: 1. Screen all pregnant women with vaginal & rectal swab for GBS at 35–37 wks gestation (unless other indications for prophylaxis exist: GBS bacteriuria during this pregnancy or previously delivered infant with invasive GBS disease; even then cultures may be useful for susceptibility testing). Use transport medium; GBS survive at room temp. up to 96 hrs. **Rx during labor if swab culture positive.** 2. Rx during labor if previously delivered infant with invasive GBS infection, or if any GBS bacteriuria during this pregnancy. 3. Rx if GBS status unknown but if any of the following are present: (a) delivery at <37 wks gestation [*see MMWR 59 (RR-10): 1, 2010* algorithms for preterm labor and preterm premature rupture of membranes]; or (b) duration of ruptured membranes ≥18 hrs; or (c) intrapartum temp. ≥100.4°F (≥38.0°C). If amnionitis suspected, broad-spectrum antibiotic coverage should include an agent active vs. group B streptococci. 4. Rx if positive intra-partum NAAT for GBS. 5. Rx not indicated if: negative vaginal/rectal cultures at 35-37 wks gestation or C-section performed before onset of labor with intact amniotic membranes (use standard surgical prophylaxis).		**Regimens for prophylaxis against early–onset group B streptococcal disease in neonate used during labor:** **Penicillin G** 5 million Units IV (initial dose) then 2.5 to 3 million Units IV q4h until delivery Alternative: **Ampicillin** 2 gm IV (initial dose) then 1 gm IV q4h until delivery Penicillin-allergic patients: • Patient not at high risk for anaphylaxis: **Cefazolin** 2 gm IV (initial dose) then 1 gm IV q8h until delivery • Patient at high risk for anaphylaxis from β-lactams: □ If organism is both clindamycin- and erythromycin-susceptible, **or** is erythromycin-resistant, but clindamycin-susceptible confirmed by D-zone test (or equivalent) showing lack of inducible resistance: **Clindamycin** 900 mg IV q8h until delivery □ If susceptibility of organism unknown, lack of inducible resistance to clindamycin has not been excluded, or patient is allergic to clindamycin: **Vancomycin** 1 gm IV q12h until delivery
Neonate of mother given prophylaxis	*See detailed algorithm in MMWR 59 (RR-10):1, 2010.*	
Preterm, premature rupture of the membranes in Group B strep-negative women	(IV **ampicillin** 2 gm q6h + IV **erythromycin** 250 mg q6h) for 48 hrs followed by po **amoxicillin** 250 mg q8h + po **erythromycin** base 333 mg q8h for 5 days. Decreases infant morbidity. *(JAMA 278:989, 1997)* (*Note:* May require additional antibiotics for therapy of specific existing infections)	Antibiotic rx reduced infant respiratory distress syndrome (50.6% to 40.8%, $p = 0.03$), necrotizing enterocolitis (5.8% to 2.3%, $p = 0.03$) and prolonged pregnancy (2.9 to 6.1 days, $p < 0.001$) vs placebo. In 1 large study (4809 pts), po erythromycin rx improved neonatal outcomes vs placebo (11.2% vs 14.4% poor outcomes, $p=0.02$ for single births) but not co-AM-CL or both drugs in combination (both assoc. with ↑ necrotizing enterocolitis) *(Ln 357:979, 2001)*. *(See ACOG discussion, Ob Gyn 102:875, 2003; Practice Bulletin in Ob Gyn 109:1007, 2007; Rev Obstet Gynecol 1:11, 2008; J Obstet Gynecol Can 31:863 & 868, 2009).*
Post-splenectomy bacteremia. Likely agents: Pneumococci (90%), meningococci , H. influenzae type b. Bacteremia due to Enterobacteriaceae, S. aureus, Capnocytophaga spp. and rarely P. aeruginosa described. Also at ↑ risk for fatal malaria, severe babesiosis. Ref: *Redbook Online, 2009. Amer Acad Pediatrics.*	**Immunizations:** Ensure admin. of pneumococcal vaccine, H. influenzae B, & quadrivalent meningococcal vaccines at recommended times. In addition, asplenic children with sickle cell anemia, thalassemia, & perhaps others, daily antimicrobial prophylaxis until at least age 5—*see Comments and Sickle-cell disease (below).* Sepsis due to susceptible organisms may occur despite daily prophylaxis *(J Clin Path 54:214, 2001).*	Antimicrobial prophylaxis until age 5: Amox 20 mg/kg/day or Pen V-K 125 mg bid. Over age 5: Consider Pen V-K 250 mg bid for at least 1 yr in children post-splenectomy. Some recommend prophylaxis for a minimum of 3 yrs or until at least age 18. Maintain immunizations plus self-administer AM-CL with any febrile illness while seeking physician assistance. For self-administered therapy, cefuroxime axetil can be used in the penicillin-allergic pt who is not allergic to cephalosporins; alternatively, respiratory FQ can be considered in beta lactam-allergic pt in appropriate populations. Pen. allergy: TMP-SMX or clarithro are options, but resistance in *S. pneumo* may be significant in some areas, particularly among pen-resistant isolates.

TABLE 15A (2)

CLASS OF ETIOLOGIC AGENT/DISEASE/CONDITION	PROPHYLAXIS AGENT/DOSE/ROUTE/DURATION	COMMENTS
Sexual Exposure		
Sexual assault survivor [likely agents and risks, see *MMWR 59 (RR-12):1, 2010*]. For review of overall care: *NEJM 365:834, 2011*.	[(**Ceftriaxone** 250 mg IM)] + (**Metronidazole** 2 gm po as single dose) + [(**Azithromycin** 1 gm po once) or (**Doxycycline** 100 mg po bid for 7 days)]	• Obtain expert advice re: forensic exam & specimens, pregnancy, physical trauma, psychological support. • Test for gonococci and chlamydia (NAAT) at appropriate sites. Check wet mount for T. vaginalis (and culture), check specimen for bacterial vaginosis and Candida if appropriate. • Serologic evaluation for syphilis, HIV, HBV; HCV not easily transmitted from sexual activity, but consider test in high-risk circumstances *(MMWR 60:945, 2011)*. • Initiate post-exposure protocols for HBV vaccine, HIV post-exposure prophylaxis as appropriate *(see Table 15D)*. • Follow-up exam for STDs in 1-2 weeks; retest if prophylaxis not given initially or if symptomatic. • Follow-up serologies for syphilis, HIV, HBV (and HCV if done) at 6 wks, 3 mos and 6 mos. Notes: Ceftriaxone is preferred over cefixime for treatment of gonorrhoea; the latter is less effective for pharyngeal infection and strains with decreased susceptibility to cephalosporins are beginning to appear: those with decreased susceptibility to cefixime are more prevalent than those with decreased susceptibility to ceftriaxone *(MMWR 60:873, 2011)*. Cefixime 400 mg po once can be used in place of ceftriaxone, if the latter is unavailable *(Derived from CDC STD treatment update MMWR 61:590, 2012)*. Azithromycin is preferred to doxycycline because it also provides activity against some GC with reduced susceptibility to cephalosporins *(MMWR 60:873, 2011)*. In patients highly allergic to cephalosporins, azithromycin 2 gm po once can be used in place of ceftriaxone.
Contact with specific sexually transmitted diseases	See comprehensive guidelines for specific pathogens in *MMWR 59 (RR-10): 1, 2010.*	
Syphilis exposure		Presumptive rx for exposure within 3 mos., as tests may be negative. *See Table 1, page 24.* If exposure occurred > 90 days prior, establish dx or treat empirically *(MMWR 59 (RR-12): 1, 2010)*.
Sickle-cell disease. Likely agent: S. pneumoniae *(see post-splenectomy, above)* Ref.: *2009 Red Book Online, Amer Acad Pediatrics*	Children <5 yrs: **Penicillin V** 125 mg po bid ≥5 yrs: **Penicillin V** 250 mg po bid. (Alternative in children: Amoxicillin 20 mg per kg per day)	Start prophylaxis by 2 mos. *(Pediatrics 106:367, 2000)*; continue until at least age 5. When to d/c must be individualized. Age-appropriate vaccines, including pneumococcal, Hib, influenza, meningococcal. Treating infections, consider possibility of penicillin non-susceptible pneumococci.

TABLE 15B – ANTIBIOTIC PROPHYLAXIS TO PREVENT SURGICAL INFECTIONS IN ADULTS*

2013 Guidelines: Am J Health Syst Pharm 70:195, 2013

General Comments:

- To be optimally effective, antibiotics must be started within 60 minutes of the surgical incision. Vancomycin and FQs may require 1-2 hr infusion time, so start dose 2 hrs before the surgical incision.
- Most applications employ a single preoperative dose or continuation for less than 24 hrs.
- For procedures lasting > 2 half-lives of prophylactic agent, intraoperative supplementary dose(s) may be required.
- Dose adjustments may be desirable in pts with BMI > 30.
- Prophylaxis does carry risk: e.g., C. difficile colitis, allergic reactions
- Active screening for S. aureus nasal colonization and application of chlorhexidine washes and intranasal mupirocin reported as a strategy that decreases surgical site infection
- In general, recommendations are consistent with those of the Surgical Care Improvement Project (SCIP)

Use of Vancomycin:

- For many common prophylaxis indications, vancomycin is considered an alternative to β-lactams in pts allergic to or intolerant of the latter.
- Vancomycin use may be justifiable in centers where rates of post-operative infection with methicillin-resistant staphylococci are high or in pts at high risk for these.

TABLE 15B (2)

- Unlike β-lactams in common use, vancomycin has no activity against gram-negative organisms. **When gram-negative bacteria are a concern following specific procedures, it may be necessary or desirable to add a second agent with appropriate in vitro activity.** This can be done using cefazolin with vancomycin in the non-allergic pt, or in pts intolerant of β-lactams using vancomycin with another gram-negative agent (e.g., aminoglycoside, fluoroquinolone, possibly aztreonam, if pt not allergic; local resistance patterns and pt factors would influence choice).
- Infusion of vancomycin, especially too rapidly, may result in hypotension or other manifestations of histamine release (red person syndrome). Does not indicate an allergy to vancomycin.

TYPE OF SURGERY	PROPHYLAXIS	COMMENTS
Cardiovascular Surgery Antibiotic prophylaxis in cardiovascular surgery has been proven beneficial in the following procedures: • Reconstruction of abdominal aorta • Procedures on the leg that involve a groin incision • Any vascular procedure that inserts prosthesis/foreign body • Lower extremity amputation for ischemia • Cardiac surgery • Permanent Pacemakers *(Circulation 121:458, 2010)* • Heart transplant	**Cefazolin** 1–2 gm IV as a single dose or q8h for 1–2 days or **cefuroxime** 1.5 gm IV as a single dose or q12h for total of 6 gm or **vancomycin** 1 gm IV as single dose or q12h for 1–2 days. For pts weighing > 90 kg, use vanco 1.5 gm IV as a single dose or q12h for 1-2 days. Consider **intranasal mupirocin** evening before, day of surgery & bid for 5 days post-op in pts with pos. nasal culture for S. aureus. Mupirocin resistance has been encountered.	**Timing & duration:** Single infusion just before surgery as effective as multiple doses. No prophylaxis needed for cardiac catheterization. For prosthetic heart valves, customary to stop prophylaxis either after removal of retrosternal drainage catheters or just a 2nd dose after coming off bypass. **Vancomycin** may be preferable in hospitals with ↑ freq of MRSA, in high-risk pts, those colonized with MRSA or for Pen-allergic pts. Clindamycin 900 mg IV is another alternative for Pen-allergic or Vanco-allergic pt.
Gastric, Billiary and Colonic Surgery **Gastroduodenal/Biliary** Gastroduodenal, includes percutaneous endoscopic gastrostomy (high risk only), pancreaticoduodenectomy (Whipple procedure)	**Cefazolin** (1-2 gm IV) or **cefoxitin** (1-2 gm IV) or **cefotetan** (1-2 gm IV) or **ceftriaxone** (2 gm IV) as a single dose (some give additional doses q12h for 2–3 days).	Gastroduodenal (PEG placement): High-risk is marked obesity, obstruction, ↓ gastric acid or ↓ motility.
Biliary, includes laparoscopic cholecystectomy	Low risk, laparoscopic: No prophylaxis Open cholecystectomy: **cefazolin, cefoxitin, cefotetan, ampicillin-sulbactam**	Biliary high-risk or open procedure: age >70, acute cholecystitis, non-functioning gallbladder, obstructive jaundice or common duct stones. With cholangitis, treat as infection, not prophylaxis.
Endoscopic retrograde cholangiopancreatography	No rx without obstruction. If obstruction: **Ciprofloxacin** 500–750 mg po or 400 mg IV 2 hrs prior to procedure or **PIP-TZ** 4.5 gm IV 1 hr prior to procedure	Most studies show that **achieving adequate drainage** will prevent post-procedural cholangitis or sepsis and no further benefit from prophylactic antibiotics; greatest benefit likely when complete drainage cannot be achieved. *See Gastroint Endosc 67:791, 2008; Gut 58:868, 2009.*
Colorectal Recommend combination of: • Mechanical bowel prep • PO antibiotic (See Comment) • IV antibiotic	**Parenteral regimens** (emergency or elective): [**Cefazolin** 1-2 gm IV + **metronidazole** 0.5 gm IV] *(see Comment)* or **cefoxitin** or **cefotetan** 1-2 gm IV (if available) or **Ceftriaxone** 2 gm IV + **Metro** 0.5 gm IV or **ERTA** 1 gm IV Beta-lactam allergy, *see Comment*	**Oral regimens: Neomycin + erythromycin.** Pre-op day: (1) 10 am 4L polyethylene glycol electrolyte solution (Colyte, GoLYTELY) po over 2 hr. (2) Clear liquid diet only. (3) 1 pm, 2 pm & 11 pm, neomycin 1 gm + erythro base 1 gm po. (4) NPO after midnight. Alternative regimens have been less well studied; GoLYTELY 1–6 pm, then neomycin 2 gm po + metronidazole 2 gm po at 7 pm & 11 pm. Oral regimen as effective as parenteral; parenteral in addition to oral not required but often used *(Am J Surg 189:395, 2005)*. Study found **Ertapenem** more effective than cefotetan, but associated with non-significant ↑ risk of C. difficile *(NEJM 355:2640, 2006)*. **Beta lactam allergy: Clindamycin** 900 mg IV + (**Gentamicin** 5 mg/kg or **Aztreonam** 2 gm IV or **Ciprofloxacin** 400 mg IV)
Ruptured viscus: *See Peritoneum/Peritonitis, Secondary, Table 1, page 47.*		

TABLE 15B (3)

TYPE OF SURGERY	PROPHYLAXIS	COMMENTS
Head and Neck Surgery		
	Cefazolin 2 gm IV (Single dose) (some add **metronidazole** 500 mg IV) **OR** **Clindamycin** 600-900 mg IV (single dose) ± **gentamicin** 5 mg/kg IV (single dose) *(See Table 10D for weight-based dose calculation).*	Antimicrobial prophylaxis in head & neck surg appears efficacious only for procedures involving oral/ pharyngeal mucosa (e.g., laryngeal or pharyngeal tumor) but even with prophylaxis, wound infection rate can be high. **Clean, uncontaminated head & neck surg does not require prophylaxis.**
Neurosurgical Procedures		
Clean, non-implant; e.g., elective craniotomy	**Cefazolin** 1-2 gm IV once. Alternative: **vanco** 1 gm IV once; for pts weighing > 90 kg, use vanco 1.5 gm IV as single dose.	Clindamycin 900 mg IV is alternative for vanco-allergic or beta-lactam allergic pt.
Clean, contaminated (cross sinuses, or naso/oropharynx)	**Clindamycin** 900 mg IV (single dose)	British recommend amoxicillin-clavulanate 1.2 gm IV[NUS] or (cefuroxime 1.5 gm IV + metronidazole 0.5 gm IV)
CSF shunt surgery, intrathecal pumps:	**Cefazolin** 1-2 gm IV once. Alternative: **vanco** 1 gm IV once; for pts weighing > 90 kg, use vanco 1.5 gm IV as single dose OR **Clindamycin** 900 mg IV.	Randomized study in a hospital with high prevalence of infection due to methicillin-resistant staphylococci showed vancomycin was more effective than cefazolin in preventing CSF shunt infections *(J Hosp Infect 69:337, 2008).*
Obstetric/Gynecologic Surgery		
Vaginal or abdominal hysterectomy	**Cefazolin** 1–2 gm or **cefoxitin** 1–2 gm or **cefotetan** 1–2 gm or **ampicillin-sulbactam** 3 gm IV 30 min. before surgery.	Alternative: (**Clindamycin** 900 mg IV or **Vancomycin** 1 gm IV) + (**Gentamicin** 5 mg/kg x 1 dose or **Aztreonam** 2 gm IV or **Ciprofloxacin** 400 mg IV) OR (**Metronidazole** 500 mg IV + **Ciprofloxacin** 400 mg IV)
Cesarean section for premature rupture of membranes or active labor	**Cefazolin** 1-2 gm IV *(See Comments).* Alternative: **Clindamycin** 900 mg IV + (**Gentamicin** 5 mg/kg IV or **Tobramycin** 5 mg/kg IV) x 1 dose	Prophylaxis decreases risk of endometritis and wound infection. Traditional approach had been to administer antibiotics after cord is clamped to avoid exposing infant to antibiotic. However, recent studies suggest that administering prophylaxis before the skin incision results in fewer surgical site infections *(Obstet Gynecol 115:187, 2010; Amer J Obstet Gynecol 199:301.e1 and 310:e1, 2008)* and endometritis *(Amer J Obstet Gynecol 196:455.e1, 2007).*
Surgical Abortion (1st trimester)	1st trimester: **Doxycycline** 300 mg po: 100 mg 1 hr before procedure + 200 mg post-procedure.	Meta-analysis showed benefit of antibiotic prophylaxis in all risk groups.
Orthopedic Surgery		
Hip arthroplasty, spinal fusion	Same as cardiac surgery	Customarily stopped after "Hemovac" removed. 2013 Guidelines recommend stopping prophylaxis within 24 hrs of surgery *(Am J Health Syst Pharm 70:195, 2013).*
Total joint replacement (other than hip)	**Cefazolin** 1–2 gm IV pre-op (± 2nd dose) or **vancomycin** 1 gm IV. For pts weighing > 90 kg, use vanco 1.5 gm IV as single dose or **Clindamycin** 900 mg IV.	2013 Guidelines recommends stopping prophylaxis within 24 hrs of surgery *(Am J Health Syst Pharm 70:195, 2013).* Usual to administer before tourniquet inflation. Intranasal mupirocin if colonized with S. aureus.
Open reduction of closed fracture with internal fixation	**Ceftriaxone** 2 gm IV once	3.6% (ceftriaxone) vs 8.3% (for placebo) infection found in Dutch trauma trial *(Ln 347:1133, 1996).* Several alternative antimicrobials can ↓ risk of infection *(Cochrane Database Syst Rev 2010: CD 000244).*

TABLE 15B (4)

TYPE OF SURGERY	PROPHYLAXIS	COMMENTS
Orthopedic Surgery, cont'd prophylaxis to protect prosthetic joints from hematogenous infection related to distant procedures (patients with plates, pins and screws only are not considered to be at risk)	• In 2003, the American Academy of Orthopedic Surgeons (AAOS), in conjunction with the American Dental Association and the American Urological Association, developed *Advisory Statements* on the use of antibiotic prophylaxis to prevent infection of implanted joint prostheses for procedures that may cause bacteremia. (*J Am Dental Assn 134:895, 2003; J Urol 169:1796, 2003*). These documents stratified procedures for risk of bacteremia, described patient factors that might place joints at ↑ risk of infection (incl. all pts in first 2 years after insertion), and offered antibiotic options. *(See also Med Lett 47:59, 2005 and review in Infect Dis Clin N Amer 19:931, 2005).* • A February 2009 *Information Statement* from the AAOS listed patient factors that may ↑ risk of infection, but recommended that antibiotic prophylaxis *be considered* for any invasive procedure that may cause bacteremia in all patients with a joint replacement (*http://aaos.org/about/papers/advistmt/1033.asp*). • The editors believe that the latter approach is excessively broad and exposes many to the risks of antibiotics without definite evidence of benefit. As pointed out in guidelines for prevention of endocarditis, transient bacteremias occur with routine daily activities *(Circulation 2007; 116:1736).* • **A recent prospective, case-control study concluded that antibiotic prophylaxis for dental procedures *did not* decrease the risk of hip or knee prosthesis infection *(Clin Infect Dis 50:8, 2010).*** • For patients with prosthetic joints, infections involving tissue to be manipulated surgically should be treated before surgery whenever possible. Prophylaxis with an anti-staphylococcal β-lactam or vancomycin (according to susceptibility of the organism) for procedures involving tissues colonized by staphylococci would be appropriate, as these organisms are common causes of prosthetic joint infections. In other circumstances, decisions must be based on individual judgment; for now, the 2003 documents cited above appear to provide the best information on which to base such decisions.	
Peritoneal Dialysis Catheter Placement	**Vancomycin** single 1 gm IV dose 12 hrs prior to procedure	Effectively reduced peritonitis during 14 days post-placement in 221 pts: vanco 1%, cefazolin 7%, placebo 12% (p=0.02) *(Am J Kidney Dis 36:1014, 2000).*
Urologic Surgery/Procedures • *See Best Practice Policy Statement* of Amer. Urological Assoc. (AUA) *(J Urol 179:1379, 2008)* and 2013 Guidelines *(Am J Health Syst Pharm 70:195, 2013).* • Selection of agents targeting urinary pathogens may require modification based on local resistance patterns; ↑ TMP-SMX and/or fluoroquinolone (FQ) resistance among enteric gram-negative bacteria is a concern.		
Cystoscopy	• Prophylaxis generally not necessary if urine is sterile (however, AUA recommends FQ or TMP-SMX for those with several potentially adverse host factors (e.g., advanced age, immunocompromised state, anatomic abnormalities, etc.) • Treat patients with UTI prior to procedure using an antimicrobial active against pathogen isolated	
Cystoscopy with manipulation	**Ciprofloxacin** 500 mg po (**TMP-SMX** 1 DS tablet po may be an alternative in populations with low rates of resistance)	Procedures mentioned include ureteroscopy, biopsy, fulguration, TURP, etc. Treat UTI with targeted therapy before procedure if possible.
Transrectal prostate biopsy	**Ciprofloxacin** 500 mg po 12 hrs prior to biopsy and repeated 12 hrs after 1st dose. *See Comment.*	Bacteremia 7% with **CIP** vs 37% with **gentamicin** *(JAC 39:115, 1997).* **Levofloxacin** 500 mg 30-60 min before procedure was effective in low risk pts; additional doses were given for ↑ risk *(J Urol 168:1021, 2002).* Serious bacteremias due to FQ-resistant organisms have been encountered in patients receiving FQ prophylaxis. Clinicians should advise patients to immediately report symptoms suggesting infection. Pre-operative prophylaxis should be determined on an institutional basis based on susceptibility profiles of prevailing organisms. Although 2nd or 3rd generation Cephalosporins or addition of single-dose gentamicin has been suggested, infections due to ESBL-producing and gent-resistant organisms have been encountered *(Urol 74:332, 2009).*
Other		
Breast surgery, herniorrhaphy	**Cefazolin** 1-2 gm IV x 1 dose or **Ampicillin-sulbactam** 3 gm IV x 1 dose or **Clindamycin** 900 mg IV x 1 dose or **Vancomycin** 1 gm IV x 1 dose (1.5 gm if wt > 90 kg)	Benefits of prophylaxis for clean surgical procedures not clear. Antibiotics may reduce risk of surgical site infection in breast cancer surgery (studies not examining immediate reconstruction), but great variability in regimens selected *(Cochrane Database Syst Rev 2006; (2): CD 005360).* For inguinal hernia repair, one analysis found prophylaxis to be beneficial in repairs with mesh *(J Hosp Infect 62: 427, 2006),* while another concluded that antibiotics may reduce risk of infection in pooled population or in those repaired with prosthetic material (mesh), but that the data were not sufficiently strong to make firm recommendations for or against their use universally *(Cochrane Database Syst Rev 2007; (3): CD 003769).*

TABLE 15C – ANTIMICROBIAL PROPHYLAXIS FOR THE PREVENTION OF BACTERIAL ENDOCARDITIS IN PATIENTS WITH UNDERLYING CARDIAC CONDITIONS*

In 2007, the American Heart Association guidelines for the prevention of bacterial endocarditis were updated. The resulting document *(Circulation 2007; 116:1736-1754 and http://circ.ahajournals.org/cgi/reprint/116/15/1736)*, which was also endorsed by the Infectious Diseases Society of America, represents a significant departure from earlier recommendations.

- Antibiotic prophylaxis for dental procedures is now directed at individuals who are likely to suffer the most devastating consequences should they develop endocarditis. Prophylaxis to prevent endocarditis is no longer specified for gastrointestinal or genitourinary procedures. The following is adapted from and reflects the new AHA recommendations. *See original publication for explanation and precise details.*

SELECTION OF PATIENTS FOR ENDOCARDITIS PROPHYLAXIS

FOR PATIENTS WITH ANY OF THESE HIGH-RISK CARDIAC CONDITIONS ASSOCIATED WITH ENDOCARDITIS:	WHO UNDERGO DENTAL PROCEDURES INVOLVING:	WHO UNDERGO INVASIVE RESPIRATORY PROCEDURES INVOLVING:	WHO UNDERGO INVASIVE PROCEDURES OF THE GI OR GU TRACTS:	WHO UNDERGO PROCEDURES INVOLVING INFECTED SKIN AND SOFT TISSUES:
Prosthetic heart valves Previous infective endocarditis Congenital heart disease with any of the following: • Completely repaired cardiac defect using prosthetic material (Only for 1st 6 months) • Partially corrected but with residual defect near prosthetic material • Uncorrected cyanotic congenital heart disease • Surgically constructed shunts and conduits Valvulopathy following heart transplant	Any manipulation of gingival tissue, dental periapical regions, or perforating the oral mucosa. **PROPHYLAXIS RECOMMENDED‡** *(see Dental Procedures Regimens table below)* (Prophylaxis is *not* recommended for routine anesthetic injections (unless through infected area), dental x-rays, shedding of primary teeth, adjustment of orthodontic appliances or placement of orthodontic brackets or removable appliances.)	Incision of respiratory tract mucosa **CONSIDER PROPHYLAXIS** *(see Dental Procedures Regimens table)* Or For treatment of established infection **PROPHYLAXIS RECOMMENDED** *(see Dental Procedures Regimens table for oral flora, but include anti-staphylococcal coverage when S. aureus is of concern)*	PROPHYLAXIS is no longer recommended solely to prevent endocarditis, **but the following approach is reasonable:** For patients with enterococcal UTIs • treat before elective GU procedures • include enterococcal coverage in perioperative regimen for non-elective procedures† For patients with existing GU or GI infections or those who receive peri-operative antibiotics to prevent surgical site infections or sepsis • it is reasonable to include agents with anti-enterococcal activity in perioperative coverage†.	Include coverage against staphylococci and β-hemolytic streptococci in treatment regimens

† Agents with anti-enterococcal activity include penicillin, ampicillin, amoxicillin, piperacillin, vancomycin and others. Check susceptibility if available. *(See Table 5 for highly resistant organisms.)*
‡ 2008 AHA/ACC focused update of guidelines on valvular heart disease use term "is reasonable" to reflect level of evidence *(Circulation 118:887, 2008)*.

PROPHYLACTIC REGIMENS FOR DENTAL PROCEDURES

SITUATION	AGENT	REGIMEN[1]
Usual oral prophylaxis	Amoxicillin	Adults 2 gm, children 50 mg per kg; orally, 1 hour before procedure
Unable to take oral medications	Ampicillin[2]	Adults 2 gm, children 50 mg per kg; IV or IM, within 30 min before procedure.
Allergic to penicillins	Cephalexin[3] OR	Adults 2 gm, children 50 mg per kg; orally, 1 hour before procedure
	Clindamycin OR	Adults 600 mg, children 20 mg per kg; orally, 1 hour before procedure
	Azithromycin or clarithromycin	Adults 500 mg, children 15 mg per kg; orally, 1 hour before procedure
Allergic to penicillins and unable to take oral medications	Cefazolin[3] OR	Adults 1 gm, children 50 mg per kg; IV or IM, within 30 min before procedure
	Clindamycin	Adults 600 mg, children 20 mg per kg; IV or IM, within 30 min before procedure

1 Children's dose should not exceed adult dose. AHA document lists all doses as 30-60 min before procedure.
2 AHA lists cefazolin or ceftriaxone (at appropriate doses) as alternatives here.
3 Cephalosporins should not be used in individuals with immediate-type hypersensitivity reaction (urticaria, angioedema, or anaphylaxis) to penicillins or other β-lactams. AHA proposes ceftriaxone as potential alternative to cefazolin; and other 1st or 2nd generation cephalosporin in equivalent doses as potential alternatives to cephalexin.

TABLE 15D – MANAGEMENT OF EXPOSURE TO HIV-1 AND HEPATITIS B AND C*

OCCUPATIONAL EXPOSURE TO BLOOD, PENILE/VAGINAL SECRETIONS OR OTHER POTENTIALLY INFECTIOUS BODY FLUIDS OR TISSUES WITH RISK OF TRANSMISSION OF HEPATITIS B/C AND/OR HIV-1 (E.G., NEEDLESTICK INJURY)

Free consultation for occupational exposures, call (PEPline) 1-888-448-4911. *[Information also available at www.aidsinfo.nih.gov]*

General steps in management:

1. Wash clean wounds/flush mucous membranes immediately (use of caustic agents or squeezing the wound is discouraged; data lacking regarding antiseptics).
2. Assess risk by doing the following: (a) Characterize exposure; (b) Determine/evaluate source of exposure by medical history, risk behavior, & testing for hepatitis B/C, HIV; (c) Evaluate and test exposed individual for hepatitis B/C & HIV.

Hepatitis B Occupational Exposure Prophylaxis

Exposed Person Vaccine Status	Exposure Source		
	HBs Ag+	**HBs Ag–**	**Status Unknown or Unavailable for Testing**[†]
Unvaccinated	Give HBIG 0.06 mL per kg IM & initiate HB vaccine	Initiate HB vaccine	Initiate HB vaccine
Vaccinated (antibody status unknown)	Do anti-HBs on exposed person: If titer ≥10 milli-International units per mL, no rx If titer <10 milli-International units per mL, give HBIG + 1 dose HB vaccine**	No rx necessary	Do anti-HBs on exposed person: If titer ≥10 milli-International units per mL, no rx If titer <10 milli-International units per mL, give 1 dose of HB vaccine**

[§] Persons previously infected with HBV are immune to reinfection and do not require postexposure prophylaxis.

For known vaccine series responder (titer ≥10 milli-International units per mL), monitoring of levels or booster doses not currently recommended. Known non-responder (<10 milli-International units per mL) to 1° series HB vaccine & exposed to either HBsAg+ source or suspected high-risk source—rx with HBIG & re-initiate vaccine series **or** give 2 doses HBIG 1 month apart. For non-responders after a 2nd vaccine series, 2 doses HBIG 1 month apart is preferred approach to new exposure.

If known high risk source, treat as if source were HBsAG positive
** Follow-up to assess vaccine response or address completion of vaccine series.

Hepatitis B Non-Occupational Exposure & Reactivation of Latent Hepatitis B

Non-Occupational Exposure *(MMWR 59(RR-10):1, 2010)*

- Exposure to blood or sexual secretion of HBsAg-positive person
  - Percutaneous (bite, needlestick)
  - Sexual assault
- Initiate immunoprophylaxis within 24 hrs or sexual exposure & no more than 7 days after parenteral exposure
- Use Guidelines for occupational exposure for use of HBIG and HBV vaccine

TABLE 15D (2)

Hepatitis B Non-Occupational Exposure & Reactivation of Latent Hepatitis B *(continued)*

Reactivation of Latent HBV *(Eur J Cancer 49:3486, 2013; Seminar of Liver Dis 33:167, 2013; Crit Rev Oncol-Hematol 87:12, 2013)*

- Patients requiring administration of anti-CD 20 monoclonal antibodies as part of treatment selected malignancies, rheumatoid arthritis and vasculitis are at risk for reactivation of latent HBV
- Two FDA-approved anti-CD 20 drugs: ofatumumab (Arzerra) & rituximab (Rituxan)
- Prior to starting anti-CD 20 drug, test for latent HBV with test for HBsAg and Anti IgG HB core antibody
- If pt has latent HBV & anti-CD 20 treatment is necessary, treatment should include an effective anti-HBV drug

Hepatitis C Exposure

Determine antibody to hepatitis C for both exposed person &, if possible, exposure source. If source + or unknown and exposed person negative, follow-up HCV testing for HCV RNA (detectable in blood in 1-3 weeks) and HCV antibody (90% who seroconvert will do so by 3 months) is advised. **No recommended prophylaxis;** immune serum globulin not effective. Monitor for early infection, as therapy may ↓ risk of progression to chronic hepatitis. Persons who remain viremic 8-12 weeks after exposure should be treated with a course of pegylated interferon *(Gastro 130:632, 2006 and Hpt 43:923, 2006). See Table 14G*. Case-control study suggested risk factors for occupational HCV transmission include percutaneous exposure to needle that had been in artery or vein, deep injury, male sex of HCW, & was more likely when source VL >6 log10 copies/mL.

HIV: Occupational exposure management *[Adapted from CDC recommendations, MMWR 54 (RR9), 2005, available at www.cdc.gov/mmwr/indrr_2005.html]*

- The decision to initiate postexposure prophylaxis (PEP) for HIV is a clinical judgment that should be made in concert with the exposed healthcare worker (HCW). It is based on:
  1. Likelihood of the source patient having HIV infection: ↑ with history of high-risk activity—injection drug use, sexual activity with known HIV+ person, unprotected sex with multiple partners (either hetero- or homosexual), receipt of blood products 1978–1985. ↑ with clinical signs suggestive of advanced HIV (unexplained wasting, night sweats, thrush, seborrheic dermatitis, etc.).
  2. Type of exposure (approx. 1 in 300–400 needlesticks from infected source will transmit HIV).
  3. Limited data regarding efficacy of PEP *(Cochrane Database Syst Rev. Jan 24; (1):CD002835, 2007).*
  4. Significant adverse effects of PEP drugs & potential for drug interactions.

     Substances considered potentially infectious include: blood, tissues, semen, vaginal secretions, CSF, synovial, pleural, peritoneal, pericardial and amniotic fluids; and other visibly bloody fluids. Fluids normally considered low risk for transmission, unless visibly bloody, include: urine, vomitus, stool, sweat, saliva, nasal secretions, tears and sputum.
- If source person is **known positive for HIV** or **likely to be infected** and **status of exposure warrants PEP,** antiretroviral drugs should be started **immediately.** If source person is HIV antibody negative, drugs can be stopped **unless source is suspected of having acute HIV infection.** The HCW should be re-tested at **3–4 weeks, 3 & 6 months whether PEP is used or not** (the vast majority of seroconversions will occur by 3 months; delayed conversions after 6 months are exceedingly rare). Tests for HIV RNA should not be used for dx of HIV infection in HCW because of false-positives (esp. at low titers) & these tests are only approved for established HIV infection [a possible exception is if pt develops signs of acute HIV (mononucleosis-like) syndrome within the 1st 4–6 wks of exposure when antibody tests might still be negative.]
- PEP for HIV is usually given for **4 wks** and monitoring of adverse effects recommended: baseline **complete blood count, renal and hepatic panel** to be **repeated at 2 weeks.** 50–75% of HCW on PEP demonstrates mild side-effects (nausea, diarrhea, myalgias, headache, etc.) but in up to ½ severe enough to discontinue PEP. Consultation with infectious diseases/ HIV specialist valuable when questions regarding PEP arise. **Seek expert help in special situations, such as pregnancy, renal impairment, treatment-experienced source.**

TABLE 15D (3)

3 Steps to HIV Postexposure Prophylaxis (PEP) After Occupational Exposure: *[Latest CDC recommendations available at www.aidsinfo.nih.gov]*

Step 1: Determine the exposure code (EC)

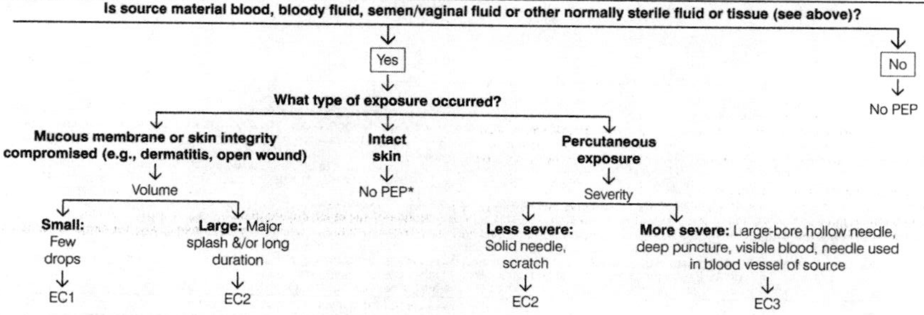

Is source material blood, bloody fluid, semen/vaginal fluid or other normally sterile fluid or tissue (see above)?

→ Yes → **What type of exposure occurred?**

- **Mucous membrane or skin integrity compromised (e.g., dermatitis, open wound)** → Volume
  - **Small:** Few drops → EC1
  - **Large:** Major splash &/or long duration → EC2
- **Intact skin** → No PEP*
- **Percutaneous exposure** → Severity
  - **Less severe:** Solid needle, scratch → EC2
  - **More severe:** Large-bore hollow needle, deep puncture, visible blood, needle used in blood vessel of source → EC3

→ No → No PEP

* *Exceptions can be considered when there has been prolonged, high-volume contact.*

Step 2: Determine the HIV Status Code (HIV SC)

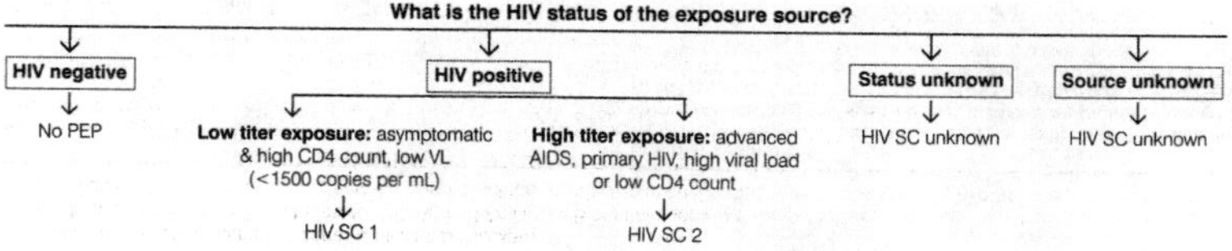

What is the HIV status of the exposure source?

- **HIV negative** → No PEP
- **HIV positive**
  - **Low titer exposure:** asymptomatic & high CD4 count, low VL (<1500 copies per mL) → HIV SC 1
  - **High titer exposure:** advanced AIDS, primary HIV, high viral load or low CD4 count → HIV SC 2
- **Status unknown** → HIV SC unknown
- **Source unknown** → HIV SC unknown

TABLE 15D (4)

3 Steps to HIV Postexposure Prophylaxis (PEP) After Occupational Exposure *(continued)*

Step 3: Determine Postexposure Prophylaxis (PEP) Recommendation

EC	HIV SC	PEP
1	1	Consider basic regimen[a]
1	2	Recommend basic regimen[a,b]
2	1	Recommend basic regimen[b]
2	2	Recommend expanded regimen
3	1 or 2	Recommend expanded regimen
1, 2, 3	Unknown	If exposure setting suggests risks of HIV exposure, consider basic regimen[c]

[a] Based on estimates of ↓ risk of infection after mucous membrane exposure in occupational setting compared with needlestick.
[b] Or, consider expanded regimen[1].
[c] In high risk circumstances, consider expanded regimen[1] on case-by-case basis.

Around the clock, urgent expert consultation available from: National Clinicians' Postexposure Prophylaxis Hotline (PEPline) at 1-888-448-4911 (1-888-HIV-4911) and on-line at http://www.ucsf.edu/hivcntr

Regimens: (Treat for 4 weeks; monitor for drug side-effects every 2 weeks)

Basic regimen: ZDV + 3TC, or **FTC + TDF**, or as an alternative **d4T + 3TC.**

Expanded regimen: Basic regimen + one of the following: lopinavir/ritonavir *(preferred)*, or *(as alternatives)* atazanavir/ritonavir or fosamprenavir/ritonavir. Efavirenz can be considered (except in pregnancy or potential for pregnancy—**Pregnancy Category D**), but CNS symptoms might be problematic. [**Do not use nevirapine;** serious adverse reactions including hepatic necrosis reported in healthcare workers.]

Other regimens can be designed. If possible, use antiretroviral drugs for which resistance is unlikely based on susceptibility data or treatment history of source pt (if known). Seek expert consultation if ART-experienced source or in pregnancy or potential for pregnancy.

NOTE: Some authorities feel that an expanded regimen should be employed whenever PEP is indicated. Expanded regimens are likely to be advantageous with ↑ numbers of ART-experienced source pts or when there is doubt about exact extent of exposures in decision algorithm. Mathematical model suggests that under some conditions, completion of full course basic regimen is better than prematurely discontinued expanded regimen. However, while expanded PEP regimens have ↑ adverse effects, there is not necessarily ↑ discontinuation.

POSTEXPOSURE PROPHYLAXIS FOR NON-OCCUPATIONAL EXPOSURES TO HIV-1
[Adapted from CDC recommendations, MMWR 54 (RR2), 2005, available at www.cdc.gov/mmwr/indrr_2005.html]

Because the risk of transmission of HIV via sexual contact or sharing needles by injection drug users may reach or exceed that of occupational needlestick exposure, it is reasonable to consider PEP in persons who have had a non-occupational exposure to blood or other potentially infected fluids (e.g., genital/rectal secretions, breast milk) from an HIV+ source. Risk of HIV acquisition per exposure varies with the act (for needle sharing and receptive anal intercourse, ≥0.5%; approximately 10-fold lower with insertive vaginal or anal intercourse, 0.05–0.07%). Overt or occult traumatic lesions may ↑ risk in survivors of sexual assault.

For pts at risk of HIV acquisition through non-occupational exposure to HIV+ source material having occurred ≤72 hours before evaluation, DHHS recommendation is to treat for 28 days with an antiretroviral **expanded regimen,** using preferred regimens [efavirenz *(not in pregnancy or pregnancy risk—Pregnancy Category D)* + (3TC or FTC) + (ZDV or TDF)] **or** [lopinavir/ritonavir + (3TC or FTC) + ZDV] or one of several alternative regimens *[see Table 14D & MMWR 54(RR-2):1, 2005]*. Failures of prophylaxis have been reported, and may be associated with longer interval from exposure to start of PEP; this supports prompt initiation of PEP if it is to be used.

Areas of uncertainty: (1) expanded regimens are not proven to be superior to 2-drug regimens, (2) while PEP not recommended for exposures >72 hours before evaluation, it may possibly be effective in some cases, (3) when HIV status of source patient is unknown, decision to treat and regimen selection must be individualized based on assessment of specific circumstances.

Evaluate for exposures to Hep B, Hep C *(see Occupational PEP above)*, and bacterial sexually-transmitted diseases *(see Table 15A)* and treat as indicated. DHHS recommendations for sexual exposures to HepB and bacterial pathogens are available in *MMWR 55(RR-11), 2006*. Persons who are unvaccinated or who have not responded to full HepB vaccine series should receive hepB immune globulin preferably within 24-hours of percutaneous or mucosal exposure to blood or body fluids of an HBsAg-positive person, along with hepB vaccine, with follow-up to complete vaccine series. Unvaccinated or not-fully-vaccinated persons exposed to a source with unknown HepBsAg-status should receive vaccine and complete vaccine series. See *MMWR 55(RR-11), 2006* for details and recommendations in other circumstances.

TABLE 15E – PREVENTION OF SELECTED OPPORTUNISTIC INFECTIONS IN HUMAN HEMATOPOIETIC CELL TRANSPLANTATION (HCT) OR SOLID ORGAN TRANSPLANTATION (SOT) IN ADULTS WITH NORMAL RENAL FUNCTION.

General comments: Medical centers performing transplants will have detailed protocols for the prevention of opportunistic infections which are appropriate to the infections encountered, patients represented and resources available at those sites. Regimens continue to evolve and protocols adopted by an institution may differ from those at other centers. Care of transplant patients should be guided by physicians with expertise in this area.

References:

For HCT: Expert guidelines endorsed by the IDSA, updating earlier guidelines *(MMWR 49 (RR-10):1, 2000)* in: *Biol Blood Marrow Transpl 15:1143, 2009.* These guidelines provide recommendations for prevention of additional infections not discussed in this table and provide more detailed information on the infections included here.

For SOT: Recommendations of an expert panel of The Transplantation Society for management of CMV in solid organ transplant recipients in: *Transplantation 89:779, 2010.* Timeline of infections following SOT in: *Amer J Transpl 9 (suppl 4):S3, 2009.*

OPPORTUNISTIC INFECTION	TYPE OF TRANSPLANT	PROPHYLACTIC REGIMENS
CMV (Recipient + **or** Donor +/Recipient –) Ganciclovir resistance: risk, detection, management *(CID 56:1018, 2013)*	SOT	**Prophylaxis: Valganciclovir** 900 mg po q24h Alternatives include **Ganciclovir** 1000 mg po 3 x/day, **Ganciclovir** 5 mg/kg IV 1 x/day, **Valacyclovir** 2 gm po 4 x/day *(kidney only, see comment)*, CMV IVIG or IVIG. Also consider preemptive therapy (monitor weekly for CMV viremia by PCR (or antigenemia) for 3-6 months post transplant. If viremia detected, start Valganciclovir 900 mg po bid or Ganciclovir 5 mg/kg IV q12h until clearance of viremia, but for not less than 2 weeks followed by secondary prophylaxis or preemptive approach. CMV hyperIVIG can be considered as an adjunct to prophylaxis in high-risk lung, heart/lung, heart, or pancreas organ transplant recipients. Dosing: 150 mg/kg within 72 hrs of transplant and at 2, 4, 6 and 8 weeks; then 100 mg/kg at weeks 12 and 16.
	HCT	Preemptive Strategy: Monitor weekly for CMV viremia by PCR (or antigenemia) for 3-6 months post transplant with consideration for more prolonged monitoring in patients at risk for late-onset CMV disease (chronic GVHD, requiring systemic treatment, patients receiving high-dose steroids, T-cell depleted or cord blood transplant recipients, and CD4 < 100 cells/mL). Start treatment with identification of CMV viremia or antigenemia as above. Consider prophylaxis (beginning post-engraftment) with **Valganciclovir** 900 mg po q24h. National Comprehensive Cancer Network Guidelines on Prevention and Treatment of Cancer-Related Infections, Version 1.2013, Blood 113:5711, 2009, and Biol Blood Marrow Transpl 15:1143, 2009.
Hepatitis B	SOT	For anti-viral agents with activity against HBV, see *Table 14B, page 172 to 173.* For discussion of prevention of HBV re-infection after transplantation and prevention of donor-derived infection *see Am J Transplant 9: S116, 2013*
	HCT	Patients who are anti-HBC positive and anti-HBs positive, but without evidence of active viral replication, can be monitored for ↑LFTs and presence of +HBV-DNA, and given pre-emptive therapy at that time. Alternatively, prophylactic anti-viral therapy can be given, commencing before transplant. *(See guidelines for other specific situations: Biol Blood Marrow Transpl 15:1143, 2009.)* These guidelines recommend Lamivudine 100 mg po q24h as an anti-viral.
Herpes simplex	SOT	**Acyclovir** 400 mg po bid, starting early post-transplant *(Clin Microbiol Rev 10:86, 1997)*
	HCT	**Acyclovir** 250 mg per meter-squared iv q12h **or Acyclovir** 400 mg to 800 mg po bid, from conditioning to engraftment or resolution or mucositis. For those requiring prolonged suppression of HSV, the higher dose (Acyclovir 800 mg po bid) is recommended to minimize the risk of emerging resistance.
Aspergillus spp.	SOT	Lung and heart/lung transplant: Inhaled **Amphotericin B** and/or a mold active oral azole are commonly used, but optimal regimen not defined. Aerosolized **Amphotericin B** 6 mg q8h (or 25 mg/day) OR aerosolized **LAB** 25 mg/day OR **Voriconazole** 200 mg po bid OR **Itraconazole** 200 mg po bid. 59% centers employ universal prophylaxis for 6 months in lung transplant recipients with 97% targeting Aspergillus. Most use Voriconazole alone or in combination with inhaled Amphotericin B *(Am J Transplant 11:361, 2011).* Consider restarting prophylaxis during periods of intensified immune suppression. Liver transplant: Consider only in high-risk, re-transplant and/or those requiring renal-replacement therapy. Recommendations on aspergillus prophylaxis in SOT can be found at *(Am J Transplant 13:228, 2013)*
	HCT/Heme malignancy	Indications for prophylaxis against aspergillus include AML and MDS with neutropenia and HCT with GVHD. Posaconazole 200 mg po tid approved this indication *(NEJM 356:335, 2007 and NEJM 356:348,2007)* Retrospective analysis suggests that Voriconazole would have efficacy in steroid-treated patients with GVHD *(Bone Marrow Transpl 45:662, 2010),* but is not approved for this indication. Amphotericin B and echinocandins are alternatives as well.
Candida spp.	SOT	Consider in select, high risk patients (liver, small bowel, pancreas): Consider in select, high-risk patients (re-transplants, dialysis). **Fluconazole** 400 mg daily for 4 weeks post-transplant. *(Amer J Transpl 13:200, 2013)*
	HCT	**Fluconazole** 400 mg po or iv once daily from day 0 to engraftment or when ANC consistently >1000, or **Posaconazole** 200 mg po tid approved for high-risk patients (e.g., with GVHD or prolonged neutropenia), or Micafungin 50 mg iv once daily.

TABLE 15E (2)

OPPORTUNISTIC INFECTION	TYPE OF TRANSPLANT	PROPHYLACTIC REGIMENS
Coccidioides immitis	Any	**Fluconazole** 200-400 mg po q24h *(Transpl Inf Dis 5:3, 2003; Am J Transpl 6:340. 2006)*. See *COID 21:45, 2008* for approach at one center in endemic area; e.g., for positive serology without evidence of active infection, Fluconazole 400 mg q24h for first year post-transplant, then 200 mg q24h thereafter.
Pneumocystis jiroveci	SOT	**TMP-SMX:** 1 single-strength tab po q24h or 1 double-strength tab po once daily for 3 to 7 days per week. Duration: kidney: 6 mos to 1 year *(Amer J Transpl 9 (suppl 3): S59, 2009)*; heart, lung, liver: ≥ 1 year to life-long *(Amer J Transpl 4 (suppl 10): 135, 2004)*.
	HCT	**TMP-SMX:** 1 single-strength tab po q24h or 1 double-strength tab po once daily or once a day for 3 days per week, from engraftment to ≥ 6 mos post transplant.
Toxoplasma gondii	SOT	**TMP-SMX** (1 SS tab po q24h or 1 DS tab po once daily) x 3-7 days/wk for 6 mos post-transplant. *(See Clin Micro Infect 14:1089, 2008)*.
	HCT	**TMP-SMX:** 1 single-strength tab po q24h or 1 double-strength tab po once daily or once a day for 3 days per week, from engraftment to ≥ 6 mos post transplant for seropositive allogeneic transplant recipients.
Trypanosoma cruzi	Heart	May be transmitted from organs or transfusions *(CID 48:1534, 2009)*. Inspect peripheral blood of suspected cases for parasites *(MMWR 55:798, 2006)*. Risk of reactivation during immunosuppression is variable *(JAMA 298:2171, 2007; JAMA 299:1134, 2008; J Cardiac Fail 15:249, 2009)*. If known Chagas disease in donor or recipient, contact CDC for treatment options *(phone 770-488-7775 or in emergency 770-488-7100)*. *Am J Transplant 11:672, 2011*

TABLE 16 – PEDIATRIC DOSAGES OF SELECTED ANTIBACTERIAL AGENTS*

Adapted from: (1) Nelson's Pocket Book of Pediatric Antimicrobial Therapy 2009, J. Bradley & J. Nelson, eds., American Academy of Pediatrics, 2009.

DRUG	DOSES IN MG PER KG PER DAY OR MG PER KG AT FREQUENCY INDICATED[1]				
	BODY WEIGHT <2000 gm		BODY WEIGHT >2000 gm		>28 DAYS OLD
	0–7 days	8–28 days	0–7 days	8–28 days	
Aminoglycosides, IV or IM (check levels; some dose by gestational age + wks of life; *see Nelson's Pocket Book, p. 25)*					
Amikacin	7.5 q18–24h	7.5 q12h	10 q12h	10 q12h	10 q8h
Gent/tobra	2.5 q18–24h	2.5 q12h	2.5 q12h	2.5 q12h	2.5 q8h
Aztreonam, IV	30 q12h	30 q8h	30 q8h	30 q6h	30 q6h
Cephalosporins					
Cefaclor					20–40 div tid
Cefadroxil					30 div bid (max 2 gm per day)
Cefazolin	25 q12h	25 q12h	25 q12h	25 q8h	25 q8h
Cefdinir					7 q12h or 14 q24h
Cefepime	30 q12h	30 q12h	30 q12h	30 q12h	150 div q8h
Cefixime					8 as q24h or div bid
Cefotaxime	50 q12h	50 q8h	50 q12h	50 q8h	50 q8h (75 q6h for meningitis)
Cefoxitin			20 q12h		80–160 div q6h
Cefpodoxime					10 div bid (max 400 mg per day)
Cefprozil					15–30 div bid (max 1 gm per day)
Ceftazidime	50 q12h	50 q8h	50 q12h	50 q8h	50 q8h
Ceftibuten					4.5 bid
Ceftizoxime					33–66 q8h
Ceftriaxone	25 q24h	50 q24h	25 q24h	50 q24h	50 q24h (meningitis 100)
Cefuroxime IV	50 q12h	50 q8h	50 q8h	50 q8h	50 q8h (80 q8h for meningitis)
po					10–15 bid (max 1 gm per day)
Cephalexin					25–50 div q6h (max 4 gm per day)
Loracarbef					15–30 div bid (max 0.8 gm per day)
Chloramphenicol IV	25 q24h	25 q24h	25 q24h	15 q12h	12.5–25 q6h (max 2–4 gm per day)
Clindamycin IV	5 q12h	5 q8h	5 q8h	5 q6h	7.5 q6h
po					
Ciprofloxacin[2] po					20–30 div bid (max 1.5 gm per day)
Ertapenem IV	No data	No data	No data	No data	15 q12h (max. 1g/day)
Imipenem[3] IV			25 q12h	25 q8h	15–25 q6h (max 2–4 gm per day)
Linezolid	10 q12h	10 q8h	10 q8h	10 q8h	10 q8h to age 12
Macrolides					
Erythro IV & po	10 q12h	10 q8h	10 q12h	13 q8h	10 q6h
Azithro po/IV	5 q24h	10 q24h	5 q24h	10 q24h	10 q24h
Clarithro po					7.5 q12h (max. 1 gm per day)
Meropenem IV	20 q12h	20 q8h	20 q12h	20 q8h	60–120 div q8h (120 for meningitis)
Metro IV & po	7.5 q24h	7.5 q12h	7.5 q12h	15 q12h	7.5 q6h
Penicillins					
Ampicillin	50 q12h	50 q8h	50 q8h	50 q6h	50 q6h
AMP-sulbactam					100–300 div q6h
Amoxicillin po				30 div bid	25–50 div tid
Amox-Clav po			30 div bid	30 div bid	45 or 90 (AM/CL-HD) div bid if over 12wks
Dicloxacillin					12–25 div q6h
Mezlocillin	75 q12h	75 q8h	75 q12h	75 q8h	75 q6h
Nafcillin, oxacillin IV	25 q12h	25 q8h	25 q8h	37 q6h	37 q6h (to max. 8–12 gm per day)
Piperacillin, PIP-tazo IV	50 q12h	100 q12h	100 q12h	100 q8h	100 q6h
Ticarcillin, TC/CL IV	75 q12h	75 q8h	75 q8h	75 q6h	75 q6h
Tinidazole					> Age 3: 50 mg/kg for 1 dose
Penicillin G, U/kg IV	50,000 q12h	75,000 q8h	50,000 q8h	50,000 q6h	50,000 units/kg per day
Penicillin V					25–50 mg per kg per day div q6–8h
Rifampin IV, po	10 q24h	10 q24h	10 q24h	10 q24h	10 q24h
Sulfisoxazole po					120–150 mg/kg per day div q4–6h
TMP-SMX po, IV; UTI: 8–12 TMP component div bid; Pneumocystis: 20 TMP component div q6h					
Tetracycline po (age 8 or older)					25–50 div q6h (>7yr old)
Doxycycline po, IV (age 8 or older)					2–4 div bid to max of 200 (>7yr old)
Vancomycin IV	12.5 q12h	15 q12h	18 q12h	22 q12h	40 div q6–8h [some start with 15 mg/kg IV q6h (normal renal function)]; 60 for meningitis.

[1] May need higher doses in patients with meningitis: *see CID 39:1267, 2004.*
[2] With exception of cystic fibrosis, anthrax, and complicated UTI, not approved for use under age 18.
[3] Not recommended in children with CNS infections due to risk of seizures.
* *See page 2 for abbreviations*

TABLE 17A – DOSAGE OF ANTIMICROBIAL DRUGS IN ADULT PATIENTS WITH RENAL IMPAIRMENT

- For listing of drugs with NO need for adjustment for renal failure, *see Table 17B*.
- Adjustments for renal failure are based on an estimate of creatinine clearance (CrCl) which reflects the glomerular filtration rate.
- **Different methods for calculating estimated CrCl are suggested for non-obese and obese patients.**
  - o Calculations for ideal body weight (IBW) in kg:
    - *Men:* 50 kg plus 2.3 kg/inch over 60 inches height.
    - *Women:* 45 kg plus 2.3 kg/inch over 60 inches height.
  - o Obese is defined as 20% over ideal body weight or body mass index (BMI) >30

- Calculations of estimated CrCl *(References, see (NEJM 354:2473, 2006 (non-obese), AJM 84:1053, 1988 (obese))*
  - o **Non-obese patient**—
    - Calculate ideal body weight (IBW) in kg (as above)
    - Use the following formula to determine estimated CrCl

$$\frac{\text{(140 minus age)(IBW in kg)}}{\text{72 x serum creatinine}} = \begin{array}{c}\text{CrCl in mL/min for men.}\\ \text{Multiply answer by 0.85}\\ \text{for women (estimated)}\end{array}$$

  - o **Obese patient**—
    - Weight ≥20% over IBW or BMI >30
    - Use the following formulas to determine estimated CrCl

$$\frac{\text{(137 minus age) x [(0.285 x wt in kg) + (12.1 x ht in meters}^2\text{)]}}{\text{51 x serum creatinine}} = \text{CrCl (obese male)}$$

$$\frac{\text{(146 minus age) x [(0.287 x wt in kg) + (9.74 x ht in meters}^2\text{)]}}{\text{60 x serum creatinine}} = \text{CrCl (obese female)}$$

- If estimated CrCl ≥90 mL/min, *see Tables 10A and 10D for dosing.*
- What weight should be used to calculate dosage on a mg/kg basis?
  - o If less than 20% over IBW, use the patient's actual weight for all drugs.
  - o **For obese patients** (≥20% over IBW or BMI >30).
    - **Aminoglycosides:** (IBW plus 0.4(actual weight minus IBW) = adjusted weight.
    - **Vancomycin:** actual body weight whether non-obese or obese.
    - **All other drugs:** insufficient data *(Pharmacotherapy 27:1081, 2007)*.

- For slow or sustained extended daily dialysis **(SLEDD)** over 6-12 hours, adjust does as for CRRT. For details, *see CID 49:433, 2009; CCM 39:560, 2011.*
- General reference: Drug Prescribing in Renal Failure, 5th ed., Aronoff, et al. (eds) *(Amer College Physicians, 2007 and drug package inserts).*

TABLE 17A (2)

ANTIMICROBIAL	HALF-LIFE (NORMAL/ ESRD) hr	DOSE FOR NORMAL RENAL FUNCTION	METHOD (see footer)	ADJUSTMENT FOR RENAL FAILURE Estimated creatinine clearance (CrCl), mL/min			HEMODIALYSIS, CAPD	COMMENTS & DOSAGE FOR CRRT
				>50–90	10–50	<10		
ANTIBACTERIAL ANTIBIOTICS								
Aminoglycoside Antibiotics: Traditional multiple daily doses—adjustment for renal disease								
Amikacin	1.4–2.3/17–150	7.5 mg per kg q12h or 15 mg per kg once daily (see below)	I	7.5 mg/kg q24h or 15 mg/kg once daily	30-50: 7.5 mg/kg q24h **Same dose for CRRT** 10-30: 7.5 mg/kg q48h	7.5 mg/kg q72h	HEMO: 7.5 mg/kg AD CAPD: 15–20 mg lost per L dialysate per day *(see Comment)*	**High flux hemodialysis** membranes lead to unpredictable aminoglycoside clearance, measure post-dialysis drug levels for efficacy and toxicity. With **CAPD,** pharmacokinetics highly variable—**check serum levels.** Usual method for CAPD: 2 liters of dialysis fluid placed qid or 8 liters per day (give 8Lx20 mg lost per L = 160 mg of amikacin supplement IV per day) Adjust dosing weight for obesity: [ideal body weight + 0.4 (actual body weight – ideal body weight)] *(CID 25:112, 1997)*. **Gent SLEDD dose** in critically ill: 6 mg/kg IV q48h starting 30 min before start of SLEDD (daily SLEDD; q48h Gent) *(AAC54:3635, 2010)*.
Gentamicin, Tobramycin (Monitor levels)	2–3/20–60	1.7 mg per kg q8h. Once daily dosing below	I	5-7 mg/kg once daily or 1.7-2.3 mg/kg q8h	1.7 mg/kg q12-48h **Same dose for CRRT** *See Comment for SLEDD dose*	1.7 mg/kg q48-72h	HEMO: 3 mg/kg AD. Monitor levels. CAPD: 3–4 mg lost per L dialysate per day	
Netilmicin[NUS]	2–3/35–72	2 mg per kg q8h. Once daily dosing below	I	2 mg/kg q8h or 6.5 mg/kg once daily	2 mg/kg q12-24h **Same dose for CRRT**	2 mg/kg q48h	HEMO3 mg/kg AD CAPD: 3–4 mg lost per L dialysate per day	
Streptomycin	2–3/30–80	15 mg per kg (max. of 1 gm) q24h. Once daily dosing below	I	15 mg/kg q24h	15 mg/kg q24-72h **Same dose for CRRT**	15 mg/kg q72-96h	HEMO: 7.5 mg/kg AD CAPD: 20–40 mg lost per L dialysate per day	

ONCE-DAILY AMINOGLYCOSIDE THERAPY: ADJUSTMENT IN RENAL INSUFFICIENCY *(see Table 10D for OD dosing/normal renal function)*

Creatinine Clearance (mL per min.)	>80	60–80	40–60	30–40	20–30	10–20	<10–0
Drug	Dose q24h (mg per kg)					Dose q48h (mg per kg)	Dose q72h and AD
Gentamicin/Tobramycin	5.1	4	3.5	2.5	4	3	2
Amikacin/kanamycin/streptomycin	15	12	7.5	4	7.5	4	3
Isepamicin[NUS]	8	8	8	8 q48h	8	8 q72h	8 q96h
Netilmicin[NUS]	6.5	5	4	2	3	2.5	2

ANTIMICROBIAL	HALF-LIFE (NORMAL/ ESRD) hr	DOSE FOR NORMAL RENAL FUNCTION	METHOD	>50–90	10–50	<10	HEMODIALYSIS, CAPD	COMMENTS & DOSAGE FOR CRRT
Carbapenem Antibiotics								
Doripenem	1/18	500 mg IV q8h	D&I	500 mg IV q8h	**≥30 – ≤50:** 250 mg IV q8h **>10 – <30:** 250 mg IV q12h	No data	No data. CRRT ref: *AAC 55:1187, 2011.*	
Ertapenem	4/>4	1 gm q24h	D	1 gm q24h	0.5 gm q24h (CrCl <30)	0.5 gm q24h	HEMO: Dose as for CrCl <10; if dosed <6 hrs prior to HD, give 150 mg supplement AD	
Imipenem *(see Comment)*	1/4	0.5 gm q6h	D&I	250–500 mg q6–8h	250 mg q6–12h **Dose for CRRT: 0.5–1 gm bid** *(AAC 49:2421, 2005)*	125–250 mg q12h	HEMO: Dose AD CAPD: Dose for CrCl <10	↑ potential for seizures if recommended doses exceeded in pts with CrCl <20 mL per min. See pkg insert, esp. for pts <70 kg
Meropenem	1/6–8	1 gm q8h	D&I	1 gm q8h	1 gm q12h **Same dose for CRRT**	0.5 gm q24h	HEMO: Dose AD CAPD: Dose for CrCl <10	

Abbreviation Key: Adjustment Method: **D** = dose adjustment, **I** = interval adjustment; **CAPD** = continuous ambulatory peritoneal dialysis; **CRRT** = continuous renal replacement therapy; **HEMO** = hemodialysis; **AD** = after dialysis; **"Supplement"** or **"Extra"** is to replace drug lost during dialysis – additional drug beyond continuation of regimen for CrCl < 10 mL/min.

TABLE 17A (3)

ANTIMICROBIAL	HALF-LIFE (NORMAL/ ESRD) hr	DOSE FOR NORMAL RENAL FUNCTION	METHOD *(see footer)*	ADJUSTMENT FOR RENAL FAILURE Estimated creatinine clearance (CrCl), mL/min			HEMODIALYSIS, CAPD	COMMENTS & DOSAGE FOR CRRT
				>50–90	**10–50**	**<10**		
ANTIBACTERIAL ANTIBIOTICS *(continued)*								
Cephalosporin Antibiotics: DATA ON SELECTED **PARENTERAL** CEPHALOSPORINS								
Cefazolin	1.9/40–70	1-2 gm q8h	I	q8h	q12h **Same dose for CRRT**	q24–48h	HEMO: Extra 0.5–1 gm AD CAPD: 0.5 gm q12h	
Cefepime	2.2/18	2 gm q8h (max. dose)	D&I	2 gm q8h	2 gm q12–24h **Same dose for CRRT**	1 gm q24h	HEMO: Extra 1 gm AD CAPD: 1–2 gm q48h	
Cefotaxime, Ceftizoxime	1.7/15–35	2 gm q8h	I	q8–12h	q12–24h **Same dose for CRRT**	q24h	HEMO: Extra 1 gm AD CAPD: 0.5–1 gm q24h	Active metabolite of cefotaxime in ESRD. ↓ dose further for hepatic & renal failure.
Cefotetan	3.5/13–25	1–2 gm q12h	D	100%	1-2 gm q24h **Same dose for CRRT**	1-2 gm q48h	HEMO: Extra 1 gm AD CAPD: 1 gm q24h	CRRT dose: 750 mg q12h
Cefoxitin	0.8/13–23	2 gm q8h	I	q8h	q8–12h **Same dose for CRRT**	q24–48h	HEMO: Extra 1 gm AD CAPD: 1 gm q24h	May falsely increase serum creatinine by interference with assay.
Ceftaroline	1.6/–	600 mg IV q12h	D	600 mg q12h	30-50: 400 mg q12h 15-30: 300 mg q12h	< 15: 200 mg q12h	HEMO: 200 mg q12h	1-hr infusion for all doses
Ceftazidime	1.2/13–25	2 gm q8h	I	q8–12h	Q12–24h **Same dose for CRRT**	q24-48h	HEMO: Extra 1 gm AD CAPD: 0.5 gm q24h	Since 1/2 dose is dialyzed, post-dialysis dose is max. of 3 gm.
Ceftobiprole	2.9–3.3/21	500 mg IV q8-12h	I	500 mg IV q8-12h	**≥30 & ≤50:** 500 mg q12h over 2 hrs **≥10 & <30:** 250 mg q12h over 2 hrs	No data	No data	
Cefuroxime sodium	1.2/17	0.75–1.5 gm q8h	I	q8h	q8–12h **Same dose for CRRT**	q24h	HEMO: Dose AD CAPD: Dose for CrCl <10	
Fluoroquinolone Antibiotics								
Ciprofloxacin	3-6/6–9	500–750 mg po (or 400 mg IV) q12h	D	100%	50–75% CRRT 400 mg IV q24h	50%	HEMO: 250 mg po or 200 mg IV q12h CAPD: 250 mg po or 200 mg IV q8h	
Gatifloxacin[NUS]	7–14/11-40	400 mg po/IV q24h	D	400 mg q24h	400 mg, then 200 mg q24h Same dose for CRRT	400 mg, then 200 mg q24h	HEMO: 200 mg q24h AD CAPD: 200 mg q24h	
Gemifloxacin	7/>7	320 mg po q24h	D	320 mg q24h	160 mg q24h	160 mg q24h	HEMO: 160 mg q24h AD CAPD: 160 mg q24h	
Levofloxacin	6–8/76	750 mg q24h IV, PO	D&I	750 mg q24h	**20-49:** 750 q48h	**<20:** 750 mg once, then 500 mg q48h	HEMO/CAPD: Dose for CrCl <20	CRRT 750 mg once, then 500 mg q48h, although not FDA-approved.
Ofloxacin	7/28-37	200-400 mg q12h	D	200-400 mg q12h	200-400 mg q24h **Same dose for CRRT**	200 mg q24h	HEMO: Dose for CrCl <10, AD CAPD: 300 mg q24h	
Macrolide Antibiotics								
Clarithromycin	5–7/22	500-1000 mg q12h	D	500 mg q12h	500 mg q12-24h	500 mg q24h	HEMO: Dose AD CAPD: None	CRRT as for CrCl 10-50
Erythromycin	1.4/5–6	250–500 mg q6h	D	100%	100%	50–75%	HEMO/CAPD/CRRT: None	Ototoxicity with high doses in ESRD

Abbreviation Key: Adjustment Method: **D** = dose adjustment, **I** = interval adjustment; **CAPD** = continuous ambulatory peritoneal dialysis; **CRRT** = continuous renal replacement therapy; **HEMO** = hemodialysis; **AD** = after dialysis; **"Supplement"** or **"Extra"** is to replace drug lost during dialysis – additional drug beyond continuation of regimen for CrCl < 10 mL/min.

TABLE 17A (4)

ANTIMICROBIAL	HALF-LIFE (NORMAL/ ESRD) hr	DOSE FOR NORMAL RENAL FUNCTION	METHOD (*see footer*)	ADJUSTMENT FOR RENAL FAILURE Estimated creatinine clearance (CrCl), mL/min			HEMODIALYSIS, CAPD	COMMENTS & DOSAGE FOR CRRT
				>50–90	**10–50**	**<10**		
ANTIBACTERIAL ANTIBIOTICS *(continued)*								
Miscellaneous Antibacterial Antibiotics								
Colistin (Polymyxin E) Based on 105 pts *(AAC 55:3284, 2011)*. All doses refer to Colistin "base" in mg	<6/≥48	*See Table 10A, page 100* for loading dose and maintenance dose	D & I	**3.5 x [(1.5 x CrCln) + 30] x (pt BSA in m2/1.73m²) =** total daily dose of Colistin base. Divide and give q12h **CrCln** = normalized CrCl based on body surface area (BSA): Pt BSA in m²/1.73m².			**Intermittent Hemodialysis:** • Calculation of dose: 3.5 (30) = 105 mg (CrCl is zero). • On days with no hemodialysis, give total daily dose of 105 mg divided bid. • On dialysis days, need to supplement the dose by 50 % due to colistimethate filtration by the dialysis membrane. • So, on dialysis days the total dose is 150 mg; divide and give half the dose during the last hour of hemodialysis and the second half 12 hours later.	**CAPD:** • 160 mg q24h (unable to locate modern CAPD data) **CRRT:** • For average serum steady state concentration of 3.5 µg/mL, the total daily dose is 672 mg; the dose is divided and given q12h. **The dose is necessarily high due to removal of drug by the dialysis membranes.** Rationale: 3.5 µg/mL as the targeted serum level X 192 mg for each 1 µg/mL of targeted serum level = total daily dose, i.e., 3.5 x 192 = 672. *See AAC 55: 3284, 2011 for data.*
Daptomycin	9.4/30	4–6 mg per kg per day	I	4–6 mg per kg per day	CrCl <30, 6 mg per kg q48h CRRT: 8 mg/kg q48h *(CCM 39:19, 2011)*		HEMO & CAPD: 6 mg per kg q48h (during or after q48h dialysis if possible). If next planned dialysis is 72 hrs away, give 9 mg/kg *(AAC 57:864, 2013; JAC 69:200, 2014)*.	
Linezolid	5-6/6-8	600 mg po/IV q12h	None	600 mg q12h	600 mg q12h **Same dose for CRRT**	600 mg q12h AD	HEMO: As for CrCl <10 CAPD & CRRT: No dose adjustment	Accumulation of 2 metabolites—risk unknown *(JAC 56:172, 2005)*
Metronidazole	6–14/7–21	7.5 mg per kg q6h	D	100%	100% **Same dose for CRRT**	50%	HEMO: Dose as for CrCl <10 AD CAPD: Dose for CrCl <10	
Nitrofurantoin	0.5/1	50–100 mg	D	100%	Avoid	Avoid	Not applicable	
Sulfamethoxazole (SMX)	10/20–50	1 gm q8h	I	q12h	q18h Same dose for CAVH	q24h	HEMO: Extra 1 gm AD CAPD: 1 gm q24h	
Teicoplanin[NUS]	45/62–230	6 mg per kg per day	I	q24h	q48h **Same dose for CRRT**	q72h	HEMO: Dose for CrCl <10 CAPD: Dose for CrCl <10	
Telithromycin	10/15	800 mg q24h	D	800 mg q24h	600 mg q24h (<30 mL per min.)	600 mg q24h	HEMO: 600 mg AD CAPD: No data	If CrCl <30, reduce dose to 600 mg once daily. If both liver and renal failure, dose is 400 mg once daily
Telavancin	7-8/17.9	10 mg/kg q24h	D&I	10 mg/kg q24h	**30-50:** 7.5 mg/kg q24h	**<30:** 10 mg/kg q48h	No data	No data
Temocillin		1-2 gm q12h	I	1-2 gm q12h	1-2 gm q24h	1 gm q48h	HEMO: 1 gm q48h AD CAPD: 1 gm q48h	

Abbreviation Key: Adjustment Method: **D** = dose adjustment, **I** = interval adjustment; **CAPD** = continuous ambulatory peritoneal dialysis; **CRRT** = continuous renal replacement therapy; **HEMO** = hemodialysis; **AD** = after dialysis; **"Supplement"** or **"Extra"** is to replace drug lost during dialysis – additional drug beyond continuation of regimen for CrCl < 10 mL/min.

TABLE 17A (5)

ANTIMICROBIAL	HALF-LIFE (NORMAL/ ESRD) hr	DOSE FOR NORMAL RENAL FUNCTION	METHOD *(see footer)*	ADJUSTMENT FOR RENAL FAILURE Estimated creatinine clearance (CrCl), mL/min			HEMODIALYSIS, CAPD	COMMENTS & DOSAGE FOR CRRT
				>50–90	10–50	<10		
ANTIBACTERIAL ANTIBIOTICS *(continued)*								
Trimethoprim (TMP)	11/20–49	100–200 mg q12h	I	q12h	**>30:** q12h **10-30:** q18h **Same dose for CRRT**	q24h	HEMO: Dose AD CAPD: q24h	CRRT dose: q18h
Trimethoprim-sulfamethoxazole-DS (Doses based on TMP component)								
Treatment (based on TMP component)	*As for TMP*	5–20 mg/kg/day divided q6-12h	D	No dose adjustment	**30–50:** No dose adjustment **10–29:** Reduce dose by 50%	Not recommended; but if used: 5–10 mg/kg q24h	Not recommended; but if used: 5–10 mg/kg q24h AD CRRT: 5-7.5 mg/kg q8h	
TMP-SMX Prophylaxis	*As for TMP*	1 tab po q24h or 3 times per week	No change	100%	100%	100%		
Vancomycin[1]	6/200–250	1 gm q12h	D&I	15-30 mg/kg q12h	15 mg/kg q24-96h	7.5 mg/kg q2-3 days	HEMO: For trough conc of 15-20 µg/mL, give 15 mg/kg if next dialysis in 1 day; give 25 mg/kg if next dialysis in 2 days; give 35 mg/kg if next dialysis in 3 days *(CID 53:124, 2011)*.	CAVH/CVVH: 500 mg q24–48h. New hemodialysis membranes ↑ clear. of vanco; **check levels**
Penicillins								
Amoxicillin Ampicillin	1/5–20 1/7–20	250–500 mg q8h 250 mg–2 gm q6h	I I	q8h q6h	q8–12h q6–12h	q24h q12–24h	HEMO: Dose AD CAPD: 250 mg q12h	IV amoxicillin not available in the U.S. CRRT: dose for CrCl 10-50
Amoxicillin/ Clavulanate[2]	1.3 AM/1 5–20/4	500/125 mg q8h *(see Comments)*	D&I	500/125 mg q8h	250–500 mg AM component q12h	250–500 mg AM component q24h	HEMO: As for CrCl <10; extra dose after dialysis	**If CrCl ≤30 per mL, do not use 875/125 or 1000/62.5 AM/CL**
Amoxicillin ext. rel. tabs	1.5/?	775 mg once daily		Once daily	CrCl <30, no data, avoid usage			
Ampicillin (AM/ Sulbactam(SB)	1 (AM)/1 (SB) 9 (AM)/10 (SB)	2 gm AM + 1 gm SB q6h	I	q6h	q8–12h	q24h	HEMO: Dose AD CAPD: 2 gm AM/1 gm SB q24h	CRRT dose: 1.5 AM/0.75 SB q12h
Aztreonam	2/6–8	2 gm q8h	D	100%	50–75% **Same dose for CRRT**	25%	HEMO: Extra 0.5 gm AD CAPD: Dose for CrCl <10	Technically is a β-lactam antibiotic.
Penicillin G	0.5/6–20	0.5–4 million U q4h	D	0.5-4 million U q4h	0.5-4 million U q8h **Same dose for CRRT**	0.5-4 million U q12h	HEMO: Dose AD CAPD: Dose for CrCl <10	1.7 mEq potassium per million units. ↑s potential of seizure. 10 million units per day max. dose in ESRD.
Piperacillin	1/3.3–5.1	3–4 gm q4–6h	I	q4–6h	q6–8h **Same dose for CRRT**	q8h	HEMO: 2 gm q8h plus 1 gm extra AD CAPD: Dose for CrCl <10	1.9 mEq sodium per gm

[1] If renal failure, use EMIT assay to measure levels; levels overestimated by RIA or fluorescent immunoassay.
[2] Clavulanate cleared by liver, not kidney. Hence as dose of combination decreased, a deficiency of clavulanate may occur *(JAMA 285:386, 2001)*.

Abbreviation Key: Adjustment Method: **D** = dose adjustment, **I** = interval adjustment; **CAPD** = continuous ambulatory peritoneal dialysis; **CRRT** = continuous renal replacement therapy; **HEMO** = hemodialysis; **AD** = after dialysis; **"Supplement"** or **"Extra"** is to replace drug lost during dialysis – additional drug beyond continuation of regimen for CrCl < 10 mL/min.

TABLE 17A (6)

ANTIMICROBIAL	HALF-LIFE (NORMAL/ ESRD) hr	DOSE FOR NORMAL RENAL FUNCTION	METHOD (*see footer*)	ADJUSTMENT FOR RENAL FAILURE Estimated creatinine clearance (CrCl), mL/min			HEMODIALYSIS, CAPD	COMMENTS & DOSAGE FOR CRRT
				>50–90	10–50	<10		
ANTIBACTERIAL ANTIBIOTICS *(continued)*								
Pip (P)/Tazo(T)	0.71-1.2 (both)/2-6	3.375 – 4.5 gm q6-8h	D&I	100%	2.25 gm q6h **<20:** q8h **Same dose for CRRT**	2.25 gm q8h	HEMO: Dose for CrCl <10 + extra 0.75 gm AD CAPD: 4.5 gm q12h; CRRT: 2.25 gm q6h	
Ticarcillin	1.2/13	3 gm q4h	D&I	1–2 gm q4h	1–2 gm q8h **Same dose for CRRT**	1–2 gm q12h	HEMO: Extra 3.0 gm AD CAPD: Dose for CrCl <10	5.2 mEq sodium per gm
Ticarcillin/ Clavulanate[2]	1.2/11-16	3.1 gm q4h	D&I	3.1 gm q4h	3.1 gm q8-12h **Same dose for CRRT**	2 gm q12h	HEMO: Extra 3.1 gm AD CAPD: 3.1 gm q12h	*See footnote*[2]
Tetracycline Antibiotics								
Tetracycline	6–10/57–108	250–500 mg qid	I	q8–12h	q12–24h **Same dose for CRRT**	q24h	HEMO/CAPD/CAVH: None	Avoid in ESRD
ANTIFUNGAL ANTIBIOTICS								
Amphotericin B & Lipid-based ampho B	24h-15 days//unchanged	Non-lipid: 0.4–1 mg/kg/day ABLC: 5 mg/kg/day LAB: 3–5 mg/kg/day	I	q24h	q24h **Same dose for CRRT**	q24h	HEMO/CAPD/CRRT: No dose adjustment	For ampho B, toxicity lessened by saline loading; risk amplified by concomitant cyclosporine A, aminoglycosides, or pentamidine
Fluconazole	37/100	100–400 mg q24h	D	100%	50%	50%	HEMO: 100% of recommended dose AD CAPD: Dose for CrCl <10	CRRT: 200-400 mg q24h
Flucytosine	3–6/75–200	37.5 mg per kg q6h	I	q12h	q12–24h **Same dose for CRRT**	q24h	HEMO: Dose AD CAPD: 0.5–1 gm q24h	Goal is peak serum level >25 mcg per mL and <100 mcg per mL
Itraconazole, po soln	21/25	100–200 mg q12h	D	100%	100% **Same dose for CRRT**	50%	HEMO/CAPD: oral solution: 100 mg q12-24h	
Itraconazole, IV	21/25	200 mg IV q12h	–	200 mg IV bid	Do not use IV itra if CrCl <30 due to accumulation of carrier: cyclodextrin			
Terbinafine	36–200/?	250 mg po per day	–	q24h	Use has not been studied. Recommend avoidance of drug.			
Voriconazole, IV	Non-linear kinetics	6 mg per kg IV q12h times 2, then 4 mg per kg q12h	–	No change	If CrCl <50 mL per min., accum. of IV vehicle (cyclodextrin). Switch to po or DC **For CRRT:** 4 mg/kg po q12h			
ANTIPARASITIC ANTIBIOTICS								
Pentamidine	3-12/73-18	4 mg per kg per day	I	q24h	q24h **Same dose for CRRT**	q24–36h	HEMO: 4 mg/kg q48h AD CAPD: Dose for CrCl<10	
Quinine	5–16/5–16	650 mg q8h	I	650 mg q8h	650 mg q8–12h **Same dose for CRRT**	650 mg q24h	HEMO: Dose AD CAPD: Dose for CrCl <10	Marked tissue accumulation

Abbreviation Key: Adjustment Method: **D** = dose adjustment, **I** = interval adjustment; **CAPD** = continuous ambulatory peritoneal dialysis; **CRRT** = continuous renal replacement therapy; **HEMO** = hemodialysis; **AD** = after dialysis; **"Supplement"** or **"Extra"** is to replace drug lost during dialysis – additional drug beyond continuation of regimen for CrCl < 10 mL/min.

TABLE 17A (7)

ANTIMICROBIAL	HALF-LIFE (NORMAL/ ESRD) hr	DOSE FOR NORMAL RENAL FUNCTION	METHOD (*see footer*)	ADJUSTMENT FOR RENAL FAILURE Estimated creatinine clearance (CrCl), mL/min			HEMODIALYSIS, CAPD	COMMENTS & DOSAGE FOR CRRT
				>50–90	**10–50**	**<10**		
ANTITUBERCULOUS ANTIBIOTICS (*See http://11ntcc.ucsd.edu/TB*)								
Amikacin/ Streptomycin (*see page 211*)								
Bedaquiline	24-30	400 mg po qd x 2 wks, then 200 mg tiw x 22 wks		No adjustment for mild-moderate renal impairment; **use with caution if severe renal impairment or ESRD**				
Capreomycin		15 mg/kg q24h	I	15 mg/kg q24h	15 mg/kg q24h CRRT: 25 mg/kg q24h (max 2.5 gm q24h)	15 mg/kg AD 3x/wk	HEMO: 15 mg/kg AD 3x/wk	
Cycloserine		10-15 mg/kg/day in 2 div doses	I	10-15 mg/kg/day in 2 div doses	CrCl 10-20: 10-15 mg/kg q12-24h	10-15 mg/kg q24h	HEMO: 10-15 mg/kg AD 3x/wk	
Ethambutol	4/7–15	15–25 mg per kg q24h	I	15-25 mg/kg q24h	**CrCl 30-50:**15 mg/kg q24–36h **Same dose for CRRT** **For CrCl 10-20:** 15-25 mg/kg q24-48h	15-25 mg/kg q48h	HEMO: 20 mg/kg 3x/wk AD CAPD: 25 mg/kg q48h	If possible, do serum levels on dialysis pts.
Ethionamide	2/9	250–500 mg q12h	D	500 mg bid	500 mg bid	250 mg bid	HEMO/CAPD/CRRT: No dosage adjustment	
Isoniazid	0.7–4/8–17	5 mg per kg per day (max. 300 mg)	D	100%	100% **Same dose for CRRT**	100%	HEMO: Dose AD CAPD/: Dose for CrCl <10	
Pyrazinamide	9/26	25 mg per kg q24h (max. dose 2.5 gm q24h)	D	25 mg/kg q24h	**CrCl 21-90:** 25 mg/kg q24h **Same dose for CRRT** **For CrCl 10-20:** 25 mg/kg q48h	12-25 mg per kg 3x/wk	HEMO: 25 mg/kg 3x/wk AD CAPD: No reduction	
Rifampin	1.5–5/1.8–11	600 mg per day	D	600 mg q24h	300–600 mg q24h **Same dose for CRRT**	300–600 mg q24h	HEMO: No adjustment CAPD/: Dose for CrCl <10	Biologically active metabolite
ANTIVIRAL/ANTIRETROVIRAL AGENTS								
Acyclovir, IV	2-4/20	5–12.4 mg per kg q8h	D&I	100% q8h	100% q12–24h	50% q24h	HEMO: Dose AD CAPD: Dose for CrCl <10	Rapid IV infusion can cause ↑ Cr. CRRT dose: 5-10 mg/kg q24h
Adefovir	7.5/15	10 mg po q24h	I	10 mg q24h	10 mg q48–72h[3]	10 mg q72h[3]	HEMO: 10 mg q week AD	CAPD: No data; CRRT: Dose?
Amantadine	12/500	100 mg po bid	I	q12h	q24-48h	q 7 days	HEMO/CAPD: Dose for CrCl<10/	CRRT: Dose for CrCl 10-50
Atripla	See each drug	200 mg emtricitabine + 300 mg tenofovir + 600 mg efavirenz	I	Do not use if CrCl <50				
Cidofovir: **Complicated dosing**—*see package insert*								

[3] Ref: *Transplantation 80:1086, 2005*

Abbreviation Key: Adjustment Method: **D** = dose adjustment, **I** = interval adjustment; **CAPD** = continuous ambulatory peritoneal dialysis; **CRRT** = continuous renal replacement therapy; **HEMO** = hemodialysis; **AD** = after dialysis; **"Supplement"** or **"Extra"** is to replace drug lost during dialysis – additional drug beyond continuation of regimen for CrCl < 10 mL/min.

TABLE 17A (8)

ANTIMICROBIAL	HALF-LIFE (NORMAL/ ESRD) hr	DOSE FOR NORMAL RENAL FUNCTION	METHOD *(see footer)*	ADJUSTMENT FOR RENAL FAILURE Estimated creatinine clearance (CrCl), mL/min			HEMODIALYSIS, CAPD	COMMENTS & DOSAGE FOR CRRT
				>50–90	**10–50**	**<10**		
ANTIVIRAL/ANTIRETROVIRAL AGENTS *(continued)*								
Induction	2.5/unknown	5 mg per kg once per wk for 2 wks	–	5 mg per kg once per wk	Contraindicated in pts with CrCl ≤ 55 mL/min.			Major toxicity is renal. No efficacy, safety, or pharmacokinetic data in pts with moderate/severe renal disease.
Maintenance	2.5/unknown	5 mg per kg q2wks	–	5 mg per kg q2wks	Contraindicated in pts with CrCl ≤ 55 mL/min.			
Didanosine tablets[4]	0.6–1.6/4.5	125–200 mg q12h buffered tabs	D	200 mg q12h	200 mg q24h	<60 kg: 150 mg q24h >60 kg: 100 mg q24h	HEMO: Dose AD CAPD/CRRT: Dose for CrCl <10	Based on incomplete data. Data are estimates.
		400 mg q24h enteric-coated tabs	D	400 mg q24h	125–200 mg q24h	**Do not use EC tabs**	HEMO/CAPD: Dose for CrCl <10	**If <60 kg & CrCl <10 mL per min, do not use EC tabs**
Emtricitabine (CAPS)	10/>10	200 mg q24h	I	200 mg q24h	**30–49:** 200 mg q48h **10–29:** 200 mg q72h	200 mg q96h	HEMO: Dose for CrCl <10	*See package insert for oral solution.*
Emtricitabine + Tenofovir	See each drug	200-300 mg q24h	I	No change	**30–50:** 1 tab q48h	**CrCl <30:** Do not use		
Entecavir	128–149/?	0.5 mg q24h	D	0.5 mg q24h	0.15–0.25 mg q24h	0.05 mg q24h	HEMO/CAPD: 0.05 mg q24h	Give after dialysis on dialysis days
Famciclovir	2.3–3/10–22	500 mg q8h	D&I	500 mg q8h	500 mg q12–24h	250 mg q24h	HEMO: Dose AD CAPD: No data	CRRT: Not applicable

ANTIMICROBIAL	HALF-LIFE (NORMAL/ ESRD) hr	CrCl (mL/min per kg body weight—only for Foscarnet								COMMENTS & DOSAGE FOR CRRT
			>1.4	**>1-1.4**	**>0.8-1**	**>0.6-0.8**	**>0.5-0.6**	**>0.4-0.5**	**<0.4**	
Foscarnet (CMV dosage). Dosage adjustment based on est. CrCl divided by wt (kg)	Normal half-life (T½) 3 hrs with terminal T½ of 18-88 hrs. T½ very long with ESRD	Induction: 60 mg/kg IV q8h x 2-3 wks	60 q8h	45 q8h	50 q12h	40 q12h	60 q24h	50 q24h	Do not use	*See package insert for further details*
		Maintenance: 90-120 mg/kg/day IV	120 q24h	90 q24h	65 q24h	105 q48h	80 q48h	65 q48h	Do not use	

ANTIMICROBIAL	HALF-LIFE (NORMAL/ ESRD) hr	DOSE FOR NORMAL RENAL FUNCTION	METHOD *(see footer)*	>50–90	10–50	<10	HEMODIALYSIS, CAPD	COMMENTS & DOSAGE FOR CRRT
Ganciclovir	3.6/30 IV:	Induction 5 mg per kg q12h IV	D&I	**70-90:** 5 mg per kg q12h **50-60:** 2.5 mg/kg q12h	**25-49:** 2.5 mg per kg q24h **10-24:** 1.25 mg/kg q24h	1.25 mg per kg 3 times per wk	HEMO: Dose AD CAPD: Dose for CrCl <10	
		Maintenance 5 mg per kg q24h IV	D&I	2.5–5.0 mg per kg q24h	0.6–1.25 mg per kg q24h	0.625 mg per kg 3 times per wk	HEMO: 0.6 mg per kg AD CAPD: Dose for CrCl <10	
	po:	1 gm tid po	D&I	0.5–1 gm tid	0.5–1 gm q24h	0.5 gm 3 times per week	HEMO: 0.5 gm AD	
Maraviroc	14–18/No data	300 mg bid		300 mg bid				Risk of side effects increased if concomitant CYP3A inhibitor
Lamivudine	5–7/15–35	300 mg po q24h	D&I	300 mg po q24h	50–150 mg q24h	25–50 mg q24h	HEMO: Dose AD; CAPD: Dose for CrCl<10. CRRT: 100 mg 1st day, then 50 mg/day.	

[4] Ref: for NRTIs and NNRTIs: *Kidney International 60:821, 2001*

Abbreviation Key: Adjustment Method: **D** = dose adjustment, **I** = interval adjustment; **CAPD** = continuous ambulatory peritoneal dialysis; **CRRT** = continuous renal replacement therapy; **HEMO** = hemodialysis; **AD** = after dialysis; **"Supplement"** or **"Extra"** is to replace drug lost during dialysis – additional drug beyond continuation of regimen for CrCl < 10 mL/min.

TABLE 17A (9)

ANTIMICROBIAL	HALF-LIFE (NORMAL/ ESRD) hr	DOSE FOR NORMAL RENAL FUNCTION	METHOD *(see footer)*	ADJUSTMENT FOR RENAL FAILURE Estimated creatinine clearance (CrCl), mL/min			HEMODIALYSIS, CAPD	COMMENTS & DOSAGE FOR CRRT
				>50–90	10–50	<10		
ANTIVIRAL/ANTIRETROVIRAL AGENTS *(continued)*								
Oseltamivir, therapy	6-10/>20	75 mg po bid – treatment	I	75 mg q12h	**30-50:** 75 mg bid **<30:** 75 mg once daily	No data	HEMO: 30 mg qd non-dialysis days[5]; CAPD: 30 mg once per week	Dose for prophylaxis if CrCl <30: 75 mg once daily CRRT: 75 mg po bid
Peramivir		600 mg once daily	P&I	600 mg q24h	**31-49:** 150 mg q24h **10-30:** 100 mg q24h	100 mg (single dose) then 15 mg q24h	HEMO: 100 mg (single dose) then 100 mg 2 hrs AD (dialysis days only)	CRRT: *http://www.cdc.gov/h1n1flu/eva/peramivir.htm*
Ribavirin	Use with caution in patients with creatinine clearance <50 mL per min.							
Rimantadine	13–65/Prolonged	100 mg bid po	I	100 mg bid	100 mg q24h–bid	100 mg q24h	HEMO/CAPD: No data	Use with caution, little data
Stavudine, po	1–1.4/5.5–8	30–40 mg q12h	D&I	100%	50% q12–24h	≥60 kg: 20 mg per day <60 kg: 15 mg per day	HEMO: Dose as for CrCl <10 AD CAPD: No data CRRT: Full dose	
Stribild		1 tab daily		If CrCl < 70: contraindicated	If CrCl < 50: discontinue			
Telbivudine	40-49/No data	600 mg po daily	I	600 mg q24h	**30-49:** 600 mg q48H **<30:** 600 mg q72h	600 mg q96h	HEMO: As for CrCl <10 AD	
Tenofovir, po	17/?	300 mg q24h		300 mg q24h	**30-49:** 300 mg q48h **10-29:** 300 mg q72-96h	No data	HEMO: 300 mg q7d or after 12 hrs of HEMO.[6]	
Valacyclovir	2.5–3.3/14	1 gm q8h	D&I	1 gm q8h	1 gm q12–24h **Same dose for CRRT**	0.5 gm q24h	HEMO: Dose AD CAPD: Dose for CrCl <10	CAVH dose: As for CrCl 10–50
Valganciclovir	4/67	900 mg po bid	D&I	900 mg po bid	450 mg q24h to 450 mg every other day	DO NOT USE	See package insert	
Zalcitabine	2/>8	0.75 mg q8h	D&I	0.75 mg q8h	0.75 mg q12h **Same dose for CRRT**	0.75 mg q24h	HEMO: Dose AD CAPD: No data	CRRT dose: As for CrCl 10–50
Zidovudine	1.1–1.4/1.4–3	300 mg q12h	D&I	300 mg q12h	300 mg q12h **Same dose for CRRT**	100 mg q8h	HEMO: Dose for CrCl <10 AD CAPD: Dose for CrCl <10	

[5] HEMO wt-based dose adjustments for children age >1 yr (dose after each HEMO): ≤15 kg: 7.5 mg; 16-23 kg: 10 mg; 24-40 kg: 15 mg; > 40 kg: 30 mg *(CID 50:127, 2010)*.
[6] Acute renal failure and Fanconi syndrome reported.

Abbreviation Key: Adjustment Method: **D** = dose adjustment, **I** = interval adjustment; **CAPD** = continuous ambulatory peritoneal dialysis; **CRRT** = continuous renal replacement therapy; **HEMO** = hemodialysis; **AD** = after dialysis; **"Supplement"** or **"Extra"** is to replace drug lost during dialysis – additional drug beyond continuation of regimen for CrCl < 10 mL/min.

TABLE 17B – NO DOSAGE ADJUSTMENT WITH RENAL INSUFFICIENCY BY CATEGORY

Antibacterials		Antifungals	Anti-TBc	Antivirals	
Azithromycin	Minocycline	Anidulafungin	Bedaquiline	Abacavir	
Ceftriaxone	Moxifloxacin	Caspofungin	Ethionamide	Atazanavir	Nelfinavir
Chloramphenicol	Nafcillin	Itraconazole oral solution	Isoniazid	Darunavir	Nevirapine
Ciprofloxacin XL	Polymyxin B	Ketoconazole	Rifampin	Delavirdine	Raltegravir
Clindamycin	Pyrimethamine	Micafungin	Rifabutin	Efavirenz	Ribavirin
Doxycycline	Rifaximin	Voriconazole, **po only**	Rifapentine	Enfuvirtide[1]	Saquinavir
Linezolid	Tigecycline			Fosamprenavir	Simeprevir[2]
				Indinavir	Sofosbuvir[2]
				Lopinavir	Tipranavir

[1] Enfuvirtide: Not studied in patients with CrCl <35 mL/min. DO NOT USE
[2] No data for CrCl <30 mL/min

TABLE 17C – ANTIMICROBIAL DOSING IN OBESITY

The number of obese patients is increasing. Intuitively, the standard doses of some drugs may not achieve effective serum concentrations. Pertinent data on anti-infective dosing in the obese patient is gradually emerging. Though some of the data needs further validation, the following table reflects what is currently known. **Obesity is defined as ≥ 20% over Ideal Body Weight (Ideal BW) or Body Mass Index (BMI) > 30. Dose** = suggested body weight (BW) for dose calculation in obese patient, or specific dose if applicable. In general, the absence of a drug in the table indicates a lack of pertinent information in the published literature.

Drug	Dose	Comments
Acyclovir	Use **Ideal BW** Example: for HSV encephalitis, give 10 mg/kg of Ideal BW q8h	Unpublished data from 7 obese volunteers *(Davis, et al., ICAAC abstract, 1991).*
Aminoglycosides	Use **Adjusted BW** Example: Critically ill patient, Gentamicin or Tobramycin (not Amikacin) 7 mg/kg of Adjusted BW IV q24h *(See Comment)*	Adjusted BW = Ideal BW + 0.4(Actual BW – Ideal BW). Ref: *Pharmacother 27:1081, 2007.* Follow levels so as to lower dose once hemodynamics stabilize.
Cefazolin (surgical prophylaxis)	No dose adjustment needed: 2 gm x 1 dose (repeat in 3 hours?)	Conflicting data; unclear whether dose should be repeated, or if an even higher dose is required. Patients with BMI 40-80 studied. Refs: *Surg 136:738, 2004; Eur J Clin Pharmacol 67:985, 2011; Surg Infect 13:33, 2012.*
Cefepime	Modest dose increase: 2 gm IV q8h instead of the usual q12h	Data from 10 patients (mean BMI 48) undergoing bariatric surgery; regimen yields free T > MIC of 60% for MIC of 8μg/mL. Ref: *Obes Surg 22:465, 2012.*
Daptomycin	Use **Actual BW** Example: 4-12 mg/kg of Actual BW IV q24h	Data from a single-dose PK study in 7 obese volunteers. Ref: *Antimicrob Ag Chemother 51:2741, 2007.*
Flucytosine	Use **Ideal BW** Example: Crypto meningitis, give 25 mg/kg of Ideal BW po q6h	Date from one obese patient with cryptococcal disease. Ref: *Pharmacother 15:251, 1995.*
Levofloxacin	**No dose adjustment** required Example: 750 mg po/IV q24h	Data from 13 obese patients; variability in study findings renders conclusion uncertain. Refs: *Antimicrob Ag Chemother 55:3240, 2011; J Antimicrob Chemother 66:1653, 2011.*
Linezolid	**No dose adjustment required** Example: 600 mg po/IV q12h	Data from 20 obese volunteers up to 150 kg body weight suggest standard doses provide AUC values similar to nonobese subjects. In a recent case report, standard dosing in a 265 kg male with MRSA pneumonia seemed to have reduced clinical effectiveness. Refs: *Antimicrob Ag Chemother 57:1144, 2013; Ann Pharmacother 47: e25, 2013.*
Moxifloxacin	**No dose adjustment** required Example: 400 mg po/IV q24h	Data from 12 obese patients undergoing gastric bypass. Ref: *J Antimicrob Chemother 66:2330, 2011.*
Oseltamivir	**No dose adjustment** required Example: 75 mg po q12h	Data from 10 obese volunteers, unclear if applicable to patients >250 kg (OK to give 150 mg po q12h). Ref: *J Antimicrob Chemother 66:2083, 2011.*
Piperacillin-tazobactam	6.75 gm IV over 4 hours and dosed every 8 hours. No data for pt with impaired renal function	Data need confirmation. Based on 14 obese patients with actual BW >130 kg and BMI >40 kg/m^2. Ref: *Int J Antimicrob Ag 41:52, 2013.* High dose to optimize dose for pathogens with MIC ≤16 mcg/mL. May enhance bleeding propensity in uremic patients.

[1] Ref. for NRTIs and NNRTIs: *Kidney International 60:821, 2001*

See page 2 for other abbreviations

TABLE 17C (2)

Drug	Dose	Comments
Vancomycin	Use **Actual BW** Example: in critically ill patient give 25-30 mg/kg of Actual BW IV load, then 15-20 mg/kg of Actual BW IV q8h-12h (infuse over 1.5-2 hr). No single dose over 2 gm. Check trough levels.	Data from 24 obese patients; Vancomycin half-life appears to decrease with little change in Vd. Ref: *Eur J Clin Pharmacol 54:621, 1998.*
Voriconazole po	**No dose adjustment** required Example: 400 mg po q12h x2 doses then 200 mg po q12h. Check trough concentrations (underdosing common with Voriconazole).	Data from a 2-way crossover study of oral voriconazole in 8 volunteers suggest no adjustment required, but data from one patient suggest use of adjusted BW. Recommended IV voriconazole dose based on actual BW (no supporting data). Refs: *Antimicrob Ag Chemother 55:2601, 2011; Clin Infect Dis 53:745, 2011.*

TABLE 18 – ANTIMICROBIALS AND HEPATIC DISEASE: DOSAGE ADJUSTMENT*

The following alphabetical list indicates antibacterials excreted/metabolized by the liver **wherein a dosage adjustment may be indicated** in the presence of hepatic disease. Space precludes details; consult the PDR or package inserts for details. List is **not** all-inclusive:

Antibacterials		Antifungals	Antivirals[§]	
Ceftriaxone	Nafcillin	Caspofungin	Abacavir	Indinavir
Chloramphenicol	Rifabutin	Itraconazole	Atazanavir	Lopinavir/ritonavir
Clindamycin	Rifampin	Voriconazole	Darunavir	Nelfinavir
Fusidic acid	Synercid**		Delavirdine	Nevirapine
Isoniazid	Telithromycin[++]		Efavirenz	Rimantadine
Metronidazole	Tigecycline		Enfuvirtide	Ritonavir
	Tinidazole		Fosamprenavir	Stribild

[§] Ref. on antiretrovirals: *CID 40:174, 2005* ** Quinupristin/dalfopristin [++] Telithro: reduce dose in renal & hepatic failure

TABLE 19 – TREATMENT OF CAPD PERITONITIS IN ADULTS*

(Periton Dial Intl 30:393, 2010)[1]

EMPIRIC Intraperitoneal Therapy: Culture Results Pending *(For MRSA see footnote[2])*

Drug		Residual Urine Output	
		<100 mL per day	**>100 mL per day**
(Cefazolin or Vanco) +	Can mix in same bag	1 gm per bag, q24h	20 mg per kg BW per bag, q24h
Ceftazidime		1 gm per bag, q24h	20 mg per kg BW per bag, q24h

Drug Doses for SPECIFIC Intraperitoneal Therapy—Culture Results Known. NOTE: Few po drugs indicated

Drug	Intermittent Dosing (once per day)		Continuous Dosing (per liter exchange)	
	Anuric	**Non-Anuric**	**Anuric**	**Non-Anuric**
Amphotericin B	NA	NA	MD 1.5 mg	NA
Ampicillin	250–500 mg po bid	ND	No LD, MD 125 mg	ND
Amp-sulbactam	2 gm q12h	ND	LD 1 gm, MD 100 mg	LD 1 gm, MD ↑ 25%
Cefazolin	15 mg per kg	20 mg per kg	LD 500 mg, MD 125 mg	LD 500 mg, ↑ MD 25%
Cefepime	1 gm in one exchange/day	1.25 gm	LD 500 mg, MD 125 mg	LD 500 mg, ↑ MD 25%
Ceftazidime	1000–1500 mg	ND	LD 500 mg, MD 125 mg	LD 500 mg; ↑ MD 25%
Ciprofloxacin	500 mg po bid	ND	LD 50 mg, MD 25 mg	ND
Daptomycin			LD 100 mg, MD 20 mg	LD 500 mg, ↑ MD 25%
Fluconazole	200 mg q24h	ND	200 mg q24h	ND
Gentamicin	0.6 mg per kg	↑ dose 25%	Not recommended	Not recommended
Imipenem	1 gm in one exchange q12h		LD 250 mg, MD 50 mg	LD 250 mg, ↑ MD 25%
Itraconazole	100 mg q12h	100 mg q12h	100 mg q12h	100 mg q12h
Metronidazole	250 mg po bid	ND	250 mg po bid	ND
TMP-SMX	160/800 mg po bid	ND	LD 320/1600 mg po, MD 80/400 mg po q24h	ND
Vancomycin	15–30 mg per kg q3–7 days	↑ dose 25%	LD 1 gm; MD 25 mg	LD 1 gm, ↑ MD 25%

CAPD = continuous ambulatory peritoneal dialysis

Indications for catheter removal: 1) Relapse with same organism within 1 mo; 2) Failure to respond clinically within 5 days; 3) Exit site and tunnel infection; 4) Fungal peritonitis; 5) Fecal flora peritonitis (suggests bowel perforation).

[1] **All doses IP unless indicated otherwise.**
LD = loading dose, **MD** = maintenance dose, **ND** = no data; **NA** = not applicable—dose as normal renal function.
Anuric = <100 mL per day, **non-anuric** = >100 mL per day

[2] **Does not provide treatment for MRSA.** If gram-pos cocci on gram stain, include vanco.

See page 2 for other abbreviations

TABLE 20A – ANTI-TETANUS PROPHYLAXIS, WOUND CLASSIFICATION, IMMUNIZATION

WOUND CLASSIFICATION		
Clinical Features	**Tetanus Prone**	**Non-Tetanus Prone**
Age of wound	> 6 hours	≤ 6 hours
Configuration	Stellate, avulsion	Linear
Depth	> 1 cm	≤ 1 cm
Mechanism of injury	Missile, crush, burn, frostbite	Sharp surface (glass, knife)
Devitalized tissue	Present	Absent
Contaminants (dirt, saliva, etc.)	Present	Absent
(From ACS Bull. 69:22,23, 1984, No. 10)		

IMMUNIZATION SCHEDULE				
History of Tetanus Immunization	**Dirty, Tetanus-Prone Wound**		**Clean, non-Tetanus-Prone Wound**	
	Td[1,2]	Tetanus Immune Globulin	Td[1,2]	Tetanus Immune Globulin
Unknown or < 3 doses[3]	Yes	Yes	Yes	No
3 or more doses	No[4]	No	No[5]	No

References: *MMWR 39:37, 1990; MMWR 46 (SS-2):15, 1997; MMWR 61:468, 2012; general vaccine considerations, MMWR 60 (RR-2):1, 2011; and general immunization schedule, MMWR Surveill Summ 62(13):256, 2013; www.cdc.gov/vaccines/schedules/hcp/adult.html*

[1] Td = Tetanus & diphtheria toxoids, adsorbed (adult). For adult who has not received Tdap previously, substitute one dose of Tdap for Td when immunization is indicated *(MMWR 61::468, 2012)*.
[2] For children < 7 years, use DTaP unless contraindicated; for persons ≥ 7 years, Td is preferred to tetanus toxoid alone, but single dose of Tdap can be used if required for catch-up series.
[3] Individuals who have not completed vaccine series should do so.
[4] Yes, if >5 years since last booster.
[5] Yes, if >10 years since last booster.

TABLE 20B – RABIES POSTEXPOSURE PROPHYLAXIS

All wounds should be cleaned immediately & thoroughly with soap & water. This has been shown to protect 90% of experimental animals![1]

Postexposure Prophylaxis Guide, United States, 2012

(MMWR 57 (RR-3): 1, 2008; http://wwwnc.cdc.gov/travel/yellowbook/2012/chapter-3-infectious-diseases-related-to-travel/rabies.htm)

Animal Type	Evaluation & Disposition of Animal	Recommendations for Prophylaxis
Dogs, cats, ferrets	Healthy & available for 10-day observation	Don't start unless animal develops sx, then immediately begin HRIG + vaccine
	Rabid or suspected rabid	Immediate HRIG + vaccine
	Unknown (escaped)	Consult public health officials
Skunks, raccoons, bats,* foxes, coyotes, most carnivores	Regard as rabid	Immediate vaccination
Livestock, horses, rodents, rabbits; includes hares, squirrels, hamsters, guinea pigs, gerbils, chipmunks, rats, mice, woodchucks	Consider case-by-case	Consult public health officials. Bites of squirrels, hamsters, guinea pigs, gerbils, chipmunks, rats, mice, other small rodents, rabbits, and hares **almost never** require rabies post-exposure prophylaxis.

* Most recent cases of human rabies in U.S. due to contact (not bites) with silver-haired bats or rarely big brown bats but risk of acquiring rabies from non-contact bat exposure is exceedingly low *(CID 48:1493, 2009)*. For more detail, *see CID 30:4, 2000; JAVMA 219:1687, 2001; CID 37:96, 2003 (travel medicine advisory); Ln 363:959, 2004; EID 11:1921, 2005; MMWR 55 (RR-5), 2006.*

Postexposure Rabies Immunization Schedule

IF NOT PREVIOUSLY VACCINATED

Treatment	Regimen[2]
Local wound cleaning	**All postexposure treatment should begin with immediate, thorough cleaning of all wounds with soap & water.**
Human rabies immune globulin (HRIG)	20 units per kg body weight given once on day 0. If anatomically feasible, the full dose should be infiltrated around the wound(s), the rest should be administered IM in the gluteal area. If the calculated dose of HRIG is insufficient to inject all the wounds, it should be diluted with normal saline to allow infiltration around additional wound areas. HRIG should **not** be administered in the **same syringe**, **or** into the **same anatomical site** as vaccine, or more than 7 days after the initiation of vaccine. Because HRIG may partially suppress active production of antibody, no more than the recommended dose should be given.[3]
Vaccine	Human diploid cell vaccine (HDCV), rabies vaccine adsorbed (RVA), or purified chick embryo cell vaccine (PCECV) 1 mL **IM (deltoid area[4])**, one each days 0, 3, 7, 14[5].

IF PREVIOUSLY VACCINATED[6]

Treatment	Regimen[2]
Local wound cleaning	All postexposure treatment should begin with immediate, thorough cleaning of all wounds with soap **&** water.
HRIG	HRIG should **not** be administered
Vaccine	HDCV or PCEC, 1 mL **IM (deltoid area[4])**, one each on days 0 & 3

CORRECT VACCINE ADMINISTRATION SITES

Age Group	Administration Site
Children & adults	**DELTOID[4]** only (**NEVER** in gluteus)
Infants & young children	Outer aspect of thigh (anterolateral thigh) may be used (**NEVER** in gluteus)

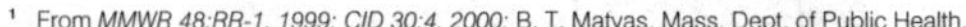

1 From *MMWR 48:RR-1, 1999; CID 30:4, 2000;* B. T. Matyas, Mass. Dept. of Public Health.

2 These regimens are applicable for all age groups, including children.

3 In most reported post-exposure treatment failures, only identified deficiency was failure to infiltrate wound(s) with HRIG *(CID 22:228, 1996)*. However, several failures reported from SE Asia in patients in whom WHO protocol followed *(CID 28:143, 1999)*.

4 The **deltoid** area is the **only** acceptable site of vaccination for adults & older children. For infants & young children, outer aspect of the thigh (anterolateral thigh) may be used. Vaccine should **NEVER** be administered in gluteal area.

5 Note that this is a change from previous recommendation of 5 doses (days 0, 3, 7, 14 & 28) based on new data & recommendations from ACIP. Note that the number of doses for persons with altered immunocompetence remains unchanged (5 doses on days 0, 3, 7, 14 & 28) and recommendations for pre-exposure prophylaxis remain 3 doses administered on days 0, 7 and 21 or 28 *(MMWR 59 (RR-2), 2010)*.

6 Any person with a history of pre-exposure vaccination with HDCV, RVA, PCECV; prior post-exposure prophylaxis with HDCV, PCEC or rabies vaccine adsorbed (RVA); or previous vaccination with any other type of rabies vaccine & a documented history of antibody response to the prior vaccination.

TABLE 21 SELECTED DIRECTORY OF RESOURCES

ORGANIZATION	PHONE/FAX	WEBSITE(S)
ANTIPARASITIC DRUGS & PARASITOLOGY INFORMATION *(CID 37:694, 2003)*		
CDC Drug Line	Weekdays: 404-639-3670 Evenings, weekends, holidays: 404-639-2888	http://www.cdc.gov/ncidod/srp/drugs/drug-service.html
DPDx: Lab ID of parasites		www.dpd.cdc.gov/dpdx/default.htm
Gorgas Course Tropical Medicine		http://info.dom.uab.edu/gorgas
Malaria	daytime: 770-488-7788 other: 770-488-7100 US toll free: 855-856-4713	www.cdc.gov/malaria
Expert Compound. Pharm.	800-247-9767/818-787-7256	www.uniquerx.com
World Health Organization (WHO)		www.who.int
Parasites & Health		www.dpd.cdc.gov/dpdx/HTML/Para_Health.htm
BIOTERRORISM		
Centers for Disease Control & Prevention	770-488-7100	www.bt.cdc.gov
Infectious Diseases Society of America	703-299-0200	www.idsociety.org
Johns Hopkins Center Civilian Biodefense		www.jhsph.edu
Center for Biosecurity of the Univ. of Pittsburgh Med. Center		www.upmc-biosecurity.org
US Army Medical Research Institute of Inf. Dis.		www.usamriid.army.mil
HEPATITIS B		
Hepatitis B Foundation		www.hepb.org, www.natap.org
HEPATITIS C *(CID 35:754, 2002)*		
CDC		www.cdc.gov/ncidod/diseases/hepatitis/C
Individual		http://hepatitis-central.com www.natap.org
Medscape		www.medscape.com
HIV		
General		
HIV InSite		http://hivinsite.ucsf.edu
Johns Hopkins AIDS Service		www.hopkins-aids.edu www.natap.org
Drug Interactions		
Johns Hopkins AIDS Service		www.hopkins-aids.edu
Liverpool HIV Pharm. Group		www.hiv-druginteractions.org
Other		http://AIDS.medscape.com
Prophylaxis/Treatment of Opportunistic Infections; HIV Treatment		www.aidsinfo.nih.gov
IMMUNIZATIONS *(CID 36:355, 2003)*		
CDC, Natl. Immunization Program	404-639-8200	www.cdc.gov/vaccines/
FDA, Vaccine Adverse Events	800-822-7967	www.fda.gov/cber/vaers/vaers.htm
National Network Immunization Info.	877-341-6644	www.immunizationinfo.org
Influenza vaccine, CDC	404-639-8200	www.cdc.gov/vaccines/
Institute for Vaccine Safety		www.vaccinesafety.edu
OCCUPATIONAL EXPOSURE, BLOOD-BORNE PATHOGENS (HIV, HEPATITIS B & C)		
National Clinicians' Post-Exposure Hotline	888-448-4911	www.ucsf.edu/hivcntr
Q-T$_c$ INTERVAL PROLONGATION BY DRUGS		www.qtdrugs.org
SEXUALLY TRANSMITTED DISEASES		www.cdc.gov/std/treatment/TOC2002TG.htm Slides: http://www.phac-aspc.gc.ca/slm-maa/slides/index.html
TRAVELERS' INFO: Immunizations, Malaria Prophylaxis, More		
Amer. Soc. Trop. Med. & Hyg.		www.astmh.org
CDC, general	877-394-8747/888-232-3299	http://wwwn.cdc.gov/travel/default.asp
CDC, Malaria:		www.cdc.gov/malaria
Prophylaxis		http://wwwn.cdc.gov/travel/default.asp
Treatment	770-488-7788	www.who.int/health_topics/malaria
MD Travel Health		www.mdtravelhealth.com
Pan American Health Organization		www.paho.org
World Health Organization (WHO)		www.who.int/home-page
VACCINE & IMMUNIZATION RESOURCES *(CID 36:355, 2003)*		
American Academy of Pediatrics		www.cispimmunize.org
CDC, National Immunization Program		www.cdc.gov/vaccines/
National Network for Immunization Information		www.immunizationinfo.org

TABLE 22A – ANTI-INFECTIVE DRUG-DRUG INTERACTIONS

Importance: ± = theory/anecdotal; + = of probable importance; ++ = of definite importance
To check for interactions between more than 2 drugs, *see: http://www.drugs.com/drug_interactions.html and http://www.healthline.com/druginteractions*

ANTI-INFECTIVE AGENT (A)	OTHER DRUG (B)	EFFECT	IMPORT
Abacavir	Methadone	↓ levels of B	++
Amantadine (Symmetrel)	Alcohol	↑ CNS effects	+
	Anticholinergic and anti-Parkinson agents (ex. Artane, scopolamine)	↑ effect of B: dry mouth, ataxia, blurred vision, slurred speech, toxic psychosis	+
	Trimethoprim	↑ levels of A & B	+
	Digoxin	↑ levels of B	±
Aminoglycosides—parenteral (amikacin, gentamicin, kanamycin, netilmicin, sisomicin, streptomycin, tobramycin)	Amphotericin B	↑ nephrotoxicity	++
	Cis platinum (Platinol)	↑ nephro & ototoxicity	+
	Cyclosporine	↑ nephrotoxicity	+
	Neuromuscular blocking agents	↑ apnea or respiratory paralysis	+
	Loop diuretics (e.g., furosemide)	↑ ototoxicity	++
	NSAIDs	↑ nephrotoxicity	+
	Non-polarizing muscle relaxants	↑ apnea	+
	Radiographic contrast	↑ nephrotoxicity	+
	Vancomycin	↑ nephrotoxicity	+
Aminoglycosides—oral (kanamycin, neomycin)	**Warfarin**	↑ prothrombin time	+
Amphotericin B and ampho B lipid formulations	Antineoplastic drugs	↑ nephrotoxicity risk	+
	Digitalis	↑ toxicity of B if K^+ ↓	+
	Nephrotoxic drugs: aminoglycosides, cidofovir, cyclosporine, foscarnet, pentamidine	↑ nephrotoxicity of A	++
Ampicillin, amoxicillin	Allopurinol	↑ frequency of rash	++
Artemether-lumefantrine	CYP3A inhibitors: amiodarone, atazanavir, itraconazole, ritonavir, voriconazole	↑ levels of A; ↑ QTc interval	++
	CYP2D6 substrates: flecainide, imipramine, amitriptyline	↑ levels of B; ↑ QTc interval	++
Atazanavir	*See protease inhibitors and Table 22B*		
Atovaquone	Rifampin (perhaps rifabutin)	↓ serum levels of A; ↑ levels of B	+
	Metoclopramide	↓ levels of A	+
	Tetracycline	↓ levels of A	++

Azole Antifungal Agents [**Flu** = fluconazole; **Itr** = itraconazole; **Ket** = ketoconazole; **Posa** = posaconazole **Vor** = voriconazole; **+** = occurs; **blank space** = either studied & no interaction OR no data found (may be in pharm. co. databases)]

Flu	Itr	Ket	Posa	Vor	OTHER DRUG (B)	EFFECT	IMPORT
+	+				Amitriptyline	↑ levels of B	+
+	+	+		+	Calcium channel blockers	↑ levels of B	++
	+			+	Carbamazepine (vori contraindicated)	↓ levels of A	++
+	+	+	+	+	Cyclosporine	↑ levels of B, ↑ risk of nephrotoxicity	+
	+	+			Didanosine	↓ absorption of A	+
	+	+	+	+	Efavirenz	↓ levels of A, ↑ levels of B	++ **(avoid)**
	+	+	+		H_2 blockers, antacids, sucralfate	↓ absorption of A	+
+	+	+	+	+	Hydantoins (phenytoin, Dilantin)	↑ levels of B, ↓ levels of A	++
	+	+			Isoniazid	↓ levels of A	+
	+	+	+	+	Lovastatin/simvastatin	Rhabdomyolysis reported; ↑ levels of B	++
				+	Methadone	↑ levels of B	+
+	+	+	+	+	Midazolam/triazolam, po	↑ levels of B	++
+	+			+	Warfarin	↑ effect of B	++
+	+			+	Oral hypoglycemics	↑ levels of B	++
			+	+	Pimozide	↑ levels of B—**avoid**	++
	+	+		+	Protease inhibitors	↑ levels of B	++
	+	+	+	+	Proton pump inhibitors	↓ levels of A, ↑ levels of B	++
+	+	+	+	+	Rifampin/rifabutin (vori contraindicated)	↑ levels of B, ↓ serum levels of A	++
	+				Rituximab	Inhibits action of B	++
			+	+	Sirolimus (vori and posa contraindicated)	↑ levels of B	++
+		+	+	+	Tacrolimus	↑ levels of B with toxicity	++
+		+			Theophyllines	↑ levels of B	+
		+			Trazodone	↑ levels of B	++
+					Zidovudine	↑ levels of B	+

TABLE 22A (2)

ANTI-INFECTIVE AGENT (A)	OTHER DRUG (B)	EFFECT	IMPORT
Bedaquiline	Rifampin	↓ levels of A	++
	Ketoconazole	↑ levels of A	
Caspofungin	Cyclosporine	↑ levels of A	++
	Tacrolimus	↓ levels of B	++
	Carbamazepine, dexamethasone, efavirenz, nevirapine, phenytoin, rifamycin	↓ levels of A; ↑ dose of caspofungin to 70 mg/d	++
Chloramphenicol	Hydantoins	↑ toxicity of B, nystagmus, ataxia	++
	Iron salts, Vitamin B12	↓ response to B	++
	Protease inhibitors—HIV	↑ levels of A & B	++
Clindamycin (Cleocin)	Kaolin	↓ absorption of A	++
	Muscle relaxants, e.g., atracurium, baclofen, diazepam	↑ frequency/duration of respiratory paralysis	++
	St John's wort	↓ levels of A	++
Cobicistat	*See Stribild, below*		
Cycloserine	Ethanol	↑ frequency of seizures	+
	INH, ethionamide	↑ frequency of drowsiness/dizziness	+
Dapsone	Atazanavir	↑ levels of A - Avoid	++
	Didanosine	↓ absorption of A	+
	Oral contraceptives	↓ effectiveness of B	+
	Pyrimethamine	↑ in marrow toxicity	+
	Rifampin/Rifabutin	↓ serum levels of A	+
	Trimethoprim	↑ levels of A & B (methemoglobinemia)	+
	Zidovudine	May ↑ marrow toxicity	+
Daptomycin	HMG-CoA inhibitors (statins)	Consider DC statin while on dapto	++
Delavirdine (Rescriptor)	*See Non-nucleoside reverse transcriptase inhibitors (NNRTIs) and Table 22B*		
Didanosine (ddI) (Videx)	Allopurinol	↑ levels of A—**AVOID**	++
	Cisplatin, dapsone, INH, metronidazole, nitrofurantoin, stavudine, vincristine, zalcitabine	↑ risk of peripheral neuropathy	+
	Ethanol, lamivudine, pentamidine	↑ risk of pancreatitis	+
	Fluoroquinolones	↓ absorption 2° to chelation	+
	Drugs that need low pH for absorption: dapsone, indinavir, itra/ ketoconazole, pyrimethamine, rifampin, trimethoprim	↓ absorption	+
	Methadone	↓ levels of A	++
	Ribavirin	↑ levels ddI metabolite—**avoid**	++
	Tenofovir	↑ levels of A **(reduce dose of A)**	++
Doripenem	Probenecid	↑ levels of A	++
	Valproic acid	↓ levels of B	++
Doxycycline	Aluminum, bismuth, iron, Mg^{++}	↓ absorption of A	+
	Barbiturates, hydantoins	↓ serum t/2 of A	+
	Carbamazepine (Tegretol)	↓ serum t/2 of A	+
	Digoxin	↑ serum levels of B	+
	Warfarin	↑ activity of B	++
Efavirenz (Sustiva)	*See non-nucleoside reverse transcriptase inhibitors (NNRTIs) and Table 22B*		
Elvitegravir	*See Stribild, below*		
Ertapenem (Invanz)	Probenecid	↑ levels of A	++
	Valproic acid	↓ levels of B	++
Ethambutol (Myambutol)	Aluminum salts (includes didanosine buffer)	↓ absorption of A & B	+
Etravirine	*See non-nucleoside reverse transcriptase inhibitors (NNRTIs) and Table 22B*		

Fluoroquinolones (**Cipro** = ciprofloxacin; **Gati** = gatifloxacin; **Gemi** = gemifloxacin; **Levo** = levofloxacin; **Moxi** = moxifloxacin; **Oflox** = ofloxacin)

NOTE: Blank space = *either studied and no interaction OR no data found*

Cipro	Gati	Gemi	Levo	Moxi	Oflox	OTHER DRUG (B)	EFFECT	IMPORT
	+		+	+		**Antiarrhythmics (procainamide, amiodarone)**	↑ Q-T interval (torsade)	++
+	+		+	+	+	Insulin, oral hypoglycemics	↑ & ↓ blood sugar	++
+						Caffeine	↑ levels of B	+
+					+	Cimetidine	↑ levels of A	+
+					+	Cyclosporine	↑ levels of B	±
+	+		+	+	+	Didanosine	↓ absorption of A	++
+	+	+	+	+	+	**Cations: Al+++, Ca++, Fe++, Mg++, Zn++ (antacids, vitamins, dairy products), citrate/citric acid**	↓ absorption of A (some variability between drugs)	++
+						Methadone	↑ levels of B	++
+			+		+	**NSAIDs**	↑ risk CNS stimulation/seizures	++
+						Phenytoin	↑ or ↓ levels of B	+

TABLE 22A (3)

ANTI-INFECTIVE AGENT (A)	OTHER DRUG (B)	EFFECT	IMPORT
Fluoroquinolones *(continued)*			

Cipro	Gati	Gemi	Levo	Moxi	Oflox	OTHER DRUG (B)	EFFECT	IMPORT
						NOTE: Blank space = either studied and no interaction OR no data found		
+	+	+			+	Probenecid	↓ renal clearance of A	+
+						Rasagiline	↑ levels of B	++
				+		Rifampin	↓ levels of A *(CID 45:1001, 2007)*	++
+	+	+	+		+	**Sucralfate**	**↓ absorption of A**	**++**
+						Theophylline	↑ levels of B	++
+						Thyroid hormone	↓ levels of B	++
+						Tizanidine	↑ levels of B	++
+			+	+	+	Warfarin	↑ prothrombin time	+

ANTI-INFECTIVE AGENT (A)	OTHER DRUG (B)	EFFECT	IMPORT
Ganciclovir (Cytovene) & **Valganciclovir** (Valcyte)	Imipenem	↑ risk of seizures reported	+
	Probenecid	↑ levels of A	+
	Zidovudine	↓ levels of A, ↑ levels of B	+
Gentamicin	*See Aminoglycosides—parenteral*		
Imipenem & Meropenem	BCG	↓ effectiveness of B – avoid combination	++
	Divalproex	↓ levels of B	++
	Ganciclovir	↑ seizure risk	++
	Probenecid	↑ levels of A	++
	Valproic acid	↓ levels of B	++
Indinavir	*See protease inhibitors and Table 22B*		
Isoniazid	**Alcohol, rifampin**	**↑ risk of hepatic injury**	++
	Aluminum salts	↓ absorption (take fasting)	++
	Carbamazepine, phenytoin	↑ levels of B with nausea, vomiting, nystagmus, ataxia	++
	Itraconazole, ketoconazole	↓ levels of B	+
	Oral hypoglycemics	↓ effects of B	+
Lamivudine	Zalcitabine	**Mutual interference—do not combine**	++
Linezolid (Zyvox)	Adrenergic agents	Risk of hypertension	++
	Aged, fermented, pickled or smoked foods —↑ tyramine	Risk of hypertension	+
	Clarithromycin	↑ levels of A	++
	Rasagiline (MAO inhibitor)	Risk of serotonin syndrome	+
	Rifampin	↓ levels of A	++
	Serotonergic drugs (SSRIs)	Risk of serotonin syndrome	++
Lopinavir	*See protease inhibitors*		

Macrolides [**Ery** = erythromycin; **Azi** = azithromycin; **Clr** = clarithromycin; **+** = occurs; **blank space** = either studied and no interaction OR no data]

Ery	Azi	Clr	OTHER DRUG (B)	EFFECT	IMPORT
	+		Calcium channel blockers	↑ serum levels of B	++
+		+	Carbamazepine	↑ serum levels of B, nystagmus, nausea, vomiting, ataxia	++ (avoid w/ erythro)
+		+	Cimetidine, **ritonavir**	↑ levels of B	+
+			Clozapine	↑ serum levels of B, CNS toxicity	+
		+	**Colchicine**	**↑ levels of B (potent, fatal)**	++(avoid)
+			Corticosteroids	↑ effects of B	+
+	+	+	Cyclosporine	↑ serum levels of B with toxicity	+
+	+	+	Digoxin, digitoxin	↑ serum levels of B (10% of cases)	+
		+	Efavirenz	↓ levels of A	++
+		+	Ergot alkaloids	↑ levels of B	++
		+	Linezolid	↑ levels of B	++
+		+	Lovastatin/simvastatin	↑ levels of B; rhabdomyolysis	++
+			Midazolam, triazolam	↑ levels of B, ↑ sedative effects	+
+		+	Phenytoin	↑ levels of B	+
+	+	+	Pimozide	**↑ Q-T interval**	++
+		+	Rifampin, rifabutin	↓ levels of A	+
+		+	Tacrolimus	↑ levels of B	++
+		+	Theophylline	↑ serum levels of B with nausea, vomiting, seizures, apnea	++
+		+	Valproic acid	↑ levels of B	+
+		+	Warfarin	May ↑ prothrombin time	+
		+	Zidovudine	↓ levels of B	+

TABLE 22A (4)

ANTI-INFECTIVE AGENT (A)	OTHER DRUG (B)	EFFECT	IMPORT
Maraviroc	Clarithromycin	↑ serum levels of A	++
	Delavirdine	↑ levels of A	++
	Itraconazole/ketoconazole	↑ levels of A	++
	Nefazodone	↑ levels of A	++
	Protease inhibitors (not tipranavir/ritonavir)	↑ levels of A	++
	Anticonvulsants: carbamazepine, phenobarbital, phenytoin	↓ levels of A	++
	Efavirenz	↓ levels of A	++
	Rifampin	↓ levels of A	++
Mefloquine	β-adrenergic blockers, calcium channel blockers, quinidine, quinine	↑ arrhythmias	+
	Divalproex, valproic acid	↓ level of B with seizures	++
	Halofantrine	Q-T prolongation	**++ (avoid)**
	Calcineurin inhibitors	Q-T prolongation (avoid)	++
Meropenem	*See Imipenem*		
Methenamine mandelate or hippurate	Acetazolamide, sodium bicarbonate, thiazide diuretics	↓ antibacterial effect 2° to ↑ urine pH	++
Metronidazole Tinidazole	**Alcohol**	Disulfiram-like reaction	+
	Cyclosporin	↑ levels of B	++
	Disulfiram (Antabuse)	Acute toxic psychosis	+
	Lithium	↑ levels of B	++
	Warfarin	↑ anticoagulant effect	++
	Phenobarbital, hydantoins	↑ levels of B	++
Micafungin	Nifedipine	↑ levels of B	+
	Sirolimus	↑ levels of B	+
Nafcillin	Warfarin	↓ Warfarin effect	++
Nelfinavir	*See protease inhibitors and Table 22B*		
Nevirapine (Viramune)	*See non-nucleoside reverse transcriptase inhibitors (NNRTIs) and Table 22B*		
Nitrofurantoin	Antacids	↓ absorption of A	+

Non-nucleoside reverse transcriptase inhibitors (NNRTIs): For interactions with protease inhibitors, *see Table 22B*.
Del = delavirdine; **Efa** = efavirenz; **Etr** = etravirine; **Nev** = nevirapine

Del	Efa	Etr	Nev	**Co-administration contraindicated** *(See package insert)*:		
+		+		Anticonvulsants: carbamazepine, phenobarbital, phenytoin		++
+		+		Antimycobacterials: rifabutin, rifampin		++
+				Antipsychotics: pimozide		++
+	+	+		Benzodiazepines: alprazolam, midazolam, triazolam		++
+	+			Ergotamine		++
+	+	+		HMG-CoA inhibitors (statins): lovastatin, simvastatin, atorvastatin, pravastatin		++
+		+		St. John's wort		++
				Dose change needed:		
+				Amphetamines	↑ levels of B—**caution**	++
+		+	+	Antiarrhythmics: amiodarone, lidocaine, others	↓ or ↑ levels of B—**caution**	++
+	+	+	+	Anticonvulsants: carbamazepine, phenobarbital, phenytoin	↓ levels of A and/or B	++
+	+	+	+	Antifungals: itraconazole, ketoconazole, voriconazole, posaconazole	Potential ↓ levels of B, ↑ levels of A	++ **(avoid)**
+			+	Antirejection drugs: cyclosporine, rapamycin, sirolimus, tacrolimus	↑ levels of B	++
+			+	Calcium channel blockers	↑ levels of B	++
+		+	+	Clarithromycin	↑ levels of B metabolite, ↑ levels of A	++
+		+	+	Cyclosporine	↑ levels of B	++
+		+		Dexamethasone	↓ levels of A	++
+	+	+	+	Sildenafil, vardenafil, tadalafil	↑ levels of B	++
+			+	Fentanyl, methadone	↑ levels of B	++
+				Gastric acid suppression: antacids, H-2 blockers, proton pump inhibitors	↓ levels of A	++
	+		+	Mefloquine	↓ levels of B	++
	+	+	+	Methadone, fentanyl	↓ levels of B	++
	+		+	Oral contraceptives	↑ or ↓ levels of B	++
+	+	+	+	Protease inhibitors—*see Table 22B*		
+	+	+	+	**Rifabutin, rifampin**	↑ or ↓ levels of rifabutin; ↓ levels of A—**caution**	++
+	+	+	+	St. John's wort	↓ levels of B	
+		+	+	Warfarin	↑ levels of B	++

ANTI-INFECTIVE AGENT (A)	OTHER DRUG (B)	EFFECT	IMPORT
Pentamidine, IV	Amphotericin B	↑ risk of nephrotoxicity	+
	Pancreatitis-assoc drugs, eg, alcohol, valproic acid	↑ risk of pancreatitis	+
Piperacillin	Cefoxitin	Antagonism vs pseudomonas	++
Pip-tazo	Methotrexate	↑ levels of B	++
Polymyxin B	Curare paralytics	Avoid: neuromuscular blockade	++

TABLE 22A (5)

ANTI-INFECTIVE AGENT (A)	OTHER DRUG (B)	EFFECT	IMPORT
Polymyxin E (Colistin)	Curare paralytics	Avoid: neuromuscular blockade	++
	Aminoglycosides, Ampho B, Vanco	↑ nephrotoxicity risk	++
Primaquine	Chloroquine, dapsone, INH, probenecid, quinine, sulfonamides, TMP/SMX, others	**↑ risk of hemolysis in G6PD-deficient patients**	++

Protease Inhibitors—Anti-HIV Drugs. (**Atazan** = atazanavir; **Darun** = darunavir; **Fosampren** = fosamprenavir; **Indin** = *indinavir;* **Lopin** = lopinavir; **Nelfin** = nelfinavir ; **Saquin** = saquinavir; **Tipran** = tipranavir). For interactions with antiretrovirals, *see Table 22B* **Only a partial list—check package insert**

Atazan	Darun	Fosampren	Indin	Lopin	Nelfin	Saquin	Tipran	**Also see http://aidsinfo.nih.gov** To check for interactions between more than 2 drugs, see: http://www.drugs.com/drug_interactions.html and http://www.healthline.com/druginteractions		
								Analgesics:		
							+	1. Alfentanil, fentanyl, hydrocodone, tramadol	↑ levels of B	+
	+			+		+	+	2. Codeine, hydromorphone, morphine, methadone	↓ levels of B *(JAIDS 41:563, 2006)*	+
+	+	+	+	+	+		+	**Anti-arrhythmics: amiodarone, lidocaine, mexiletine, flecainide**	↑ levels of B; **do not co-administer or use caution** *(See package insert)*	++
	+		+	+	+	+		**Anticonvulsants: carbamazepine, clonazepam, phenobarbital**	↓ levels of A, ↑ levels of B	++
+		+	+				+	Antidepressants, all tricyclic	↑ levels of B	++
+	+						+	Antidepressants, all other	↑ levels of B; do not use pimozide	++
	+							Antidepressants: SSRIs	↓ levels of B - avoid	++
							+	Antihistamines	**Do not use**	++
+	+	+	+	+	+		+	**Benzodiazepines, e.g., diazepam, midazolam, triazolam**	**↑ levels of B—do not use**	++
+	+			+				Boceprevir	↓ levels of A & B	++
+	+	+	+	+	+	+	+	Calcium channel blockers (all)	↑ levels of B	++
+	+			+	+	+	+	Clarithro, erythro	↑ levels of B if renal impairment	+
+	+			+	+		+	Contraceptives, oral	↓ levels of A & B	++
	+	+		+		+		Corticosteroids: prednisone, dexamethasone	↓ levels of A, ↑ levels of B	+
+	+	+	+	+	+	+	+	Cyclosporine	↑ levels of B, monitor levels	+
						+		Digoxin	↑ levels of B	++
+	+	+	+	+	+	+	+	Ergot derivatives	**↑ levels of B—do not use**	++
		+	+		+	+		Erythromycin, clarithromycin	↑ levels of A & B	+
			+		+	+		Grapefruit juice (>200 mL/day)	↓ indinavir & ↑ saquinavir levels	++
+	+	+	+	+	+	+		H2 receptor antagonists	↓ levels of A	++
+	+	+	+	+	+	+	+	**HMG-CoA reductase inhibitors (statins): lovastatin, simvastatin**	**↑ levels of B—do not use**	++
+								Irinotecan	**↑ levels of B—do not use**	++
	+	+	+	+	+	+	+	Ketoconazole, itraconazole, ? vori.	↑ levels of A, ↑ levels of B	+
	+	+	+	+	+	+	+	Posaconazole	↑ levels of A, no effect on B	++
				+			+	Metronidazole	Poss. disulfiram reaction, alcohol	+
				+				Phenytoin *(JAIDS 36:1034, 2004)*	↑ levels of A & B	++
+	+	+	+	+	+	+	+	**Pimozide**	**↑ levels of B—do not use**	++
+	+		+	+	+	+		Proton pump inhibitors	↓ levels of A	++
+	+	+	+	+	+	+	+	Rifampin, rifabutin	↓ levels of A, ↑ levels of B **(avoid)**	++ **(avoid)**
+	+	+	+	+	+	+	+	Sildenafil (Viagra), tadalafil, vardenafil	Varies, some ↑ & some ↓ levels of B	++
+	+	+	+	+	+	+	+	**St. John's wort**	**↓ levels of A—do not use**	++
+	+	+	+	+	+	+	+	**Sirolimus, tracrolimus**	**↑ levels of B**	++
+								Tenofovir	↓ levels of A—add ritonavir	++
	+		+	+				Theophylline	↓ levels of B	+
+		+		+			+	Warfarin	↑ levels of B	+

ANTI-INFECTIVE AGENT (A)	OTHER DRUG (B)	EFFECT	IMPORT
Pyrazinamide	INH, rifampin	May ↑ risk of hepatotoxicity	±
Pyrimethamine	Lorazepam	↑ risk of hepatotoxicity	+
	Sulfonamides, TMP/SMX	↑ risk of marrow suppression	+
	Zidovudine	↑ risk of marrow suppression	+
Quinine	Digoxin	↑ digoxin levels; ↑ toxicity	++
	Mefloquine	↑ arrhythmias	+
	Warfarin	↑ prothrombin time	++
Quinupristin- dalfopristin (Synercid)	Anti-HIV drugs: NNRTIs & PIs	↑ levels of B	++
	Antineoplastic: vincristine, docetaxel, paclitaxel	↑ levels of B	++
	Calcium channel blockers	↑ levels of B	++
	Carbamazepine	↑ levels of B	++
	Cyclosporine, tacrolimus	↑ levels of B	++

TABLE 22A (6)

ANTI-INFECTIVE AGENT (A)	OTHER DRUG (B)	EFFECT	IMPORT
Quinupristin-dalfopristin (Synercid) *(continued)*	Lidocaine	↑ levels of B	++
	Methylprednisolone	↑ levels of B	++
	Midazolam, diazepam	↑ levels of B	++
	Statins	↑ levels of B	++
Raltegravir	**Rifampin**	**↓ levels of A**	++
Ribavirin	Didanosine	↑ levels of B → toxicity—**avoid**	++
	Stavudine	↓ levels of B	++
	Zidovudine	↓ levels of B	++
Rifamycins (rifampin, rifabutin)	Al OH, ketoconazole, PZA	↓ levels of A	+
	Atovaquone	↑ levels of A, ↓ levels of B	+
Ref.: *ArIM 162:985, 2002*	Beta adrenergic blockers (metoprolol, propranolol)	↓ effect of B	+
The following is a partial list of drugs with rifampin-induced ↑ metabolism and hence lower than anticipated serum levels: ACE inhibitors, dapsone, diazepam, digoxin, diltiazem, doxycycline, fluconazole, fluvastatin, haloperidol, moxifloxacin, nifedipine, progestins, triazolam, tricyclics, voriconazole, zidovudine *(Clin Pharmacokinetic 42:819, 2003).*	Caspofungin	↓ levels of B—increase dose	++
	Clarithromycin	↑ levels of A, ↓ levels of B	++
	Corticosteroids	↑ replacement requirement of B	++
	Cyclosporine	↓ effect of B	++
	Delavirdine	**↑ levels of A, ↓ levels of B—avoid**	++
	Digoxin	↓ levels of B	++
	Disopyramide	↓ levels of B	++
	Fluconazole	↑ levels of A	+
	Amprenavir, indinavir, nelfinavir, ritonavir	↑ levels of A (↓ dose of A), ↓ levels of B	++
	INH	Converts INH to toxic hydrazine	++
	Itraconazole, ketoconazole	↓ levels of B, ↑ levels of A	++
	Linezolid	↓ levels of B	++
	Methadone	↓ serum levels (withdrawal)	+
	Nevirapine	**↓ levels of B—avoid**	++
	Warfarin	Suboptimal anticoagulation	++
	Oral contraceptives	↓ effectiveness; spotting, pregnancy	+
	Phenytoin	↓ levels of B	+
	Protease inhibitors	**↓ levels of A, ↑ levels of B—CAUTION**	++
	Quinidine	↓ effect of B	+
	Raltegravir	↓ levels of B	++
	Sulfonylureas	↓ hypoglycemic effect	+
	Tacrolimus	**↓ levels of B**	++
	Theophylline	↑ levels of B	+
	TMP/SMX	↓ levels of A	+
	Tocainide	↓ effect of B	+
Rimantadine	*See Amantadine*		
Ritonavir	*See protease inhibitors and Table 22B*		
Saquinavir	*See protease inhibitors and Table 22B*		
Stavudine	Dapsone, INH	May ↑ risk of peripheral neuropathy	±
	Ribavirin	↓ levels of A—**AVOID**	++
	Zidovudine	Mutual interference—do not combine	++
Stribild (Elvitegravir & Cobicistat components) *(See Emtricitabine & Tenofovir for other components)*			
Elvitegravir	Antacids	↓ levels of A	++
Cobicistat	Antiarrhythmics & digoxin	↑ levels of B	++
Cobicistat	Clarithromycin, telithromycin	↑ levels of B	++
Cobicistat & Elvitegravir	Carbamazepine, phenobarbital, phenytoin	↓ levels of A – **AVOID**	++
Cobicistat	SSRIs, TCAs, trazodone, antidepressants	↓ levels of A – **AVOID**	++
Cobicistat	Itraconazole, ketoconazole, voriconazole	↑ levels of B	++
Cobicistat	Colchicine	↑ levels of B – lower dose	++
Elvitegravir & Cobicistat	Rifabutin, rifapentine	↓ levels of A – **AVOID**	++
Cobicistat	Beta blockers	↑ levels of B	++
Cobicistat	Calcium channel blockers	↑ levels of B	++
Cobicistat & Elvitegravir	Dexamethasone	↓ levels of A	++
Cobicistat	Bosentan	↑ levels of B	++
Cobicistat	HMG-CoA reductase inhibitor, sirolimus	↑ levels of B	++
Cobicistat	Cyclosporine, tacrolimus	↑ levels of B	++
Cobicistat	Neuroleptics	↑ levels of B	++
Cobicistat	PDE5 inhibitors, e.g., Sildenafil, vardenafil, tadalafil	↑ levels of B – **AVOID**	++
Cobicistat	Benzodiazepines	↑ levels of B	++
Cobicistat	Ergot derivatives	↑ levels of B – **AVOID**	++
Cobicistat	Cisapride	↑ levels of B – **AVOID**	++
Cobicistat & Elvitegravir	St. John's wort	↑ levels of B – **AVOID**	++

TABLE 22A (7)

ANTI-INFECTIVE AGENT (A)	OTHER DRUG (B)	EFFECT	IMPORT
Sulfonamides	Beta blockers	↑ levels of B	++
	Cyclosporine	↓ cyclosporine levels	+
	Methotrexate	↑ antifolate activity	+
	Warfarin	↑ prothrombin time; bleeding	+
	Phenobarbital, rifampin	↓ levels of A	+
	Phenytoin	↑ levels of B; nystagmus, ataxia	+
	Sulfonylureas	↑ hypoglycemic effect	+
Telithromycin (Ketek)	Carbamazine	↓ levels of A	++
	Digoxin	↑ levels of B—do digoxin levels	++
	Ergot alkaloids	**↑ levels of B—avoid**	++
	Itraconazole; ketoconazole	↑ levels of A; no dose change	+
	Metoprolol	↑ levels of B	++
	Midazolam	↑ levels of B	++
	Warfarin	↑ prothrombin time	+
	Phenobarbital, phenytoin	↓ levels of A	++
	Pimozide	**↑ levels of B; QT prolongation—AVOID**	++
	Rifampin	**↓ levels of A—avoid**	++
	Simvastatin & other "statins"	↑ levels of B (↑ risk of myopathy)	++
	Sotalol	↓ levels of B	++
	Theophylline	↑ levels of B	++
Tenofovir	Atazanavir	↓ levels of B—add ritonavir	++
	Didanosine (ddI)	**↑ levels of B (reduce dose)**	++
Terbinafine	Cimetidine	↑ levels of A	+
	Phenobarbital, rifampin	↓ levels of A	+
Tetracyclines	*See Doxycycline, plus:*		
	Atovaquone	↓ levels of B	+
	Digoxin	↑ toxicity of B (may persist several months—up to 10% pts)	++
	Methoxyflurane	↑ toxicity; polyuria, renal failure	+
	Sucralfate	↓ absorption of A (separate by ≥2 hrs)	+
Thiabendazole	Theophyllines	↑ serum theophylline, nausea	+
Tigecycline	Oral contraceptives	↓ levels of B	++
Tinidazole (Tindamax)	*See Metronidazole—similar entity, expect similar interactions*		
Tobramycin	*See Aminoglycosides*		
Trimethoprim	Amantadine, dapsone, digoxin, methotrexate, procainamide, zidovudine	↑ serum levels of B	++
	Potassium-sparing diuretics	↑ serum K⁺	++
	Repaglinide	↑ levels of B (hypoglycemia)	++
	Thiazide diuretics	↓ serum Na⁺	+
Trimethoprim-Sulfamethoxazole	Ace inhibitors	↑ serum K+	++
	Amantadine	↑ levels of B (toxicity)	++
	Azathioprine	Reports of leukopenia	+
	Cyclosporine	↓ levels of B, ↑ serum creatinine	+
	Loperamide	↑ levels of B	+
	Methotrexate	Enhanced marrow suppression	++
	Oral contraceptives, pimozide, and 6-mercaptopurine	↓ effect of B	+
	Phenytoin	↑ levels of B	+
	Rifampin	↑ levels of B	+
	Warfarin	↑ activity of B	+
Valganciclovir (Valcyte)	*See Ganciclovir*		
Vancomycin	Aminoglycosides	↑ frequency of nephrotoxicity	++
Zalcitabine (ddC) (HIVID)	Valproic acid, pentamidine (IV), alcohol, lamivudine	↑ pancreatitis risk	+
	Cisplatin, INH, metronidazole, vincristine, nitrofurantoin, d4T, dapsone	↑ risk of peripheral neuropathy	+
Zidovudine (ZDV) (Retrovir)	Atovaquone, fluconazole, methadone	↑ levels of A	+
	Clarithromycin	↓ levels of A	±
	Indomethacin	↑ levels of ZDV toxic metabolite	+
	Nelfinavir	↓ levels of A	++
	Probenecid, TMP/SMX	↑ levels of A	+
	Rifampin/rifabutin	↓ levels of A	++
	Stavudine	**Interference—DO NOT COMBINE!**	++
	Valproic Acid	↑ levels of A	++

TABLE 22B – DRUG-DRUG INTERACTIONS BETWEEN NON-NUCLEOSIDE REVERSE TRANSCRIPTASE INHIBITORS (NNRTIS) AND PROTEASE INHIBITORS
(Adapted from Guidelines for the Use of Antiretroviral Agents in HIV-Infected Adults & Adolescents; *see www.aidsinfo.nih.gov*)

NAME (Abbreviation, Trade Name)	**Atazanavir (ATV, Reyataz)**	**DARUNAVIR (DRV, Prezista)**	**Fosamprenavir (FOS-APV, Lexiva)**	**Indinavir (IDV, Crixivan)**	**Lopinavir/Ritonavir (LP/R, Kaletra)**	**Nelfinavir (NFV, Viracept)**	**Saquinavir (SQV, Invirase)**	**Tipranavir (TPV)**
Delavirdine (DLV, Rescriptor)	No data	No data	**Co-administration not recommended**	IDV levels ↑ 40%. Dose: IDV 600 mg q8h, DLV standard	Expect LP levels to ↑. No dose data	NFV levels ↑ 2X; DLV levels ↓ 50%. Dose: No data	SQV levels ↑ 5X. Dose: SQV 800 mg q8h, DLV standard	No data
Efavirenz (EFZ, Sustiva)	ATV AUC ↓ 74%. Dose: EFZ standard; ATA/RTV 300/100 mg q24h with food	Standard doses of both drugs	FOS-APV levels ↓. Dose: EFZ standard; FOS-APV 1400 mg + RTV 300 mg q24h or 700 mg FOS-APV + 100 mg RTV q12h	Levels: IDV ↓ 31%. Dose: IDV 1000 mg q8h. EFZ standard	Level of LP ↓ 40%. Dose: LP/R 533/133 mg q12h, EFZ standard	Standard doses	Level: SQV ↓ 62%. Dose: SQV 400 mg + RTV 400 mg q12h	No dose change necessary
Etravirine (ETR, Intelence)	↑ ATV & ↑ ETR levels.	Standard doses of both drugs	↑ levels of FOS-APV.	↓ level of IDV.	↑ levels of ETR, ↓ **levels of LP/R.**	↑ levels of NFV.	↓ ETR levels 33%; SQV/R no change. Standard dose of both drugs.	↓ levels of ETR, ↑ levels of TPV & RTV. **Avoid combination.**
Nevirapine (NVP, Viramune)	Avoid combination. ATZ increases NVP concentrations > 25%; NVP decreases ATZ AUC by 42%	Standard doses of both drugs	Use with caution. NVP AUC increased 14% (700/100 Fos/rit; NVP AUC inc 29% (Fos 1400 mg bid).	IDV levels ↓ 28%. Dose: IDV 1000 mg q8h or combine with RTV; NVP standard	LP levels ↓ 53%. Dose: LP/R 533/133 mg q12h; NVP standard	Standard doses	Dose: SQV + RTV 400/400 mg, both q12h	**Standard doses**

TABLE 23 – LIST OF GENERIC AND COMMON TRADE NAMES

GENERIC NAME: TRADE NAMES	GENERIC NAME: TRADE NAMES	GENERIC NAME: TRADE NAMES
Abacavir: Ziagen	Efavirenz: Sustiva	Nitazoxanide: Alinia
Abacavir + Lamivudine: Epzicom	Efavirenz/Emtricitabine/Tenofovir: Atripla	Nitrofurantoin: Macrobid, Macrodantin
Abacavir + Lamivudine + Zidovudine: Trizivir	Elvitegravir + Cobicistat + Emtricitabine + Tenofovir: Stribild	Nystatin: Mycostatin
Acyclovir: Zovirax	Emtricitabine: Emtriva	Ofloxacin: Floxin
Adefovir: Hepsera	Emtricitabine + tenofovir: Truvada	Olysio: Simeprevir
Albendazole: Albenza	Emtricitabine + tenofovir + rilpivirine: Complera	Oseltamivir: Tamiflu
Amantadine: Symmetrel	Enfuvirtide (T-20): Fuzeon	Oxacillin: Prostaphlin
Amikacin: Amikin	Entecavir: Baraclude	Palivizumab: Synagis
Amoxicillin: Amoxil, Polymox	Ertapenem: Invanz	Paromomycin: Humatin
Amoxicillin extended release: Moxatag	Etravirine: Intelence	Pentamidine: NebuPent, Pentam 300
Amox./clav.: Augmentin, Augmentin ES-600; Augmentin XR	Erythromycin(s): Ilotycin	Piperacillin: Pipracil
Amphotericin B: Fungizone	*Ethyl succinate:* Pediamycin	Piperacillin/tazobactam: Zosyn, Tazocin
Ampho B-liposomal: AmBisome	*Glucoheptonate:* Erythrocin	Piperazine: Antepar
Ampho B-lipid complex: Abelcet	*Estolate:* Ilosone	Podophyllotoxin: Condylox
Ampicillin: Omnipen, Polycillin	Erythro/sulfisoxazole: Pediazole	Polymyxin B: Poly-Rx
Ampicillin/sulbactam: Unasyn	Ethambutol: Myambutol	Posaconazole: Noxafil
Artemether-Lumefantrine: Coartem	Ethionamide: Trecator	Praziquantel: Biltricide
Atazanavir: Reyataz	Famciclovir: Famvir	Primaquine: Primachine
Atovaquone: Mepron	Fidaxomicin: Dificid	Proguanil: Paludrine
Atovaquone + proguanil: Malarone	Fluconazole: Diflucan	Pyrantel pamoate: Antiminth
Azithromycin: Zithromax	Flucytosine: Ancobon	Pyrimethamine: Daraprim
Azithromycin ER: Zmax	Fosamprenavir: Lexiva	Pyrimethamine/sulfadoxine: Fansidar
Aztreonam: Azactam, Cayston	Foscarnet: Foscavir	Quinupristin/dalfopristin: Synercid
Bedaquiline: Sirturo	Fosfomycin: Monurol	Raltegravir: Isentress
Boceprevir: Victrelis	Fusidic acid: Taksta	Retapamulin: Altabax
Caspofungin: Cancidas	Ganciclovir: Cytovene	Ribavirin: Virazole, Rebetol
Cefaclor: Ceclor, Ceclor CD	Gatifloxacin: Tequin	Rifabutin: Mycobutin
Cefadroxil: Duricef	Gemifloxacin: Factive	Rifampin: Rifadin, Rimactane
Cefazolin: Ancef, Kefzol	Gentamicin: Garamycin	Rifapentine: Priftin
Cefdinir: Omnicef	Griseofulvin: Fulvicin	Rifaximin: Xifaxan
Cefditoren pivoxil: Spectracef	Halofantrine: Halfan	Rilpivirine: Edurant
Cefepime: Maxipime	Idoxuridine: Dendrid, Stoxil	Rimantadine: Flumadine
Cefixime[NUS]: Suprax	INH + RIF: Rifamate	Ritonavir: Norvir
Cefoperazone-sulbactam: Sulperazon[NUS]	INH + RIF + PZA: Rifater	Saquinavir: Invirase
Cefotaxime: Claforan	Interferon alfa: Intron A	Spectinomycin: Trobicin
Cefotetan: Cefotan	Interferon, pegylated: PEG-Intron, Pegasys	Stavudine: Zerit
Cefoxitin: Mefoxin	Interferon + ribavirin: Rebetron	Stibogluconate: Pentostam
Cefpodoxime proxetil: Vantin	Imipenem + cilastatin: Primaxin, Tienam	Silver sulfadiazine: Silvadene
Cefprozil: Cefzil	Imiquimod: Aldara	Sulfamethoxazole: Gantanol
Ceftaroline: Teflaro	Indinavir: Crixivan	Sulfasalazine: Azulfidine
Ceftazidime: Fortaz, Tazicef, Tazidime	Itraconazole: Sporanox	Sulfisoxazole: Gantrisin
Ceftibuten: Cedax	Iodoquinol: Yodoxin	Telaprevir: Incivek
Ceftizoxime: Cefizox	Ivermectin: Stromectol, Sklice	Telavancin: Vibativ
Ceftobiprole: Zeftera	Kanamycin: Kantrex	Telbivudine: Tyzeka
Ceftriaxone: Rocephin	Ketoconazole: Nizoral	Telithromycin: Ketek
Cefuroxime: Zinacef, Ceftin	Lamivudine: Epivir, Epivir-HBV	Temocillin: Negaban, Temopen
Cephalexin: Keflex	Lamivudine + abacavir: Epzicom	Tenofovir: Viread
Cephradine: Anspor, Velosef	Levofloxacin: Levaquin	Terbinafine: Lamisil
Chloroquine: Aralen	Linezolid: Zyvox	Thalidomide: Thalomid Thiabendazole: Mintezol
Cidofovir: Vistide	Lomefloxacin: Maxaquin	Ticarcillin: Ticar
Ciprofloxacin: Cipro, Cipro XR	Lopinavir/ritonavir: Kaletra	Tigecycline: Tygacil
Clarithromycin: Biaxin, Biaxin XL	Loracarbef: Lorabid	Tinidazole: Tindamax
Clindamycin: Cleocin	Mafenide: Sulfamylon	Tipranavir: Aptivus
Clofazimine: Lamprene	Maraviroc: Selzentry	Tobramycin: Nebcin
Clotrimazole: Lotrimin, Mycelex	Mebendazole: Vermox	Tretinoin: Retin A
Cloxacillin: Tegopen	Mefloquine: Lariam	Trifluridine: Viroptic
Colistimethate: Coly-Mycin M	Meropenem: Merrem	Trimethoprim: Primsol
Cycloserine: Seromycin	Mesalamine: Asacol, Pentasa	Trimethoprim/sulfamethoxazole: Bactrim, Septra
Daptomycin: Cubicin	Methenamine: Hiprex, Mandelamine	Valacyclovir: Valtrex
Darunavir: Prezista	Metronidazole: Flagyl	Valganciclovir: Valcyte
Delavirdine: Rescriptor	Micafungin: Mycamine	Vancomycin: Vancocin
Dicloxacillin: Dynapen	Minocycline: Minocin	Voriconazole: Vfend
Didanosine: Videx	Moxifloxacin: Avelox	Zalcitabine: HIVID
Diethylcarbamazine: Hetrazan	Mupirocin: Bactroban	Zanamivir: Relenza
Diloxanide furoate: Furamide	Nafcillin: Unipen	Zidovudine (ZDV): Retrovir
Dolutegravir: Tivicay	Nelfinavir: Viracept	Zidovudine + 3TC: Combivir
Doripenem: Doribax	Nevirapine: Viramune	Zidovudine + 3TC + abacavir: Trizivir
Doxycycline: Vibramycin		

TABLE 23 (2)
LIST OF COMMON TRADE AND GENERIC NAMES

TRADE NAME: GENERIC NAME	TRADE NAME: GENERIC NAME	TRADE NAME: GENERIC NAME
Abelcet: Ampho B-lipid complex	Halfan: Halofantrine	Rifadin: Rifampin
Albenza: Albendazole	Hepsera: Adefovir	Rifamate: INH + RIF
Aldara: Imiquimod	Herplex: Idoxuridine	Rifater: INH + RIF + PZA
Alinia: Nitazoxanide	Hiprex: Methenamine hippurate	Rimactane: Rifampin
Altabax: Retapamulin	HIVID: Zalcitabine	Rocephin: Ceftriaxone
AmBisome: Ampho B-liposomal	Humatin: Paromomycin	Selzentry: Maraviroc
Amikin: Amikacin	Ilosone: Erythromycin estolate	Septra: Trimethoprim/sulfa
Amoxil: Amoxicillin	Ilotycin: Erythromycin	Seromycin: Cycloserine
Ancef: Cefazolin	Incivek: Telaprevir	Silvadene: Silver sulfadiazine
Ancobon: Flucytosine	Intelence: Etravirine	Sirturo: Bedaquiline
Anspor: Cephradine	Intron A: Interferon alfa	Sklice: Ivermectin lotion
Antepar: Piperazine	Invanz: Ertapenem	Spectracef: Cefditoren pivoxil
Antiminth: Pyrantel pamoate	Invirase: Saquinavir	Sporanox: Itraconazole
Aptivus: Tipranavir	Isentress: Raltegravir	Stoxil: Idoxuridine
Aralen: Chloroquine	Kantrex: Kanamycin	Stribild: Elvitegravir + Cobicistat + Emtricitabine + Tenofovir
Asacol: Mesalamine	Kaletra: Lopinavir/ritonavir	Stromectol: Ivermectin
Atripla: Efavirenz/emtricitabine/tenofovir	Keflex: Cephalexin	Sulfamylon: Mafenide
Augmentin, Augmentin ES-600	Ketek: Telithromycin	Sulperazon[NUS]: Cefoperazone-sulbactam
Augmentin XR: Amox./clav.	Lamisil: Terbinafine	Suprax: Cefixime[NUS]
Avelox: Moxifloxacin	Lamprene: Clofazimine	Sustiva: Efavirenz
Azactam: Aztreonam	Lariam: Mefloquine	Symmetrel: Amantadine
Azulfidine: Sulfasalazine	Levaquin: Levofloxacin	Synagis: Palivizumab
Bactroban: Mupirocin	Lexiva: Fosamprenavir	Synercid: Quinupristin/dalfopristin
Bactrim: Trimethoprim/ sulfamethoxazole	Lorabid: Loracarbef	Taksta: Fusidic acid
Baraclude: Entecavir	Macrodantin, Macrobid: Nitrofurantoin	Tamiflu: Oseltamivir
Biaxin, Biaxin XL: Clarithromycin	Malarone: Atovaquone + proguanil	Tazicef: Ceftazidime
Biltricide: Praziquantel	Mandelamine: Methenamine mandel	Teflaro: Ceftaroline
Cancidas: Caspofungin	Maxaquin: Lomefloxacin	Tegopen: Cloxacillin
Cayston: Aztreonam (inhaled)	Maxipime: Cefepime	Tequin: Gatifloxacin
Ceclor, Ceclor CD: Cefaclor	Mefoxin: Cefoxitin	Thalomid: Thalidomide
Cedax: Ceftibuten	Mepron: Atovaquone	Ticar: Ticarcillin
Cefizox: Ceftizoxime	Merrem: Meropenem	Tienam: Imipenem
Cefotan: Cefotetan	Minocin: Minocycline	Timentin: Ticarcillin-clavulanic acid
Ceftin: Cefuroxime axetil	Mintezol: Thiabendazole	Tinactin: Tolnaftate
Cefzil: Cefprozil	Monocid: Cefonicid	Tindamax: Tinidazole
Cipro, Cipro XR: Ciprofloxacin & extended release	Monurol: Fosfomycin	Tivicay: Dolutegravir
Claforan: Cefotaxime	Moxatag: Amoxicillin extended release:	Trecator SC: Ethionamide
Coartem: Artemether-Lumefantrine	Myambutol: Ethambutol	Trizivir: Abacavir + ZDV + 3TC
Coly-Mycin M: Colistimethate	Mycamine: Micafungin	Trobicin: Spectinomycin
Combivir: ZDV + 3TC	Mycobutin: Rifabutin	Truvada: Emtricitabine + tenofovir
Complera: Emtricitabine + tenofovir + rilpivirine	Mycostatin: Nystatin	Tygacil: Tigecycline
Crixivan: Indinavir	Nafcil: Nafcillin	Tyzeka: Telbivudine
Cubicin: Daptomycin	Nebcin: Tobramycin	Unasyn: Ampicillin/sulbactam
Cytovene: Ganciclovir	NebuPent: Pentamidine	Unipen: Nafcillin
Daraprim: Pyrimethamine	Nizoral: Ketoconazole	Valcyte: Valganciclovir
Dificid: Fidaxomicin	Norvir: Ritonavir	Valtrex: Valacyclovir
Diflucan: Fluconazole	Noxafil: Posaconazole	Vancocin: Vancomycin
Doribax: Doripenem	Olysio: Simeprevir	Vantin: Cefpodoxime proxetil
Duricef: Cefadroxil	Omnicef: Cefdinir	Velosef: Cephradine
Dynapen: Dicloxacillin	Omnipen: Ampicillin	Vermox: Mebendazole
Edurant: Rilpivirine	Pediamycin: Erythro. ethyl succinate	Vfend: Voriconazole
Emtriva: Emtricitabine	Pediazole: Erythro. ethyl succinate + sulfisoxazole	Vibativ: Telavancin
Epivir, Epivir-HBV: Lamivudine	Pegasys, PEG-Intron: Interferon, pegylated	Vibramycin: Doxycycline
Epzicom: Lamivudine + abacavir	Pentam 300: Pentamidine	Victrelis: Boceprevir
Factive: Gemifloxacin	Pentasa: Mesalamine	Videx: Didanosine
Famvir: Famciclovir	Pipracil: Piperacillin	Viracept: Nelfinavir
Fansidar: Pyrimethamine + sulfadoxine	Polycillin: Ampicillin	Viramune: Nevirapine
Flagyl: Metronidazole	Polymox: Amoxicillin	Virazole: Ribavirin
Floxin: Ofloxacin	Poly-Rx: Polymyxin B	Viread: Tenofovir
Flumadine: Rimantadine	Prezista: Darunavir	Vistide: Cidofovir
Foscavir: Foscarnet	Priftin: Rifapentine	Xifaxan: Rifaximin
Fortaz: Ceftazidime	Primaxin: Imipenem + cilastatin	Yodoxin: Iodoquinol
Fulvicin: Griseofulvin	Primsol: Trimethoprim	Zerit: Stavudine
Fungizone: Amphotericin B	Prostaphlin: Oxacillin	Zeftera: Ceftobiprole
Furadantin: Nitrofurantoin	Rebetol: Ribavirin	Ziagen: Abacavir
Fuzeon: Enfuvirtide (T-20)	Rebetron: Interferon + ribavirin	Zinacef: Cefuroxime
Gantanol: Sulfamethoxazole	Relenza: Zanamivir	Zithromax: Azithromycin
Gantrisin: Sulfisoxazole	Rescriptor: Delavirdine	Zmax: Azithromycin ER
Garamycin: Gentamicin	Retin A: Tretinoin Retrovir: Zidovudine (ZDV)	Zovirax: Acyclovir
	Reyataz: Atazanavir	Zosyn: Piperacillin/tazobactam
		Zyvox: Linezolid

INDEX OF MAJOR ENTITIES

PAGES (page numbers bold if major focus)

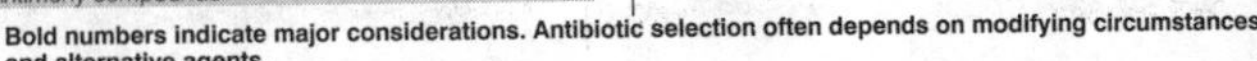
Bold numbers indicate major considerations. Antibiotic selection often depends on modifying circumstances and alternative agents.

PAGES (page numbers bold if major focus)

PAGES (page numbers bold if major focus)

PAGES (page numbers bold if major focus)

F

G

H

PAGES (page numbers bold if major focus)

PAGES (page numbers bold if major focus)

PAGES (page numbers bold if major focus)

PAGES (page numbers bold if major focus)

PAGES (page numbers bold if major focus)

PAGES (page numbers bold if major focus)

U

V

W

X

Y

Z